Bronchology and Bronchoesophagology: State of the Art

Bronchology and Bronchoesophagology: State of the Art

Proceedings of the 11th World Congress for Bronchology (WCB) & the 11th World Congress for Bronchoesophagology (WCBE), held in Yokohama, Japan on the 7th–10th June, 2000.

Editors:

Hirokuni Yoshimura
Kitasato University
Kanagawa, Japan

Akinori Kida
Nihon University
School of Medicine
Tokyo, Japan

Takashi Arai
National Hospital Tokyo
Disaster Medical Center
Tokyo, Japan

Seiji Niimi
Tokyo Medical University
Tokyo, Japan

Masahiro Kaneko
National Cancer Center
Central Hospital
Tokyo, Japan

Satoshi Kitahara
National Defence
Medical College
Saitama, Japan

2001

ELSEVIER

Amsterdam – London – New York – Oxford – Paris – Shannon – Tokyo

ELSEVIER SCIENCE B.V.
Sara Burgerhartstraat 25
P.O. Box 211, 1000 AE Amsterdam, The Netherlands

First edition 2001

Library of Congress Cataloging in Publication Data
A catalog record from the Library of Congress has been applied for.

ISBN: 0-444-50592-X
ISSN: 0531-5131
International Congress Series No. 1217

∞ The paper used in this publication meets the requirements of ANSI/NISO Z39.48-1992 (Permanence of Paper).

Printed in the Netherlands

Preface

The 11th World Congresses for Bronchology and Bronchoesophagology (WCB & WCBE) were held in Yokohama, Japan for 4 days from 7 to 10 June 2000, under the main theme of "State of the Art in the Digital Age".

These congresses addressed all aspects of bronchology and bronchoesophagology and also included sessions on other area of interventional pulmonology, such as thoracoscopy.

A total of 778 participants, giving 413 presentations, gathered from 37 countries around the world from various backgrounds (pulmonology, pediatrics, ENT, gastroenterology, surgery, anesthesiology, radiology, etc.).

The scientific program consisted of two special lectures, 32 invited lectures, 11 symposia with 51 presentations, 164 oral presentations, 158 poster presentations, 6 luncheon seminars, 19 video presentations, two hands-on workshops and one teleconference.

We believe that these conferences provided an exciting opportunity for all participants to exchange the most up-to-date scientific information, knowledge, ideas and skills on modern bronchology and bronchoesophagology, and also to obtain a view of what the future has in store through in-depth discussion. It is, therefore, my great pleasure to publish those presentations in a proceedings volume.

We are confident that this volume which has just been published in the first year of the 21st century will pave the way to new vistas in bronchology and bronchoesophagology in the 21st century.

September, 2000

Hirokuni Yoshimura MD
President of the 11th World Congress for Bronchology
Chair of the World Association for Bronchology

Foreword

It gives me a great honor to be the President of the 11th World Congress for Bronchoesophagology at Yokohama in the commemorative millennium. It has been just 10 years since the 6th World Congress for Bronchoesophagology (WCBE) was held in Tokyo. I trust that the Proceedings of the 11th *WCB/WCBE* will contribute to the development of this field in the 21st century.

The Japan Broncho-esophagological Society is an interdisciplinary society, which consists of otolaryngologists, head and neck surgeons, pulmonary surgeons, esophageal surgeons, pulmonologists, and radiologists, who are specialists of the airway or upper digestive tract. The WCBE is sponsored by the International Broncho-eesophagological Society (IBES Executive Secretary/Treasurer, Prof Sanderson). I, as the President, with the general help of the Japan Broncho-esophagological Society planned the Program, Luncheon Seminars and Social Program with Prof Yoshimura, who is the President of WCB. As a result, the 11th WCB/WCBE proved to be a major meeting, with 796 participants from 36 countries gathering in Yokohama.

Two special lectures, namely “Micromachine” by Mr Mizuno (Japan) and “Gastroesophageal Reflux Disease” by Prof Dent (Australia), gave us a vision of the future, and impressed us with their advanced knowledge. We invited 13 speakers from Asia, Europe and the USA; and they gave excellent talks about topics in bronchoesophagology. Six symposia, namely “Cancer of the Esophagus”, “Phonosurgery”, “Tracheo-esophageal Fistulae”, “Laryngeal Cancer”, “Gastroesophageal Reflux Disease”, and “Dysphagia”. These talks led us to expand and deepen our knowledge of the field. In addition, 54 papers in a free Oral Session, and 61 papers in a Poster Session were presented. Among the papers in the Poster Session, three were selected and awarded in the Banquet.

The social program included an Opening Ceremony, Welcome Party, Dinner Cruise, Closing Ceremony, and Banquet. The Closing Ceremony and Banquet were held on the evening of 9 June. At this time, three poster awards were selected from each field: the airway, esophagus, and larynx/hypopharynx were presented. At the end of the ceremony, the Banner of the WCBE was given to Prof Shapshay, who will be the President of the 12th WCBE in Boston in 2002.

The congress was successfully coordinated by the members of the Organizing Committee. The Committee would like to extend their thanks to all participants for having contributed to the success of the meeting. I am looking forward to meeting you again in Boston in 2002.

Akinori Kida
President of 11th WCBE
Editor-in-Chief for Proceedings of 11th WCB/WCBE

Address by His Imperial Highness, Prince Akishino

I would like to congratulate the organizers of the 11th World Congress for Bronchology and the 11th World Congress for Bronchoesophagology in this momentous year 2000. I would also like to welcome all of you here to this important occasion.

I was told that there are representatives from 44 different countries at this meeting, all specializing in either diseases of the airway or the esophagus or both; and I am sure that there will be many significant reports on state-of-the-art progress in these fields.

In Japan, malignant diseases affecting the airway and esophagus are increasing, and particularly in the past few years there seems to be a worldwide resurgence of tuberculosis and other infectious diseases.

Against this background, it is extremely significant that you are holding these joint meetings on bronchology and bronchoesophagology in Japan, the country in which the fiberoptic bronchoscope was developed; and I hope that with this international cooperation, it will be possible to make significant strides in not only the diagnosis and treatment of disease but also prevention, and I would like to express my heartfelt best wishes for your endeavors.

In closing, I would like to express my hope that everybody taking part in these events will be able to make use of the results and findings presented here in order to improve the health and condition of society in their own countries and regions.

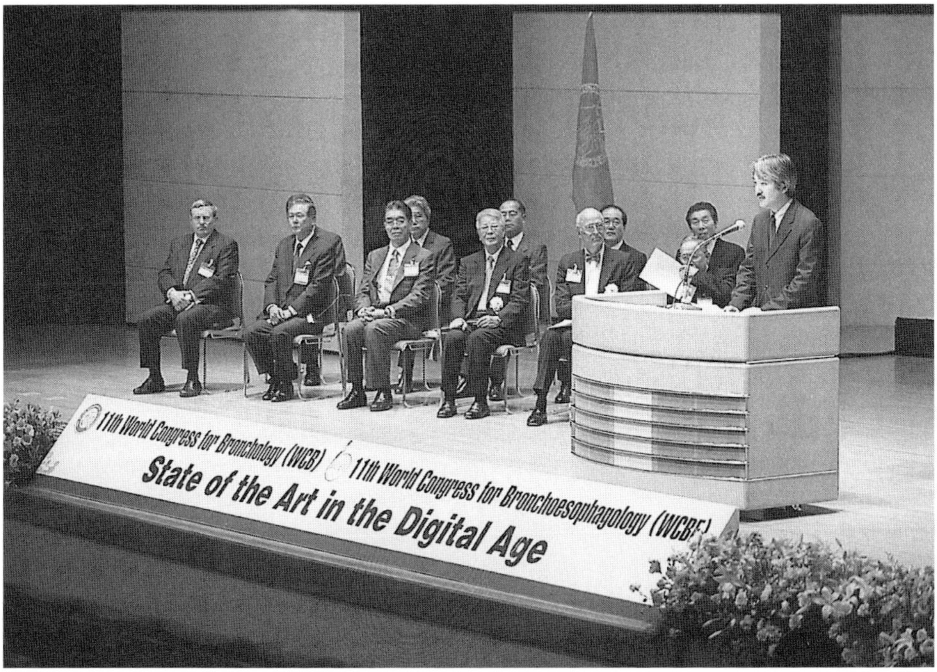

President's message

Your Imperial Highnesses Prince and Princess Akishino, members and guests, ladies and gentlemen.

It is not only a great pleasure but also a great honor to be able to welcome their imperial highnesses Prince and Princess Akishino and also all participants from many countries throughout the world, to the 11th World Congress for Bronchology and the 11th World Congress for Bronchoesophagology in this momentous year, 2000. Our Congress has gathered more than 600 papers and presentations from 41 countries and we will have more than 1500 participants.

We believe that these congresses will provide an exciting opportunity for all participants from around the world to explore their special interests in the fields of bronchology and bronchoesophagology through in-depth discussion and by exchanging the most up-to-date scientific information, knowledge, ideas and skills. One of the most recent major developments in the field, the integration of CCD chip technology to produce video endoscopes, has definitely ushered in the digital age in our specialties. Combined with the push for minimally invasive diagnosis and therapeutic procedures, this will have far-reaching effects in the fields of bronchology and bronchoesophagology. We hope our congresses will allow you to obtain a view of what the future has in store.

In particular, the Intercontinental Tele-Video Conference will highlight future possibilities for the combination of telecommunications and medicine in the rapidly developing fields of telemedicine and e-health.

We are confident that these combined meetings in the last year of the 20th century will pave the way to new vistas in bronchology and bronchoesophagology in the 21st century.

We look forward to spending time with you in wonderful Yokohama, a beautiful bay-front city offering some of the best convention facilities in the world.

Hirokuni Yoshimura, MD
President of the 11th WCB/WCBE

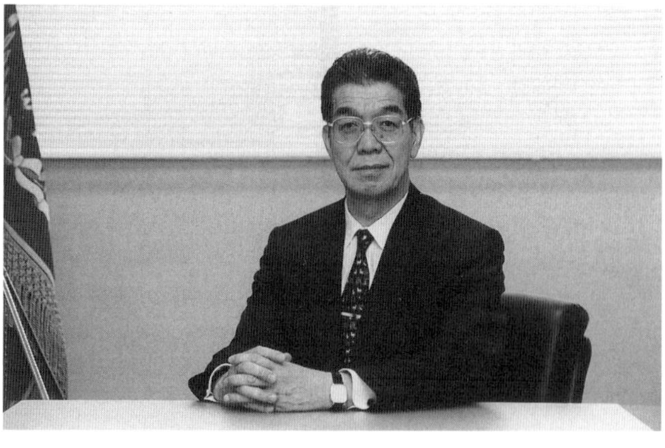

Address

It is my pleasure and privilege to welcome you, with the presence of their Imperial Highnesses Prince and Princess Akishinomiya, to the 11th World Congress for Bronchology and the 11th World Congress for Bronchoesophagology.

The principal regions of bronchology and bronchoesophagology are hypopharynx, larynx, trachea, bronchus and esophagus; and the function of these regions are the pathway of air and foods, as well as phonation. These functions will be disturbed by infection, trauma, tumor, nerve paralysis and disorder of the central nervous system.

The World Congress is the major gathering of our multidisciplinary specialists. It is an opportunity for various specialists and different interest work groups to meet and exchange ideas in a mono- or multidisciplinary format.

In addition to being stimulated by the Congress, I hope you will be able to enjoy the beautiful surroundings of the city of Yokohama, and bring back memories of Yokohama and the Japanese hospitality. Thank you.

Akinori Kida
President of the 11th WCBE

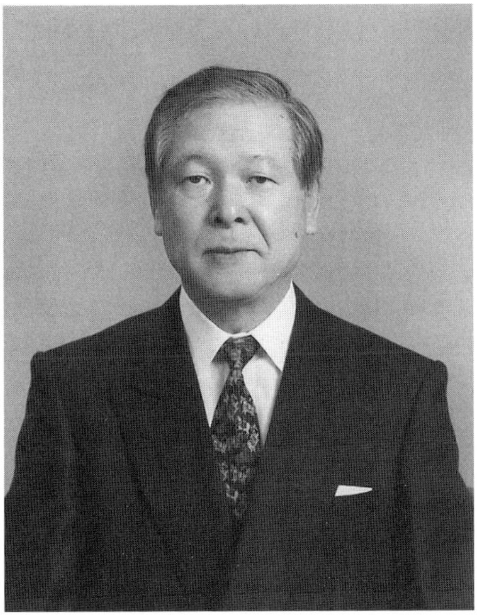

Contents

Symposia

Bronchoscopy in nontumorous pulmonary disorders

Controversies in stenting

Diagnosis and treatment of early stage central type lung cancer

Video, oral and poster presentations

Airway stenosis

Asthma

Brachytherapy

Endobronchial tumors

Esophageal cancer

Gene diagnosis and therapy

Head and neck cancer

Imaging

Thyroid cancer

Ultrasound

Invited lectures

Bronchology and Bronchoesophagology: State of the Art.
H. Yoshimura et al., editors.

Bronchoscopy: the present trend in Indonesia

Nirwan Arief
Department of Pulmonology, Faculty of Medicine, University of Indonesia, Jakarta, Indonesia

Abstract. *Introduction.* Flexible fiberoptic bronchoscopy (FB) has been practiced in Indonesia since 1975. It has been used ever since as an important method in the diagnosis and management of pulmonary disease. According to the Indonesian Association of Bronchology (IAB or Perbronki) Annual Report, 44 pulmonologists perform bronchoscopy routinely for diagnostic, therapeutic and perioperative purposes, in three large cities in Indonesia: Jakarta, Surabaya and Medan. Meanwhile, ear, nose, and throat (ENT) physicians prefer the rigid bronchoscope for most foreign body cases.

Materials and Methods. We retrospectively reviewed the reports of five university hospitals (UHs) since 1977 until 1999 in Jakarta (Persahabatan General Hospital, Cipto Mangunkusumo General Hospital, Dharmais Cancer hospital), Surabaya (Dr Soetomo General Hospital) and Medan (Pirngadi General Hospital). Other data were also obtained from the annual report of the IAB and questionnaires mailed to the five centers. Unfortunately, some of the data cannot be compiled in this article due to improper and incomplete reports.

Results. Between 1997 and 1999, 3,533 bronchoscopy procedures were carried out in five centers. Bronchogenic carcinoma was found as a major indication for bronchoscopy followed by hemoptysis and infection. The procedure was most often performed in the bronchoscopy suite, except for the complicated cases which were carried out in the operating theater. The technique applied (including anesthetic procedure) was generally the same in the five centers. O_2 supplement, transoral insertion, chest X-ray prior to the procedure, and coagulation test were applied in most of the cases. Recently, rigid bronchoscopy was carried out more frequently for laser and stent application. Due to the lack of facilities, it is performed only in Jakarta.

Conclusion. It appears that FB is mostly performed by pulmonologists, and that the technique of RB is retrained among bronchoscopists in workshops organized by the IAB. Bronchogenic carcinoma was revealed as the main indication for bronchoscopy in our study. Presently, RB is performed again in the pulmonology department since laser and stent application have recently increased.

Keywords: flexible fiberoptic bronchoscopy (FB), rigid bronchoscopy (RB).

Introduction

Diseases of the respiratory tract are still a large problem in Indonesia. According to the National Household Survey in 1986, 1992, and 1995, respiratory disease ranked second, third, and third, respectively, among morbidity [1]. Besides tuberculosis, the number of bronchogenic carcinoma cases has recently been increasing significantly. Cigarette smoking is considered to be one of the risk factors. More than 50% of male adults in Indonesia are smokers, who usually started smoking in their youth. Perhaps this factor contributes to the high incidence of

Address for correspondence: Nirwan Arief, Department of Pulmonology, Faculty of Medicine, University of Indonesia, Kalibata Timur IV/34 Jakarta 12740, Indonesia. Tel.: +62-21-799-1054. Fax: +62-21-470-5684.

the bronchogenic carcinoma in Indonesia.

The bronchoscopy procedure plays an important role in the diagnosis and management of pulmonary disease. The procedure is mainly performed by a pulmonologist. Ear, nose and throat (ENT) specialists have also practiced this procedure, particularly in the removal of a foreign body using rigid bronchoscopy (RB). Flexible fiberoptic bronchoscopy (FB) started to be performed after a staff member at the Pulmonology Department of the Medical Faculty, University of Indonesia, was sent to Japan (sponsored by JICA) to undergo the training for flexible fiberoptic bronchoscopy. He was trained and supervised by Dr Shigeto Ikeda himself and a few other bronchoscopists. Since then, FB has replaced the practice of RB in Indonesia. More than 120 residents in Pulmonology and ENT, who come from different parts of the Indonesia, have now been trained in Jakarta. After the training, these residents practice the FB procedure in their home institution or hospital. According to the Indonesian Association of Bronchology (IAB or Perbronki), there are 44 pulmonologists who perform bronchoscopy routinely for diagnostic, therapeutic, and perioperative purposes in three large cities in Indonesia, namely Jakarta, Surabaya and Medan. Meanwhile, there are five ENT specialists who practice RB and reside in Jakarta. In fact, there are 365 pulmonologists throughout Indonesia, and about 40% of them perform bronchoscopy in hospitals.

Materials and Methods

We retrospectively reviewed the reports of five university hospitals (UHs) from 1997 until 1999 in three large cities. These were Persahabatan General Hospital (Jakarta), Dharmais Cancer Hospital (Jakarta), Dr Soetomo General Hospital (Surabaya), Pingardi General Hospital (Medan), and Cipto Mangunkusumo General Hospital (Jakarta). Jakarta is the largest city in Indonesia with 11 million inhabitants, while Surabaya and Medan have populations of 6 million and 4 million, respectively. The Pulmonology Department was the source of the data from the first four above-mentioned hospitals, while the fifth UH sent the data from ENT Department. Other data were obtained from the Annual Report of the IAB and questionnaires mailed to the five UHs. The questionnaire consisted of 25 questions addressing the following aspects: the personnel involved, category of manpower, standard bronchoscopy procedure, facilities, clinical setting, training system, interventional bronchoscopy, number of nurses, number of residents, length of practice, etc. Data from the Bronchoscopy Division were excluded, as the procedure is not performed routinely in this department. Routinely is defined as "performing the procedure at least once a week" for the Pulmonology Department, and "performing the procedure at least once in 2 weeks" for the ENT Department. Centers outside the five UHs were also excluded from the study since they only run the service and do not have the educational aspect of the UHs. The questionnaires were directed to the institutions and not to individuals.

Table 1. Demographic data.

	n	%
Physician category		
Pulmonologists	20	80
ENT	5	20
Length of practice		
> 10 years	10	40
5 10 years	10	40
< 5 years	5	20
Procedure number		
UH1	1910	54
UH2	350	9.9
UH3	668	18.9
UH4	467	13.2
UH5	138	3.9

UH: University Hospital.

Results

In total, 25 active bronchoscopists, consisting of 20 pulmonologists and 5 ENT specialist, were involved in these five UHs. Of the bronchoscopists, 10 have been working for longer than 10 years, the other 10 have practiced the procedure for about 5–10 years, and five physicians have been doing the job for less than 5 years (Table 1). The total number of procedures between 1997 and 1999 is 3,533. Of these procedures, 95% were performed using FB (3,433 cases), and RB was used in 100 cases (5%) of the whole procedures. The reported patients are from both the out-patient and in-patient departments. ENT specialists carried out 72% of all of the RB procedures, mainly for the removal of foreign bodies. Meanwhile, pulmonologists used FB to remove the foreign bodies in all cases.

There are 20 bronchoscopes (11 flexible fiber bronchoscopes, six rigid bronchoscopes, and three pediatric bronchoscopes) available in five UHs (Table 2). Surprisingly, we have more than enough bronchoscopes for RB considering

Table 2. Type of instrument.

	n	%
Bronchoscope		
FB	5 UH	100
RB	3 UH	60
Pediatric bronchoscope	3 UH	60
Fluoroscope	3	60
Oximetry	5	100
Videobronchoscope	4	80

its low utility (only 5%) compared to FB having utilized in 95% of the cases. Oximetry was found in all five UHs. It is of no surprise that the five centers reported its use in every procedure, as well as oxygen supplement.

Fluoroscopes are available in three UHs, all kept in the operating theater, where transbronchial lung biopsy (TBLB) and transbronchial needle aspiration biopsy (TBNA) are performed. A videobronchoscope was found in four UHs. Obviously, the purpose of its use was educational, as mentioned by three UHs. In one UH, this instrument had not been used since last year, and the reason was not mentioned.

The bronchoscopy examination in our study was performed in various places. In general, it was performed in the bronchoscopy suite, as reported by all centers. Sometimes the procedure was carried out in the emergency unit, at the patient's bedside or in the operating theater. The TBNA procedure was found to be performed only in two UHs, TBLB in four UHs, and bronchoalveolar lavage (BAL) was carried out in all five UHs.

A minimum of two nurses assisted in every procedure. The nurses are reported by all UHs as having more than 5 years of experience in their work. As part of an education module, in four UHs two residents were usually trained in the Bronchoscopy division for at least 3 months. The making of a "model bronchial tree" was mandatory for these residents in one UH. To meet the requirement, residents needed to perform more than 20 procedures independently in three UHs, while two other UHs gave a figure between 10 and 15 procedures.

Bleeding was the most common complication of the procedure reported in our study. The amount was usually less than 50 cc. Atropine 0.5–1 mg is given intramuscularly as premedication, reported by all UHs. A chest X-ray and coagulation test are required before the procedure in all UHs, while blood gas analysis, complete blood count and spirometry are additional tests in two UHs (Table 3).

Three UHs indicate the requirement of an ECG test for patients older than 40 years, whereas the remaining two UHs mentioned this test only by certain indications such as history of cardiac disease or if the patient was confirmed as a cardiac patient.

The major indication in our study is bronchogenic carcinoma, as found in 1,939 cases. Out of the 1,939 malignancy cases, TBLB was carried out in 190 cases with 74% positivity. TBNA was performed in 43 cases but the result was

Table 3. Prebronchoscopy tests.

Prebronchoscopy test	n	%
Chest X-ray	5	100
Blood gas analysis	2	40
Complete blood count	2	40
Coagulation test	5	100
ECG	3	60
Spirometry	2	40

Table 4. Number of procedures and indication in five University Hospitals from 1997 to 1999.

Indication	UH1	UH2	UH3	UH4	UH5	Total
Mass/nodule/tumor	927	220	520	260	12	1939
Hemoptysis	221	9	10	112	27	379
Infection	270	20	43	36	0	369
Atelectasis	49	9	30	44	15	147
Foreign bodies	14	5	4	2	72	97
Pneumothorax	56	10	20	2		88
Interstitial Lung disease	3	3	4	—	—	10
Other	370	74	37	11	12	504
Total	1910	350	668	467	138	3533

not mentioned. Other indications are hemoptysis and determination of the etiologic microorganism in infections such as bronchiectasis, pneumonia and other lower respiratory tract infections, as shown in Table 4.

A large number of the cases (504) found in our study were classified under "other" as indication for the procedure. When asked verbally, the institution classified this "other" classification as sputum retention, postoperative lung surgery, difficult intubation, and in order to evaluate the position of the endotracheal tube.

We found 379 cases of hemoptysis, of which 65 cases developed fully into massive hemoptysis (Table 5). All UHs agreed in defining massive hemoptysis as bleeding of more than 200 cc and up to 600 cc in a 24-h period, or between 250 and 600 cc in a 48-h period without a tendency to stop. Of 65 cases, 26 patients underwent the FB procedure while the remaining patients refused the procedure for various reasons. The origin of the bleeding was identified in 20 cases. Due to a number of reasons, only 12 cases agreed to undergo the surgery. The 39

Table 5. Bronchoscopy procedure in massive hemoptysis.

	n	%
Category of hemoptysis		
Nonmassive	314	83
Massive	65	17
Procedure for massive case		
Yes	26	40
No	39	60
Result		
Identified	20	77
Cannot be identified	6	23
Underwent surgery		
Yes	12	60
No	8	40

patients who refused the bronchoscopy procedure were treated conservatively. The oral route was found to be the favorite way for bronchoscope insertion in our study. The insertion of the bronchoscope by the nasal route is practiced in very rare cases, such as with an uncooperative patient in order to prevent, for instance, the instrument being bitten by the patient.

Most of the FB procedures were performed under local anesthesia. All centers used 2% lidocain for the upper airway (pharynx area) and this was given by gargling. Then, lidocain (10%) was sprayed in the larynx and epiglottis area. Finally, xylocaine (2%) was instillated to the glottis and trachea. General anesthesia was employed by one UH for laser and stent application. Unfortunately due to the lack of facilities, up until now, only two UHs perform these modalities. The supine position was reported in most cases (almost 99%).

Interventional bronchoscopy has entered our field since 1996. Laser therapy was applied in 25 cases in one UH, while stent placement was employed in 15 cases. In one-half of the cases, GRZ stent was applied due to the fact that only this type of stent was available during that time. Since 1997 we have had access to the Dumont stent, this stent, however, has replaced the use of the former type. Although most procedures are preformed using FB, residents in one UH are still taught and trained in rigid bronchoscopy. In order to anticipate the progressive development of interventional bronchoscopy, all centers suggested that the IAB should organize more training and workshops in this aspect.

Discussion

Recently, lots of publications have presented the topic of bronchoscopy practice worldwide [2–5], but there is a lack of information on bronchoscopic practice in Indonesia, as publications on this subject are rare. Improper and incomplete reporting by the UHs also caused difficulties in compiling data, as indicated by some items of the question that were left unanswered.

There were 365 pulmonologists throughout Indonesia, but only around 40% of them practiced the bronchoscopy procedure due to very limited facilities. All flexible fiber bronchoscopes and rigid bronchoscopes as well as the supporting instrumentation belonged to the hospital. Bronchoscopes are available in 32 cities in Indonesia and the procedure is only performed in hospitals. Private practices outside the hospital with facilities for performing this procedure do not exist. This might explain why the number of procedures in our country are very low considering the large population of the country. Actually, outside the three main cities, the procedure is also carried out in 29 other cities, but not as frequently as in these three cities. The lack of supporting facilities and access to thoracic surgeons were given as reasons.

This study indicates that at present the procedure is performed mainly using the flexible fiberoptic bronchoscope, as found by Nanjundiah, Colt and Prakash [2,4,5]. In fact only one UH still teaches RB. Unlike in the Netherlands where there is free access to health care [3], in Indonesia unfortunately, people are very limited in medical insurance. Approximately only 10–20% of the population have access to health insurance. The majority of this group consists of government employees. Since most patients must bear the cost of procedures by themselves (which is very expensive when taking into account the level of general income), this causes many patients to refuse procedures. Therefore, the number of procedures is found to be very low in our study. We found that oximetry and oxygen supplement were used routinely for each procedure, even though the use of oxygen supplement by nasal canula did not increase the PO_2 level significantly as did O_2 supplement given through the bronchoscope, as reported by Hidayat et al. [6].

The main indication of the procedure (lung tumor) is in agreement with other authors. The requirement of a chest X-ray as bronchoscope test was similar to those reported by Suteja et al. [3] in small and large hospitals.

As for the technical procedures, there were similarities in nearly all institutions including: premedication, anesthesia, route of insertion, the routine use of O_2 supplement, prior chest X-ray, etc. Perhaps this occurred because most of the medical professionals who performed the procedures received their skills from one center, namely the Department of Pulmonology, Medical Faculty, University of Indonesia.

Conclusion

At present, FB is mostly performed in Indonesia with the main indication being bronchogenic carcinoma. This technique and other standard procedures in five UHs are similar, as they are taught by the same trainer. Since the introduction of interventional bronchoscopy, the use of RB has increased remarkably. Therefore, to anticipate this change, the IAB has annually organized courses and workshops in rigid bronchoscopy since 1998 in the hope of improving the skills of the members.

Acknowledgements

The author would like to thank the heads of the Pulmonology Department, Medical Faculty, University of Indonesia, the Pulmonology Department of Dharmais Cancer Hospital, the ENT Department, Medical Faculty, University of Indonesia, the Pulmonology Department Medical Faculty, University of Airlangga and the Pulmonology Department, University of North Sumatra for their support in answering the questionnaire and providing other additional data.

References

1. Department of Health, Republic of Indonesia: Profile of Health, 1996.
2. Colt HG, Prakash UBS, Offund KP. Bronchoscopy. N Am J Bronchol 2000;7:8–25.
3. Suteja T, Festen J, Vanderschueren R, Janster J, Postmus P. A postal survey of bronchoscopic

practice in the Netherlands. J Bronchol 1996;3:17–21.
4. Prakash USB, Offord KP, Stubbs SE. Bronchoscopy in North America: the ACCP Survey. Chest 1991;100:1668–1675.
5. Nanjudiah S. Bronchoscopy in India. J Bronchol 1999;6:257–262.
6. Hidayat S, Arief N, Rasmin M, Supsiyar Toto S. The comparison of changing between delivery oxygen by nasal canula and modified BF_2 TR bronchoscope channel. Paru 1993;13(3):15–19.

Bronchology and Bronchoesophagology: State of the Art.
H. Yoshimura et al., editors.

Pediatric bronchography in 2000

György Baktai
Pediatric Institute 'Svábhegy' Department of Bronchology, Budapest, Hungary

Abstract. Bronchography (BG) is a traditional method used to assess patients with suspected pathological processes of the peripheral bronchi, in whom bronchoscopy alone is not sufficient to make a proper diagnosis. In our practice, BG studies are carried out after rigid bronchoscopy through a rigid filling tube and the contrast medium is filled with overpressure during apnea. The contrast medium used is a radio opaque contrast dye, which contains chemically bound iodine. X-ray pictures, called bronchograms, are done in medium inspiration from three directions. Sagittal and frontal views are taken to show the situation of the bronchi in the thoracic cavity and a semioblique view is taken for punctual segmental analysis.

During the last decade about 300 BGs were performed yearly in our bronchologic lab. The greatest difficulty in doing a BG was the temporary lack of a proper contrast medium in the past. BGs of good quality resulted from the use of Hytrast (BYK G), beginning about 5 years ago. After this, Omnipaque (Nycomed) was applied (from August 1997 to January 1999 in 187 cases) and proved not to be very suitable for BG. Currently, i.e., from January 1999, Broncholux (Goldham Bioglan, Pharma GmbH) is available, and we used it for 154 BGs until December 1999. Our experiences with Hytrast (used for the last 160 BGs performed between June 1996 and August 1997), Omnipaque and Broncholux will be compared in this presentation.

BG is essential for the diagnosis of bronchiectasis and bronchial deformation. It is also an important tool for diagnosing developmental disorders of the bronchi, useful for finding pulmonary sequestrations. In addition, BG is mandatory for the accurate segmental assessment for preoperative planning.

During the last 10 years we have never experienced any complications like pneumothorax, severe pneumonia, or allergic reactions. However, slow clearance of the contrast medium and hyperthermia occurring within 24 h of the BG was observed in some rare cases.

In summary, BG is still an essential, and in certain respects unavoidable, part of pediatric pulmonary diagnostics.

Keywords: bronchial deformation, bronchiectasis, bronchography, bronchoscopy, contrast material, pediatrics.

Introduction

Bronchography (BG) is a traditional method used to assess patients with suspected pathological processes of the peripheral bronchi, in whom bronchoscopy alone is not sufficient for a proper diagnosis. The pioneers of this method were Sicard and Forestier, and BG became extensively used in the 1950s. The significance of BG was questioned in the 1970s, e.g., Avery wrote an article on BG

Address for correspondence: György Baktai MD, Pediatric Institute 'Svábhegy' ('Szabadsághegy'), Department of Bronchology, P.O. Box 939, 1535 Budapest, Hungary. Tel.: +36-1-3954922 (ext. 130). Fax: +36-1-3957649. E-mail: bak8070@helka.iif.hu entitled, "Outmoded procedure?" [1]. In a book published on pediatric pulmonary diseases, BG was characterised as a method that, "produces clear radiographs," but, "has never been popular among paediatricians" [2]. BG in adults also came under speculation; "the procedure has not gained a wide acceptance because of the technical difficulties" [3]. The apparent desire to visualise the peripheral bronchi can be gleaned from statements such as, "Bronchograms performed using a flexible bronchoscope are quick, and provide an easy method to obtain information unavailable by direct visual bronchoscopy..." [4].

Briefly described, BG entails the direct instillation of radio opaque contrast material into the bronchi. X-rays are subsequently taken, and these produce clear radiographs called bronchograms. In our practice a bronchogram is considered unilateral to, and performed in conjunction with, rigid bronchoscopy under general anaesthesia. In a normal bronchogram the filling of the bronchi is uniform and this allows normal arborization of the bronchial tree. X-ray pictures, called bronchograms, are performed in medium inspiration, from three directions. Sagittal and frontal views show the situation of the bronchi in the thoracic cavity and the semioblique view is needed in order to carry out punctual segmental analysis of the bronchi [5].

Equipment

In our practice, Storz or Friedel rigid bronchoscopes are used. It is also worth mentioning the specific metallic cannula created by Thal. The distal end of this canulla closes the distal end of the bronchoscope. Special catheters like Metras should provide a positive contrast under the fluoroscope. In older children, the Carlens double lumen catheter enables us to fill one lung.

Instillation, amount of contrast material

We apply overpressure during apnea. We follow the filling on the screen and discontinue it when two additional branchings, after the subsegments, are visible (6th order bronchi). Filling is routinely controlled on video screen and recorded on videotape. Normally, the motion of the bronchi occurs in parallel with ventilation.

Contrast material

The existence of an ideal contrast material is essential for a good quality BG. The positive contrast with the chest X-ray (CXR) is provided by a high atom mass number, in our practice, iodine. Absolute innocuity, i.e., no irritating effects, proper elimination, homogeneity and stability, proper viscosity, adherence to the bronchial wall, and mixing with the secretions are our requirements. No contrast material satisfies all.

In the past we have had to face the lack of proper contrast material. Hytrast

(BYK G) was withdrawn for commercial reasons. We applied Omnipaque (Nycomed), however, it was not perfect for bronchography. Those who perform bronchography through the flexible bronchoscope have the same problem. As Wood summarizes in his book, "Unfortunately, Dionosyl has been taken off the market, and so it is difficult to perform bronchograms these days. Alternative contrast material may be developed, but at present, I cannot give any specific recommendation" [6]. Today Broncholux (Goldham) is available; it contains 250 mg/ml iodine. Broncholux will probably be available until 2002.

Indications

Bronchial deformation (BD) and bronchiectasis (BE), either suspected or known, are essential indications for BG. BG is an examination of primary importance prior to a thoracotomy for resection of ectatic bronchi (it is important to underline the BG of the presumed normal side). Other important fields for BG are localized narrowing, obstruction or displacement of the bronchi, and suspicion of congenital abnormalities, especially anomalous distribution of the bronchi [7].

Contraindications

Contraindications include all those for bronchoscopy, as well as acute pulmonary inflammations, impaired lung function, pulmonary hemorrhage, untreated pulmonary tuberculosis. Age alone is not a contraindication to BG; however, it is an essential factor in building up an indication.

Complications

In general, we did not experience complications in the practice. However, we did observe slow clearance of the contrast material in certain cases, mainly after BGs done by Hytrast, and mild hyperthermia occurring on the afternoon after a BG was also occasionally observed. Following a BG, asthmatics sometimes suffered from wheezing and in some rare cases children contracted pneumonia. Pneumothorax, severe pneumonia, allergic reactions were also described as possible after effects in the literature, but they did not occur in our patients.

Study design

A retrospective study was carried out to compare BGs performed, in our practice, using Hytrast (160 BGs), Omnipaque (187 BGs) and Broncholux (154 BGs). The proportion of boys (65.1%) and girls (34.9%) was found to correspond with that of children suffering from chronic chest symptoms. Indications for BG were mainly recurrent pneumonias (45.9%) and wheeze or bronchial asthma, that were not responding to conventional therapy (48.7%). The symptoms observed in the three examined groups were similar.

CXRs were positive in 75.4% of the cases. Out of these positive CXR cases, 61 and 59% had perfect positive BGs using Hytrast and Broncholux, respectively. Out of the positive CXR cases who had BGs performed using Omnipaque only 46% of the cases were positive. All contrast studies performed using Hytrast or Broncholux were valuable. There were 21 (11%) invaluable BGs performed using Omnipaque.

Bronchial deformation and bronchiectasis

BD was diagnosed by Hytrast, Broncholux and Omnipaque in 33, 26 and 20% of cases, respectively. BE was verified by Hytrast, Broncholux and Omnipaque in 11, 10 and 5% of cases, respectively. Consequently, we can conclude that Omnipaque is less sensitive when compared to Hytrast or Broncholux in demonstrating bronchial diseases in children.

The use of Hytrast and Broncholux provides a sharp outline of the bronchi and allows us to make a precise evaluation of the shape of the bronchi. The diagnosis of BD is rather difficult, and sometimes impossible if using Omnipaque. It must be added that BG is essential for the follow up of BD.

In our experience, BD is frequently found in bronchial asthma. We can diagnose BD after the removal of aspirated or endogenous (plastic cast) foreign bodies. There are plenty of questions concerning BD that still remain. Is BD a separate medical condition? Is it a symptom of bronchial asthma? Is it one of the stages of progression towards BE?

The appearance of BE, when using Hytrast, Omnipaque and Broncholux, was also demonstrated. On the basis of the BGs that we performed, Omnipaque was, to a certain degree, sufficient for the diagnosis of BE. However, upon thorough evaluation Omnipaque was discovered to be more flawed than suspected, especially prior to lung resection for the diagnosis of BE. Whereas, the normal and ectatic bronchi branch off clearly in pictures obtained using Hytrast or Broncholux, this difference cannot be distinguished in pictures obtained from BGs using Omnipaque.

In summary, the most substantial difference between BD and BE is their reversibility. The primary diagnostic tool of both conditions is bronchography, although it is not always possible to differentiate between the two with only the help of one BG. Thoroughly following up patients and repeated BGs is the only solution to being able to make a clear distinction between the two conditions (Fig. 1).

Developmental disorders

We speak about bronchial aplasia when there is a blind bronchus without adjacent lung tissue. In general, reduced development of the bronchi and adjacent lung tissue results in lung hypoplasia. However, there is a special definition for bronchographically diagnosed lung hypoplasia, namely lobular filling after the

	BRONCHIAL DEFORMATION (Bronchial dilatation)	BRONCHIECTASIS
	dilated	dilated
➚	Uneven	DESTRUCTION
Bronchi➔	walls	OF THE
➘	Tortuous course	BRONCHIAL WALL
	REVERSIBLE diagnosis with bronchography	IRREVERSIBLE diagnosis mainly with bronchography

Fig. 1. Bronchial deformation/dilatation, bronchiectasis.

fifth order bronchi. Exclusively, BG can diagnose this condition, however, it is not possible to demonstrate it using Omnipaque, only Hytrast or Broncholux.

Disturbance in organ rotation during the embryonic development results in situs inversus. Consequently, there is right type bronchial branching in the left and left type branching in the right side. In Karatgener syndrome, bronchiectasis maxillary sinusitis and primary ciliary dyskinesia complete the condition.

Other applications of BG

Other applications for BG include proving cavity filling after pneumonia. BG also shows the length and shape of stenosis caused by scarification. Last but not least BG reveals the condition of the bronchi, which are situated behind the stenosis. Due to this, we can follow the displacement of the bronchi caused by an inflammatory pseudotumor.

Conclusion

To conclude, there is an ever-growing desire to visualize the peripheral bronchi. In the hands of experienced bronchoscopists, BG is a safe procedure practiced either through rigid or flexible bronchoscopes. A problem that always arises is the availability and suitability of contrast material. In well-selected patients, BG is still an essential, and in certain respects unavoidable, part of pediatric pulmonary diagnostics. There is a place for BG even in the age of CT scans and MRI. However, the application of these techniques and BG depends on skill, knowledge and the availability of the correct instrumentation, and last but not least on whether it is advantageous to the patient.

References

1. Avery ME. Bronchography: outmoded procedure? – commentary. Pediatrics 1970;46(3): 333–334.
2. Lewiston NJ. Bronchiectasis. Hillmanns' Pediatric Respiratory Disease WB. Saunders Company, 1993;225.
3. Morcos SK. Airways and lung: bronchography through the fiberoptic bronchoscope. Radiology 1996;200:612.
4. Bramson RT et al. Pediatric bronchography performed through the flexible bronchoscope. Eur J Radiol 1993;16:158–161.
5. Székely E, Farkas E. Pediatric Bronchology – Akadémia Kiadó-Budapest. Philadelphia: Baltimore Park Press, 1978;116–131.
6. Wood RE. Pediatric flexible bronchoscopy. A Postgraduate Course at Davos Congress Center, Davos, Switzerland 1999. Bronchography, Chapter 12, 10–11.
7. Committee on therapy American thoracic society. Bronchography. Am Rev Resp Dis 1970;101: 815.

Bronchology and Bronchoesophagology: State of the Art.
H. Yoshimura et al., editors.

Dumon-Novatech Y-stents: a 4-year experience with 50 tracheobronchial tumors involving the carina

J.F. Dumon
Centre Laser du CHU Sud et Service d'endoscopie Bronchique, Marseille, France

Abstract. This article reports a 4-year experience in using a new silicone Y-stent, which is characterized by the elasticity of its construction material, optimal inner diameter, and nonstick surface quality. Fifty patients with malignant disease involving the carina were treated by rigid bronchoscopy, including laser therapy and mechanical dilatation, followed by Y-stent insertion. Mean survival was only 109 days due to the severity of illness, but quality of life was good. Survival in 19 patients with esophageal cancer was particularly significant. For the eight patients with invasion or compression of the airway without fistula, mean duration of survival was 138 days. In the 11 patients presenting esotracheal fistulas in the vicinity of the carina, survival was only 71 days. Good life quality was directly related to good tolerance and complete re-establishment of respiratory function.

Introduction

Since the end of the 1980s, endobronchial stents have allowed palliative treatment of patients with extrinsic airway compression which was formerly beyond the reach of any other therapeutic modality [1]. The silicone stent that we designed in cooperation with the Novatech Company in France (Dumon-Novatech stent) features a patented studded outer surface. These studs hold the stent in place by fitting between the cartilaginous rings, and limit contact between the silicone tube and tracheobronchial mucosa. A major advantage of silicone stents is easy removal regardless of the duration of implantation.

Since the introduction of the first Dumon-Novatech stents, many improvements have been made to reduce complications observed during early experience. The rim edge has been beveled to limit irritation of the mucosa. As a result of this change, the problem of granuloma formation has practically been eliminated. Silicone quality has been upgraded to enhance elasticity and the range of standard sizes has been widened. These changes have reduced events involving migration. The surface of the stent has been treated to reduce adherence of secretions. This improvement greatly lowers the risk of obstruction which used to be a major drawback.

Straight stents have been shown to be highly effective for indications in midsections of the trachea and main stem bronchi [2–7]. However, they were not well-suited to lesions located on or near the carina. In view of these problems, we designed and produced a Y-stent. The purpose of this report is to describe our

Address for correspondence: J.F. Dumon, Centre Laser du CHU Sud et Service d'Endoscopie Bronchique, 270 Bd de Sainte Marguerite, 13009 Marseille, France. E-mail: jdumon@mail.ap-hm.fr initial experience in a series of 50 patients treated using the Dumon-Novatech Y-stent for tumor-related obstruction involving the carina.

Materials and Methods

Stent design

Design of the Dumon-Novatech Y-stent was based on over 10 years of experience with the straight stent. This experience showed that tolerance depends mainly on three factors: elasticity of the construction material, optimal inner diameter, and nonstick surface quality. Other important factors in stent design include total length, rim design, and wall thickness.

Adjusting elasticity is a major problem in stent design. The stent must be strong enough to withstand extrinsic compressive forces without being overly rigid. By trial and error, we determined that a wall thickness of 1.3 mm was sufficient to maintain the normal diameter of the carina by the vault effect. In this regard it should be underlined that we have never observed secondary stent compression in our experience of over 1,000 cases. Stents may be slightly compressed immediately after insertion, but always return to their original round shape within 3 days.

The inner diameter of the stent should be as close as possible to that of the normal airway lumen, i.e., 15—16 mm for the trachea and 12—13 mm for the main stem bronchi. This size requirement further underlines the importance of elasticity which must be great enough to allow insertion into the airways. This is also the reason why it is important to re-establish original airway diameter by resection and/or dilatation prior to insertion.

Surface quality is an essential factor for long-term placement. In addition to being smooth, the surface of the stent must be specially treated to prevent accumulation of secretions which can lead to obstruction.

Several features of the Y-stent have been studied to facilitate placement. Rim edges have been beveled to the inside and finely polished to allow smooth sliding over mucosa. A wide range of sizes have been provided so that the lesion can be completely covered without excessive projection onto healthy mucosa. The stent has been designed to permit identification of the front and back before deployment.

Figure 1A shows the most commonly used Y-stent model, $16 \times 13 \times 13$. These numbers indicate that the diameter of the tracheal leg is 16 mm while those of the right and left legs are both 13 mm. Only the front and sides of the tracheal leg of the stent are studded. The back of the prosthesis can thus be identified by the absence of studs. Studs were left off the bronchial legs to facilitate insertion. A Y-stent with a short slant-cut right leg can be used to preserve ventilation of the right upper lobe bronchus. Models are available with longer branches and slightly smaller diameters ($15 \times 12 \times 12$) (Fig. 1B).

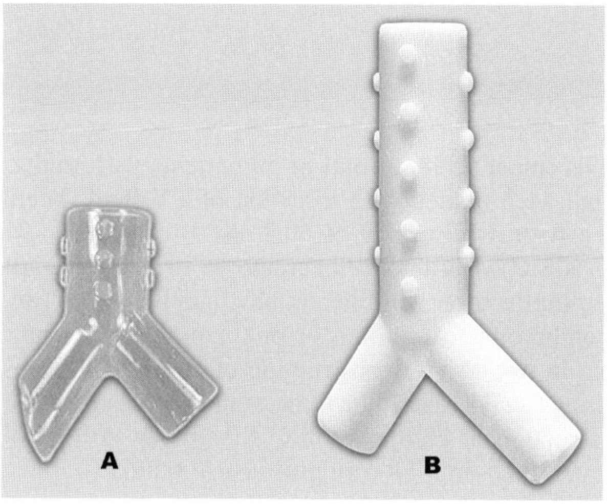

Fig. 1. **A:** Short Y-stent, 16/13/13 (these numbers indicate that the diameter of the tracheal leg is 16 mm while those of the right and left legs are both 13 mm). Only the front and sides of the tracheal leg of the stent are studded. **B:** Longer Y-stent, 15/12/12. This stent can be trimmed as needed.

Placement

Y-stent placement must be performed using a rigid therapeutic bronchoscope under general anesthesia. The first step in placement is to re-establish normal airway diameter by means of mechanical dilatation with or without laser-assisted resection. This reopening step is a prerequisite for placement of any type of stent.

Placement is performed using a large-diameter tracheal rigid tube (12 mm). The stent is loaded into a stent applicator and pushed out into the trachea just above the carina. After turning the prosthesis to the proper front/back position using foreign body forceps, the stent is seated on the carina. Beginning endoscopists sometimes have difficulty in deploying the legs, especially into the left main stem, but this problem is quickly overcome with experience.

Stent removal

Stent removal is always possible regardless of the duration of placement. The upper rim is seized using foreign body forceps and the prosthesis is twisted so that the walls collapse. The collapsed stent is then jammed against the tip of the bronchoscope and withdrawn.

Results

Patients

Between 1 July 1994 and 31 December 1998, a total of 50 patients with malignant lesions involving the carina were treated with insertion of a Y-stent. There were seven women and 43 men with a mean age of 60.3 years (range: 20–91 years). The histological diagnosis was squamous cell carcinoma in 32 cases, adenocarcinoma in seven, cylindroma in three, undifferentiated carcinoma in two, small cell carcinoma in two, embryonal carcinoma in one, lymphoma in one, melanoma in one, and sarcoma in one. Airway obstruction or compression was the indication for Y-stent placement in 44 cases. The remaining six cases involved esotracheal fistula with no obstruction or compression of the airway. A total of 19 patients had esophageal cancer, including 11 with esotracheal fistula.

Type of stent

The following Y-stent models were used: Y $16 \times 13 \times 13$ short in 40 patients, Y $1 \times 12 \times 12$ long in nine, and Y $18 \times 13 \times 13$ in one. In 23 patients with extensive tumors, Y-stents were combined with a straight tracheal (17 cases) or bronchial (six cases) stent. In all these cases short Y-stents ($16 \times 13 \times 13$) were used. Short Y-stents were used alone in only 17 cases. Straight stents were attached by telescoping with the Y-stent.

Removal

Removal of the Y-stent was performed in six cases. In one case, immediate removal was necessary because tumor compression resulted in such extensive deformation of tracheobronchial geometry that the Y-stent was almost completely flattened into a T-shape. In the five other cases, removal was carried out 43, 55, 78, 222, and 1,259 days after placement. Two Y-stents are still in place at 108 and 304 days after insertion.

Survival

Forty-two patients died during follow-up. This high mortality rate attests to the terminal nature of disease in patients indicated for palliative stenting. Mean survival was 109 days (139 days for patients still alive more than 1 month after placement). Three patients survived between 12 and 18 months.

Survival in 19 patients with esophageal cancer was particularly significant. For the eight patients with invasion or compression of the airway without fistula, mean duration of survival was 138 days. This is longer than for patients with isolated tracheobronchial tumors. In the 11 patients presenting esotracheal fistulas in the vicinity of the carina, survival was only 71 days. However, it should be pointed out that one of these patients survived for longer than 1 year after placement and another was still alive at 3 months after placement.

Case reports

The outcome of Y-stenting is well-illustrated by the following five cases.

Case 1: DEM Jeanine

In 1998, a 64-year-old woman undergoing treatment for melanoma developed severe dyspnea. Endoscopic examination revealed a tumor involving the carina. Therapeutic endoscopy using a rigid bronchoscope under general anesthesia was performed on 2 March 1998. A large tumor was found growing on the carina with complete obstruction of the right main stem bronchus and 90% obstruction of the left main stem bronchus. Histological study confirmed metastasis of melanoma. Laser-assisted resection was performed and the airways were re-established. To maintain the new carina, a Y-stent ($16 \times 13 \times 13$) was inserted. Full examination of the tracheobronchial tree revealed black metastatic lesions in most segmental bronchi with obstruction of the left upper division bronchus. Dyspnea improved dramatically, but the patient complained of chronic coughing which she attributed to the stent. At her request, the stent was removed on 26 April 1998. However, immediate replacement was required due to collapse of the carina after removal. Coughing was controlled by medical treatment using antitussive and sedative drugs. The cause of this complication is unclear, but was probably linked to extensive peripheral bronchial metastatic involvement. Subsequent follow-up was uneventful and the patient returned to a practically normal lifestyle. She was still alive 8 months after stent placement (Fig. 2).

Case 2: JOU Michel

In November 1994, a 48-year-old man was sent to our department from Toulon (France) for emergency treatment of acute respiratory distress due to extrinsic compression by a mediastinal tumor. The tumor caused 75% narrowing of the distal end of the trachea and 80% narrowing of the right main stem bronchus. Therapeutic endoscopy using a rigid bronchoscope under general anesthesia allowed re-establishment of the airway lumen. To prevent recurrence, a Dumon-Novatech Y-stent ($16 \times 13 \times 13$) was inserted. Respiratory function immediately improved and the patient was sent back to the referring physician 24 h later. Histological study of biopsy specimens obtained during therapeutic endoscopy demonstrated adenocarcinoma. The patient underwent high-dose radiation therapy in Toulon and was not re-examined. In April 1998, the patient returned to our department complaining of slight breathing disturbance. Thoracic CT-scan showed that the stent was still in place and that the mediastinal tumor had disappeared. The patient reported that he had never used the aerosol sprays

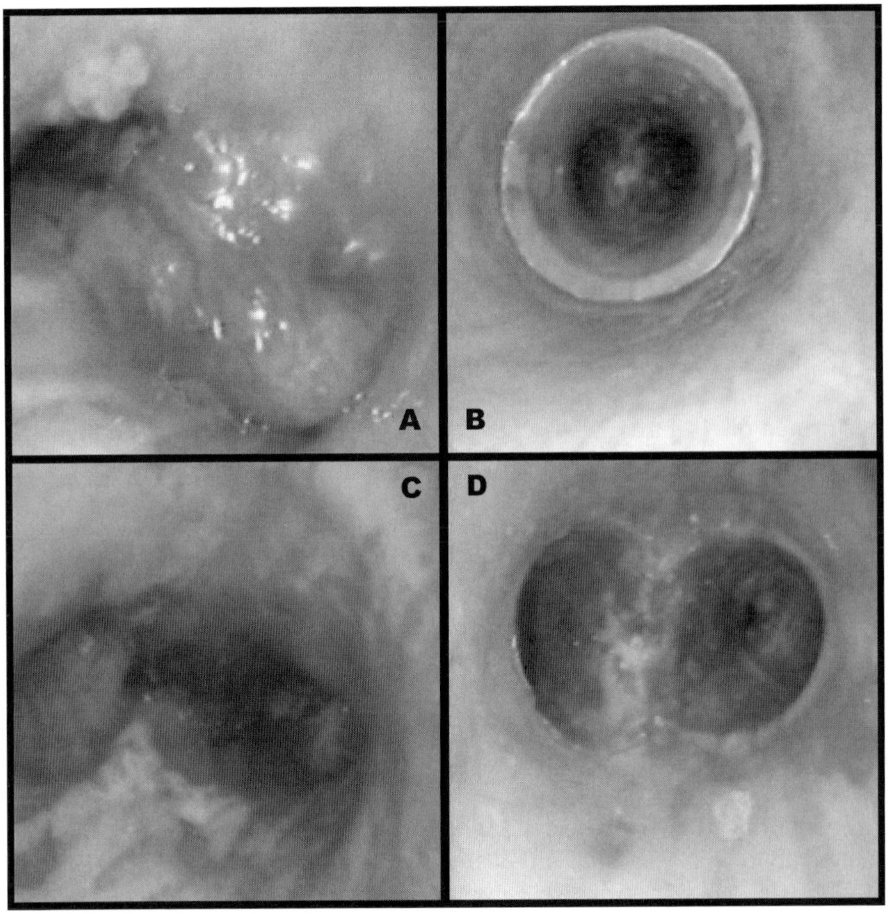

Fig. 2. Metastasis of melanoma. **A:** Large tumor astride the carina. **B:** Dumon-Novatech Y-stent in the trachea. **C:** Result after endoscopic YAP laser resection and dilatation. **D:** Close-up showing the carina covered by the Y-stent.

advised to reduce accumulation of secretions and that he had lived a practically normal life. On 5 May 1998 (Fig. 3), i.e., 41 months after placement, the stent was removed. Removal was easy. The stent was clean. Inspection of the airway showed that the mucosa was almost normal with only the presence of a small benign granuloma at the upper rim of the stent on the left side of the prosthesis. The patient was re-examined for 3 months after removal and then was again lost from follow-up.

Case 3: TRI André

A 69-year-old patient with cancer in the middle third of the esophagus with eso-tracheal fistula was sent to our department for emergency treatment. Five days

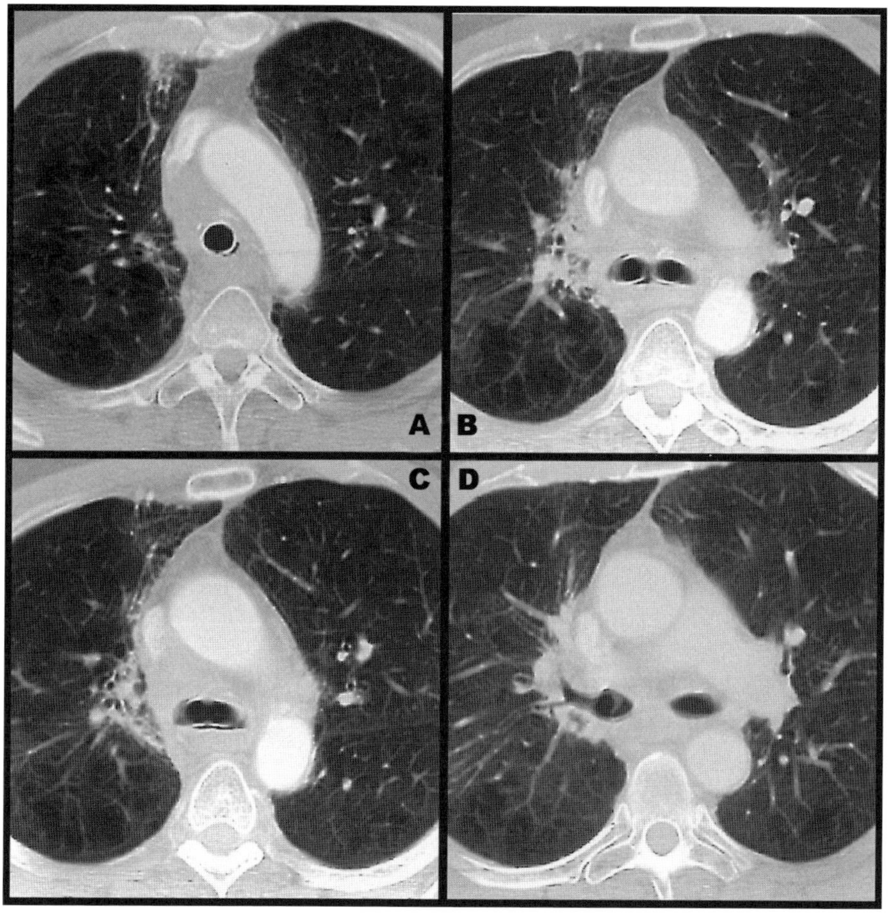

Fig. 3. Long-term follow-up of a Y-stent. CT scan 41 months after Y-stent placement for adenocarcinoma treated by radiation therapy and chemotherapy. The stent is visible at the level of: the trachea (**A**); the two main stem bronchi (**B**); the carina (**C**); the right upper lobe bronchus (**D**). The short slant-cut right leg preserves ventilation of the right upper lobe bronchus.

earlier, he had undergone placement of a partially covered Ultraflex esophageal stent. Endoscopic examination revealed the presence of two fistulas. The first was located in the middle third of the trachea over the uncovered metallic segment of the esophageal stent. More distally another fistula extending 3 cm down to the carina was found over the covered segment of the stent. Insertion of two stents was required to cover and seal the fistulas. A Y-stent (16 × 13 × 13) was inserted into the carina and a straight stent (18/60) was then telescoped into the tracheal leg of the Y-stent. The patient was able to eat the next day but died suddenly 11 days later (Fig. 4).

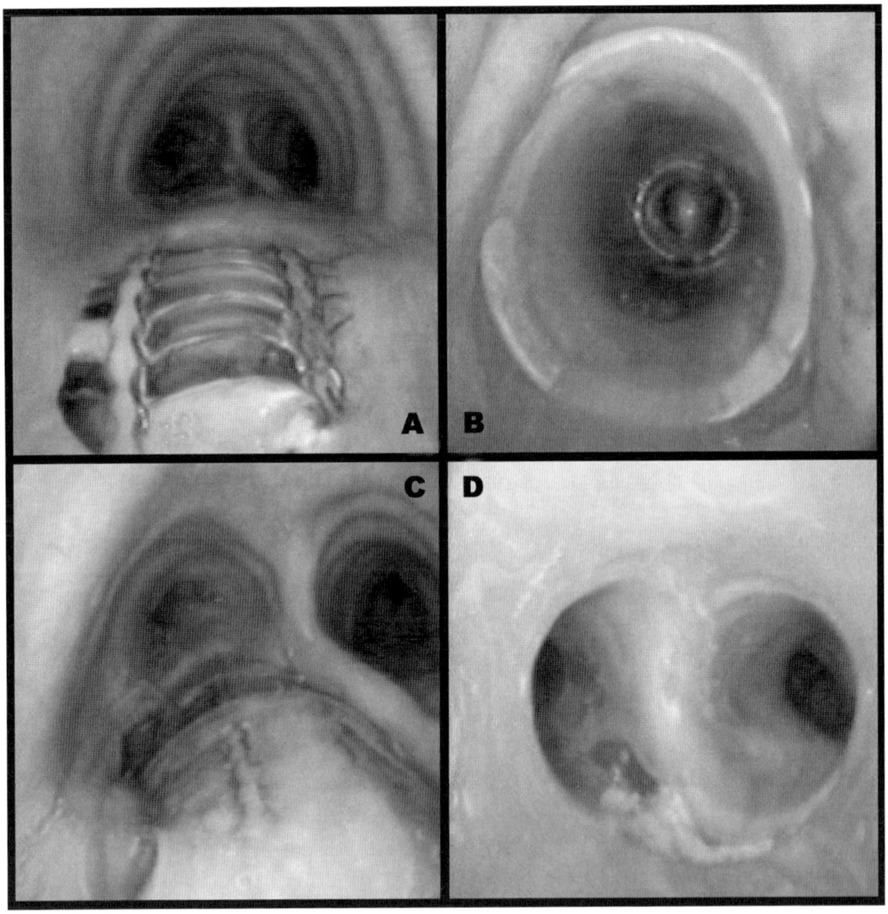

Fig. 4. Iatrogenic esotracheal fistula. **A:** Upper esotracheal fistula revealing uncovered segment of an Ultraflex esophageal stent. **B:** Straight stent (18/60) covering the upper fistula. **C:** Lower fistula extending 3 cm down to the carina and revealing the covered segment of the same stent. **D:** Y-stent (16 × 13 × 13) covering the lower fistula at the level of the carina. The two stents have been telescoped together.

Case 4: DRO Joel

A 53-year-old patient presenting an obstructive tumor in the middle third of the esophagus underwent placement of an uncovered Ultraflex stent. Ten days after placement, erosion of the mucosa led to fistula with exposure of the stent through the posterior wall of the trachea. The patient was referred to our department for treatment. Endoscopic examination revealed a fistula located 1 cm above the carina with no extrinsic compression. A Dumon-Novatech Y-sent (16 × 13 × 13) was inserted since the proximity of the fistula to the carina ruled out placement of a straight stent. Coverage and sealing was satisfactory. The patient was able to

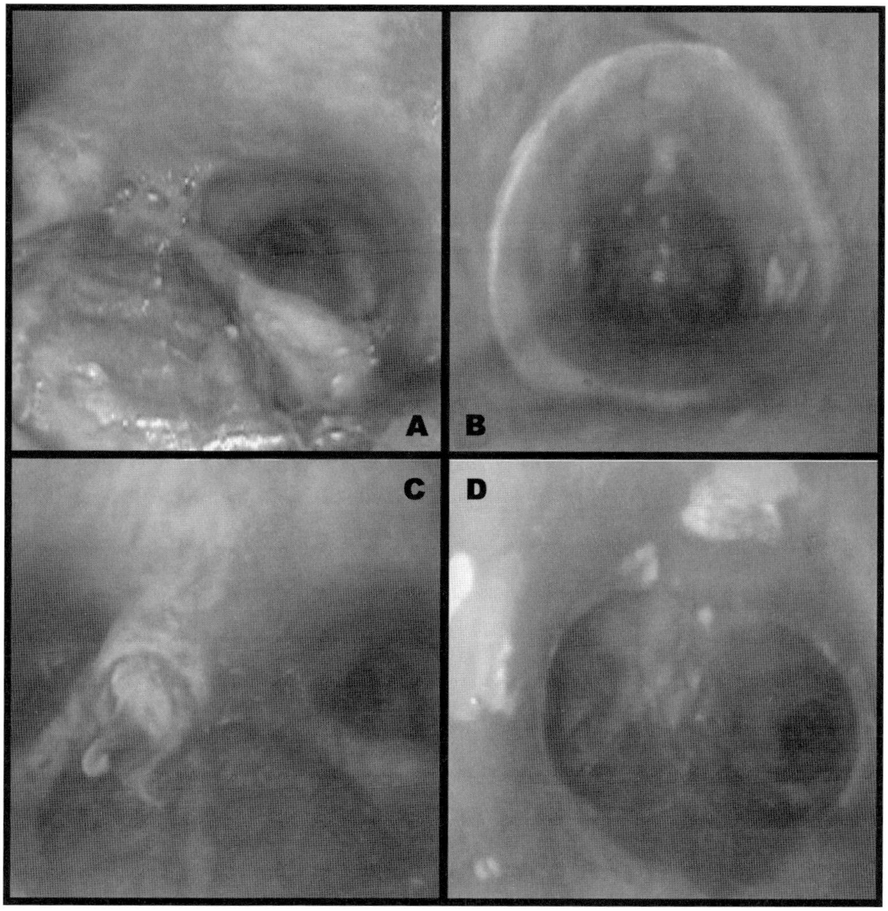

Fig. 5. Iatrogenic esotracheal fistula. **A:** Large fistula located 1 cm above the carina with no extrinsic compression. **B:** Y-stent covering the fistula. **C:** Close-up showing the carina. **D:** The fistula is visible through the stent.

eat again the next day. Survival with almost normal lifestyle lasted for 2 months (Fig. 5).

Case 5: GIAN Vincent

A 66-year-old patient was referred to our department for treatment of esotracheal fistula following radiation therapy. Tracheobronchial endoscopy revealed a fistula located 1 cm above the carina in association with extrinsic compression of the lower third of the trachea and high-grade stenosis of the left main stem bronchus. After therapeutic endoscopy to re-establish the airway lumen, a Y-stent (16 × 13 × 13) was inserted. Inspection of the esophagus revealed a tumor starting 20 cm below the dental arches and extending 10 cm. An Atkinson prosthesis was inserted into the esophagus. The two stents achieved effective sealing of the fistula and the patient was able to eat normally for three months. He was still alive 108 days later.

Discussion

Several findings deserve further discussion. The first is the short mean survival time after placement, which was only slightly longer than 3 months, i.e., 109 days. This finding must be correlated with the poor prognosis of patients indicated for palliative Y-stent placement. Survival without stenting would probably have been much shorter and the quality of life dramatically lower. Most patients with esotracheal fistula, die within one week after occurrence under extremely difficult conditions. Mean survival after placement of a Y-stent in these patients was 71 days with good quality of life.

Another interesting observation was the remarkably good tolerance to these stents. Stenting was successful without migration in all but one case in which placement failed due to compressive deformation of tracheobronchial geometry. One patient complained of persistent coughing following placement but this symptom disappeared and tolerance has been good for 8 months. Obstruction due to accumulation of secretions was not observed. Granulomas were uncommon and always of small size.

Insertion was easy provided that the lumen of two main stem bronchi was re-established to a diameter greater than 13 mm prior to placement. Removal was always easy even after almost 3½ years in one case. High-dose radiation therapy did not affect the integrity of the stent.

The large Y-stent ($16 \times 13 \times 13$) was used most frequently. The length of this stent is 4 cm which is excellent in terms of ease of insertion and coverage of the carina. However, in 23 of the 40 cases performed using this model, extensions using straight stents were necessary either proximally in the trachea (17 cases) or distally in the main stem bronchi (six cases). Based on this initial experience, we asked the manufacturer (Novatech) to make models with longer legs.

Conclusion

Over a period of 54 months, we placed a total of 50 Dumon-Novatech stents in patients with tracheobronchial or mediastinal tumors. The diameter of the bronchial legs of these stents is greater than 12 mm in all models. This feature probably accounts for the remarkably good tolerance. In all cases therapeutic endoscopy was performed to re-establish normal tracheobronchial diameter before placement and allow complete deployment of the stent. Mean survival was relatively short due to the severity of illnesses, but quality of life was good. Good life quality was directly related to good tolerance and complete re-establishment of respiratory function.

References

1. Dumon JF. A dedicated tracheobronchial stent. Chest 1990;97(2):328–332.
2. Bolliger CT, Probst R, Tschopp K, Soler M, Perruchoud AP. Silicone stents in the management of inoperable tracheobronchial stenoses. Indications and limitations. Chest 1993;104(6): 1653–1659.
3. Martinez-Ballarin JI, Diaz-Jimenez JP, Castro MJ, Moya JA. Silicone stents in the management of benign tracheobronchial stenoses. Tolerance and early results in 63 patients. Chest 1996;109 (3):626–629.
4. Cavaliere S, Venuta F, Foccoli P, Toninelli C, La Face B. Endoscopic treatment of malignant airway obstructions in 2,008 patients. Chest 1996;110(6):1536–1542.
5. Colt HG, Harrell JH. Therapeutic rigid bronchoscopy allows level of care changes in patients with acute respiratory failure from central airways obstruction. Chest 1997;112(1):202–206.
6. Miyazawa T, Arita K. Airway stenting in Japan. Respirology 1998;3(4):229–234.
7. Abdullah V, Yim AP, Wormald PJ, van Hasselt CA. Dumon silicone stents in obstructive tracheobronchial lesions: the Hong Kong experience. Otolaryngol Head Neck Surg 1998;118(2): 256–260.

Address of Novatech which manufactures the stent:
144, chemi de Saint Marc
06130 Plan de Grasse
France
E-mail b.ferreyrol@novatech.fr

Bronchology and Bronchoesophagology: State of the Art.
H. Yoshimura et al., editors.

Zenker's diverticulum: the endoscopic approach

Karl Hoermann and Cathrine Mattinger
Department of Otorhinolaryngology, Head and Neck Surgery, University Hospital Mannheim, Mannheim, Germany

Abstract. *Background.* Two approaches can be used for the operative therapy of Zenker's diverticulum: the external approach or the endoscopic technique.

Methods. The records of 52 patients who had an endoscopic operation of Zenker's diverticulum were evaluated retrospectively. Twenty-two patients were treated with endoscopic scissors and 30 patients by carbon dioxide laser resection. The therapeutic concept of rigid endoscopic diverticulotomy was appraised concerning the intraoperative and postoperative management for treatment and prevention of complications.

Results. Of 52 patients, 46 were free of symptoms, whereas eight patients (15.4%) had recurrence, four of these patients within 4 months. Except for two cases the recurrences could be reoperated endoscopically. The complication rate was 11.5%, haemorrhage was the most often occurring complication (three cases). Two cases required an external approach to control severe bleeding.

Conclusions. The endoscopic technique is a safe and effective procedure to operate Zenker's diverticulum, if the surgeon is prepared to handle extraordinary complications like severe haemorrhage quickly and sufficiently.

Keywords: carbon dioxide laser, endoscopic diverticulotomy, pharyngeal pouch, Zenker's diverticulum.

Introduction

Zenker's diverticulum can be treated surgically either by an open external approach with diverticulectomy or diverticulopexy and cricopharyngeal myotomy, or by the endoscopic technique [1]. In 1917, Mosher was the first surgeon to operate on Zenker's diverticulum endoscopically. He divided the mucosal and muscular wall between the diverticulum and the oesophagus by using the blade of a long knife, but he abandoned the method after his seventh patient had died of mediastinitis [2]. In the 1930s, Seiffert developed a similar endoscopic technique using scissors through a tubular instrument [3]. At the same time Dohlman introduced the endoscopic management of Zenker's diverticulum in Scandinavia [4]. He developed a specially designed hypopharyngoscope with a horizontal slit at its distal end, inserting the longer upper lip into the oesophagus and the shorter lower end in the diverticulum expanding the diverticular oesophageal wall as a horizontal bar in the middle. The wall was coagulated with isolated forceps

Address for correspondence: Prof Dr Med Karl Hoermann, Direktor der Univsität, HNO-Klinik, Universitätsklinikum Mannheim, 68135 Mannheim, Germany. Tel.: +49-621-383-2249. Fax: +49-621-383-3827. E-mail: karl.hoermann@hno.ma.uni-heidelberg.de and divided with a diathermic knife. In 1960 he published his results of more than 100 patients without having had any major complications and residual diverticulum was observed in 7% only [5]. Following this, the endoscopic resection of Zenker's diverticulum has also been called Dohlman's procedure and even though modifications have been introduced the basic technique remains the same. Different rigid endoscopes have been developed, for instance, the modified Dohlman's endoscope by van Overbeek (Medin, Groningen, the Netherlands) to introduce light conductors [6], or the Holinger–Benjamin endoscope (Karl Storz, Tuttlingen, Germany) to facilitate laser diverticulotomy [7] or the spreadable diverticuloscope designed by Weerda (Karl Storz, Tuttlingen, Germany) [8].

A variety of methods have been applied to divide the muscular bridge between the diverticulum and the oesophagus: electrocoagulation [5,6], carbon dioxide laser [6–10], endoscopic scissors [11,12], KTP-Laser (potassium titanyl phosphate) [13] or the endoscopic stapling technique which has the advantage of cutting the bridge and closing the pharyngeal mucosa at the same time [14–16].

In contrast to the above-mentioned rigid techniques, the division of the diverticulum can also be carried out via the flexible endoscope [17]. General anaesthesia is not necessary to perform the operation, but patients usually need more than one procedure to have a complete relief of symptoms [18,19].

Many surgeons still prefer the external approach as there are two life-threatening complications associated with endoscopic resection: the increased intraoperative risk of severe haemorrhage and the postoperative risk of mediastinitis. However, mediastinitis has also been observed after external diverticulectomy.

With the endoscopic technique, the number and type of complications vary to a great extent in the literature [6,9,10,12,13,20–22].

This prompted us to evaluate the value of our therapeutic concept of rigid endoscopic diverticulotomy using either endoscopic scissors or the carbon dioxide laser. We mainly focused on the intraoperative and postoperative management for prevention and treatment of complications.

Patients and Methods

We retrospectively reviewed the records of 52 patients who had been operated endoscopically on a Zenker's diverticulum. Twenty-two patients (1974–1984) were treated with endoscopic scissors and 30 patients (1994–1998) using carbon dioxide laser resection. The main symptoms of all patients were regurgitation, dysphagia, foetor ex ore and weight loss. The diagnosis was achieved with a barium swallow radiograph and/or by flexible oesophagoscopy, which ameliorates the assessment of the diverticulum by air insufflation [23,24]. The average age of the patients was 68.4 years, ranging from 39 to 89 years.

All operations were performed under general anaesthesia. First, a nasogastric tube was inserted through one nostril. The diverticulum was exposed and cleaned either through Dohlman's hypopharyngoscope (in the years from 1974 to 1984) or through Weerda's spreadable diverticuloscope. The wall between the diverticulum and the oesophagus was then expanded between the blades of the diverticuloscope (Fig. 1). The operations were performed either with endoscopic scissors or with the carbon dioxide laser (ESC Medical Systems, Sharplan™, USA) under the operating microscope (400-mm objective, Zeiss®, Oberkochen, Germany).

The cricopharyngeal muscle was separated step by step (Fig. 2) until all muscle fibers were separated completely and the mediastinal fat could be seen through the thin layer of oesophageal adventitia (Fig. 3). All patients received iv antibiotics (2 g Cefamandol or 2 g Cefazolin) intraoperatively and after 8 h. On the day of surgery temperature was controlled 3 times and the neck was checked for subcutaneous emphysema. Full blood count and sedimentation rate were determined on the 1st postoperative and consecutive days. Feeding over the nasogastric tube was started on the 1st postoperative day. In cases of coughing, antitussival medication was applied.

The nasogastric tube was only removed when the wound to the mediastinum was covered with a layer of fibrin tissue. Therefore, a nonbarium water-soluble iodinated contrast media (Gastrografin®) radiograph was performed on the 4th postoperative day. If the mediastinum was free of contrast media the nasogastric tube was removed and a soft diet could be started orally. Regular diet was started as tolerated. All patients could be discharged within 14 days, the earliest was after 5 days with an average stay of 7.2 days.

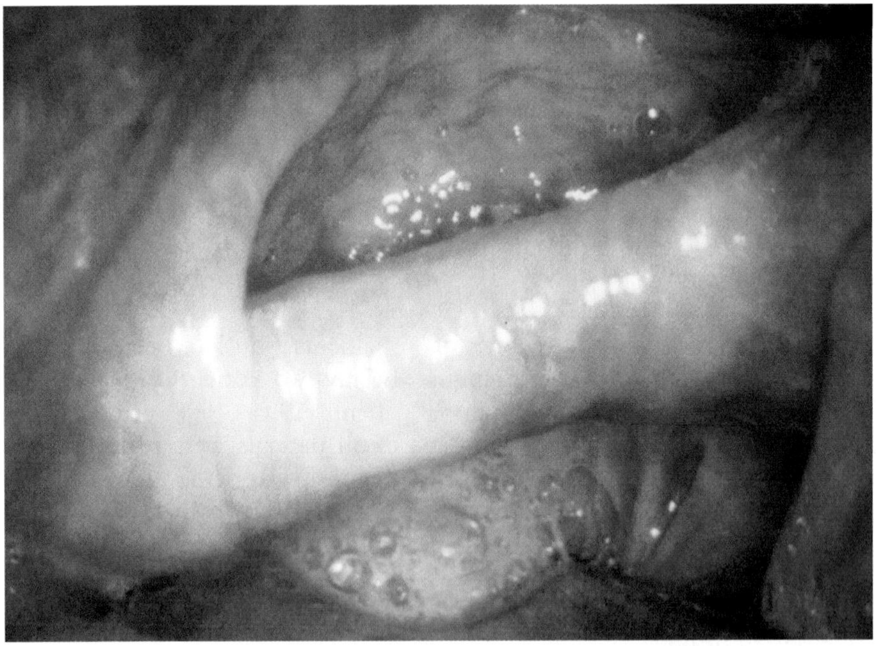

Fig. 1. The muscular bridge of Zenker's diverticulum is exposed between the blades of Weerda's spreadable hypopharyngoscope under the operating microscope.

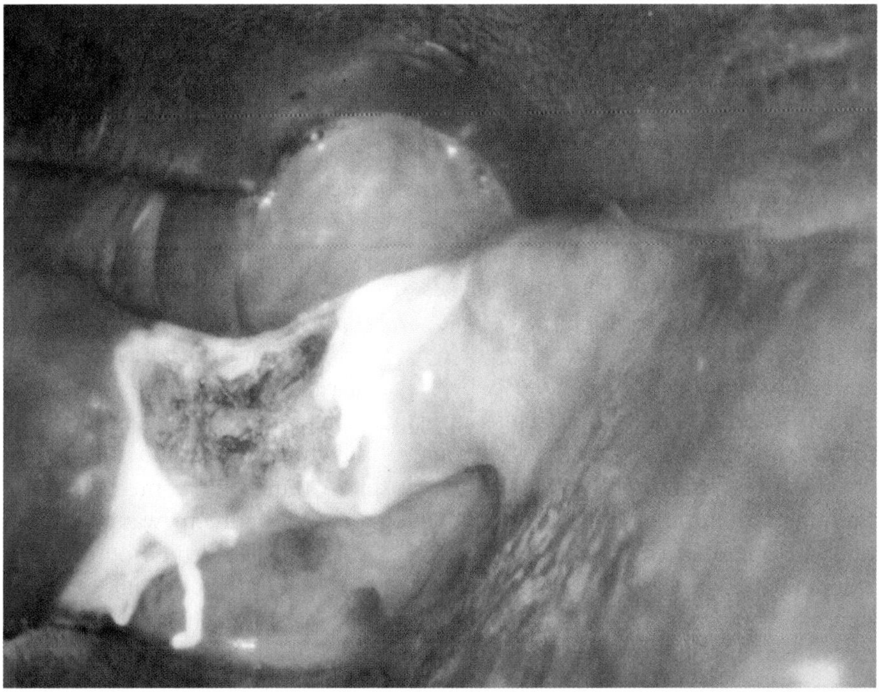

Fig. 2. The muscular bridge is divided step by step with the carbon dioxide laser.

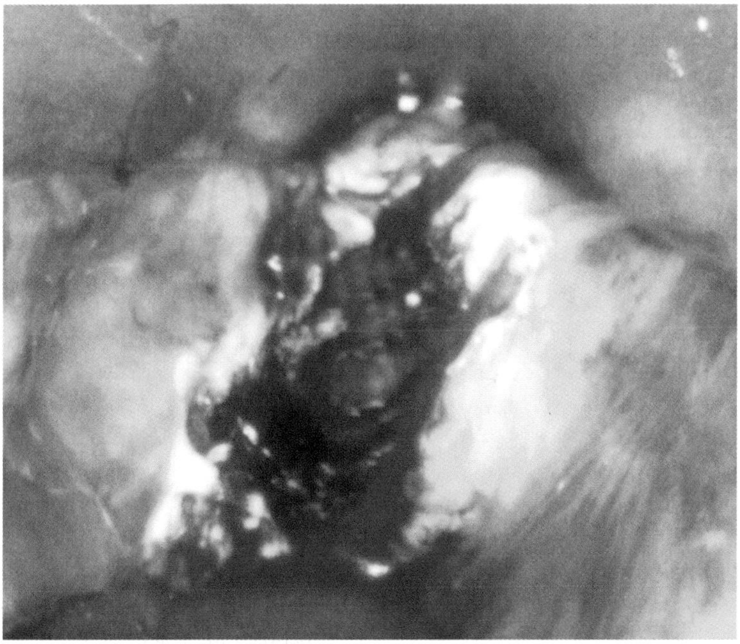

Fig. 3. The muscle fibers retract and a rhomboid window to the mediastinum is created.

The patient charts were evaluated retrospectively focusing particularly on intra- and postoperative complications.

Results

52 patients with Zenker's diverticulum were treated. From 1974 to 1984, 22 patients received an endoscopic dissection of the cricopharyngeal muscle with endoscopic scissors, and from 1994 to 1998, 30 patients were treated by carbon dioxide laser resection. 84.6% were disease-free after the intervention, eight patients had a recurrence of symptoms (15.4%), four of these patients within 4 months. Two patients with an early recurrence could be reoperated successfully with the endoscopic technique. One patient had a second recurrence of symptoms 2 years after the endoscopic revision, which was then treated by an external diverticulectomy. The fourth patient with early recurrence was reoperated successfully by an external approach in another hospital.

During the evaluation period four patients appeared with a recurrent diverticulum that was operated earlier (2, 4, 20 and 22 years previously). Three patients were reoperated successfully endoscopically, one patient with an external approach.

The overall complication rate was 11.5% (six out of 52 cases). None of the complications lead to long-standing problems or lethal outcome. An 84-year-old female patient died of myocardial infarction on the 8th postoperative day.

Four complications were noted perioperatively. Severe haemorrhage occurred intraoperatively during carbon dioxide laser resection in two cases and moderate haemorrhage in one case. The moderate bleeding could be controlled endoscopically by electrocoagulation. An external approach was necessary to stop the bleeding in those cases with severe haemorrhage. One patient experienced bleeding from an atypical inferior thyroid artery located just next to the cricopharyngeal muscle. The other patient bled from the inferior pole of the thyroid gland. Blood substitution was not necessary.

One vocal fold paralysis was observed postoperatively, which resolved spontaneously after 2 months.

Most of the patients had elevated body temperature, leucocyte counts and a raised sedimentation rate on postoperative days 1–4 independent of the method that was used to cut the diverticulum. The body temperature ranged from 36.6°C up to 39.0°C, with a mean temperature of 37.6 ± 0.6°C. The mean sedimentation rate in the 1st hour was 33.0 ± 22.1 mm (ranging from 5 to 75 mm), and 51.6 ± 26.5 mm during the 2nd hour (ranging from 9 to 90 mm). The leucocyte count ranged from $3{,}950 \times 10^6/l$ to $1{,}8800 \times 10^6/l$ with a mean leucocyte count of $11{,}429 \pm 4{,}620 \times 10^6/l$.

Despite these findings only two patients showed clinical signs of mediastinitis. They had the highest postoperative temperature of all of the patients (38.8 and 39.0°C) and complained of pain between the shoulder blades. One of these patients developed a subcutaneous cervical emphysema on the 2nd postoperative day until the 6th postoperative day. In both patients the complication could be managed conservatively with iv antibiotics (metronidazol; mezlocilline) and prolonged nasogastric feeding. Oral diet was started on the 6th and 8th postoperative day, and both patients could be discharged within 10 days with normal clinical and laboratory findings.

Discussion

Zenker's diverticulum can either be operated by an external approach or by the endoscopic approach with rigid or flexible endoscopes. In our evaluation haemorrhage was the complication that occurred the most often using the endoscopic technique. Twice the bleeding could only be controlled using the external approach. Wouters and van Overbeek have operated on the largest series of patients in the world with the endoscopic technique. Out of 544 patients treated with electrocoagulation or carbon dioxide laser, only five cases had severe intraoperative haemorrhage. The bleeding could be stopped endoscopically by electrocoagulation in four cases, in one case a packing was necessary for 24 h [20]. Bradwell had one major bleeding complication in 11 cases that could be handled by electrocoagulation and transfusion [10]. Other authors do not mention any intraoperative haemorrhages using the same technique as we use [9,11,21,22]. Considering the literature, severe haemorrhage is not the most frequent complication using the carbon dioxide laser. Steps to avoid major bleeding are to dissect exactly in the middle of the muscular bridge, to exclusively laser the muscle fibers and to avoid cutting into the mediastinal fat, that appears in a rhomboid window after complete incision of the muscular bridge (Fig. 3). However, if the bleeding cannot be controlled by electrocoagulation, a large and sufficient packing should be applied and the surgeon should not hesitate to use an external approach to ligate the vessel. Life-threatening arterial bleeding arises in most cases either from a lusory artery or from the inferior thyroid artery. The lusory artery is an abnormal right subclavian artery, which runs between the vertebral column and the oesophagus coming from the aortic arch. This vessel anomaly is apparently seen in 0.4% of cases. Legler lost a patient by cutting into the lusory artery, which can obstruct the oesophagus similar to the cricopharyngeal muscle and presents like a Zenker's diverticulum [25]. If the patient has a goitre, the risk for haemorrhage is increased as the inferior thyroid artery is pushed medially between the vertebral column and the oesophagus [26]. Weerda therefore proposes performing a preoperative angiogram [27]. We recommend to do a B-scan ultrasound of the thyroid gland preoperatively to locate atypical enlargements of the gland.

The overall complication rate in our cases was 11.5% using the endoscopic technique. We have used two different methods to divide the diverticulum, endoscopic scissors and later the carbon dioxide laser. The complication rate remains the same with both cutting methods. However, severe bleeding occurred with the carbon dioxide laser. It could be presumed that dividing the bridge with the scissors is safer than using the carbon dioxide laser, but we think that this outcome is incidental. The use of the carbon dioxide laser allows a better view of the diverticular bridge (Fig. 2), as the view through the endoscope is not impeded by the instrument.

Many surgeons prefer the external approach to avoid the risk of mediastinitis. There is no risk for mediastinitis when the myotomy is performed solely or in combination with diverticulopexy. Following diverticulectomy, mediastinitis can also occur. Lippert compared the complications after transcutaneous operation (n = 76) to the complications after endoscopic laser resection (n = 37). A purulent mediastinitis was observed in three cases after transcervical diverticulectomy and simultaneous myotomy, whereas only one mediastinitis was observed after the endoscopic technique [28].

Welch and Stafford compared 28 patients undergoing primary resection of Zenker's diverticulum with 32 cases undergoing endoscopic diathermy. 82% of the patients were asymptomatic after primary resection compared to 52% following endoscopic diathermy. The complication rate was lower in the endoscopic diathermy group, even though two patients developed mediastinitis, which was fatal in one case. No mediastinitis was seen in the other group. They propose to use the endoscopic technique only as an alternative in patients with small diverticula or with multiple diseases [29]. Parker and Hawthorne, on the other hand, saw significantly fewer complications after the endoscopic technique (n = 24) than after the external diverticulectomy (n = 16) and no significant differences between the recurrence rate. Of their patients, two developed a minor chest infection after Dohlman's procedure, whereas four chest infections were observed after diverticulectomy. Mediastinitis was apparently not observed [30]. Maran does not favour the endoscopic technique over the external approach because it failed in 30% of the patients with a complication rate of 17% and had to be repeated in 20%. One case of mediastinitis was observed [31]. Todd compared the external diverticulectomy with the endoscopic diathermy division in 121 patients. The complication rate was much higher in the diverticulectomy group with 52% (two cases of mediastinitis, one mediastinal abscess) compared to the endoscopic group with 9% (one mediastinitis). The success rate was 88% in the diverticulectomy group and 84% in the endoscopic group, but some patients needed two procedures [32].

Most of these studies report at least one case of mediastinitis even in a small series of patients. The nasogastric tube in our concept is the main tool with which to prevent infectious complications. When the muscular bridge between the oesophagus and the diverticulum is separated completely, the muscle fibers retract and a rhomboid window to the mediastinum is created (Fig. 3). In this window the mediastinal fat can be seen through the thin layer of oesophageal adventitia. The separation of the upper oesophageal sphincter and the negative inspiratory oesophageal pressure allow air to be swallowed during inspiration. If the patient is coughing, a positive oesophageal pressure will be created and the air can be pushed through the rhomboid opening into the mediastinum. The clinical result is a mediastinal and subcutaneous emphysema. Furthermore, air-resident bacteria can follow the same way causing life-threatening complications such as mediastinitis. The nasogastric tube is the main therapeutic concept for preventing these complications. It inhibits the elevation of the oesophageal pressure, serves as a track for the saliva to pass through the oesophagus and is necessary to nourish the patient.

A thorough postoperative follow-up can help identify the patients who are developing a mediastinitis and early therapy can prevent the worst. All our patients underwent a control iodinated contrast media oesophagogram before oral intake was allowed. Regular control for signs of infection can help to detect any developing mediastinitis. However, our results also demonstrate that most patients do have elevated body temperature, leucocyte counts and sedimentation rates even when they clinically do not present any symptoms. Lippert, who has seen temperatures up to 40°C on the 1st postoperative day after carbon dioxide laser resection, supposes that this could be due to mediastinal irritation rather than mediastinal infection [33]. Nevertheless, our patient with the highest temperature of 39.0°C presented clinical signs of mediastinitis. One has to be aware that the mediastinum is opened up when the endoscopic resection of Zenker's diverticulum, either by diathermy, endoscopic scissors or by carbon dioxide laser, is performed properly. In the future the endoscopic stapling technique could help to prevent these problems at least in those cases where the size of the diverticular bridge is suitable for use of the stapler [34].

Summarizing our results, we conclude that the surgeon operating on Zenker's diverticulum endoscopically should be sufficiently prepared to handle extraordinary complications like severe haemorrhage quickly and sufficiently. All precautions should be taken to prevent postoperative mediastinitis. When these requirements are fulfilled the endoscopic resection is a safe, quick and effective procedure for Zenker's diverticulum.

References

1. Grégoire J, Duranceau A. Surgical Management of Zenker's Diverticulum. Hepato Gastroenterol 1991;39:132–138.
2. Mosher HP. Webs and pouches of the esophagus, their diagnosis and treatment. Surg Gynecol Obstet 1917;25:175–187.
3. Seiffert A. Operation endoscopique d'un gros diverticule de pulsion. Bronchoscop Oesophagoscop Gastroscop 1937;3:232–234.
4. Dohlman G. Endoscopic operations for hypopharyngeal diverticula. Proc Fourth Int Congr Otolaryngol London 1949:715–717.
5. Dohlman G, Mattsson O. The endoscopic operation for hypopharyngeal diverticula. A roentgencinematographic study. Arch Otolaryngol Head Neck Surg 1960;71:744–752.
6. Van Overbeek JJM, Hoeksema PE, Edens ET. Microendoscopic surgery of the hypopharyngeal diverticulum using the electrocoagulation or carbon dioxide laser. Ann Otol Rhinol Laryngol 1984;93:34–36.
7. Holinger LD, Benjamin B. New endoscope for (laser) endoscopic diverticulotomy. Ann Otol Rhinol Laryngol 1987;96:658–660.
8. Weerda H, Schlenter WW. Neues Divertikuloskop zur Schwellendurchtrennung des Zenkerschen

Divertikels mit dem CO_2-Laser. Arch Otorhinolaryngol 1988;(Suppl. II):269–271.
9. Knegt PP, de Jong PC, van der Schans EJ. Endoscopic treatment of the hypopharyngeal diverticulum with the CO_2 laser. Endoscopy 1985;17:205–206.
10. Bradwell RA, Bieger AK, Strachan DR, Homer JJ. Endoscopic laser myotomy in the treatment of pharyngeal diverticula. J Laryngol Otol 1997;111:627–630.
11. Laubert A, Lehnhardt E. Die endoskopische Schwellenspaltung, eine Alternative bei der operativen Behandlung von Zenkerschen Divertikeln. HNO 1989;37:211–215.
12. Von Doersten PG, Byl FM. Endoscopic Zenker's diverticulotomy (Dohlman procedure): forty cases reviewed. Otolaryngol Head Neck Surg 1997;116:209–212.
13. Kuhn FA, Bent JP. Zenker's diverticulotomy using the KTP/532 Laser. Laryngoscope 1992; 102:946–950.
14. Martin-Hirsch DP, Newbegin CJR. Autosuture GIA gun: a new application in the treatment of hypopharyngeal diverticula. J Laryngol Otol 1993;107:723–725.
15. Scher RL, Richtsmeier WJ. Long-term experience with endoscopic staple-assisted esophagodiverticulostomy for Zenker's diverticulum. Laryngoscope 1998;108:200–205.
16. Baldwin DL, Toma AG. Endoscopic stapled diverticulotomy: a real advance in the treatment of hypopharyngeal diverticulum. Clin Otolaryngol 1998;23:244–247.
17. Feussner H. Reducing treatment of Zenker's diverticulum to the essentials: the flexible endoscopic approach. Endoscopy 1995;27:445.
18. Ishioka S, Sakai P, Maluf Filho F, Melo JM. Endoscopic incision of Zenker's diverticula. Endoscopy 1995;27:433–437.
19. Mulder CJJ, den Hartog G, Robijn RJ, Thies JE. Flexible endoscopic treatment of Zenker's diverticulum: a new approach. Endoscopy 1995;27:438–442.
20. Wouters B, van Overbeek JJM. Endoscopic treatment of the hypopharyngeal (Zenker's) diverticulum. Hepato Gastroenterol 1992;39:105–108.
21. Flamenbaum M, Becaud P, Genes J, Cassan P. Traitement endoscopique du diverticule de Zenker associé au laser CO_2. Gastroenterol Clin Biol 1997;21:950–954.
22. Gehanno P, Delattre J, Depondt J, Guedon C, Barry B. Traitement endoscopique des diverticules de Zenker. Press Med 1997;26:1228–1231.
23. Hörmann K, Schmidt H. Flexible Endoskopie im HNO-Bereich. HNO 1998;46:654–659.
24. Schmidt H, Hörmann K, Stasche N, Steiner W. Tracheobronchoskopie und Ösophagoskopie in der Hals-Nasen-Ohren-Heilkunde. HNO 1998;46:643–650.
25. Legler U. Untersuchungen vor und nach endoskopischer Operation kleiner und großer Hypopharynxdivertikel. Archiv Ohr-usw Heilk u Z Hals-usw Heilk 1952;160:547–560.
26. Ungerecht K. Ösophagus. In: Berendes J, Link R, Zöllner FS (eds) Hals-Nasen-Ohren Heilkunde in Praxis und Klinik. Stuttgart: Georg Thieme Verlag, 1978;15,27.
27. Weerda H, Ahrens KH, Schlenter WW. Maßnahmen zur Verringerung der Komplikationsrate bei der endoskopischen Operation des Zenkerschen Divertikels. Laryngo Rhino Otol 1989;68: 675–677.
28. Lippert BM, Folz BJ, Gottschlich S, Werner JA. Microendoscopic treatment of the hypopharyngeal diverticulum with the CO_2 laser. Lasers Surg Med 1997;20:394–401.
29. Welch AR, Stafford F. Comparison of endoscopic diathermy and resection in the surgical treatment of pharyngeal diverticula. J Laryngol Otol 1985;99:179–182.
30. Parker AJ, Hawthorne MR. Endoscopic diverticulectomy versus external diverticulectomy in the treatment of pharyngeal pouch. J R Coll Surg Edin 1985;33:61–64.
31. Maran AGH, Wilson JA, Al Muhanna AH. Pharyngeal diverticula. Clin Otolaryngol 1986;11: 219–225.
32. Todd GB. The treatment of pharyngeal pouch. J Laryngol Otol 1974;88:307–315.
33. Lippert BM, Werner JA. Ergebnisse und operative Erfahrungen bei der Schwellendurchtrennung des Hypopharynx- (Zenker-) Divertikels mit dem CO_2-Laser. HNO 1995;43:605–610.
34. Omote K, Feussner H, Stein HJ, Ungeheuer A, Siewert RJ. Endoscopic stapling diverticulostomy for Zenker's diverticulum. Surg Endosc 1999;13:535–538.

Bronchology and Bronchoesophagology: State of the Art.
H. Yoshimura et al., editors.

Foreign bodies of the aerodigestive tract: a 5-year Philippine General Hospital experience

Joselito C. Jamir, Samantha R. Soriano, David Paul M. Guirao, Jackeline M. Lim-Santos and Vincent M. Jardin
Department of Ear, Nose & Throat, University of the Philippines, College of Medicine, Philippine General Hospital, Manila, Philippines

Abstract. Foreign bodies of the aerodigestive tract have been commonly encountered in most hospitals nowadays. This study reviewed the charts of patients with foreign body aspiration or ingestion from January 1995 to December 1999 to determine trends concerning this problem. Most foreign body ingestions were noted in the pediatric age group (3- to 6-year-olds) and usually involved coins. In the adult age group, the most common ingestion is of dentures. Most were located in the cricopharyngeal area and were removed by rigid esophagoscopy. There were minimal morbidities such as abrasions and lacerations. Length of stay in the hospital was usually only 1 to 2 days. Ingestion of balut white was given special attention due to the rising number of patients with this problem. Most of the patients encountered were in the adult age group and the majority were males. All were located in the cricopharynx and were removed by forceps although three were pushed down to the stomach. No major complications were noted. Foreign body aspirations were also mostly in the pediatric age group and involved seeds. Rigid bronchoscopy was used. Patients stayed for a longer period of time (> 7 days). This study hopes to enlighten parents and hospital personnel about the growing problem of foreign body aspiration and ingestion and thus minimize its occurrence.

Keywords: aerodigestive tract, balut, foreign bodies.

Introduction

Foreign bodies are objects whether edible or inedible, animate or inanimate, metallic or nonmetallic which are found in areas where they should not normally be found. The obstruction of air and food passages by foreign bodies is a problem that physicians have to contend with in the daily practice of otolaryngology. In fact, the ingestion or aspiration of foreign bodies is one of the leading causes of pediatric accidents. Some would even claim that it is the leading cause of accidents in children, after traffic accidents. Confounding the problem is the fact that it occurs mostly in the two extremes of age, the pediatric and geriatric age groups, thereby making the presence of a clear history of ingestion or inhalation virtually impossible to elicit. This is even more so if the patient is in a depressed state of sensorium. More fortunate is the situation where a definite history is elicited from the patient. Even in the presence of a definite history, it may be con-

Address for correspondence: Joselito C. Jamir, Department of Ear, Nose & Throat, Ward 10, Philippine General Hospital, Taft Avenue, Manila 1004, Philippines. Tel.: +63-2-526-43-60. Fax: +63-2-522-09-46. E-mail: psohns@skyinet.net cealed by the person involved, be it the patient himself or the caregiver, in order to cover up the failure of the nursemaid taking care of or looking after the patient to exercise due care and diligence required.

Foreign bodies may or may not be life threatening for the patient, but all cases are distressing, not only for the patient but also for the caregivers and family involved. Thus, immediate medical attention is required.

The problem of foreign body ingestion and aspiration, both in the adult and pediatric age group, has been recognized since ancient times. Since Chevalier Jackson's description of endoscopic techniques for removal of foreign bodies in the aerodigestive tract in 1936, this has remained the most trusted method of treatment, however, morbidity and mortality have still been reported. The US National Safety Council reports that there are approximately 1,000 deaths per year due to foreign body aspiration and ingestion [1]. A study by Stroud estimated that 1,500 deaths occur annually due to foreign body ingestion and 3,000 due to aspiration [2]. Even though this is a familiar topic for most otolaryngologists, a review is warranted due to the significant morbidity and mortality associated with it. Special focus has been placed on the ingestion of balut white, a native delicacy among Filipinos, due to the rising number of patients encountered with this problem and the difficulties associated with its extraction. The increase in exports of food products and the presence of Filipino communities may also give rise to problems of this nature in other parts of the world, as yet unfamiliar with it.

This study was undertaken to relate the Philippine General Hospital experience on foreign body ingestion and aspiration from 1995 to 1999. The objectives of the study are as follows:

1. To determine the prevalence of foreign body ingestion and aspiration among Philippine General Hospital patients from 1995 to 1999.
2. To identify trends concerning foreign bodies of the aerodigestive tract in terms of:
   - patient profile (age and gender);
   - the most common foreign body ingested and aspirated in the pediatric and adult age group;
   - the most common site of lodgment of the foreign body;
   - the methods of extraction of the foreign body;
   - the most common morbidity; and
   - the average length of stay in the hospital.
3. To describe cases of ingestion of balut white in terms of:
   - patient profile (age and sex);
   - the factors predisposing to lodgment;
   - the most common site of lodgment; and
   - the methods of extraction.

Methodology

The study is a comprehensive review of charts of patients with foreign body ingestion or aspiration from January 1995 to December 1999. The following aspects were noted in the review of charts: the age and sex of the patient; the type of foreign body ingested or aspirated; management; complications; and length of stay in hospital. The ingestion of balut white was specifically reviewed, using the above parameters. Data gathered were tabulated nominally and descriptive statistics were used.

Results

Case records of 407 patients seen at Philippine General Hospital for foreign body ingestion and aspiration within the study period, i.e., from 1995 to 1999, were reviewed. Of these, 278 (68.3%) were males and 129 (31.7%) were females, with a male to female ratio of 2.1:1. The majority of cases, 268 out of 407 (65.85%), were less than 14 years of age. Table 1 summarizes the incidence of foreign body ingestion or aspiration per age group.

Coins are the most common type of foreign body encountered, with an incidence of 214 or 52.58%. In about 16% of the cases reviewed, the type of foreign body was not specified. Dentures follow in frequency of ocurrence with 46 cases or 11.30%. The next most frequent occurrences are balut white, chicken bone, metal objects, pins and seeds. Table 2 lists the type of foreign body with the corresponding incidence per age group.

Most of the cases were ingestion, not aspiration. Of the 407 cases reviewed, 389 or 95.58% were lodged in the esophagus while the remaining 18 or 4.42% were lodged in the bronchus.

There were two age groups noted to have peaks in incidence of esophageal foreign bodies, namely the 3- to 6-year-olds and the 14- to 54-year-olds. Bronchial foreign bodies, on the other hand, occurred more commonly in the 7- to 13-year-old age group followed by the 0- to 2-year old age group (see Table 2B). It is important to note, in Tables 2A and 3, that the peak in incidence in the age group of 3- to 6-year-olds was attributable to coin ingestion while in the 14- to 54-year-

Table 1. Incidence of foreign bodies ingested/aspirated per age group.

Age range in years	No. of patients
0–2	95 (23.34%)
3–6	13 (32.19%)
7–13	42 (10.32%)
14–54	125 (30.71%)
55+	14 (3.43%)
Total	289

Table 2A. The types of foreign bodies lodged in the esophagus per age group.

Foreign body	0–2 years	3–6 years	7–13 years	14–54 years	> 54
Coin	72	113	23	6	
Metal Object	4	2		4	
Pin	2	1	3	2	
Seed			1	2	1
Thumbtack			3		
Dentures		1		45	
Balut White				15	1
Meat Chunk				8	2
Chicken Bone				10	4
Other	8	14	3	30	6

Table 2B. The types of foreign bodies lodged in the bronchus per age group.

Foreign body	0–2 years	7–13 years	14–54 years
Pin	1	2	
Seed	1	9	1
Metal object			
Peanut	1	1	
Plastic object			1
Crab shell			1

old age group it was due to denture ingestion.

Further review of charts of foreign body cases from 1997 to 1999 showed that most foreign bodies were lodged in the cricopharynx, both in the adult and pediatric population (see Tables 4 and 5).

Foreign bodies in the airway were found to be more commonly lodged in the left mainstem bronchus followed by right mainstem bronchus, as shown in Table 6.

The most common duration of hospital stay usually ranged from 1 to 2 days, followed by 3 to 4 days, as shown in Table 7.

Some extractions of foreign bodies were without morbidities. These include, in decreasing frequency, abrasions, lacerations, nasogastric tube (NGT) insertion, edema, lateral pharyngotomy and pneumothorax. Table 8 lists the morbidity cases attributable to extraction procedures.

Table 3. The lodging locations of foreign bodies per age group.

Age range in years	Esophagus	Bronchus
0–2	89	6
3–6	131	0
7–13	33	9
14–54	122	3
54+	14	0
Total	389	18

Table 4. The level at which esophageal foreign bodies have been found in adult patients (1997–1999).

Level	1999	1998	1997
Cricopharynx	18 (72%)	11 (73%)	1 (7%)
18–22 cm	2 (12.5%)	3 (20%)	12 (86%)
23–29 cm	1 (8%)	0	0
30–34 cm	4 (16%)	1 (7%)	1 (7%)
Total	25	15	14

In the removal of bronchial foreign bodies, there were three cases of morbidity in 1998, specifically, laceration, NGT insertion and edema. There was one reported case of pneumothorax in 1999.

Once admitted and the diagnosis established, all the patients were then prepared for esophagoscopy or bronchoscopy. The majority of foreign bodies were removed using forceps, as shown in Table 9. When the foreign body was visualized and removal using forceps failed, some foreign bodies were either pushed to the stomach or removed via lateral pharyngotomy. There were three cases of failure noted from 1997 to 1999. Of these three cases, two involved foreign bodies found in the bronchus and were transferred to other hospitals (Table 7).

Of the 429 patients with foreign body ingestion, there were 16 cases of balut white ingestion. Only 10 charts were available for review. All were in the adult age range with a male preponderance (8 males and 2 females). In general the balut white was lodged in the cricopharyngeus and was removed by rigid esophagoscopy. Three cases had to be removed piecemeal and were pushed to the stomach without any complication. Most of these patients stayed in the hospital for only a few days (Table 10).

Discussion

Most cases of foreign body aspiration and ingestion were found in the pediatric age group, specifically in the 3- to 6-year-old age group, with a second peak at

Table 5. The level at which esophageal foreign bodies have been found in pediatric patients per age group (1997–1999).

Level	< 1 year	1–3 years	4–6 years	6–10 years	11–14 years
Hypopharynx	2 (9%)	0	1 (2%)	0	0
Cricopharynx	14 (67%)	31 (76%)	34 (76%)	9 (75%)	5 (83%)
12–17 cm	4 (19%)	7 (17%)	8 (18%)	3 (25%)	0
18–28 cm	1 (5%)	1 (2%)	2 (4%)	0	1 (17%)
Stomach	0	2 (4%)	0	0	0
Total	21	41	45	12	6

Table 6. The locations at which bronchial foreign bodies have been found in patients (1998/1999).

Location	1999	1998
Right mainstem bronchus	1 (8%)	2 (67%)
Left mainstem bronchus	11 (85%)	0
Left lower bronchus	1 (8%)	0
Glottis	0	1 (33%)
Total	13	3

the 14- to 54-year-old age group. In a study by Oclarence among pediatric PGH patients from 1991 to 1995, the majority of patients with foreign body ingestion were between 1 and 5 years of age [3]. Bailey also stated that 70% of all foreign bodies ingested occur in children younger than 14 years of age, but that 55% of these occur below 4 years of age [1]. In another study by Al-Salem, 28.2% of these cases were less than 3 years of age and 57.5% less than 6 years of age [4]. A study by Stroud stipulated that the majority of foreign body aspiration and ingestion occurs in children below age of five [2]. This is because children at this age range are just beginning to explore their environment. They tend to pick up objects and put them in their mouths predisposing to foreign body ingestion [5]. The second peak, in adults, is due to alcohol use, denture wear and neurological diseases [6].

It is also important to note the rise in the number of foreign body ingestion cases from 1995 to 1999. Due to the economic crisis, women are forced to seek employment and thus have less time to watch over their children.

The majority of patients were males with a male to female ratio to 2:1. This was also noted in the studies of Oclarence [3] and Tsuiki. This could be attributed to the fact that boys are more curious and exploratory than girls of the same age.

Coins were the most common foreign body ingested in the pediatric age group. This is consistent with other studies [4,5,7,8]. In adults, dentures were the common foreign body ingested along with food items. In a study by Villarta, dentures were the most common foreign body ingested by adults [9]. The etiology of the ingestion of dentures could be due to: 1) ill-fitting dentures; 2) intoxication; 3)

Table 7. Length of hospital stay.

Length of stay (days)	No. of patients
1–2	88 (46%)
3–4	73 (38%)
5–6	13 (7%)
7 or more	14 (7%)
Transferred	2 (1%)
Total	190

Table 8. The morbidities encountered during the extraction of esophageal foreign bodies (1997–1999).

Type of morbidity	1999 (n = 127)	1998 (n = 78)	1997 (n = 50)
Abrasion	9 (26%)	20 (43%)	2 (22%)
Laceration	11 (32%)	5 (11%)	3 (33%)
NGT insertion	7 (21%)	10 (22%)	2 (22%)
Edema	6 (18%)	10 (22%)	2 (22%)
Lateral pharyngotomy	1(3%)	1 (2%)	0
Total	34 (26.77%)	46 (58.97%)	9 (18%)

breakage of denture, and 4) trauma [2,9,10]. Adults also have an increased incidence of food impaction due to decreased sensation of the oral cavity in denture wearers [2].

The most common foreign body aspirated was seed and was noted mainly in the pediatric age group. There has been a decline in the aspiration of safety pins noted in this study, however, there was an increase in ingestion instead. The rise of safety pin ingestion could be attributed to the increased use of cloth diapers.

The most common site of lodgment is at the cricopharynx. The esophagus has three areas of physiologic constriction: the cricopharynx, the crossing of the aorta and the lower esophageal sphincter. These are also the areas were most of the foreign bodies are entrapped [11]. There is a definite predilection for esophageal foreign bodies to become lodged at the level of the cricopharynx due to its inferior edge being somewhat narrowed. Others attribute this to spasm, irritation and contraction of the cricopharyngeus muscle [4]. Once the foreign body has passed through the esophagus, it usually clears the rest of the alimentary tract without difficulty [11]. Other foreign bodies have occasionally become lodged in the ileocecal valve. The only exceptions would be sharp, pointed objects or objects too long (greater than 6 cm in children and 10 cm in adults) [11,12]. The average time for a foreign body to traverse the gastrointestinal tract is 7 days [11]. Patients with pre-existing esophageal abnormalities such as stenosis or webs are likely to have foreign body impaction at the site of the abnormality [12]. In our study,

Table 9. Methods of extraction used (1997–1999).

Methods	1999	1998	1997
Forceps	76 (84%)	64 (90%)	20 (77%)
Pushed to abdomen	5 (6%)	2 (3%)	1 (3%)
Lateral Pharyngotomy	1 (1%)	1 (1%)	3 (12%)
No foreign body	5 (6%)	4 (6%)	2 (8%)
Failed	3 (3%)	0	0
Total	90	71	26

Table 10. Cases of balut white ingestion.

Location	Method of extraction	Complications	Length of stay in hospital (days)
Cricopharynx	Forceps	(–)	4
Cricopharynx	Forceps	Abrasion	3
Cricopharynx	Forceps	(–)	3
Cricopharynx	Forceps	Abrasion,NGT	5
Cricopharynx	Pushed to stomach	Edema,NGT	3
Cricopharynx	Pushed to stomach	Abrasion, NGT	4
Cricopharynx	Forceps	Abrasion	2
Cricopharynx	Forceps	Abrasion	3
29 cm	Forceps	Abrasion	2
Cricopharynx	Pushed to stomach	(–)	2

there were no cases of any esophageal abnormality observed, except for one case of esophageal stenosis due to caustic ingestion 5 years prior to consultation.

Surprisingly, the most common site of entrapment for aspirated foreign bodies in our study was the left mainstem bronchus. In a study by Giannoni, 5% of aspiration cases occurred in the hypoharynx, 12% in the larynx/trachea, and 88% in the bronchus of which 43% where in the right mainstem bronchus [6]. This is attributed to the more vertical orientation and wider diameter of the right mainstem bronchus as compared to the left. However, paroxysmal coughing as a result of the body's futile attempt to extrude the foreign body may have caused its dislodgement from the right and its entrapment in the left mainstem bronchus.

All patients underwent rigid esophagoscopy with removal of the foreign body using forceps under general anesthesia. Endoscopy is by far the most commonly used means of removal and is the procedure of choice [1,2,5,12]. Nonendoscopic techniques are frequently discussed in the literature and are considered to be less ideal and possess a significantly greater risk of complications and of failure to remove the foreign body [6,13]. No mortality was noted in this study but there were a number of morbidities. Most of the morbidities were abrasions and lacerations of the esophagus requiring NGT insertion. There were two cases that underwent lateral pharyngotomy because of the size of the denture. The success rates for endoscopic removal of foreign bodies were also noted to be high (99.9%) in a study by Hsu and and in another (98%) by Brady [13,14].

Most of the patients with foreign body ingestion stayed in hospital for only 1 to 2 days, proving the point that the endoscopic removal of foreign bodies is usually risk-free.

Rigid bronchoscopy is the procedure of choice for foreign bodies in the airway. There has been a debate about whether to use rigid or flexible bronchoscopy, but the decision depends on user-preference, the location of the foreign body and the size of the foreign body [15]. The ideal situation for rigid brochoscopy is a controlled, well-equipped and prepared operative setting [6]. Patients who underwent this procedure were observed postoperatively for possible airway distress and adjunctive treatments were given. As reported by other authors, complications of foreign bodies of the airway include airway edema and respiratory distress, postobstructive pneumonia, postobstructive hypoxemia, airway perforation, airway stenosis or scarring and a retained foreign body [6].

In the cases involving balut white ingestion, all of the patients were in the 14- to 55-year-old age group. All were males except for two patients. This could be associated with the fact that balut white is usually used as a bar chow and eaten as a whole. Balut is a hard-boiled unhatched duck egg. It has three main parts: the chick, the yolk and the balut white. It is surrounded by a liquid which is the waste material of the chick. In the vernacular, it is called "bato", which means stone, due to its firm to hard consistency. The balut white has an average dimension of 3 to 4 cm by 2 cm, depending upon the stage of development of the chick. Most people eat it by creating an opening at the top of the eggshell and sucking the liquid. The consistency being smooth, they do not chew it properly. Most of these cases were successfully treated endoscopically since most were located in the cricopharyx. Three cases were treated with piecemeal removal and the rest were pushed down into the stomach. No major morbidity was noted except for abrasions. Most patients were discharged within 5 days.

Conclusion

In summary, most of the cases were foreign body ingestion by children in the 3- to 6-year-old age group and most frequently involved coins. The adult age group usually ingested dentures. There was a male preponderance. The common lodgement area was in the cricopharyngeus and which was successfully treated by rigid esophagoscopy with minimal morbidity. Most of the patients were discharged within 2 days.

The cases of foreign body aspiration mainly involved the 7- to 13-year-old age group and the foreign body was mostly seeds. There was also a male preponderance. The common site of lodgment was the left mainstem bronchus. Removal was performed using rigid bronchoscopy. Most of the patients stayed in the hospital for more than 7 days.

The cases of ingestion of balut white involved mostly male adults and lodgement occurred in the cricopharyngeus. Rigid esophagoscopy was used to extract the balut white. Most patients were discharged after 3 or 4 days.

This study recommends that parents take special care of their children, specifically in the 3- to 6-year-old age group since they have the predisposition to put things in their mouth leading to ingestion. Parents should be aware of the dangers of swallowed foreign bodies and avoid leaving small objects lying around or avoid giving their children small objects and toys to play with [4]. Adults with dentures should have regular check-ups with their dentist to ensure a good fit of their dentures.

There has also been an increasing number of balut white ingestion. The public should be informed of this to create an awareness about this growing problem.

References

1. Bailey B. Foreign bodies in the aerodigestive tract. Department of Otolaryngology, UTMB, Grand Rounds. October 1991.
2. Stroud R. Foreign bodies of the upper aerodigestive tract. Department of Otolaryngology, UTMB, Grand Rounds. October 22, 1997.
3. Oclarence M, Jose E. Foreign body ingestion in children (esophagus): A 5-year experience at the Philippine General Hospital. Acta Med Philippina (In press).
4. Al-Salem A, Murugan A, Hammad H, Talwalker V. Swallowed foreign bodies in children: aspects of management. ASM 1995;15(4).
5. Munter D. Foreign Bodies, Gastrointestinal.
6. Giannoni C. Foreign body aspiration. BCM Otolaryngology Home Page, 12 March 2000.
7. Reilly JS, Walter MA. Consumer product aspiration and ingestion in children: analysis of emergency room reports to the National Electronic Injury Surveillance System. Ann Otol Rhinol Laryngol 1992;101(9):739–741.
8. Rimell FL, Thome A Jr, Stool S, Reilly JS, Stool D, Wilson CL. Characteristics of objects that cause choking in children. J Am Med Assoc 1995;274(22):1763–1766.
9. Villarta RL, Ureta CV, Cosalan EM, Cruz BC. Esophageal foreign bodies of dental origin – a 3-year retrospective study. Philippine J Otolaryngol Head Neck Surg 1994;271–275.
10. Tsuiki T, Abe T, Murai K, Sasamori S. Statisitcal study of 41 cases with denture foreign bodies in the air and food passages and significance of the duplicated denture model. Otolaryngol Head Neck Surg 2000;122(3):450-454.
11. Nord HJ, Brady PG. Management of esophageal and gastric foreign bodies. Mosby-Year Book Inc. Vol 2 (1) July 1994.
12. Conners GP. Pediatrics, foreign body ingestion.
13. Brady PG. Esophageal foreign bodies. Gastroenterol Clin North Am 1991;20(4):691–700.
14. Hsu WC, Sheen TS, Lin CD, Tan CT, Yeh TH, Lee SY. Clinical experiences of removing foreign bodies in the airway and esophagus with a rigid endoscope: a series of 3217 cases from 1970 to 1996. Eur J Emergency Med 1995;2(2):83–87.
15. Gelford B. Foreign bodies, trachea.

Bronchology and Bronchoesophagology: State of the Art.
H. Yoshimura et al., editors.

Adenoid cystic carcinoma of the trachea

Kwang Hyun Kim, Myung-Whun Sung, Dong-Young Kim and Jeong-Whun Kim
Department of Otolaryngology — Head and Neck Surgery, Seoul National University College of Medicine, Seoul, Korea

Abstract. *Background.* Primary adenoid cystic carcinoma of the trachea is rare, but is the second most common malignant tumor of the trachea following squamous cell carcinoma. This tumor is frequently misdiagnosed as thyroid carcinoma involving the trachea. It is, therefore, very important to make a clear distinction between this tumor and thyroid carcinoma. The purpose of this study is to describe clinical and radiological findings about the adenoid cystic carcinoma of the trachea and to provide help in order to make exact diagnoses and treatment plans possible.

Methods. Nine cases of the adenoid cystic carcinoma of the trachea were diagnosed and managed in our institute. Most of the tumors were found in the cervical trachea and the most common symptom was slowly progressing airway obstruction. These cases were mainly treated by extensive surgery such as total laryngectomy or tracheal resection followed by radiation.

Results. The overall disease-specific survival rates were 66.7% over 5 years, and 44.4% over 10 years. The disease-free periods of these patients ranged from 11 to 111 months. There were five cases of distant metastasis during the follow-up.

Conclusions. Our experience indicates that head and neck surgeons should have a high index of suspicion if they are to differentiate adenoid cystic carcinoma of the trachea from thyroid cancer.

Keywords: adenoid cystic carcinoma, thyroid cancer, trachea.

Introduction

Primary tracheal tumors are rare, with an incidence of only 0.2 per 100,000 persons per year [1]. When all series are combined, primary adenoid cystic carcinoma of the trachea is seen to be the second most common malignant tumor of the trachea following squamous cell carcinoma. The clinical and pathological features of adenoid cystic carcinoma of the trachea were first reported by Billroth in 1859 [2]. This tumor is frequently misdiagnosed as thyroid carcinoma involving the trachea and so, it is very important that we are able to differentiate between this tumor and thyroid carcinoma [3].

The purpose of this study is to describe the clinical and radiological findings about adenoid cystic carcinoma of the trachea and provide help in order to make exact diagnoses and treatment plans possible.

Address for correspondence: Kwang Hyun Kim MD, Department of Otolaryngology — Head and Neck Surgery, Seoul National University College of Medicine, 28 Yongon-Dong, Chongno-Gu, Seoul 110-744, Korea. Tel.: +82-2-760-2286. Fax: +82-2-745-2387. E-mail: kimkwang@plaza.snu.ac.kr

Table 1. Symptom and treatment modalities.

Patient No.	Sex/Age (years)	CC/Duration[a] (months)	1° Treatment
1	F/28	Neck mass/5	TREE, thyroidectomy + RT
2	F/23	Dyspnea/6	TREE + RT
3	F/45	Dyspnea/36	RT
4	F/43	Dyspnea/4	TL, thyroidectomy + RT
5	F/42	Dyspnea/12	TL, thyroidectomy
6	F/41	Dyspnea/5	Laser bronchoscopy + RT
7	M/34	Neck mass/4	TREE, thyroidectomy + RT
8	M/49	Dyspnea/7	TL, thyroidectomy + RT
9	M/53	Hoarseness/30RT	RT

[a]Mean duration of symptoms prior to diagnosis: 12 months. CC = chief complaint; TREE = tracheal resection and end-to-end anastomosis; RT = radiation therapy; TL= total laryngectomy.

Patients and Methods

Nine patients with histologically confirmed adenoid cystic carcinoma of the trachea were treated at the Department of Otolaryngology – Head and Neck Surgery, Seoul National University Hospital, Seoul, Korea, from 1979 to 1999. All medical records were reviewed retrospectively. The age of the patients ranged from 23 to 53 years of age (mean 40 years) with a female preponderance (male:female = 3:6). The patients were followed for at least 11 months upto a maximum of 111 months (mean 60 months).

Most of the tumors were found in the cervical trachea, except in two cases. Six patients had dyspnea as their chief complaint, two neck mass and one patient had hoarseness. The duration of symptoms ranged from 4 to 36 months (mean 12 months). Five patients were treated with extensive surgery, such as total laryngectomy or tracheal resection followed by radiation, one with laser bronchoscopy and postoperative radiation, two with radiation therapy alone, and a final one with extensive surgery alone (Table 1).

The survival distributions over 5 and 10 years were calculated using Kaplan-Meier method.

Results

Primary treatment failed in six (66.7%) out of the nine patients. The causes of treatment failure were distant metastasis, local recurrence, and distant metastasis combined with local recurrence, with the number of patients succumbing to each condition being four, one and one, respectively. Out of six patients, three remained alive with the disease and three died of the disease (Table 2). There were five cases of distant metastasis during the follow-up, and the lung was the most common site for this complication to occur.

When treatment results were considered according to treatment modalities, two

Table 2. Follow-up results.

Patient No.	Recurrence of disease	DFI (months)	2nd Treatment	Status	Follow-up period (months)
1	–	111	–	NED	111
2	DM	95	RT	AWD	97
3	DM	52	RT + chemoTx	DOD	71
4	DM	27	None	AWD	69
5	LR+DM	26	Mass excision	DOD	59
6	LR	11	TREE	DOD	57
7	DM	27	None	AWD	36
8	–	24	–	NED	24
9	–	–	–	Stationary	11

DM = distant metastasis; LR = locoregional recurrence; DFI = disease-free interval; NED = no evidence of disease; AWD = alive with disease; DOD = died of disease.

patients seemed to have no evidence of disease and three out of five patients, who were treated with extensive surgery followed by radiation, remained alive with distant metastasis. However, in the cases of four patients with other treatment modalities, only one patient, who was treated with radiation alone, remained alive with distant metastasis, while the other the patients died.

The disease-free periods of these patients ranged from 11 to 111 months. The overall disease-specific survival rates were 66.7% over 5 years, and 44.4% over 10 years. Only two cases were disease-free, however, there is still the possibility that distant metastasis might occur.

Discussion

Adenoid cystic carcinoma of the trachea is not known to have any association with gender, race, or cigarette smoking [1], however, there was female predominance (M:F = 3:6) in our series. Dyspnea was the most common chief complaint. Others included neck mass or hoarseness. The symptom duration prior to diagnosis was relatively long (mean 12 months), because adenoid cystic carcinoma has a much more indolent course than squamous cell carcinoma [1].

It is difficult to differentiate adenoid cystic carcinoma of the trachea from thyroid cancer, because of its rarity and similar radiological and clinical findings, especially in exophytic mass out of the trachea [3]. Of seven patients, who had tumors in the cervical trachea, three received total laryngectomy. Due to differential diagnosis being difficult and the possibility of total laryngectomy being higher in cervical tracheal adenoid cystic carcinoma, preoperative fine needle aspiration biopsy, informed consent for laryngectomy, and in particular, clinical suspicion, are very important.

Treatment options include surgery alone, radiation alone, or a combination. Regnard et al. [4] reported that survival was significantly longer for those with complete resections than for those with incomplete resections in tracheal cancers.

Grillo et al. [5] recommended surgical resection followed by radiation as a primary choice of treatment in adenoid cystic carcinoma of the trachea on the basis of their experiences and data. In our studies, extensive surgery followed by radiation also showed the best treatment results, although the small number of cases made statistical analysis impossible.

Conclusion

Our experience indicates that head and neck surgeons need a high index of suspicion to be able to differentiate adenoid cystic carcinoma of the trachea from the thyroid cancer. We believe that extensive surgery and postoperative radiation are currently the best treatment modality and improve survival.

References

1. Azar T, Abdul-Karim FW, Tucker HM. Adenoid cystic carcinoma of the trachea. Laryngoscope 1998;108:1297–1300.
2. Maziak DE, Todd TRJ, Keshavjee SH, Winton TL, Nostrand PV, Pearson FG. Adenoid cystic carcinoma of the airway: thirty-two-year experience. J Thorac Cardiovasc Surg 1996;112: 1522–1532.
3. Kim KH, Sung MW, Kang JK, Ahn SH, Han MH. Primary adenoid cystic carcinoma of the trachea. Korean J Otolaryngol 1997;40:17–20.
4. Regnard JF, Fourquier P, Levasseur P. Results and prognostic factors in resections of primary tracheal tumors: a multicenter retrospective study. J Thorac Cardiovasc Surg 1996;111: 808–813.
5. Grillo HC, Mathisen DJ. Primary tracheal tumors: treatment and results. Ann Thorac Surg 1990;49:69–77.

Bronchology and Bronchoesophagology: State of the Art.
H. Yoshimura et al., editors.

Imaging techniques of the larynx

M. Külekçi
Ministry of Health Taksim Hospital ENT Department, Istanbul, Turkey

Evaluating the mucosal surfaces of the larynx radiologically has always been secondary to clinical examination, but we know that cross–sectional imaging plays an indispensable complementary role because it enables one to evaluate the deep structures of the larynx and extent of tumors. Disease of the larynx covers a wide spectrum of different entities that are investigated by various radiological techniques. The indications for these different radiological examinations depend on the clinical problems to be investigated. The current modalities for the treatment of head and neck cancer consist mainly of surgical removal. Both CT and MRI imaging can provide images with excellent detail of the larynx and hypopharynx. CT, the standard modality for more than a decade, has recently become further enhanced by the introduction of helical scanning, which enables much faster image acquisition. CT and MRI play important roles in endoscopy in the pretherapeutic workup of laryngeal, hypopharyngeal cancer and are very valuable for the detection of tumor recurrence after surgery. Histopathological studies also denoted that modern laryngeal imaging with high resolution CT scans or MRI images provide accurate information about primary tumor extent and the status of neck nodes. Although some substantial drawbacks of MRI, including long acquisition periods, motion artifacts and claustrophobia, still persist, MRI seems to be the optimal method of examination in cooperative patients, especially for the evaluation of their larynx before an attempted partial laryngectomy. MRI seems to be more sensitive than CT in detection of neoplastic soft tissue invasion, but seems to have a somewhat lower specificity especially concerning thyroid cartilage involvement. Therefore, MRI imaging tends to overestimate neoplastic cartilage invasion and may result in overtreatments, whereas CT tends to underestimate neoplastic cartilage invasion and may lead to inadequate therapy. We should remember that the primary goal of the diagnostic imaging of the larynx is the analysis of submucosal structures that are not visible by clinical or endoscopic means. Therefore, imaging analysis of the larynx should only be performed under knowledge of the results of clinical diagnosis.

The larynx lies deep within the soft tissues of the neck, this organ can be heard before visualized. A skilled otolaryngologist with a modern endoscope can see

Address for correspondence: M. Külekçi MD, PhD, Taksim, Müssuyu, Irönü CAD, 43/I 80090, Istanbul, Turkey. Tel.: +90-212-2929-767. Fax: +90-212-2929-763.

almost all of the mucosal surface of the larynx. Most laryngeal diseases show themselves at the mucosal level, and so diagnosis is frequently made by indirect laryngoscopic examination and biopsy by laryngoscopy. The problem for otolaryngologists is the limitations of endoscopy when planning or performing surgery. The surgeon needs much more detail about submucosal extension of the tumor. The most common mucosal lesions of the larynx to be imaged are squamous cell carcinoma. Other disease processes or clinical situations are encountered less frequently.

Anatomy

The larynx has a cartilaginous skeleton connected by muscles and ligaments. The inner luminal aspect of the larynx is covered by mucous membranes with underlying elastic tissues and muscles. The anterior surface of the epiglottis, the upper half of the posterior epiglottis, the superior margin of the aryepiglottic folds, and the margin of the vocal folds are all covered with stratified squamous epithelium. Elsewhere a ciliated columnar epithelium is seen.

Skeletal elements of the larynx

Hyoid bone
Criticea cartilage
Epiglottis
Corniculate cartilage
Arytenoid cartilage
Thyroid cartilage
Cricoid cartilage

Muscles and folds of larynx

Thyrohyoid membrane
Quadrangular membrane
Hyoepiglottic ligament
Vestibular ligament
Cricoidthyroid membrane
Cricotracheal membrane
Vocal ligament

Radiological interpretations of scans of the larynx for abnormal findings requires a good knowledge of normal radiological anatomy. Some degree of normally occurring asymmetry should be recognized in patients with suspected laryngeal abnormalities to avoid misinterpretation of scans.

Imaging

Imaging plays an indispensable role in the diagnostic evaluation of the larynx. The primary goal of the diagnostic imaging of the larynx is analysis of the submucosal structures that are not visible endoscopically. Therefore, imaging of the larynx should only be performed using knowledge of the results of clinical diagnosis. Since its discovery, the X-ray has been used for imaging the head and neck regions.

Available imaging modalities

1) Endoscopic view of laryngeal mucosal surface documented by video and photography;
2) Frontal and lateral conventional films of the neck;
3) Tomography;
4) Fluoroscopy of the larynx and barium swallow;
5) Contrast laryngography;
6) Computed tomography;
7) Magnetic resonance imaging.

High kilovolt techniques and tomography are used to give a better demonstration of the outlines of these air filled cavities by partially eliminating the overlying bony structures from the image. Fluoroscopy of the larynx and barium swallow is done with the patient in the sitting position and is complementary to all other radiological studies. Contrast laryngography provides a good view of the tomographic anatomy and a clear assessment of the functional dynamics of the larynx and hypopharynx, when combined with cineradiography. Even though there are limitations to the axial plane, neoplasms are identifiable on computed tomography as areas of increased soft tissue density that alter the normal symmetric laryngeal anatomy. Similarly, the hallmark of an abnormal larynx on an MRI is asymmetry. Recent techniques such as helical or spiral CT have enabled scanning of the entire larynx during a single held breath. Three-millimeter slices are used routinely. Thinner slices may occasionally be used if a more complete assessment of the true cord-ventricle-false cord complex is required. Iodinated contrast is administered intravenously to distinguish nonenhancing lymph nodes from enhancing vessels. Gadolinium enhanced MRI improve the delineation of margins in many lesions. Surface coils are essential in order to adequately image the larynx. Sagittal, axial, and coronal T1-weighted images best display anatomic relationships. T2-weighted images further define the signal characteristics of the tissues. Sections are usually 3- to 5-mm thick, and gaps of 1 mm between sections improve slice quality.

Clinical evaluation

Imaging is not a substitute for, but complementary to laryngoscopy. Imaging may show advanced mucosal abnormalities, but abnormalities of intrinsic motion are best studied by laryngoscopy. Rigid and flexible endoscopes are now used routinely as a complement to the laryngeal mirror examination. Basic imaging of the laryngeal pathology should be carried out by an experienced otolaryngologist. The determination of the mobility of the vocal cords and suspicious invasions of the pre-epiglottic space can be diagnosed clinically. Anatomically, the larynx is divided into the supraglottic, glottic and subglottic regions. The majority of laryngeal-cancer cases among my series were supraglottic. The second largest group of the 364 cases with squamous-cell carcinoma were detected as having transglottic carcinoma. Only 33 cases were glottic and a limited number, seven of the 364, were diagnosed with subglottic pathologies (Table 1).

Glottic carcinoma

Most of the vocal cord lesions begin on the free margin and upper surface of the vocal cord. These lesions can be diagnosed early, and clinical evaluation and detection of the spread in limited lesions may be done endoscopically. There is no need for further evaluation and imaging with CT and MRI. When the lesion crosses over to the opposite cord, anterior commissure and direct cartilage involvement may be seen. These tumors often involve the anterior commissure and invade the laryngeal surface of the thyroid cartilage at the insertion of the Broyle ligament. To detect cartilage involvement, which upstages these tumors to T4, a CT may be helpful. The primary role of imaging true cord neoplasms is the evaluation of the borderline of the cancer periglottic and subglottic spaces. CT and MRI enable the otolaryngologist to determine the extent of the cancer and what tissues are involved, and thus his or her decisions on the surgical approach. Low volume tumors limited to the midportion of the vocal cord may be treated with cordectomy. When the pathology spread to a false cord, a standard hemilaryngectomy, involving a resection of the affected vocal cord, ipsilateral false vocal cord and adjacent thyroid cartilage, was carried out. A supracricoid laryngectomy may be used to treat stage T1 and T2 glottic tumors that invade the periglottic space or cross the anterior commissure to involve the contralateral

Table 1. Cases that were evaluated and treated at Taksim Research and Education Hospital.

Glottic	33
Supraglottic	197
Transglottic	127
Subglottic	7
Total	364

vocal cord. This procedure includes resection of the supraglottis, glottis, and thyroid cartilage. Imaging to evaluate glottic carcinomas should be performed to determine which patients are suitable candidates for partial resection. MRI now give excellent coronal images. On coronal images, the ventricle may be visible. The inferior extent of a cord lesion is very important. Less extension is allowed posteriorly than anteriorly because of the shape of the cricoid cartilage. The cricoid cartilage is easily seen on CT and MRI, and so the position of the tumor relative to cricoid is also easily defined.

Subglottic carcinoma

Primary subglottic cancers are less common than other regions of the larynx susceptible to cancer. Only seven cases of subglottic carcinoma were detected among 364 laryngeal cancers. The role of imaging is to identify cartilage invasion, to demonstrate the inferior extent of a tumor, and to help to determine the extent of tracheal resection necessary for adequate margins. These tumors invade cricoid cartilage early and are detected by CT and MRI very easily.

Supraglottic carcinoma

The contents of the supraglottic region are the epiglottis, aryepiglottic folds, false vocal cords, laryngeal ventricle, and the arytenoid processes of the arytenoid cartilage. CT and MRI scans provide an excellent means for looking at the pre-epiglottic space and periglottic fat spaces. The fat spaces are an important avenue of submucosal tumor spread for infrahyoid epiglottis, false vocal cord, and true vocal cord lesions. The spread of squamous-cell carcinoma are governed by the normal anatomical barriers and infiltrate by pushing the borders of their original compartments. Supraglottic lesions do not start near the vocal cords, meaning that the involvement of the cords on their external-epithelial surface is a late phenomenon, but that submucosal extension, by way of the periglottic area, occurs earlier. When thyroid cartilage invasion occurs, it usually occurs in the ossified section of the cartilage. The posterior portions of the cartilages are more commonly ossified. The calcified or ossified portions of the laryngeal skeleton are hypointense on MRI and may be more difficult to identify than on a CT. Noncalcified cartilage such as the epiglottis is intermediate in signal intensity on MRI. On axial images, the level of the ventricle can be difficult to determine because of the horizontal orientation of the split structure. As the tumor approaches the ventricle through the periglottic space, the fat is obliterated. If a section can be found below the tumor where the periglottic fat is not obliterated, then one can be confident that the lesion is supraglottic. Early low-volume tumors, situated along the free margin of the epiglottis, are often not detected on CT and MRI, the role of imaging in these small tumors is to exclude submucosal extension that may not be identified at endoscopy. When imaging is performed to evaluate supraglottic carcinomas, one should attempt to determine which patients are candidates for a supraglottic laryngectomy. The most commonly performed laryngeal conservation technique for supraglottic carcinomas is the supraglottic laryngectomy. This technique is used to treat tumors arising from the laryngeal surface of the epiglottis, false vocal cords and aryepiglottic fold. This surgery entails resection of the false vocal cords, aryepiglottic folds, epiglottis, pre-epiglottic space, superior half of the thyroid cartilage, and hyoid bone. The inferior margin of a standard supraglottic laryngectomy is the laryngeal ventricle. We perform an extended supraglottic laryngectomy to treat tumors that involve portions of the arytenoid cartilage.

References

1. Becker M. Larynx and hypopharynx. Radiol Clin North Am 1998;36:891–920.
2. Becker M, Zbören P, Laenf H. Neoplastic invasion of the cartilage. Comparison of MR imaging and CT with histopathologic correlation. Radiology 1995;194:661–669.
3. Bloom C, Just N, Remy H, Black M, Rossignol M. Laryngeal Cancer: is computed tomography a valuable imaging technique? A retrospective analysis. Can Ass Radiol J 1998;49(6):370–377.
4. Castelijns JA, Becker M, Hermans R. The impact of cartilage invasion on treatment and prognosis of laryngeal cancer. Eur Radiol 1996;6:156–169.
5. Castelijns JA, Gerritsen GJ, Kaier MC et al. MRI of normal and cancerous laryngeal cartilages; histopathologic correlation. Laryngoscope 1997;97:1085–1093.
6. Casteljins JA, van den Brekel MW, Niekoop VA, Snow GB. Imaging of the larynx. Neuroimaging Clin North Am 1996;6(2):401–415.
7. Giovanni A, Guelfucci B, Nazarian B, Marciano S, Moulin G, Zanaret M. X-ray imaging in assessing the extent of laryngeal cancer. Rev Laryngol Otol Rhinol (Bord) 1999;120(3): 155–159.
8. Issacs JH, Mancuso AA, Wendenhall WM et al. Beep spread pa herrus in CT staging of T2-4 squamous cell laryngeal carcinoma. Otolaryngol Head Neck Surg 1998;99;455–464.
9. Kirchner JA. Invasion of the framework by laryngeal cancer. Acta otolaryngol 1984; 97:392–397.
10. Külekçi M, Kiniski M, Amatsu M, Itoh H. MRI of laryngeal carcinoma a correlation with histologic sections. Kobe J Med Sci 1987;33:215–234.
11. Lev MH, Curtin HD. Larynx. Neuroimaging Clin North Am 1998;8(1):235–56.
12. Thahet HM, Sessions DG, Gado MH et al. Comparison of clinical evaluation and computed tomographic diagnostic accuracy for tumors of the larynx and hypopharynx. Laryngoscope 1996;06:589–594.
13. Wiliams DW. Imaging of laryngeal cancer. Otolaryngol Clin North Am 1997;30:35–58.
14. Zbören P, Becker M, Laeng H. Staging of laryngeal cancer; endoscopy, computed tomography and magnetic resonance imaging versus hystopathology. Eur Arch Otolaryngol 1997;254: 117–122.

©2001 Published by Elsevier Science B.V.
Bronchology and Bronchoesophagology: State of the Art.
H. Yoshimura et al., editors.

Tracheal augmentation with autologous grafts for tracheal stenosis

Doo Yun Lee, Yoon Joo Hong and Do Hyung Kim
Department of Thoracic and Cardiovascular Surgery, Yongdong Severance Hospital, Yonsei University College of Medicine, Seoul, Korea

Abstract. Severe, long segment tracheal stenosis is a difficult to manage, life-threatening condition whose management is still debated. Many approaches and techniques have been described but the knowledge of long-term results is limited due to the rarity of disease and the lack of comparative analysis between each method demonstrating different, individual characteristics. This report summarizes our experience of surgical repair for 21 patients of tracheal stenosis between February 1990 and December 1999. The mean age was 32.7 (1–73) years and the mean follow-up period was 49 (0–77) months. The initial diagnosis was postintubation or posttracheostomy tracheal stenosis in 16 patients, endotracheal tuberculosis in two patients, adenoid cystic carcinoma in one patient and congenital tracheal stenosis in two patients. Five patients with postintubation stenosis of less than 30% of the length had undergone resection and end-to-end anastomosis resulting in a satisfactory outcome. Thirteen patients had undergone costal (11) or chonchal (2) cartilage tracheoplasty and 12 of them had required repeated treatment with bonchoscopy or laser microsurgery for removal of granulation tissue in 11 patients and two patients had undergone reoperation for restenosis. One patient with endobronchial tuberculosis, repaired by Wessex pericardial patch, suffered from restenosis only 1 month after operation. A successful intermediate result was shown in another patient with endobronchial tuberculosis, 13 months after autologous pericardial patch tracheoplasty.

A severe granulation formation and restenosis occurred in a third 15-year-old patient with adenoid cystic carcinoma after bronchial cartilage tracheoplasty, and was repaired by reoperation with autologous pericardial patch. For focal stenosis involving less than 30% of the length, resection and end-to-end anastomosis appeared to be the technique of choice. For longer stenosis, augmentation tracheoplasty using autologous cartilage or pericardial patch graft could be used. An obvious intermediate-to-long-term result of strong tendency to exuberant granulation formation and restenosis after costal or chonchal cartilage tracheoplasty resulted in our series. Although the number of our cases of pericardial patch tracheoplasty was too small to compare the operative results with the cartilage tracheoplasty, the theoretical advantages of pericardium as the augmentation patch are so well documented, that further experiments and research on pericardial patch tracheoplasty are encouraging and should be discussed further after long-term follow-up.

Keywords: cartilage, pericardium, tracheal stenosis, tracheoplasty.

Introduction

Tracheal reconstruction is necessary in patients with extensive tracheal stenosis caused by trauma, congenital disease, or benign or malignant tumor. Several

Address for correspondence: Dr Y.J. Hong, Department of Thoracic and Cardiovascular Surgery, Yongdong Severance Hospital, Yonsei University College of Medicine, Yongdong P.O. Box 1217, Seoul 135-270, Korea. Tel.: +82-2-3497-3380. Fax: +82-2-3461-8282. E-mail: dylee@yumc.yonsei.ac.kr operative techniques have been described to enlarge the tracheal lumen without predominance of a single technique, including segmental resection and end-to-end anastomosis, tracheoplasty using a variety of autologous materials such as costal cartilage, pericardial patch or bronchial cartilage and slide tracheoplasty. The primary focus for the surgical outcome of long tracheal stenosis involving more than 50% of the trachea include the incidence of granulation tissue formation at repair sites and further restenosis, the growth potential of the reconstructed trachea and the long-term functional outcomes of various types of repair. As experience is gained in this field, several procedures have been emerging but the rarity of this disease explains the lack of an accepted standard management and knowledge of long-term results. We report herein our experience with the surgical management of tracheal stenosis using several techniques at Yongdong Severance Hospital, Yonsei University Medical College.

Materials and Methods

Twenty-one patients underwent surgical repair of tracheal stenosis at Yongdong Severance Hospital, between February 1990 and December 1999. There were 13 males and eight females, whose age ranged from 1 to 73 years (mean of 32 years). The initial diagnosis was postintubation or posttracheostomy tracheal stenosis in 16 patients, endobronchial tuberculosis in two patients, adenoid cystic carcinoma of low trachea and right mainstem bronchus in one patient and congenital tracheal stenosis in two patients. Airway films were basically obtained and were most helpful in the small children. Preoperative assessment with fiberoptic bronchoscopy was essential to confirm and measure the degree and length of tracheal stenosis and was performed in all patients. Intraoperative bronchoscopic guidance was used to determine the proximal and distal ends of the tracheal narrowing validating the direct external surgical inspection. Four underwent computed tomography and 12 had direct laryngoscopy. Five patients with postintubation stenosis of less than 30% of the length had undergone resection and end-to-end anastomosis; of them, a 73-year-old female had concomitant right-sided pneumonectomy and repair of tracheoesophageal fistula, and was the only case of mortality due to postoperative respiratory failure. In 13 patients, stenosis was repaired by placement of a section of costal (11) or conchal (2) cartilage as an augmentation patch into the anterior and/or posterior surface of the trachea, which had been incised through the entire length of the stenosis. Three patients underwent pericardial patch tracheoplasty (two by autologous pericardium and one by Wessex pericardium). The patient with endobronchial tuberculosis, repaired by Wessex pericardial patch, suffered from restenosis only 1 month after operation. Another patient with long segment stenosis due to endobronchial tuberculosis underwent autologous pericardial patch tracheoplasty resulting in a satisfactory outcome. A 15-year-old boy diagnosed with adenoid cystic carcinoma of lower trachea and right mainstem bronchus underwent autologous bronchial cartilage tracheoplasty and concomitant right-sided pneumonectomy. He needed up to six sessions of bronchoscopic removal of granulation tissue at the suture lines, and eventually underwent an emergency reoperation with autologous pericardial patch due to restenosis 3 months after the initial operation. To perform a resection and end-to-end anastomosis for short-segment tracheal stenosis, the patient was placed in the supine position with the neck fully hyperextended. A generous collar incision was used for lesions involving the upper one-half to two-thirds of the trachea and right posterolateral thoracotomy incisions were required for the stenosis in the distal one-third of the trachea. The airway was divided distally just beyond the stricture. Stay sutures were placed in the midline anteriorly and posterolaterally at the junction between tracheal cartilage and membranous trachea. With the airway completely divided, the distal end was intubated with an aseptic intubation tube, which was passed alongside the jaw and under the drapes to the anesthetic connections at the head of the operating table. The stricture had been resected, stay sutures placed in the proximal tracheal margin, and the posterior layer of anastomotic sutures begun. Reasonably deep 3- to 4-mm bites were taken in the tracheal wall on each side. Interrupted sutures were placed across the entire posterior wall of the anastomosis without being tied. An absorbable suture of Vicryl 3-0 was used for the anastomosis and the sutures on the posterior wall were tied first. Then the endotracheal tube was advanced across the anastomosis into the distal trachea and the anastomosis was completed. The incisions were closed in a standard fashion, and a stitch between the chin and chest placed at the completion of the operation holds the patient's head in flexion, avoiding excessive tension in the early postoperative period. The stitches were cut on the 7th postoperative day. Cartilage tracheoplasty was mostly performed for stenotic lesions of the upper one-half to two-thirds of the trachea and carried out via the collar incision. A generous amount of costal cartilages from either the 7th or 8th rib or choncal cartilage from either external ear lobule was harvested carefully to include intact perichondrium and tailored for the meticulous alignment. A vertical midline incision was made onto the anterior and/or posterior surface of the trachea through the entire length of the stenosis, and a section of prepared costal or chonchal cartilage was placed as an augmentation patch by the interrupted sutures of Vicryl 4-0. For pericardial patch or bronchial cartilage tracheoplasty, a right posterolateral thoracotomy incision through the fourth intercostal space was performed and mobilization of the anterior pretracheal plane, avoiding injury to the lateral blood supply to the trachea, was done carefully. Also the division of the inferior pulmonary ligament and mobilization of the right hilum were performed. A rectangular piece of fresh autologous pericardium was harvested and tailored to enlarge the tracheal lumen. The pericardium was sutured to the outer three-quarters of the tracheal edge with continuous running 5-0 polydioxanone (PDS) suture. Care was taken not to place the sutures in the tracheal mucosa so as to avoid any suture material in the lumen of the airway which would stimulate granulation tissue formation. Several partial-thickness sutures were placed on the outer surface of the pericardial patch anteriorly to suspend it to the surrounding mediastinal tissues. For the case of bronchial cartilage tracheoplasty performed in a 15-year-old boy with adenoid cystic carcinoma of lower trachea and right mainstem bronchus, right-side pneumonectomy was performed first and the normal portion of bronchus intermedius was excised out and cut in the midline of the membranous portion to make an augmentation flap. It was then tailored and placed to enlarge the stenotic lesion by interrupted sutures of 3-0 Vicryl. After completion of the tracheal suture line, the anesthesiologist reinserted the endotracheal tube and increased the tracheal airway pressure temporarily to 50 mmHg to confirm an airtight anastomosis.

Results

The mean follow-up period was 49 months (ranging from 0 to 77). Five patients with postintubation stenosis of less than 30% of the length underwent end-to-end anastomosis resulting in a satisfactory outcome. In four patients no problematic granulation formation occurred. One death resulted from respiratory failure on the 2nd postoperative day in a 73-year-old female who underwent concomitant right-sided pneumonectomy and repair of tracheoesophageal fistula due to postpneumonectomy empyem thoracis, tracheoesophageal fistula and postintubation tracheal stenosis. In another 13 patients, stenosis was repaired by placement of a section of costal (11) or conchal (2) cartilage as an augmentation patch into the anterior and/or posterior surface of the trachea, which had been incised through the entire length of the stenosis. Twelve out of the 13 patients had required several treatments with a bronchoscope or laser microsurgery (LMS) for removal of granulation tissue and two of them underwent reoperation for restenosis; only one patient could permanently seal off the T-tube stoma without further evidence of granulation formation. Another three patients underwent pericardial patch tracheoplasty (two by autologous pericardium and one by Wessex pericardium). A patient with endobronchial tuberculosis, repaired by Wessex pericardial patch, suffered from restenosis only 1 month after operation. Successful intermediate result (follow-up of 13 months) with no granulation formation was shown in another patient with long segment stenosis due to endobronchial tuberculosis who had underwent autologous pericardial patch tracheoplasty (Fig. 1A and B). A 15-year-old patient who underwent autologus bronchial cartilage tracheoplasty had resulting severe and recurrent granulation formation and restenosis, with adenoid cystic carcinoma of lower trachea and right mainstem bronchus. Concomitant right-sided pneumonectomy was repaired by reoperation with autologous pericardial patch (Fig. 2A and B). Complications included exuberant granulation (11(52%)), further restenosis requiring reoperation (1(5%)), graft dehiesence (2(10%)) and bronchopleural fistula (1(5%)).

Discussion

Focal tracheal stenosis can be successfully repaired by end-to-end anastomosis but the surgical management of long segment tracheal stenosis remains a

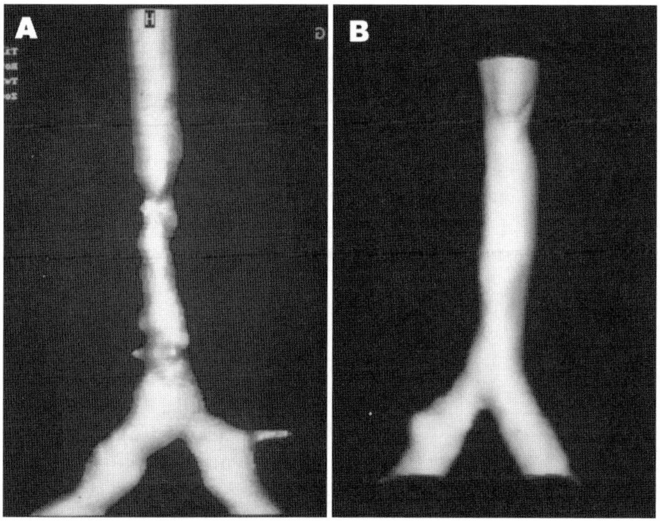

Fig. 1. **A:** Preoperative three-dimensional computed tomographic scan of tracheobronchial tree showing diffuse, long-segment narrowing of trachea by endobronchial tuberculosis. **B:** Postoperative finding of successfully enlarged tracheal lumen, scanned 3 months after autologous pericardial patch tracheoplasty.

challenging clinical problem. Formerly, operative approaches using tracheal resection and end-to-end anastomosis resulted in only up to 57% survival [1,2]. Nonoperative management such as balloon dilation, laser excision or stent is no longer considered to be optimal treatment especially not for the circumferential, cicatricial lesions or long segment stenosis [3–5]. The operative approaches have been evolved with experiencing various augmentation materials such as esophageal wall, marlex mesh, Tantalum mesh, free periosteum, dermal grafts, myocuta-

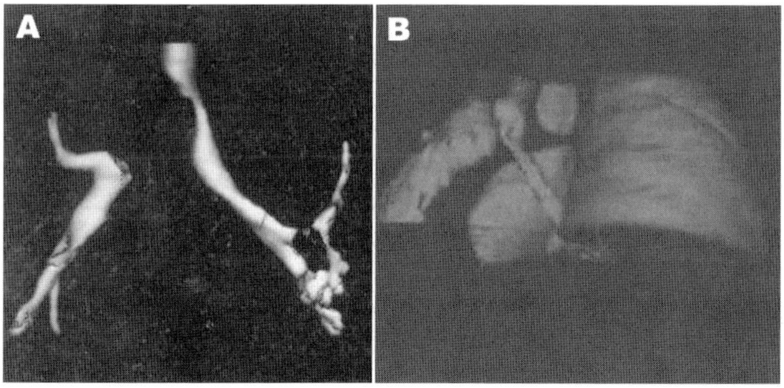

Fig. 2. **A:** A three-dimensional computed tomographic scan of adenoid cystic carcinoma, nearly obstructing the lower trachea and right mainstem bronchus in a 15-year-old boy. **B:** Postoperative scan of enlarged tracheobronchial lumen after autologous bronchial cartilage tracheoplasty, concomitant right pneumonectomy and a reoperation of autologous pericardial patch tracheoplasty.

neous island flaps and intercostal muscle pedicle flaps [6–8]. Toomes and colleagues reported on use of the Neville prosthesis for reconstruction of the trachea and its bifurcation [9]. The silicone rubber prosthesis described by Neville and Bolanwski with a nonterminal Dacron ring and telescopic sinking of the prosthesis into the tracheal lumen was ideal except for the resultant epithelialization of the prosthesis and also the erosion of the great vessel. They suggested that prosthetic reconstruction should be considered only when anastomosis or autologous material reconstruction is not feasible [10]. Eliachar and colleagues reported on the use of pectoralis myocutaneous island flaps in performing tracheal reconstruction [8]. Intercostal muscle pedicle flaps have been successfully used by Gustafson and Hrabovsky in the treatment of tracheoesophageal fistulae [6]. In 1984, Akl and colleagues described the technique of using a reversed bronchial segment for total tracheal reconstruction of the trachea of an infant [11]. A variety of more recent operative approaches, including slide tracheoplasty, rib cartilage augmentation, and anterior pericardial patch augmentation, have been proposed with encouraging early results [5,12]. Nonetheless, the optimal repair technique still remains controversial because of a lack of mid- to long-term follow-up data. The costal cartilage tracheoplasty, first described by Kimura et al. in 1982 resulted in good early and midterm outcomes having the advantage of rigid repair with no need of internal stenting, although the frequent need for repeat bronchoscopy to remove granulation tissue remains problematic [12,13]. DeLorimier and associates showed that carilagenous grafts can be absorbed and replaced by fibrous tissue within 3 months of the repair [14]. However, poor outcome of gradual degeneration with chondrocyte necrosis of grafted cartilage and replacement fibrous tissue has also been reported [15]. Proper rib harvesting with intact perichondrium and meticuous graft alignment are necessary for successful outcome [16]. Compared with costal or conchal cartilage graft, pericardial patch has several advantages for tracheal reconstruction. Pericardium is readily accessible in the surgical field and a generous amount can be harvested without compromising other adjacent structures. It molds easily, is also thin and pliable, and exhibits high tensile strength. It can be tailored to fit specific locations and forms an airtight seal [17,18]. The adherence to the surrounding soft tissue eventually gives the reconstructed segment structural support: pericardium fixes with time to the surrounding mediastinal tissues and does not require internal stenting for very long. The autologous nature of pericardium avoids problems of tissue rejection and foreign body reaction and its low metabolic rate requires a minimal blood supply. Its use avoids the introduction of a synthetic foreign body which would be more prone to infection [19]. The pericardial graft functions as a scaffold for re-epithelialization of pseudostratified ciliated epithelium. It recreates the mechanical properties of the trachea which normally has a pliable posterior membranous wall where shrinkage or adverse changes in relation to growth of the patients do not seem to appear [20]. However, pericardium lacks the structural rigidity to prevent narrowing at the graft site as the trachea grows and frequent obstruction by exuberant granulation tissue is inevitable. Excessive granulation formation on the mesenchymal surface of the tracheal substitute and the requirement for frequent postoperative bronchoscopy may be the common disadvantages of pericardial patch or costal cartilage tracheoplasy. The largest experience with the anterior pericardial patch repair was reported by the group at the Children's Hospital in Chicago [21] and described up to 16 bronchoscopic sessions in patients for debridement of excessive granulation tissue. In our series, two patients experienced severe granulation formation and early restenosis each after Wessex pericardial patch tracheoplasty and bronchial cartilage tracheoplasty. The latter case had undergone a reoperation of pericardial tracheoplasty to repair the restenosis caused by severe circumferential formation of granulation tissue at the proximal and distal suture lines (interrupted sutures of Vicryl 3-0) of the bronchial cartilage flap. For stenosis involving less than a third of the tracheal length, resection of the stenotic segment and end-to-end anastomosis of the trachea appear to be technique of choice. Delorimier reported the largest series of resection and end-to-end anastomosis with only two cases of exuberant granulation tissue formation. The five cases in our series did not experience any problematic granulation formation.

For longer stenotic lesions, augmentation tracheoplasty using autologous cartilage or pericardium may offer an attractive solution. Comparative analysis between cartilage and pericardial patch graft was not possible from our data due to the small number of pericardial patch tracheoplasty. However, the obvious intermediate-to-long-term result of a strong tendency for exuberant granulation formation and restenosis after costal cartilage tracheoplasty, and the well-documented theoretical advantages of pericardial patch, promote further experiments and research on pericardial patch tracheoplasty.

References

1. Bando K, Turrentine MW, Sun K, Sharp TG, Matt B et al. Anterior pericardial tracheoplasty for congenital tracheal stenosis: intermediate to long-term outcomes. Ann Thorac Surg 1996;62: 981–989.
2. Effman EL, Fram EK, Vock P, Kirks DR. Tracheal cross-sectional area in children; CT determination. Radiology 1983;149:137–140.
3. Jaquiss RDB, Lusk PR, Spray TL, Huddleston CB. Repair of long-segment tracheal stenosis in infancy. J Thorac Cardiovasc Surg 1995;110:1504–1512.
4. Heimansohn DA, Kesler KA, Turrentine MW et al. Anterior pericardial tracheoplasty for congenital tracheal stenosis. J Thorac Cardiovasc Surg 1991;102:710–716.
5. Nakayama DK, Harrison MR, DeLorimier AA, Brasch RC, Fishman NH. Reconstructive surgery for obstructing lesions of the intrathoracic trachea in infants and small children. J Pediatr Surg 1982;17:854–871.
6. Gustafson RA, Hrabovsky EE. Intercostal muscle and myo-osseous flaps in difficult pediatric thoracic problems. J Pediatr Surg 1982;17:541–545.
7. Cohen RC, Filler RM, Konuma K et al. The successful reconstruction of thoracic tracheal defects with free periosteal grafts. J Pediatr Surg 1985;20:852–858.
8. Eliachar I, Goldsher M, Moscona AR, Hurwitz DJ. Reconstruction of the larynx and cervical trachea with the pectoralis major myocutaneou flap reconstruction. Otolaryngol Head Neck Surg 1985;93(6):754–758.

9. Toomes H, Mickisch G, Vogt-Moykopf I. Experiences with prosthetic reconstruction of the trachea and bifurcation. Thorax 1985;40:32—37.
10. Neville WE, Bolanwski PJP. Prosthetic reconstruction of the trachea and carina. J Thorac Cardiovasc Surg 1976;72:525—538.
11. Akl BF, Yabek SM, Berman W. Total tracheal reconstruction in a three-month-old infant. Thorac Cardiovasc Surg 1987;87:543—546.
12. Kimura K, Mukohara N, Tsugawa C et al. Tracheoplasty for congenital stenosis of entire trachea. J Pediatr Surg 1982;17:869—871.
13. Tsugawa C, Kimura K, Muraji T et al. Congenital stenosis involving a long segment of the trachea: further experience in reconstructive surgery. J Pediatr Surg 1988;23:471—475.
14. DeLorimier AA, Harrison MR, Karen H, Howell LJ, Adzick NS. Trachebroncial obstructions in infants and children; experience with 45 cases. Ann Surg 1990;212:277—289.
15. Prescott CA, Laing C. Medium term fate of cartilage grafts from children after laryngo-tracheoplasty. Int J Pediatr Otorhinolaryngol 1993;27(2):163—171.
16. Van Meter CH, Lusk RM, Muntz H, Spray TL. Am Surg 1991;57(3):157—160.
17. Alan TL, Backer CL, Holinger LD, Dunham ME, Mavroudis C, Gonzalez-Crussi F. Histopathologic changes after pericardial patch tracheoplasty. Arch Otolaryngol Head Neck Surg. 1997;123:1069—1072.
18. Idriss FS, Deleon SY, Ilbawi MN, Gerson CR, Tucker GF, Holinger L. Tracheoplasty with pericardial patch for extensive tracheal stenosis in infants and children. J Thorac Cardiovasc Surg 1984;58:527—536.
19. Bryant LR. Replacement of tracheobronchial defects with autogenous pericardium. J Thorac Cardiovasc Surg 1964;48:733—740.
20. Dykes EH, Bahoric A, Smith C, Kent G, Filler RM. Reduced tracheal growth after reconstruction with pericardium. J Pediatr Surg 1990;25:25—29.
21. Dunham ME, Backer CL, Holinger LD, Mavroudis C. Management of severe congenital tracheal stenosis. Ann Otol Rhinol Laryngol 1994;103:351—356.

©2001 Published by Elsevier Science B.V.
Bronchology and Bronchoesophagology: State of the Art.
H. Yoshimura et al., editors.

Bronchoscopic cryosurgery

M.O. Maiwand
Harefield Hospital, Harefield, Middlesex, UK

Introduction

Tracheobronchial obstruction, whether malignant or benign, causes distressing symptoms including dyspnoea, cough and haemoptysis which require early and effective treatment. The majority of cases are caused by advanced malignant disease and about one-third present with central, intraluminal obstruction, which requires recanalisation of the lumen if symptoms are to be alleviated. Over the last two decades considerable interest and effort have been devoted to the development of new methods of palliation of endobronchial obstruction and restoration of airway patency. These methods can generally be categorised into those involving physical reopening of the lumen (such as cryosurgery, laser treatment, diathermy resection, blunt resection or insertion of a stent) and those causing alteration in the growth of tumours (such as brachytherapy or photodynamic therapy). Cryosurgery, the controlled application of extreme cold for the destruction of abnormal tissue, was first used for endobronchial treatment in the UK in 1986 [1].

Methods

We present the results of cryosurgery on 352, nonselected, patients with histologically confirmed malignant or benign tracheobronchial lesions and assess the effectiveness of this method of treatment for obstruction and for the relief of symptoms. Patients were assessed clinically, radiologically and for performance status before and after cryosurgery. Symptom evaluation was carried out for dyspnoea, haemoptysis, cough and chest pain as described previously [2]. Respiratory function tests, forced expiratory volume in 1 s (FEV1) and forced vital capacity (FVC) were measured using a Microlab 3000 turbine spirometer, before cryosurgery and after an average of 10 weeks. Performance status was assessed using the Karnofsky and WHO scales.

Cryosurgery was performed under general anaesthesia (propofol) using a large 9.2-mm rigid bronchoscope. Oxygenation was maintained with Venturi positive-

Address for correspondence: M.O. Maiwand, Harefield Hospital, Harefield, Middlesex UB9 6JH, UK. Tel./Fax: +44-1895-828558. E-mail: cryotherapy@rbh.nthames.nhs.uk pressure ventilation. The distal tip of the bronchoscope was placed about 0.5 cm above the lesion and the appropriate cryoprobe (straight, right-angled or flexible) inserted through the bronchoscope and applied to the tumour, which was frozen for 3 min and allowed to thaw. The probe with nitrous oxide cryogen (Joule-Thomson type, involving adiabatic expansion of compressed gas) achieved temperatures of at least –70°C at the probe tip. The selection of probe diameter, 5 or 2.2 mm, was based on the size and position of the tumour. The 2.2-mm probe was used for peripheral smaller tumours and inserted through a fibreoptic bronchoscope. The 5-mm probe was used for larger, central tumours so that a larger area was treated. Where the tumour covered wider areas of the bronchial tree, multiple cryoapplications were made during the same treatment session. Where a large mass of necrotic tumour was present after the cryoapplication, the mass was removed before the second application. It was essential that all areas involved or infiltrated by the tumour were frozen to achieve adequate tumour destruction. The use of a large rigid bronchoscope allowed a small suction catheter to be placed next to the site of treatment to remove blood and secretions throughout the procedure. Tissue samples for histological examination were taken before each cryotreatment.

Monitoring and recording of temperature during cryosurgery is important as tissue destruction is directly related to the temperature drop achieved at the treatment site. Probe temperatures were determined potentiometrically with a needle placed about 2 mm from the tip. These have been found to achieve a mean minimum temperature of –30°C (standard deviation: ±5.6) over 100 applications [3]. In the author's experience, bleeding from the site of a biopsy or cryosurgery has not been a major difficulty and moderate bleeding can be contained by the local application of epinephrine (adrenaline) 1:1,000. The majority of patients recover sufficiently well to be discharged home on the same day. By the time of rebronchoscopy, typically performed 2 weeks after the first treatment, large areas of tumour necrosis are often seen which can be removed using biopsy forceps. The procedure can be repeated when symptoms reoccur and then if necessary after a further 6 weeks.

Cryodestruction and removal of a tumour blocking a major bronchial lumen and drainage of secretions from behind the blockages followed by reventilation of a collapsed lung, not surprisingly, leads to patients reporting symptomatic relief soon after the procedure.

Results

The mean age of the 352 patients with malignant or benign tracheobronchial lesions was 65.7 years (range: 9–87 years) and the male:female ratio was 1.77:1. Histological composition for the 305 patients with malignant disease was as follows: squamous cell carcinoma 67.3%, adenocarcinoma 15.3%, large cell carcinoma 1.7%, undifferentiated 4.7% and small cell 11.0%. TNM staging of non-small cell carcinoma (NSC) patients was stage II, 6.7%; IIIa, 24.6%;

IIIb, 23.8%; and IV, 44.9%. The benign and low-malignancy patients comprised 49% granulation tissue following heart lung transplantation, 26% carcinoid, 7% sarcoid and 18% other benign tumours.

Of thc patients with malignant lesions, symptomatic improvements were seen in 83.8% of patients for haemoptysis, 69.9% for cough, 64.1% for dyspnoea and 59.7% for chest pain. Results of respiratory function tests showed that mean FEV1 improved from 1.39 to 1.52 l ($p \leq 0.001$) and FVC from 2.00 to 2.23 l ($p = 0.003$) (Fig. 1). Mean performance status, measured using the Karnofsky scale, improved from 67.5 to 74.6 and the WHO scale from 2.52 to 2.16. The Kaplan-Meier median survival time (95% CL) was 12.9 months (range: 9.8–15.1 months) (Fig. 2). Bronchoscopic findings are shown in Fig. 3.

For patients with benign lesions, symptomatic improvement was present in 69% for dyspnoea, 67% for haemoptysis and chest pain and 58% for cough, and mean performance status improved from 76.8 to 85.3 (Karnofsky) and from 2.0 to 1.53 (WHO). The mean FEV1 increased from 1.94 to 2.15 l and FVC from 2.61 to 2.80 l (Fig. 1).

Discussion

Lung cancer is the most common cancer and also the most frequent cause of death from malignant disease, leading to around 600,000 deaths per year, world-wide [4]. It is rapidly disabling and has a very poor survival rate, which has improved very little over the years. Surgical resection offers the best possibility of a cure, particularly for patients with stage I and II disease, but unfortunately most patients (over 80%) at the time of presentation are at such an advanced stage that surgery is not possible and symptom palliation is the only course of action available. Since survival rates are so poor, the issue of quality of life for

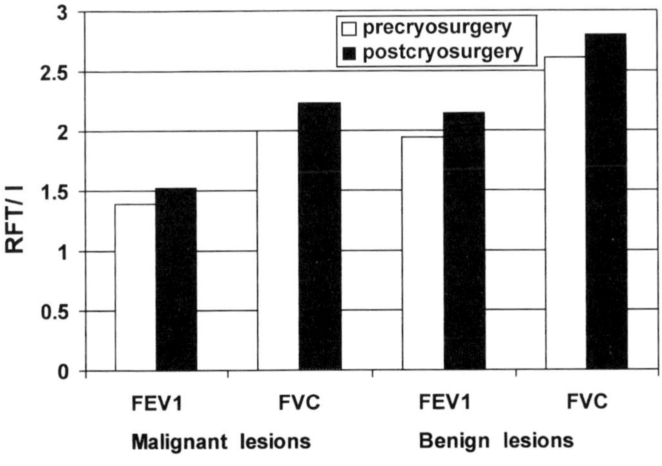

Fig. 1. Respiratory function tests before and after cryosurgery.

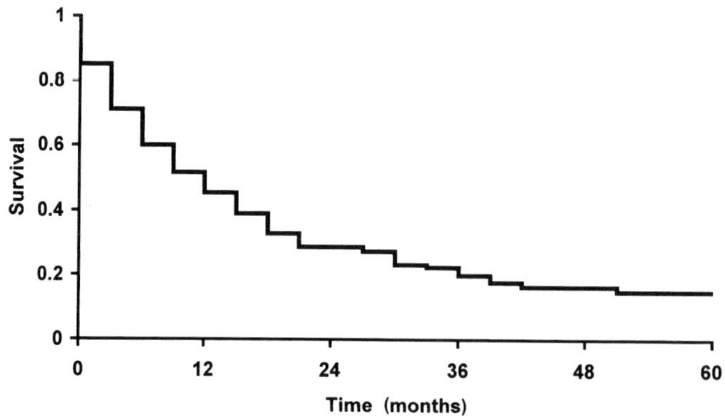

Fig. 2. Kaplan-Meier survival curve (malignant patients).

these patients becomes paramount. Around 30% of the patients present with major airway obstruction which itself causes significant morbidity and mortality [5]. Clinical symptoms include cough, breathlessness, haemoptysis and recurrent infection which in extreme cases may lead to gradual asphyxiation, where central airways are obstructed. For most patients, curative resection is not possible and the standard method of treatment of obstruction caused by lung cancer has been radiotherapy or chemotherapy. This has limited effectiveness for reopening blocked bronchial lumen and a damaging effect on surrounding healthy tissue [6].

Cryosurgery, the controlled application of extreme cold, leads to the formation of ice crystals, initially in the extracellular compartment and later in the intracellular area. Ice crystals form from pure water which causes dehydration and bio-

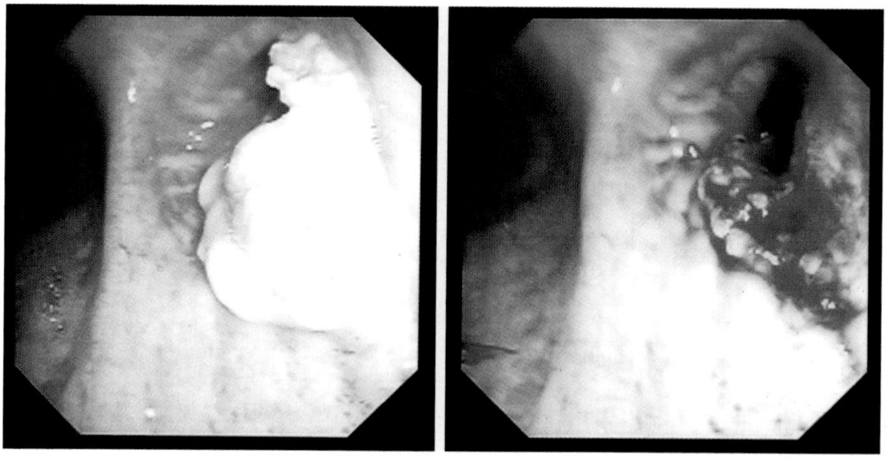

Fig. 3. Bronchoscopic findings before and after cryosurgery. Squamous cell carcinoma, right main bronchus.

chemical changes which result in cell death. Tissue destruction is almost guaranteed if the entire tumour mass is frozen to a temperature of at least −30°C.

Cryosurgery has been used in the treatment of a number of benign and low-malignancy conditions including carcinoid tumours, granulation tissue following heart/lung transplant, amyloidosis, tracheobronchopathia osteochondroplastica (TBOCP), sarcoid, lipoma, polyps, postintubation tubal stenosis, leiomyoma, haemangioma and Wegner's granulomatosis.

In a study carried out at this hospital, 12 patients with histologically proven endobronchial typical carcinoid tumours were treated with cryosurgery between 1992 and 1998. All patients, except one who died accidentally, are still alive with a mean follow-up of 49.4 months. Nine of these, treated only with cryosurgery (mean 3.4 treatments), showed no tumour present on histological and radiological examination at follow-up. For the patient who died accidentally, postmortem examination reported no residual tumour. For the other three patients, cryosurgery downstaged the tumour from the main to lobar bronchus, allowing for resection by lobectomy rather than pneumonectomy. There was a significant improvement in respiratory function tests and performance status after treatment. These results suggest that cryosurgery is an effective palliative and potentially curative treatment for carcinoid tumours deemed inoperable because of the extent of disease or comorbid conditions. Cryosurgery can also be considered as a treatment for downstaging endobronchial carcinoid tumours to allow for less radical resection.

Cryosurgery has also been used successfully in this hospital for the treatment of a case of primary localised tracheobronchial amyloidosis of the respiratory tract, which caused narrowing of the intermediate bronchus and almost complete blockage of the lower lobe. Repeated sessions of cryosurgery to the lesions, over a follow-up period of 11 years, have been found to be an effective treatment for this progressive disease [7].

Cryosurgery has also been used in this hospital as a first-line treatment for airways compromised by granulation tissue after heart/lung transplantation. In a study of 23 patients [8], results were judged as good in 15 patients and fair in six patients. There were no cryosurgery-related complications. Respiratory function tests were shown to increase significantly after treatment. The use of cryosurgery markedly reduced the percentage of patients requiring stents compared to other series.

TBOCP is a rare, benign condition that affects large airways, which become narrowed by ossified or cartilaginous nodules in the submucosa with normal overlying mucosa. In this hospital, three patients with TBOCP have been treated with cryosurgery. Patients received between three and seven sessions of cryosurgery that in all cases resulted in symptom improvement for cough and haemoptysis although haemoptysis did return at a later date in some cases.

Conclusions

Cryosurgery offers an effective method to restore the patency of blocked tracheobronchial lumen and therefore improve symptoms, respiratory function and quality of life. It is well tolerated by the patient who is discharged home the same day. Cryosurgery has the advantages of being easy to perform, not requiring expensive equipment, it does not have a risk of bronchial wall perforation, is safe for the operator, has minimal complications and the treatment can be repeated as often as is necessary. Cryosurgery often improves the patient tolerance to the stage that a further treatment such as surgery, radiotherapy or chemotherapy can be tolerated, thus providing a better outcome and improved quality of life and survival.

References

1. Maiwand MO. Cryotherapy for advanced carcinoma of the trachea and bronchi. Br Med J 1986; 293:181–182.
2. Walsh DA, Maiwand MO, Nath AR, Lockwood P, Lloyd MH, Saab M. Bronchoscopic cryotherapy for advanced bronchial carcinoma. Thorax 1990;45:509–513.
3. Maiwand MO, Homasson JP. Cryotherapy for tracheobronchial disorders. Intervent Pulmonol 1995;16:427–443.
4. Strauss GM. Bronchogenic carcinoma. In: Baum GL, Crapo JD, Celli BR, Karlinsky JB (eds) Textbook of Pulmonary Diseases. Philadelphia: Lippincott-Raven, 1998;1329–1382.
5. Bolliger CT, Solèr M, Tamm M, Perruchoud AP. Kombinierte endobronchiale und konventionelle therapie-möglichkeiten bei inoperablen zentralen lungentumoren. Schweiz Med Wochenschr 1995;125:1052–1059.
6. Murren JR, Buzaid AC. Chemotherapy and radiation for the treatment of non-small cell lung cancer. Lung Cancer 1993;14:161–171.
7. Maiwand MO, Nath AR, Kamath BSK. Cryosurgery in the treatment of tracheobronchial amyloidosis. J Bronchol (In press).
8. Maiwand MO, Zehr KJ, Dyke CM, Peralta M, Tadjkarimi S, Khagani A, Yacoub M. The role of cryotherapy for airway complications after lung and heart-lung transplantation. Eur J Cardio Thorac Surg 1997;12:549–54.

Bronchology and Bronchoesophagology: State of the Art.
H. Yoshimura et al., editors.

Management of cancer of the supraglottic larynx

Eugene N. Myers
Department of Otolaryngology, University of Pittsburgh School of Medicine, Pittsburgh, Pennsylvania, USA

Keywords: extracapsular spread, laser, organ preservation, radiation, supracricoid laryngectomy, supraglottic cancer.

The treatment of cancer of the supraglottic (SG) larynx is a treatment that is still evolving. Partial laryngeal surgery for cancer of the SG was introduced by Prof Justo Alonzo of Uruguay in 1947 [1]; however, the senior laryngeal surgeons in our country did not accept this operation because they felt that anything less than a total laryngectomy was not oncologically sound and would result in recurrence of the cancer. Dr Joseph Ogura in 1958 [2] gave special emphasis to this topic and through his own lecturing and teaching of numerous residents and fellows popularized this procedure in our country. Today these concerns have been settled and the operation is considered safe in properly selected patients. New treatment programs have been introduced in recent years and all of these have found some place in our armamentarium for treating patients with this disease. The introduction of the bioanatomic concepts of conservation laryngeal surgery have long been established and were a result of the work of Frazer, Tucker, Pressman, Kirschner, and others [3]. They all demonstrated either in the laboratory or in the clinical situation that the SG appeared to be separated embryologically and anatomically from the glottis and therefore removal of the SG is technically and oncologically feasible while leaving the glottis (voice) in place.

The treatment of SG cancer with conventional radiation therapy has proven to be curative in patients with early T stage SG cancer. However, in more advanced T stages it is not effective. Recent innovations in radiation, such as hyperfractionation, may make these treatments more efficacious. The Organ Preservation Program organized by Dr Gregory Wolf of Ann Arbor has indicated that patients with stage III and stage IV cancer of the larynx can be treated with intensive chemoradiation and that while this treatment program has the same survival rate as standard treatment with surgery and radiation, nonetheless, approximately 60% of the patients who survived this treatment retained their voice. These two innovations are now being carefully used and monitored.

Steiner and Rudert of Germany have been the major proponents of endoscopic

Address for correspondence: Eugene N. Myers, the Eye and Ear Institute, Suite 500, 200 Lothrop Street, Pittsburgh, Pennsylvania 15213, USA. Tel.: +1-412-647-2111. Fax: +1-412-647-2080.
E-mail: myersen@msx.upmc.edu

laser surgery for treatment of cancer of the SG [3]. They have shown that the advantages are good oncological control, no need for tracheotomy or nasogastric feeding tube, and early discharge from the hospital. This treatment does not eliminate the need for neck dissections. In this country, this work is slowly being adopted in various centers.

Several centers in France [3], including Paris and Lille, have given us a better understanding of supracricoid laryngectomy with cricohyoidopexy in patients with supraglottic cancer. This procedure is designed to effectively remove almost the entire larynx, with the exception of one arytenoid cartilage, with the advantage of preserving voice and being oncologically sound. In certain selected patients, this has proven to be an excellent addition to our armamentarium.

The results of the Department of Otolaryngology at the University of Pittsburgh for surgical treatment with the use of adjunctive radiation and chemotherapy based on pathological findings of perineural invasion or multiple positive lymph nodes or extracapsular spread in cervical lymph nodes has continued to produce a good cure rate. Our studies [4,5] have indicated that it is of fundamental importance to include bilateral neck dissection in the management of this disease.

I feel certain that the treatment of SG cancer will continue its evolutionary process in order to serve the best interest of the patients.

References

1. Alonzo JM. Conservative surgery of cancer of the larynx. Trans Am Acad Ophthalmol Otolaryngol 1947;51:633–642.
2. Ogura JH. Supraglottic subtotal laryngectomy and radical neck dissection for carcinoma of the epiglottis. Laryngoscope 1958;68:983–1003.
3. Myers EN, Alvi A. Management of carcinoma of the supraglottic larynx: evolution, current concepts, and future trends. Laryngoscope 1996;106:559–567.
4. Lutz CK, Johnson JT, Wagner RL, Myers EN. Supraglottic carcinoma: patterns of recurrence. Ann Otol Rhinol Laryngol 1990;99:12–17.
5. Snyderman NL, Johnson JT, Schramm VL, Myers EN, Bedetti CD, Teharle P. Extracapsular spread of carcinoma in cervical lymph nodes: impact upon survival in patients with carcinoma of the supraglottic larynx. Cancer 1985;56:1597–1599.

Bronchology and Bronchoesophagology: State of the Art.
H. Yoshimura et al., editors.

RIDTELC™ lung study: reduction of lung cancer mortality through automated sputum cytometry and autofluorescence bronchoscopy: a controlled feasibility study on lung cancer screening

J.A. Nakhosteen[1], B. Khanavkar[1], A. Muti[1], W. Marek[1], S. Philippou[2], R. Heckemann[3], K.-H. Jöckel[5], N. Kotchy-Lang[6], T. Topalidis[4] and Z. Atay[4]

[1]Department of Respiratory Disease and Allergy, Research Institute for Diagnosis and Treatment of Early Lung Cancer (RIDTELC™); [2]Institute for Pathology; [3]Department of Radiology, Augusta Teaching Hospital, Bochum; [4]Institute for Cytology, Hannover; [5]Institute for Biomathematics, Medical Informatics, and Epidemiology, University Clinics, Essen; and [6]BG-Klinik für Berufskrankheiten (Clinic for Occupational Disease), Falkenstein, Germany

Abstract. *Background.* Based on results from an intensive 5-year program for new early lung cancer (ELC) detecting methods, obtained at RIDTELC™, a multicenter ELC screening program has been developed, with patient recruitment starting on 15 May 2000. The primary aim of the RIDTELC™ Lung Study is large-scale validation of promising pilot studies on automated sputum cytometry (ASC) and autofluorescence (AF) bronchoscopy, and also to analyse a host of epidemiological data with respect to development of lung cancer.

Patients, Materials and Methods. 6,000 males and females with a 30-pack year (one pack year is one pack of cigarettes a day for one year) history of cigarette use were recruited and randomised into H-1 (treatment) and H-0 (control) groups. Induced sputum was collected and chest X-rays were taken for both groups. Prevalence chest X-rays were read for all subjects, and in tumor-positive cases, usual staging and therapy were instituted (these subjects were excluded from the study). H-1 sputa were read, and on suspicion of lung cancer, conventional and AF bronchoscopy were performed (prevalence). ASC of H-0 sputa was carried out (but not read), and then stored for 3 years. This was repeated at year 3 for a second, incidence sample. In a retroanalysis, these are jointly read. H-1 will repeat all examinations at year 3 (incidence). Results in H-1 and H-0 will be compared.

Results. Relative sensitivity and specificity will be calculated for conventional cytology + ASC compared to the former alone, and conventional bronchoscopy + AF endoscopy compared to the conventional procedure alone. Patients in both groups will be followed up for at least 5 years for survival calculations. Multivariate analysis will be performed on the large volume of epidemiological information with respect to disease development.

Conclusion. Based on results to date, this prospective study should demonstrate the following: 1) at least a doubling in the detection of dysplasia, Carcinoma-in-situ and stage I central lung cancers through automated sputum cytometry combined with conventional cytology, 2) a similar 2-fold increase in endoscopic localization of early curable cancers using AF bronchoscopy, and 3) based on a doubling in detection and localization rates of ELC, 5-year survival should increase accordingly.

The controlled design of this trial will allow for definitive recommendations regarding active diagnostic interventions in patients with a high risk for lung cancer. In addition, further knowledge about the oncogenesis of lung cancer and the dynamics of precancerous lesions are expected. Multi-

Address for correspondence: Prof Dr J.A. Nakhosteen, Director, Augusta Teaching Hospital, Bergstr. 26, D-44791 Bochum, Germany. Tel.: +49-234-517-2461. Fax: +49-245-517-2463.
E-mail: prof.nakhosteen@ridtelc.com

variate analysis will allow insights into the effects of a host of epidemiological factors involved with lung cancer development.

Introduction

During the past four decades industrialized nations have witnessed an epidemic rise in lung cancer, which for many years has been the most common cause of tumor death in men, and more recently, in women. Although the causal link between cigarette smoking and lung cancer is undisputed, many industrialized countries and certain EU agencies are lagging in legislating and implimenting effective antismoking measures. However, even in those countries where aggressive antismoking policies led to a significant decline in cigarette consumption in the 1970s, lung cancer incidence has continued to rise steeply for up to two decades, before finally flattening and declining. Furthermore, in these countries, two disturbing recent counter-trends are being observed: two groups are smoking more, adult women (e.g., 36% in France) and adolescents.

Another long-recognized fact is that the earlier a lung cancer is detected, the better the prognosis [1,2]. Based on this knowledge, five large screening trials took place in the 1970s, using various combinations of chest X-ray, sputum cytology and bronchoscopy, in an effort to increase survival in high-risk patients [3,4]. For a number of reasons (including antiquated technologies), these trials failed, and health authorities turned to antismoking measures as the only viable alternative to combat lung cancer. However, as the evidence cited above shows, these measures alone were insufficient in stemming the spread of this disease for which up to one-half of the adult population (smokers and ex-smokers) is at risk.

Hence, a two-pronged strategy against lung cancer should be implemented: on the one hand, redoubling efforts to eliminate smoking, especially among women and adolescents, and on the other, instituting carefully monitored lung cancer screening programs using promising new technologies with a higher sensitivity than those used in earlier trials [5,6]. Since 1995 at RIDTELC™ we have intensively evaluated and refined two innovative diagnostic procedures, as well as developing our own automation technology: ASC, AF bronchoscopy, and automated sputum processing [7]. Ongoing analyses of 600 AF bronchoscopies and 5,000 ASCs have shown sensitivities at least double those of conventional procedures alone. Thus, it seems justifiable to test the validity of these examinations as screening tools in a large, controlled study. This paper addresses in detail the multicenter early lung cancer study which RIDTELC™ commenced in May 2000. We calculate that the use of our new technology, combined with conventional procedures, epidemiological data, and early tumor markers, can forward-shift lung cancer stage distribution to the extent that the number of curable cancers — and thus also 5-year survival — will double.

Patients, Materials and Methods

Patients

Inclusion criteria for patients were smokers or ex-smokers (male and female) with 30 pack years (one pack year is one pack of cigarettes a day for one year), aged 50–74 years, with no other active cancer, severe chronic disease or acute broncho-pulmonary symptoms. 6,000 subjects, including 1,000 radon-exposed ex-miners, will be recruited and divided into a H-1 Treatment Group and H-0 Control Group. Both groups will submit sputum and undergo chest X-rays at year 1 and year 3. Anyone with tumor-suspect chest X-ray will be staged and treated as indicated, and excluded from the study. In the H-1 collective, sputum will be read both at year 1 (prevalence) and 3 (incidence), and in case of any tumor-suspicious findings, conventional and AF bronchoscopy will be performed. In the HO Group, ASC print-outs will be stored and read at year 3 with the incidence sample in a retro-analysis, as will cytology (Fig. 1).

The 3,000 participants in each group will include 500 very-high-risk, industrially exposed individuals. Participants with normal (tumor-negative) chest X-rays are single-blindly randomized into treatment and control groups.

Identical postal monitoring of broncho-pulmonary symptoms will be performed every 9-12 months in both H-0 and H-1 groups. The study flow-sheet is given in Fig. 2.

Materials

Standard documentation forms will be used for patient history, sputum results, X-ray findings, spirometry and endoscopies. The individual documentation form

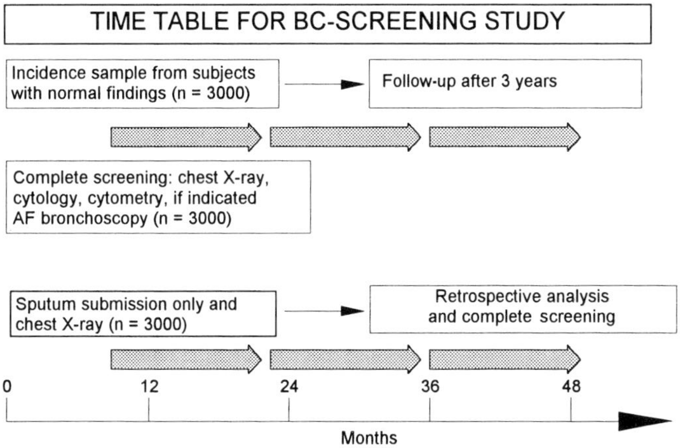

Fig. 1. Time-course for prevalence and incidence examinations of H-1 (Treatment) and H-0 (Control) groups. Results of the H-0 group will be analyzed at year 3 (retroanalysis).

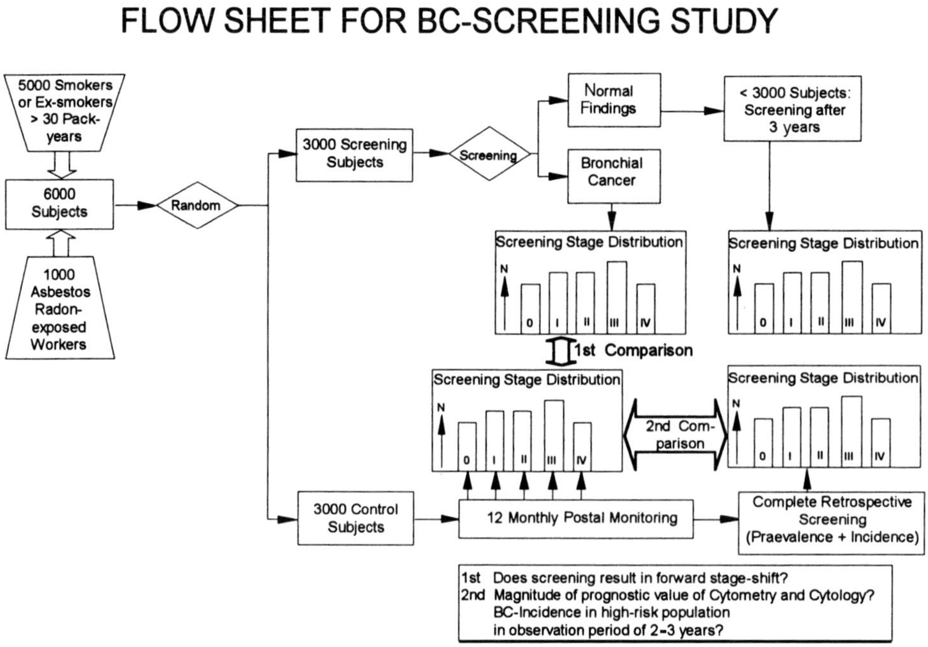

Fig. 2. Flow-sheet for the 3-year trial period.

is 12 pages long and elicits a host of epidemiological, social, economic and life-style information for multifactorial analysis with respect to lung cancer genesis. Patients will be informed in writing and personally (by the Study Co-ordinator) about the nature and scope of the RIDTELC Lung Study, being requested subsequently to sign the Informed Consent Form.

Methods

Sputum studies will include conventional cytology and ASC. For automated sputum processing, RIDTELC has developed a prototype [7] called MARATHON-S (Medical Application Robot Automation for Tissue Handling and Nuclei Separation), which is fully integrated into routine sputum work-ups. Cytometry will be carried out using the automated cytometer, Cyto-Savant®, developed by Dr Branko Palcic and co-workers at Oncometrics Corp., in collaboration with the British Columbia Research Agengy (BCCA) [8,9]. The cytometer can analyze, unattended, up to 50 mono-layer sputum slides even overnight and on week-ends. Its print-outs are then interpreted by a biologist (WM) trained specifically for this task [10]. Parallel cytology will also be carried out (AM, TT,ZA) [11]. Standard chest X-rays may be performed in any radiology unit with digital technique, but these will be read by RH. If any one of the sputum results is suspicious for lung cancer (ASC and cytology, Pap IIID,s = severe dysplasia or more), conventional and AF bronchoscopy [12–15] will be performed. Whereas ASC studies are carried out exclusively at RIDTELC, endoscopy may be undertaken at collaborating institutes. In suspicious endoscopic findings, histological samples plus two biopsies from normal sites will be performed; in normal endoscopies, only the two negative control biopsies at predetermined sites (LMB, RUL spur) will be performed. Histology will be carried out by SP.

Relative sensitivities, specificities and positive predictive values will be calculated for

ASC + cytology compared to cytology alone;
AF + conventional bronchoscopies compared to conventional alone;
chest X-ray compared to final diagnosis.

Multivariate analysis will be performed on all epidemiological data with respect to occurrence of dysplasia and ELC (Fig. 3).

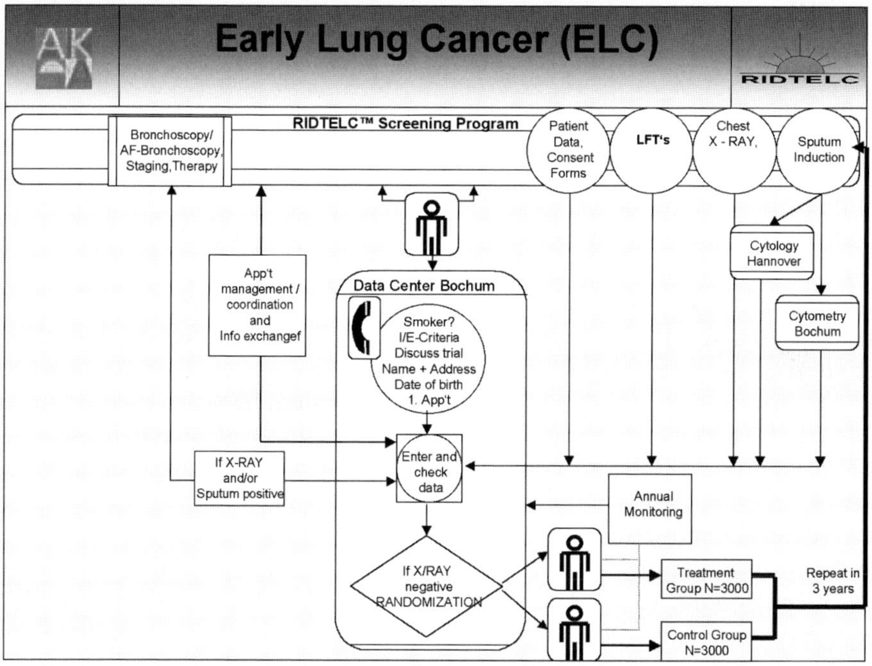

Fig. 3. RIDTELC™ Lung Study overview, developed in close collaboration with K.-H. Jöckel and coworkers. Initial contact between study candidates from all centers is via the Study Coordinator at the central phone number (shown as phone symbol). Appointments are given in prearranged blocks and exact times notified in writing to collaborating centers and participants. At local centers, the responsible doctor rechecks for inclusion/exclusion criteria, reviews the completed documentation form, collects Informed Consent Forms (center of upper block) and sends the subject to X-ray, LFT's and sputum induction (upper right). In X-ray negative cases, randomization takes place (lower right). In cases of tumor-suspicious sputum findings, conventional and AF bronchoscopy are undertaken (upper left).

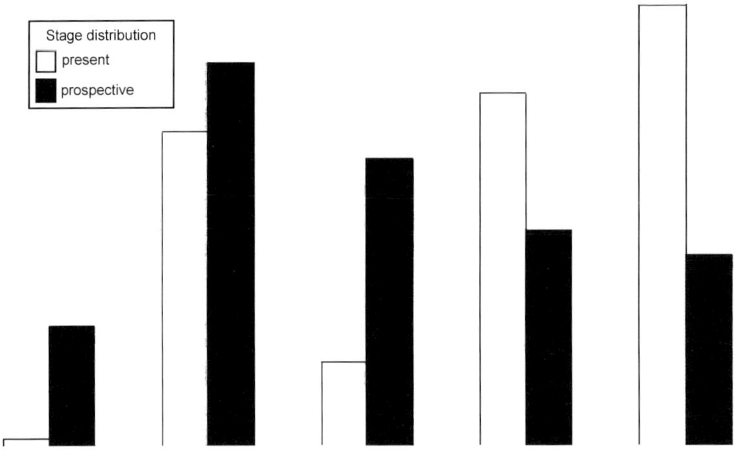

Fig. 4. Assumed stage distribution of new lung cancers in RIDTELC™ Lung Study.

In this trial we expect a forward shift in stage distribution of newly diagnosed lung cancers, as shown in Fig. 4.

Discussion

The lead time gained by modern screening procedures leads to a significant increase of early stage cancers, whose cure potential is much higher than advanced lung cancer. Integrating autofluorescence bronchoscopy and automated cytometry into screening programs could realistically be expected to double the 5-year survival from today's 10–15% to nearly 30%.

The concept expressed by QALYs, or quality-adjusted life years should also be considered. Those cured of lung cancer can return to good quality, productive lives. This is in stark contrast to patients undergoing chemotherapy, radiotherapy, and, more recently, multi-modal interventions which often reduce quality of life to an existential minimum.

A further important element of the RIDTELC™ Lung Study will be the wealth of epidemiological evidence which may elucidate the multifactorial effect of socio-economic, life-style and genetic factors on the development of lung disease, in particular, ELC and COPD,

Conclusion

In the RIDTELC™ Lung Study of 6,000 high-risk patients for lung cancer, a diagnostic rate of 2% is expected. These will be lung cancers at various stages, predominantly, however, in Stages 0-II. These ELCs do not include at least triple that amount of metaplasia and various stages of dysplasia (up to and including moderate dysplasia). These pre-cancerous findings will all be histo-cytologically verified and as such provide a fruitfull source for early tumor markers and molecular studies on oncogenesis, with a view to influencing tumor growth through chemo-preventive measures. Finally, multivariate analysis of a host of epidemiological and oncogenic data will allow insights into the multifactorial nature in the development of chronic lung disease and lung cancer. Indeed, it may be possible to identify the profile of subjects more likely to get sick from smoking than others.

References

1. Watanabe Y, Shimizu J, Okta M et al. Early Hilar lung cancer: its clinical significance. J Surg Oncol 1991;48:75–80.
2. Von Boxem TJ, Venmans BJ, Postmus PE et al. Curative endobronchial therapy in early stage non-small cell lung cancer. J Bronchol 1999;6:198–206.
3. Fontana RS, Sanderson DR, Woolner LB et al. Screening for lung cancer: a critique of the Mayo Lung Project. Cancer 1991;67:1155–1164 (Abstract).
4. Melamed MR, Flehinger BJ, Zaman MB. Impact of early detection on the clinical course of lung cancer. Surg Clin North Am 1987;67:909–924.
5. Kennedy TC, Miller YE, Prindiville S. Screening for lung cancer revisited and the role of sputum cytology and fluorescence bronchoscopy in a high-risk group. Chest 2000;117:72–79.
6. Strauss GM, Dominioni L. Meeting report on "International conference on prevention and early diagnosis of lung cancer. Varese, 1998". Lung Cancer 1999;23:171–172.
7. Nakhosteen B, Scherf B, Muti A, Marek W, Nakhosteen JA. MARATHON-S: a new fully automated cytology and cytometry sample processor for sputum and other cell suspensions. Acta Cytol 1998;42:542 (Abstract).
8. Wong HH, Fahy JV. Safety of one method of sputum induction in asthmatic subjects. Am J Respir Crit Care Med 1997;156:299–303.
9. Doudkine A, MacAulay C, Poulin N, Palcic B. Nuclear texture measurements in image cytometry. Pathologica 1995;87:286–299.
10. Marek W, Krampe S, Dickgreber NJ, Nielsen L, Muti A, Khanavkar B, Müller KM, Atay Z, Topalidis T, Nakhosteen JA. Automatisierte quantitative Image-Zytometrie bronchialer Spülflüssigkeiten bei Verdacht auf broncho-pulmonale Tumoren: Vergleich mit Zytologie, Histologie und klinischer Diagnose. Pneumologie 1999;53:583–559.
11. Woolner LB. Pathology of Cancers Detected Cytologically. NCI, NIH, US Department of Health and Human Services. Atlas of Early Lung Cancer. Tokyo: Igaku-Shoin. 1983;107–213.
12. Lam S, MacAulay C, LeRiche JC et al. Early localisation of bronchogenic carcinoma. Diagn Ther Endo 1994;1:75–78.
13. Lam S, Kennedy T, Unger M et al. Localisation of bronchial intraepithelial neoplastic lesions by fluorescence bronchoscopy. Chest 1998;113:696–702.
14. Thiberville L, Sutedja T, Vermylen P et al. Multicenter European study using the light induced fluorescence endoscopy system to detect precancerous lesions in high-risk individuals. Eur Respir J 1999;14:2475.
15. Khanavkar B. Autofluorescence bronchoscopy. J Bronchol 2000;7:60–66.

Bronchology and Bronchoesophagology: State of the Art.
H. Yoshimura et al., editors.

Cicatric stenoses of trachea: is it possible to treat patients endoscopically or not?

Alexei A. Ovchinnikov
Surgery Clinic N3, Moscow Medical Academy, Moscow, Russia

Abstract. During the last 5 years 105 endotracheal laser operations were performed for 76 patients with cicatric stenoses of the upper and middle part of trachea. To achieve stabilization of tracheal lumen, intratracheal Dumon's stents were used for 49 patients and tracheostomic Montgomery T-tubes were used for 27 patients. The stents were left in the patients for periods ranging from 3 months to 5 years. In all these cases the immediate results of laser surgery and stenting were excellent, but the long-term results were much worse. In the majority of patients (76% after Dumon's stent implantation and 41.2% after T-tubes insertion), full relapse of stenoses occurred very soon after removing stents. In 22 of these patients a radical circular resection of the upper part of trachea was performed. A full restoration of tracheal lumen, which can be considered as an excellent result, resulted in 15 patients, 68.2% of total. In another five patients (22.7%) the results were estimated as good, with clinically compensative narrowing of trachea without any symptoms. All of these 20 patients, (90% of whole group), are healthy now and have returned to their usual style of life. Thus, radical surgery is much preferable in patients with cicatric stenoses of the upper and middle part of trachea.

Keywords: laser resection, stents, tracheal stenosis, tracheal surgery.

Cicatric stenosis of the upper and middle part of the trachea is not a rare condition. It can occur as a complication after tracheostomy and prolonged intubation. The main possible causes for this are ischemia and necrosis of mucous membrane and more deep layers of tracheal wall, as a result of a too high pressure from the overinflated cuff of tracheostomy or endotracheal tubes. An important role in this situation belongs to purulent tracheobronchitis, which develops if there is no adequate tracheobronchial sanation, or if the ventilators are of inferior quality or poorly sterilized. We believe that there might be some other causes for stenosis, such as a high activity of fibroblastes in patients with severe trauma, or individual reaction of connecting tissue in some patients.

It is difficult to imagine a more dramatic situation than a progressive cicatric tracheal stenosis. The asphyxia gradually increases when the patient is fully conscious, and any drug therapy or even tracheostomy are inefficient. Long torture and suffering during life and an agonizing death from asphyxia is a fate of these patients. Most of them are young or middle-aged dynamic people, as these ages are more often injured as a result of traffic and other accidents.

Address for correspondence: Professor Alexei Ovchinnikov MD, Endoscopical department of city hospital N61, 15 Dovator Street, Moscow 119048, Russia. Tel.: +7-095-245-5228. Fax: +7-095-245-3735.

Patients with severe stenoses are often hospitalized in intensive care units with deep cyanosis and severe hypoxia. There is only one way out in this situation, that is an urgent bronchoscopy and recanalization of trachea with the help of NdYAG or CO_2 surgical laser [1–3,6,7]. However, the effect of this treatment is only temporary. The restenosis develops, as a rule, one or two weeks later. Only endotracheal stents enable patients to breathe freely for a longer time [1,4,5].

During the last 5 years, since 1995, we have performed 105 endotracheal laser operations for 76 patients with cicatric stenoses of the upper part of trachea. The age of patients ranged from 18 to 65 years. In our clinic we use the Russian NdYAG laser "Rainbow" and Sharplane NdYAG laser COMBO 1064/532 XJ with a double wavelength of 1,064 and 532 nm, working in the green part of spectrum. We also used a CO_2 Sharplane laser 1080S, combined with a special laser bronchoscope. For stabilization of tracheal lumen we used intratracheal Dumon's stents for 49 patients and tracheostomic Montgomery T-tubes for 27 patients. We used the latter only for patients with open tracheostomies. In some of the patients, we introduced different stents repeatedly, so the number of operations was more than the number of patients themselves. The stents were left in the patients for periods from 3 months to 5 years. In all these cases the immediate results of laser surgery and stenting were excellent: a full restoration of tracheal lumen immediately after operation.

These results and the data collected from medical publications, created an optimistic attitude to this treatment at the beginning. We hoped that support of tracheal wall by stents would create a new scar around the tube, which would help to stabilize the tracheal lumen. Unfortunately, the long-term results were not so promising.

We used the following criteria for the evaluation of the results:

1. Good results – a compensative stenosis with absence of stridor and dispnea. Diameter of stenosis in these cases was 8mm or more.
2. Admissible results – subcompensative stenosis: the absence of stridor and dispnea when resting. Stridor and short breath developed during physical exercises. Diameter of stenosis was between 6 and 7 mm.
3. Bad results – full relapse of stenosis with diameter of narrowed trachea less than 5 mm.

We could trace the long-term results of stenting for 46 patients during the period from 2 to 5 years after laser endoscopical operation.

Intratracheal Dumon's stents were used for 29 patients. We used the following criteria for the evaluation of results:

1. Good results – a conversion of stenosis into compensative state, found in only two patients, about 7% of total.
2. Admissible results – subcompensative stenoses, found in five patients, 17% of total.
3. Bad results – in most patients (76% of total, 22 people), unfortunately, full relapse of stenoses occurred and we had to operate on them radically or introduce stents repeatedly.

The results of using Montgomery T-tubes in the group of 17 patients were a little bit better. Good results were found in 23.5% of patients, four people. Admissible results were found in 35.3% of patients, six patients. Bad results were found in 41.2% of patients, seven people.

The worst results found in a group of patients were where Dumon's stents were used. The fact is that multiple lugs on the external surface of stents tear the delicate new tracheal mucous membrane and granulomas when stents are extracted. The process of scarring begins again. T-tubes with their smooth surface are preferable, but not all the patients have tracheostomy. Thus, even prolonged stenting of trachea after laser resection of cicatric stenoses very seldom leads to stabilization of tracheal lumen and to conversion of stenosis into a compensative state.

Since 1997 in our clinic we have performed 22 radical circular resection of the upper part of trachea from the cervical approach according to Kocher with end-to-end anastomosis. The maximum length of resection was 6 cm. The final results of surgery treatment were traced during the period from 6 months to 3 years. A full restoration of tracheal lumen, which can be estimated as an excellent result, was found in 68.2% of patients, 15 people. In another five patients (22.7% of total) the results were estimated as good, with clinically compensative narrowing of trachea without any symptoms. All of these 20 patients, (90% of all group), are healthy now and could return to their usual style of life. Only two patients suffered from short breath and stridor during physical exercises, which was estimated as an admissible result.

On the basis of our experience we had to change our curative tactics for patients with cicatric stenoses of the upper part of trachea. In severe cases with ventilatory insufficiency we used urgent laser endoscopic recanalization of the trachea (for vital indications). Four to six days later, after partial healing of burned tracheitis, we performed radical circular resection of the trachea with end-to-end anastomosis. In cases of compensative stenosis, if the diameter of narrowed zone permitted introducing a tracheal tube, minimum N 6, to provide an adequate ventilation during narcosis, we performed radical circular resection of the trachea without any attempts of endoscopical treatment. CT scanning with computer reconstruction of stenotic zone is obligatory except for tracheoscopy. It allows an accurate measurement of narrowings which is very important before the operation.

The main contraindications for the radical surgery treatment are either too long stenosis, more than 6—7 cm, multiple stenoses at different levels, or former surgery interventions on the trachea, which makes it impossible to provide adequate mobilization of the trachea. Nevertheless, tracheostomy is not a contraindication for radical surgery, it only enlarges the zone of tracheal resection. If operating is impossible, the patients must be treated endoscopically and retain stents for a long period of time, or undergo very difficult multiple plastic operations on the trachea with unpredictable results.

References

1. Cavaliere S, Beamis J. Atlas of therapeutic bronchoscopy: laser-stents. Italy, Brescia: R.I.B.E.L., 1991;93.
2. Dumon J, Meric B. Handbook of endobronchial YAG-laser surgery. Hopital Salvator, Marseille, France. 1983;97.
3. Dumon JF. YAG-laser bronchoscopy. New-York: Praeger, 1985;150.
4. Dumon JF. A dedicated tracheobronchial stent. The 6th world congress for bronchology. Program and book of abstracts. Tokyo, 1989;122.
5. Dumon JF, Cavaliere S, Diaz-Jimenez JP et al. Seven-year experience with the dumon prosthesis. J Bronchol 1996;3:6—10.
6. Nakhosteen JA, Niederle N, Zavala DC. Atlas und lehrbuch der bronchoskopie. 2 Auflage. Berlin-Heidelberg: Springer-Verlag, 1989;300.
7. Unger M. Neodymium: YAG-laser therapy for malignant and benign endo-bronchial obstruction. In: Unger M (ed) Clinics in Chest Medicine, Simposium on Laser Techniques. Philadelphia: W.B.Saunders Co., 1985;6:277—290.

Bronchology and Bronchoesophagology: State of the Art.
H. Yoshimura et al., editors.

Bronchofiberscopy in the diagnosis of endobronchial TB

Reury-Perng Perng
Chest Department, Taipei Veterans General Hospital, Taipei, Taiwan

Abstract. *Background.* Bronchofiberscopy contributes to the diagnosis of airway diseases, both malignant and benign. In this study we used bronchofiberscopy for patients with endobronchial TB and evaluated its indications, scopic findings and diagnostic rates.

Method. Patients were referred to our department for bronchofiberscopy because of exhibiting abnormal chest X-ray films or clinical pictures of suspected endobronchial lesions. Every patient's scopic finding was recorded and specimen was used for pathological or bacteriological examination. Patients with no definite diagnosis would be required to have exploratory thoracotomy.

Results. Females accounted for 56% of a total of 62 patients. The age of patients ranged from 17 to 72. Ninety-two percent of patients had examinations because of abnormal chest films, and 8% of them because of clinical suspicions. Right and left upper lobes were primary lesion sites, 30.6 and 20.9%, respectively. The left main bronchus was where the disease was most frequently extended. Ulcerogranuloma (48%) and caseation (40%) were the most frequent findings in the acute group; stenosis (83%) was the most frequent finding in the chronic group. Forty-seven out of 50 cases in the acute group had a definite diagnosis, the diagnostic rate was 94%. The diagnostic rate for the chronic group was 17%; and for the whole group 79%.

Conclusion. Bronchofiberscopy provides a valuable aid in the diagnosis of endobronchial tuberculosis (TB), especially for the acute group.

Keywords: bronchofiberscopy, diagnosis, endobronchial TB.

Introduction

Due to different approaches to obtaining samples, the incidence of endobronchial TB varies widely in literature reports. For example, in autopsy specimens it was 42% [1], in surgical specimens and rigid bronchoscopy specimens it was 40 to 50% [2,3], and 11% [4], respectively.

Due to advances in chemotherapy and public health improvements, TB is controlled effectively in the world especially in developed countries both in terms of its prevalence and population mortality rates for the past 50 years. Endobronchial TB is thus rarely seen.

Since Ikeda's invention of bronchofiberscope in 1968 [5], there has been a great improvement in diagnosing airway diseases, including endobronchial TB. For the past 30 years, TB has been under appropriate control in developed countries. Literature in English, therefore, on the use of bronchofiberscopy in the diagnosis

Address for correspondence: Reury-Perng Perng MD, Chest Department, Taipei Veterans General Hospital No. 201, Sec. 2, Shih-Pai Road, Taipei 11217, Taiwan. Tel.: +886-2-2875-7562. Fax: +886-2-2875-2380. E-mail: rpperng@vghtpe.gov.tw of endobronchial TB is very rare. Hence, we would like to present our experiences in this area.

Materials and Methods

Our study included patients referred to our department for bronchofiberscopy due to abnormal chest X-ray films or clinical pictures with suspected endobronchial lesion. We divided them into two groups according to their length of disease history. Patients with a history of less than 2 years were in an acute group, and others were in a chronic group. Every patient's bronchofiberscopic finding was recorded in detail and specimens taken by bronchofiberscopy were used for pathological or bacteriological examination to provide confirmation. Patients with no definite diagnosis by bronchofiberscopy were required to receive exploratory thoracotomy in an attempt to make a definite diagnosis.

Results

In our study, bronchofiberscopy or exploratory thoracotomy confirmed that 62 patients were had endobronchial TB. Looking at demographic data, female patients accounted for 56%, and the distribution of the ages ranged from 17 to 72 years old, covering every age group.

Ninety-two percent of our patients had bronchofiberscopy because of exhibiting abnormal chest X-ray films. Atelectasis and chronic pulmonary infiltration were the most frequent findings. Five patients (8%) had normal chest films but were examined due to clinical suspicions of having endobronchial lesions. Among these, three had localized rhonchi (Table 1).

The upper lobe bronchus was the most frequent primary lesion site. The right upper lobe accounted for 30.6%; the left upper lobe, 20.9%. The primary lesion site of patients (16.2%) could not be determined (Table 2). Lesions extending to the left main bronchus comprised 32.3%, followed by the right main bronchus 19.4%, trachea 16.1%, and right intermediate bronchus 11.3%.

From our study, a total of 50 patients were in an acute group and 12 patients were in a chronic group. In the acute group, the most common bronchofiber-

Table 1. Indication of bronchofiberscopy.

A. Abnormal chest X-ray film 57 patients (92%)	
1. Atelectasis	39
2. Chronic pulmonary infiltration	11
3. Mass shadow	5
4. Pleural effusion	1
5. Mediastinal widening	2
B. Clinical suspicion five patients (8%)	
1. Localized rhonchi	3
2. Irritating cough	1
3. Hemoptysis	1

Table 2. Primary lesion site.

	Site	%
Right	Upper lobe	30.6
	Middle lobe	3.2
	Lower lobe	9.7
Left	Upper lobe	20.9
	Lower lobe	19.4
Undetermined		16.2

scopic findings were ulcerogranuloma (48%) and caseation (40%). However, partial stenosis (83%) was the most common seen in the chronic group.

Of the 50 patients in the acute group, 47 were confirmed as having endobronchial TB pathologically or bateriologically with a diagnostic rate of 94%. In the chronic group, the diagnostic rate was 17%. For the whole group it was 79% (Table 3).

Discussion

The females tended to have a higher incidence of endobronchial TB [2,3,6,7], where female patients accounted for 56% of our study. However, females in a reported study only accounted for 33% [8] due to different inclusion/selection criteria or a smaller sample size.

The lobar or sequmental bronchus, especially both upper lobe bronchi, were frequently seen primary lesion sites [1]. Indeed our study bears this out too. The right and left upper lobe bronchus in our study were 30.6 and 20.9%, respectively. The same results have been reported recently [7].

When endobronchial TB invades bronchial wall it usually causes narrowing of bronchial lumen, even complete obstruction. This leads to the appearance of

Table 3. Diagnostic rate of bronchofiberscopy in endobronchial tuberculosis.

Group	Findings	%	Diagnostic method			Positive rate	Total
			P	B	P + B		
Acute	Submucosal infiltration	8%	1	3	0	4/4 (100%)	47/50 (94%)
(< 2 years, n = 50)	Ulcerogranuloma	48%	3	7	11	21/24 (88%)	
	Caseation necrosis	40%	0	6	14	20/20 (100%)	
	Nonspecific	4%	0	2	0	2/2 (100%)	
Chronic	Complete stenosis	17%	0	0	0	0/0 (0%)	2/21 (79%)
(> 2 years, n = 12)	Partial stenosis	83%	0	2	0	2/10 (17%)	
Total			4	20	25		49/62 (79%)

P = pathology; B = bacteriology.

atelectasis on patient's chest X-ray film. Among 62 patients in our study, 39 had this clinical manifestation for bronchofiberscopy. If chronic pulmonary infiltration, especially in both lower lung fields, is presented on the chest X-ray film, and the sputum examination for TB is confirmed positive, then endobronchial TB should be suspected [9]. In our study 11 patients had chronic pulmonary infiltration on chest X-ray films, most of them were in lower lung field.

If patients with a normal chest X-ray finding but with a long history of cough problems and localized rhonchi in auscultation, they are suspected of having endobronchial lesions and necessitate bronchofiberscopy. Three patients were diagnosed in our study under this condition.

The normal left main bronchus is 4 to 6 cm in length, longer than the right main bronchus. In other words, it becomes an easy target for being involved in the disease. The left main bronchus was 32.3% more often involved than the right main bronchus (at 19.4%) in our study, similar to other reports' findings [7].

Lee [7] classified bronchofiberscopic findings as hypertrophy with luminal narrowing, erosion and ulceration, mucosal edema and redness, and cicatricial stenosis with pseudomenbrances. Cicatricial stenosis with pseudomembrane in Lee's report was equivalent to partial or complete stenosis in our study. Furthermore, we classified our findings into submucosal infiltration, ulcerogranuloma, and caseation which were in more detail than Lee's classification as hypertrophy with luminal narrowing and erosion and ulceration.

Of 50 patients in the acute group, 47 had pathological or bacteriological proof, and the other three were in the ulcerogranuloma group. Their biopsy reports were blood clots or granulation tissue because of an insufficient quantity of specimens.

In the 12 cases of chronic group, two cases of complete stenosis stemmed from obstruction of lumen covered by membrane. Among 10 cases of partial stenosis, two cases of specimens by brush were bacteriologically proven.

References

1. Auerbach O. Tuberculosis of the trachea and major bronchi. Am Rev Tuberc 1949;60:604–620.
2. Olson DE, Jones FS, Angevine DM. Bronchial disease in lungs resected for pulmonary tuberculosis. Am Rev Tuberc 1953;68:657–677.
3. Meissner WA. Surgical pathology of endobronchial tuberculosis. Dis Chest 1954;11:18–25.
4. McIndoe RB, Steele JD, Samson PC et al. Routine bronchoscopy in patients with active pulmonary tuberculosis. Am Rev Tuberc 1939;39:617–628.
5. Ikeda S, Yanai K, Ishikawa S. Flexible bronchofiberscope. Keio J Med 1968;17:1.
6. Salkin D, Cadden AV, Edson RC. The nature history of tuberculous tracheobronchitis. Am Rev Tuberc 1943;47:351–369.
7. Lee JH, Park SS, Lee DH et al. Endobronchial tuberculosis. Clinical and bronchoscopic features in 121 cases. Chest 1992;102:990–94.
8. Ip MSM, So SY, Lam WK et al. Endobronchial tuberculosis, revisited. Chest 1986;102: 990–994.
9. Chang SC, Lee PY, Perng RP. Lower lung field tuberculosis. Chest 1987;91:230–233.

Bronchology and Bronchoesophagology: State of the Art.
H. Yoshimura et al., editors.

Bronchoesophagology in the USA – 2000

David R. Sanderson
Mayo Medical School, Mayo Clinic Scottsdale, Arizona, USA

Bronchology and esophagology have undergone remarkable changes and experienced unprecedented growth over the past three decades in the United States.

One way of approaching a report of this kind is to examine the various specialties performing these procedures, and attempt to estimate the volumes of procedures being performed. Pulmonary physicians, otolaryngologists, gastroenterologists, thoracic surgeons, and pediatric specialists in surgery, pulmonology, and gastroenterology all share expertise and responsibility for various aspects of per-oral endoscopy. Table 1 lists the numbers of Board certified specialists in those fields.

There are three principle societies with endoscopy as their main interest. The American Broncho-Esophagological Association (ABEA) was founded in 1917 by Chevalier Jackson. It is a multidisciplinary organization with a preponderance of otolaryngologists. It has an academic focus and membership is by invitation. In 2000 it has a total of 440 members, of which 285 are active members. It shares in sponsorship of the Annals of Otology, Rhinology and Laryngology.

The American Association for Bronchology (AAB) was founded in 1993 following the 7th World Congress for Bronchology and Bronchoesophagology in Rochester, Minnesota. There are 176 active members and the organization publishes the Journal of Bronchology.

The American Society for Gastrointestinal Endoscopy (ASGE) has 5,205

Table 1. Board certified physicians in the USA.

Pulmonary disease	8689
Gastroenterology	9622
Otolaryngology - HNS	6000[a]
Thoracic surgery	5785
Pediatric surgery	764[b]
Pediatric pulmonology	596
Pediatric gastroenterology	587
Total	32043

[a]Estimate; [b]1998 figure.

Address for correspondence: Prof David R. Sanderson MD, Mayo Clinic, 13400 E. Shea Boulevard, Scottsdale, AZ 85259, USA. Tel.: +1-480-301-8265. Fax: +1-480-301-4869.

members, most of whom are gastroenterologists. It was founded in 1941 as the American Gastroscopic Club. In 1946 the name was changed to the American Gastroscopic Society and the name changed again in 1961 to its present appellation. It publishes a variety of practice guidelines, standards and position papers.

In 1999 the AAB mailed a questionnaire to 2,500 members of the American College of Chest Physicians. Results were published in the January 2000 issue of the Journal of Bronchology by Colt and Prakash [1]. They had a 30% response rate, nearly all of whom (98%) were pulmonologists. Among that constituency they noted very little utilization of the rigid bronchoscope. Only 6% said they performed rigid bronchoscopy, and only 4% had done so within the preceding 12 months. Stent placement and laser bronchoscopy were also done by only a small number of individuals (5 and 8%, respectively). This would seem to suggest that those more specialized and hazardous procedures are being concentrated in higher volume, usually academic, institutions.

Data do not exist on the total number of endoscopic procedures performed annually in the US. However, a market survey in 1999 estimated there were 1,500 fiber bronchoscopes and 800 video bronchoscopes sold, and 650 flexible GI endoscopes and 8,000 GI video endoscopes [2].

Diagnostic bronchoscopy probably constitutes the most common category of that procedure with suspected neoplasm, localized infiltrates, hemoptysis, and diffuse lung disease the more common indications. Immune compromised patients, either as a result of chemotherapy or AIDS, represent an increasingly frequent indication. Therapeutic indications include atelectasis or retained secretions, localized obstructive lesions, and foreign body removal. Bronchoalveolar lavage has both clinical and research applications as a method for obtaining "medical" lung biopsy.

The future holds a number of challenges. One of these is the need to maintain high quality training, and assure that trainees have adequate numbers and variety of procedures under appropriate supervision. After training one needs to perform an adequate volume of procedures on an ongoing basis to remain proficient. Pediatric bronchoscopy and esophagoscopy are sufficiently unique and distinct from adult practice as to require special training, and probably should be concentrated in a few centers of excellence. Health care costs in the US are under increased scrutiny by both public and private payers, and appropriate utilization of scarce resources is critical to delivering quality care. Overutilization of procedures certainly is not in the best interest of patient care, or judicious expenditure of health care dollars.

References

1. Colt HG, Prakash UBS, Offord KP. Bronchoscopy in North America: survey by the American Association for Bronchology, 1999. J Bronchol 2000;7:8–25.
2. Millennium Research Group. Personal Communication. 1999.

Bronchology and Bronchoesophagology: State of the Art.
H. Yoshimura et al., editors.

Pulsed dye laser treatment of laryngeal papillomas

Stanley M. Shapshay and Tulio A. Valdez
Department of Otolaryngology Head and Neck Surgery, Tufts University School of Medicine, New England Medical Center, Boston, Massachusetts, USA

Abstract. *Background.* Microvascular targeting with the 585-nm pulsed dye laser (PDL) may provide a new form of therapy to control symptoms caused by recurrent respiratory papillomatosis (RRP).

Methods. Twelve patients with RRP underwent 15 procedures under general anesthesia with the 585 nm PDL. A micromanipulator (13 procedures) and a flexible naso-laryngoscope (two procedures) were used to deliver the laser pulses. Patients were followed postoperatively according to protocol.

Results. Clinical examination revealed regression of papillomas in all patients. Eight patients had complete regression after PDL surgery and three patients had partial response to treatment. One patient was lost to follow up. No complications were present during this prospective nonrandomized pilot study.

Conclusion. Patients treated with PDL experienced regression of their papillomas. PDL may provide patients with RRP an alternative treatment without the risks associated with CO_2 laser surgery. This procedure also has potential to be delivered on an outpatient basis with flexible fiberoptic laryngoscopes.

Introduction

Recurrent respiratory papillomatosis (RRP) is a viral disease characterized by multiple recurrences of benign tumors of the aerodigestive tract mucosa. RRP shows a marked predilection for the larynx, with the true vocal cords being the most frequently affected site [1]. No medical therapy has been found to cure RRP and surgical treatment is aimed at achieving control of the symptoms. Microsurgical ablation of the lesions with the CO_2 laser has become the standard method of treating RRP [2]. Surgical ablation with CO_2 laser can be associated with soft tissue complications such as scarring, webbing and stenosis, as well as the possibility of endotracheal tube ignition.

The PDL 585 nm has been successfully used to treat cutaneous warts, port wine stains and telangectasias because of its affinity for hemoglobin absorption [3,4].

Address for correspondence: Tulio A. Valdez MD, New England Medical Center, NEMC # 187, Department of Otolaryngology Head and Neck Surgery, 750 Washington Street, Boston, MA 02111, USA. Tel.: +1-617-636-1662. Fax: +1-617-636-1690. E-mail: Tvaldez@lifespan.org

Materials and Methods

Laser system

A 585-nm PDL (Model SPTL–1a, Candela Corporation, Wayland, MA) with a pulse duration of 300 to 500 μs was used for this study. The PDL was coupled to an operating microscope using a micromanipulator (Ultraspot CO_2, Heraeus Laser-Sonics, Inc., Milpitas, CA) that had been specially modified to deliver 585-nm PDL radiation with even energy distribution to a 2.7-mm diameter spot on the tissue surface.

A flexible naso-laryngoscope (Pentax) was used in two patients. The standard 1-mm diameter optical fiber of the PDL was replaced with a 600-μm core diameter silica fiber that was inserted in the working channel of the flexible naso-laryngoscope.

Clinical protocol

Twelve patients, aged 23 to 54 were enrolled in the protocol. Nine patients were male and three were female. The average number of years with the disease for this group ranged between 1 and 25 years. All patients presented with hoarseness at the time of surgery. A total of 15 procedures were performed with PDL including two using a flexible naso-laryngoscope. Duration of the follow-up ranged from 1 month to 30 months. Three patients underwent a second surgery with PDL.

Patients were treated under general anesthesia with the use of a standard rigid laryngoscope for exposure. Four patients received PDL treatment exclusively in nonphonatory areas of the larynx (ventricles and false cords). In this group of patients, lesions affecting the vocal cords received standard CO_2 laser treatment [5]. The remaining patients were treated with PDL in all sites compromised by papillomas, including the true vocal cords and the anterior commissure. The end point for our study was purpura or blanching of the vasculature within the papilloma (see Fig. 1).

Patients were scheduled to be seen approximately once a month to determine the course of treatment. The examination consisted of a flexible nasal laryngoscopy with video documentation. Success was defined as 1) complete or partial regression of lesions following treatment with PDL, 2) lack of significant adverse effects related to the PDL, and 3) improvement of symptoms.

Results

No peri- or postoperative complications were noted. All patients had subjective improvement of their voice after treatment. All patients treated with PDL showed clinical regression of papillomas at 1 month follow-up without evidence of soft tissue complications and good vocal cord mobility. Seven patients showed com-

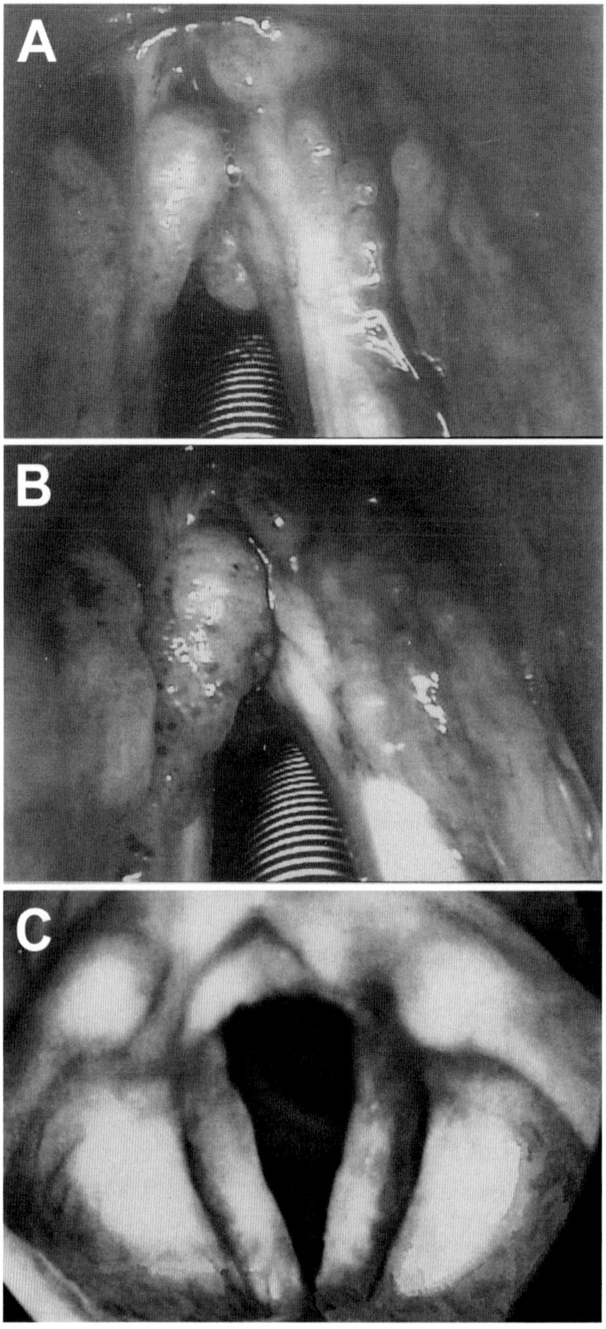

Fig. 1. **A:** Intraoperative view of laryngeal papilloma inmediately prior to PDL treatment. (Papillomas involving the anterior commissure, ventricles and false vocal cords.) **B:** Intraoperative view immediately after PDL treatment. Irradiated papillomas show darkening of vasculature. **C:** Photograph of vocal cords 1 month after surgery. Treated areas appear free of disease.

Table 1.

Age (years)	Sex	Treatment	PDL fluence (J/cm^2)	PDL No. of pulses	Outcome of PDL treatment
25	F	PDL + CO2	6, 8, 10	1–2	TR[a]
46	M	PDL + CO2	6, 8, 10	1–2	TR
37	F	PDL + CO2	6	1–2	TR
39	M	PDL + CO2	6, 8, 10	1–2	TR
40	M	PDL	8	2–5	TR
33	M	PDL	10	2–5	TR
28	M	PDL	10	2–5	PR
25	M	PDL	10	2–5	TR
43	M	PDL	10	2–5	PR
23	M	PDL	9[b]	2–5	TR
40	F	PDL	10	2–5	PR
29	M	PDL	10	2–5	TR

[a]Second PDL treatment, PR partial regression, TR total regression, LF lost to follow up; [b]flexible scope.

plete resolution of their papillomas 1 month after surgery. Two patients showed partial regression of their papilloma and one patient was lost to follow up (Table 1). The areas of papilloma that responded only partially to treatment were noted to be thicker than the rest.

Discussion

The results in our pilot study demonstrate that PDL causes clinical regression of vocal cord papillomas without evidence of soft tissue complications or changes in vocal cord function. This is important especially when providing palliative treatment for a condition, which may require multiple procedures during its course. Recently, similar results have been reported in children with RRP using a 577-nm flash pumped dye laser [6].

Although PDL treatment does not cure RRP it provides the physician with a new option for RRP treatment with no discernable side effects. The absence of exposed raw surfaces with PDL should allow treatment in areas like the anterior commissure in a single procedure with reduced risk of webbing or stenosis. We also believe that there may be a long-term benefit in mucosal preservation, since it is well known that traumatized areas such as tracheotomy sites provide a pathway for RRP dissemination. This study also validates the possibility of delivering PDL through a flexible naso-laryngoscope in the future in an outpatient setting.

References

1. Kashima H, Mounts P, Leventhal B, Hruban RH. Sites of predilection in recurrent respiratory papillomatosis. Ann Otol Rhinol Laryngol 1993;102:580–583.

2. Simpson GT, Strong MS. Recurrent respiratory papillomatosis: the role of the carbon dioxide laser. Otolaryngol Clin North Am 1983;16:887–894.
3. McMillan K, Shapshay SM, McGilligan JA, Wang Z, Rebeiz EE. A 585 Nanometer pulsed dye laser treatment of laryngeal papillomas: preliminary report. Laryngoscope 1998;108:968–972.
4. Kauvar ANB, McDaniel DH, Geronemus RG. Pulsed dye laser treatment of warts. Arch Fam Med 1995;4:1035–1040.
5. Levine VJ, Geronemus RG. Adverse effects associated with the 577 nanometer pulsed dye laser in the treatment of cutaneous vascular lesions. A study of 500 patients. J Am Acad Dermatol 1995;32:613–617.
6. Bower CM, Flock S, Waner M, Schaeffer R. Flash pump dye laser treatment of laryngeal papillomas. Ann Otol Rhinol Laryngol 1998;107:1001–1005.

Bronchology and Bronchoesophagology: State of the Art.
H. Yoshimura et al., editors.

Developmental disorders in division of the upper lobe bronchi

Edgár Székely
Pediatric Institute 'Svábhegy', Budapest, Hungary

Abstract. The normal division of the bronchial system is dichotomy. However, in 2–4,000 patients we may find other types of divisions. The most important alterations are the divisional disorders of the right and/or left upper lobe bronchi because they may promote pathological processes like recurrent infections and/or pneumonia. On the basis of the literature and 10,000 bronchoscopies on infants and children a new classification will be shown. The divisional disorders of the upper lobe bronchus are: 1) split of the right and/or left upper lobe bronchus, 2) duplication of the right and/or left upper lobe bronchus, 3) transposition of one or two right segment bronchus(i) into the trachea, 4) supernumerary tracheal bronchus, 5) duplication of the right upper lobe, and 6) trifurcation of the trachea. Bilateral disorders are rarely found. Occurrence of tracheal bronchus on the left side is extremely rare. Anatomical situations and endoscopical pictures will be discussed.

Keywords: developmental disorders of the bronchi, pediatric bronchology.

Developmental disorders of the upper lobe bronchi are very rare: about four per 1,000 patients. The question arises as to whether there is any clinical significance of these disorders or if they are only interesting aspects of the development of the bronchial system. A colleague considers these variations to be facultative only. In any case, divisional disorders are a real object of interest for doctors working every day with the bronchial system.

Usually one can see dichotomical divisions in the bronchi, i.e., in most cases the bronchi divide into two branches. Before this, the trachea divides into two main bronchi: the right main bronchus to upper lobe bronchus and stem bronchus, the left main bronchus to upper lobe and lower lobe bronchi, etc. In such a system the airflow is laminar without turbulence. In the case when the dichotomical divisions change, however, the airflow becomes turbulent. This may promote the settlement of bacteria causing recurrent infections. In our bronchological practices we found 8-fold more developmental disorders of the division in bronchi in children suffering from recurrent bronchitis than in the normal or tuberculous patients. After precise diagnosis and care, those patients who had often been severely ill due to recurrent infections became healthy. A typical example is that of a 1-year-old girl who had had many infections and resulting hospitalization. After the diagnosis of the duplication of the left upper lobe bronchus she became symptom-free and no further hospitalization was needed. Now she is 23 years of age and married. We think therefore that the

Address for correspondence: Dr E. Székely, Pediatric Institute 'Svábhegy', Budapest H-1535, Budapest Pf 939, Hungary. Tel.: +36-1-3957649. Fax: +36-1-3957649.

developmental disorders of the bronchi in division have not only anatomical importance but also clinical. The diagnosis of these alterations is based on bronchoscopy and bronchography. Modern CT techniques are not detailed enough for the visualization of these small alterations.

Developmental disorders of the upper lobe bronchi are described below.

Split of the upper lobe bronchus: in this case the orifice of the upper lobe bronchus is divided by a carina.

Duplication of the upper lobe bronchus: in this case the upper lobe bronchus originates with two orifices.

Transposition of one or two segments of the upper lobe into the trachea, i.e., tracheal duplication of the right upper lobe bronchus: here, one part of the upper lobe bronchus originates from the main bronchus and one from the trachea. We may say one segment of the upper lobe bronchus is dislocated into the trachea.

Downward transposition of one upper lobe segment: in this case there are only two segments in the upper lobe bronchus and one in the area of the middle lobe bronchus.

Supernumerary tracheal bronchus: in this case there are three segment divisions in the normal place of the upper lobe bronchus and one extra segment originating from the right side of the trachea. The tracheal bronchus has many variations in size and height. There are very small and large tracheal bronchi, or it may originate in the lower or middle part of the trachea.

Duplication of the upper lobe: in this case we can see two regular upper lobes with three segments in each. One originates from the normal place in the mainstem bronchus and the other one from the trachea. In this case the right lung has 13 segments. This is a very rare alteration, we have found only one case in 70,000 bronchoscopies.

Tracheal trifurcation: in this case the upper lobe bronchus originates from the trachea and no upper lobe bronchus is seen in the normal place in the mainstem bronchus. Thus we can speak about the trichotomy of the trachea.

Developmental disorders of the upper lobe bronchus can be found either in the left side or as a bilateral case.

A tracheal bronchus in the left side is extremely rare due to the long left mainstem bronchus. This could be because when one segment becomes transposed to the left side the dislocated bronchus cannot arrive at the trachea but remains in the mainstem bronchus. We have found left tracheal bronchus in a child with situs inversus, and two left side tracheal bronchi are cited in the references [1,2].

Conclusion

The developmental disorders in the division of the upper lobe bronchi are rare alterations but interesting for the bronchologist. They also have their clinical significance. By looking at these alterations we can gain further insight into the development of the bronchial system.

Pictures and videos on this matter can be found in the Atlas of Pediatric Bronchology CD ROM [2].

References

1. Székely E, Farkas E. Pediatric Bronchology. Baltimore and Akadémiai Kiadó Budapest: University Park Press, 1978;116–131
2. Székely E, Farkas E. Atlas of Pediatric Bronchology. Budapest: CD ROM Medicom Glaxo Wellcome, 1999.

Bronchology and Bronchoesophagology: State of the Art.
H. Yoshimura et al., editors.

Videography and digital imaging of the larynx (videotape presentation)*

Eiji Yanagisawa
Section of Otolaryngology, Yale University School of Medicine; and Southern New England Ear, Nose & Throat and Facial Plastic Surgery Group, New Haven, Connecticut, USA

Abstract. Videography is still a most effective method of documenting the anatomy, pathology and physiology of the larynx. Videography of the larynx also serves as an important source for digital imaging. Digital imaging is now possible using newer digital image capture systems or a digital still camera. It allows easy retrieval, high quality images, and long-term storage without image degradation; however, the equipment is still costly. As new technology improves and the costs of digital imaging systems decrease, the use of digital imaging for laryngeal documentation of the larynx will likely become more widespread.

The purpose of this presentation is to demonstrate various methods of videography and digital imaging of the larynx. It will describe my early experiences with laryngeal videography, my current techniques of videography in the office and in the operating room, and newer techniques of digital imaging of the larynx.

Videography of the larynx

I began to experiment with laryngeal videography in the late 1970s. In 1975, using a large bulky Magnavox CV 440 home video camera mounted on an operating microscope, I was able to document my first successful videography of the larynx of a patient with a verrucous carcinoma in April 1977. In 1981, I presented a videotape "Videolaryngoscopy Using a Rigid Telescope and a Video Home Camera" at the Annual Meeting of the American Bronchoesophagological Association. This videotape was co-authored by Casuccio and Suzuki [1]. The term videolaryngoscopy was first used and popularized by Eiji Yanagisawa.

In the early 1980s, I examined my own larynx using a flexible fiberscope, which was attached to a home video camera on the tripod placed just in front of me. I tried this technique before I used it on my patients. I learned this technique from Japanese researchers Dr K. Honda and Dr Masafumi Suzuki. In 1988, Jo Estill and I presented a video "Contribution of Aryepiglottic Constriction to Ringing Voice Quality" at the Symposium on Care of the Professional Voice in New York City [2]. In our study, we observed that aryepiglottic constriction was

Address for correspondence: Eiji Yanagisawa MD, FACS, Southern New England Ear, Nose & Throat and Facial Plastic Surgery Group, Primary and Specialist Medical Center, LLC, 98 York Street, New Haven, CT 06511, USA. Tel.: +1-203-777-2264. Fax: +1-203-624-4081.

*This article is an edited version of the videotape presentation made at the WCBE Meeting in Yokohama, Japan on 9 June 2000.

present in high-intensity vocal qualities. We confirmed Garcia's observation of 1855, associating aryepiglottic constriction with a brilliant voice.

Videography in the office

Videography in the office is the most practical and effective method of documenting the larynx and can be accomplished by either a flexible fiberscope or a rigid telescope [3–7].

Fiberscopic videolaryngoscopy (Fig. 1A) has great value in evaluating and documenting the physiological functions and pathology of the larynx. It permits simultaneous voice and video recording. There are many excellent flexible fiberscopes. The author uses the Olympus ENF-P3 and ENF-L3. The wider diameter fiberscope provides larger and clearer laryngeal images. Fiberscopic videolaryngoscopy is easier and better tolerated by both adults and children. A fiberscopic view of laryngeal polyps taken by the Olympus ENF-L3 is shown in Fig. 1B.

Telescopic videolaryngoscopy (Fig. 1C) provides larger, brighter images of the larynx with little optical distortion. A 70° telescope recommended by Yamashita, Hirose and Yanagisawa provides a large close-up image of the larynx which

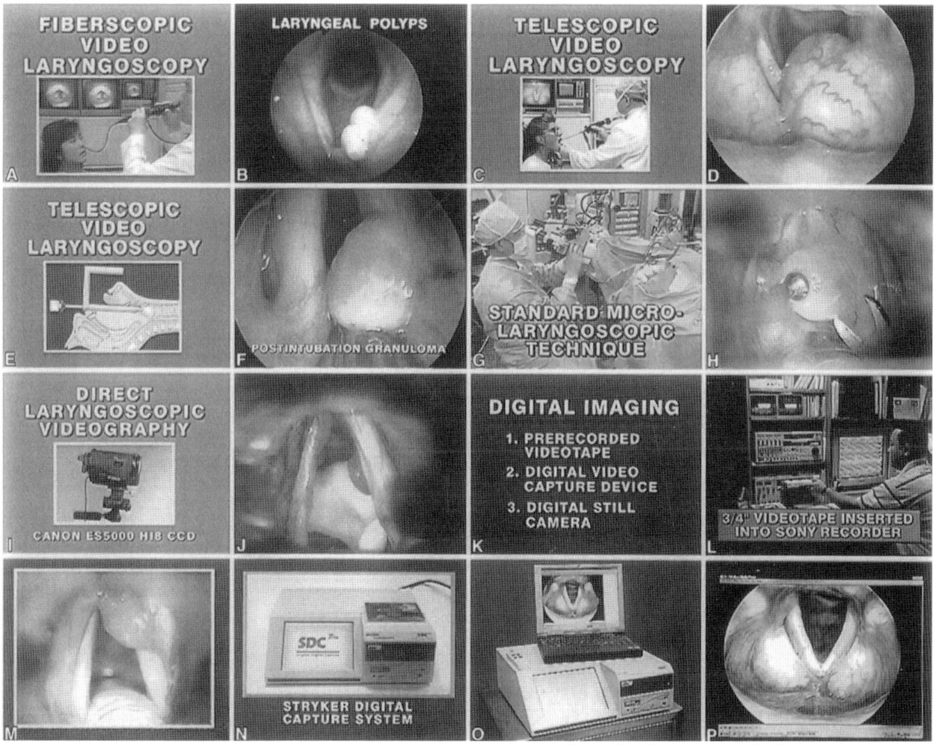

Fig. 1.

includes both anterior and posterior commissures. A large laryngocele arising from the left ventricle is shown in Fig. 1D.

Videography in the operating room

Operating room videolaryngoscopy can be accomplished using a telescope, a microscope, a Kantor/Berci tele-videomicrolaryngoscope, or direct videography through a laryngoscope [4–10].

Telescopic videolaryngoscopy (Fig. 1C) can be performed during microlaryngoscopy in the operating room. This technique will provide the clearest images of the larynx and is recommended for teaching and publication. A 0° telescopic view of a laryngeal polyp taken during suspension microlaryngoscopy in an intubated anesthetized patient is shown in Fig. 1F.

The standard microlaryngoscopic technique (Fig. 1G) is used to document laryngeal surgery. The microscopic technique has the advantage of visualizing at various magnifications, allowing for a precise surgical procedure. A microlaryngoscopic view of large obstructive polyps taken with a three-tube Hitachi camera mounted on the Zeiss operating microscope is shown in Fig. 1H. The magnification was ×25, using a 400-mm objective lens. Note the excellent clarity of the images taken with this technique.

Direct laryngoscopic videography can be performed simply (Fig. 1I). Direct laryngoscopic videography can be accomplished by using a high-power zoom home video camera placed on a tripod. I have tried several video cameras and had good results with the Canon ES-5000. After the patient was prepared for laryngoscopy, a Canon Hi8 Power Zoom video camera was placed on the tripod and the larynx videotaped. The lens was zoomed in until the full view of the vocal folds became automatically focused. The image of laryngeal papilloma is shown in Fig. 1J.

Digital imaging of the larynx

Digital imaging of the larynx can be accomplished using prerecorded videotapes, digital video capture devices, or digital still cameras (Fig. 1K). The required equipment includes: a digital or analog video camera, a computer, a digital recorder, a digital printer, and a digital still camera.

Digital imaging from prerecorded videotape

Digital imaging can be achieved from prerecorded videotape. I have used this technique for many years with very satisfactory results. The computer system we use for digital image processing is a Macintosh Quadra 950 with 64 MB of RAM and 4 GB of hard disk space with Avid Media Suite Pro and Adobe Photoshop (Fig. 1L). The prerecorded videotape is inserted into the video player. In order to convert video to prints via the computer system, the first step is to convert the image into digital information. Using the Avid Media Suite Pro software, we capture the video clip and then export a single frame of video from the video software to the hard drive. Once the image is saved on the hard drive, it is opened using image editing software, Adobe Photoshop. When the image is formatted, we make our prints using the Sony UP-5500 color digital printer. An image produced with this technique is shown in Fig. 1M.

Digital imaging with image capture system

Digital imaging can also be accomplished with newer image capture systems. Digital image capture systems currently available include: the Stryker digital capture system (SDC Pro); the Kay video recording system; and the Pentax digital electronic endoscopy system.

The Stryker digital capture system (SDC Pro) (Fig. 1N,O) is a new digital capture device that can transpose still images and moving video directly to a writable CD. It captures both still and video images from the digital Stryker camera. It can send images directly to a high-quality printer. Another advantage is that this unit is portable. The unit also allows for still images or video to be downloaded directly to the hospital network for file sharing.

Captured motion video images can be replayed using a portable PC computer (Fig. 1O). Captured images were zoomed in on the computer and the motion of the vocal folds on phonation can be viewed. A single CD may record up to 20 min of continuous video. Still images captured by the Stryker SDC Pro are shown in Fig. 1P. A single CD may hold approximately 650 images captured in bitmap format, or approximately 12,000 images in compressed JPEG format.

The Kay video recording system (DVRS) (Fig. 2A) is a newer version of its previous 9100 Stroboscopy Recording System based on VHS or S-VHS videotape recorders. Unlike its previous model, patient examinations are recorded directly to computer storage media. It captures both full-motion video and high-resolution still images with excellent quality. Audio and video are captured

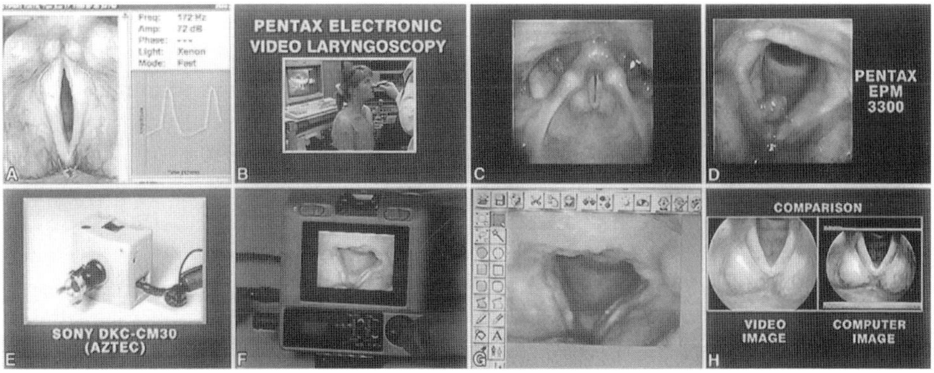

Fig. 2.

together. It also allows on-screen display of important information such as an EGG wave form. Image retrieval is easy. It allows instantaneous review of the data.

Pentax digital electronic endoscopy (Fig. 2B) is a videoendoscopic study using an electronic flexible endoscope and the Pentax EPM 3300 video processor. It has been used for evaluation of the larynx and pharynx, and has been useful for the study of swallowing disorders. The Pentax laryngoscope, which has the camera chip at the tip of the endoscope, shows remarkably clear images of both the hypopharynx and the larynx (Fig. 2C) and a close-up view of the vocal folds. An images of a laryngeal polyp captured with the EPM 3300 is shown in Fig. 2D. Note the clear image of the laryngeal polyp. A smaller, lighter processor for laryngeal examination is now available (EPM 3000).

Still digital cameras

Digital imaging can be accomplished with a digital still camera. The Sony DKC-CM30 takes only still images and does not capture video segments. The new Sony DKC-CM30 is a compact digital still camera which accepts C-mount lenses and adapters (Fig. 2E). The LCD screen for image viewing is in the back of the camera (Fig. 2F). Up to 30 images may be captured with high resolution or up to 120 images may be captured in standard resolution. During the endoscopic laryngeal examination, a series of still images are captured. A still image of chronic laryngitis with leukoplakia is shown in Fig. 2F,G. This still image captured by the Sony digital camera can be downloaded to the PC. Advantages of this camera include the following: the endoscope can be attached to the camera, the surgeon views the procedure through the camera LCD monitor, it is compact and lightweight, and it is relatively inexpensive. The major disadvantage is that the small memory records only 30 high-resolution images which must be downloaded frequently to a computer. The still digital camera is so new that it will have to be tested further before it can be recommended for laryngeal imaging.

Comparison of videographic and computer images

I compared the image acquired using the conventional videographic method and the digital image capturing device. Video images of a normal larynx taken with the Stryker 3-chip CCD camera, xenon light source and the Kay 70° rigid telescope recorded on a three-quarter inch U-matic videotape are compared with a digital image of the same patient's normal larynx captured by the Stryker SDC Pro image capture system. Both video and computer capture devices produced almost equally high quality images. A comparison of the same motion images are shown in Fig. 2H. On the left is a video image, and on the right is a digital computer image of a normal larynx.

References

1. Yanagisawa E, Casuccio JR, Suzuki M. Video laryngoscopy using a rigid telescope and video home system color camera – a useful office procedure. Ann Otol Rhinol Laryngol 1981;90: 346-350.
2. Yanagisawa E, Estill J, Kmucha ST, Leder SB. The contribution of aryepiglottic constriction to "ringing" voice quality – a videolaryngoscopic study with acoustic analysis. J Voice 1989;3: 342–350.
3. Yanagisawa E, Owens TW, Strothers G et al. Videolaryngoscopy – a comparison of fiberscopic and telescopic documentation. Ann Otol Rhinol Laryngol 1983;92:430–436.
4. Yanagisawa E, Yanagisawa R. Laryngeal Photography. Otolaryngol Clin N Am 1991;24: 999–1022.
5. Yanagisawa E. Documentation. In: Ferlito A (ed) Neoplasms of the Larynx. Edinburgh: Churchill Livingston, 1993; Chapter 21.
6. Yamashita K. Diagnostic and Therapeutic ENT Endoscopy. Tokyo: Medical View, 1988.
7. Yanagisawa E, Weaver EM. Videolaryngoscopy: equipment and documentation. In: Blitzer A et al. (eds) Office-Based Surgery in Otolaryngology. New York: Thieme, 1998; Chapter 25.
8. Yanagisawa E. Videography and laryngeal photography. In: Ferlito A (ed) Diseases of the Larynx. London: Arnold, 2000; Chapter 7.
9. Kantor E, Berci G, Partlow E et al. A completely new approach to microlaryngeal surgery. Laryngoscope 1991;101:678–679.
10. Yanagisawa E, Horowitz JB, Yanagisawa K et al. Comparison of new telescopic video microlaryngoscopic and standard microlaryngoscopic techniques. Ann Otol Rhinol Laryngol 1992; 101:51–60.

Symposia

Bronchoscopy in nontumorous pulmonary disorders

Bronchology and Bronchoesophagology: State of the Art.
H. Yoshimura et al., editors.

The value and limitation of transbronchial lung biopsy for the diagnosis of diffuse interstitial lung diseases

Arata Azuma[1], Takuo Takahashi[1], Shoji Kudoh[1], Shinobu Henmi[2] and Yu Fukuda[2]
Departments of [1]Pulmonary Medicine, and [2]Pathology, Nippon Medical School, Sendagi, Bunkyo-ku, Tokyo, Japan

Keywords: bronchoscopy, idiopathic interstitial pneumonias (IIPs), surgical lung biopsy, video-assisted thoracoscope (VATS).

The value and limitation of transbronchial lung biopsy (TBLB) for the diagnosis of interstitial lung diseases (ILDs) are discussed in this paper. The main disease will be idiopathic pulmonary fibrosis (IPF) which shows the worst prognosis and is of unknown etiology. We focused TBLB on IPF in this symposium. Caring for patients with diffuse interstitial lung diseases (DILDs) is a challenge because the etiology is often unknown and better treatment needs to be developed. Based on our experience of managing patients with DILD, I will propose the best way at present of diagnosing IPF in an actual clinical setting.

We know that the many kinds of DILD should be distinguished from each other. Since idiopathic interstitial pneumonias (IIPs) include a variety of illnesses, the name of the disease is controversial because the etiology and pathogenesis are unknown. Although the term "IIP" in Japan will be used as equivalent to both terms of acute interstitial pneumonia (AIP) and idiopathic pulmonary fibrosis (IPF), the nomenclature "IIPs" is used for all idiopathic interstitial pneumonia, including not only AIP and IPF but also desquamative interstitial pneumonia (DIP)/alveolar macrophage pneumonia (AMP), respiratory bronchiole-interstitial lung disease (RB-ILD), bronchiolitis obliterance/organizing pneumonia (BOOP)/cryptogenic organizing pneumonia (COP) and nonspecific interstitial pneumonia (NSIP) defined by Katzenstein [1]. These additional disease entities show such clinical features as subacute onset and a relatively good response to corticosteroids, resulting in a better prognosis compared with that of IPF/UIP. Cellular and fibrotic NSIP were reported with 100 and 90% of 5 years survival ratio respectively, as compared to 43% for UIP [2]. Thus we will accurately diagnose IIPs by evaluation of clinical information, radiological information and pathological information to distinguish better prognostic IPs from worse ones.

Usual interstitial pneumonia (UIP) is a typical pathological feature of IPF, cryptogenic fibrosing alveolitis (CFA). Diffuse alveolar damage (DAD) is a fea-

Address for correspondence: Arata Azuma MD, PhD, 1-1-5 Sendagi, Bunkyo-ku, Tokyo, 113-8603, Japan. Tel.: +81-3-5814-6266. Fax: +81-3-5685-3075. E-mail: azuma/med4@nms.ac.jp ture of AIP, however, it is difficult to get pathological diagnoses because of a severe clinical setting. These categorizations are according to the American Thoracic Society (ATS) / European Respiratory Society (ERS) consensus statement of IPF [3]. "RB-ILD" which is commonly seen in heavy smokers and shows fibrosis with alveolar macrophage pneumonia (AMP) being similar to desquamative interstitial pneumonia (DIP) is an uncommon nomenclature in Japan. Lymphoid interstitial pneumonia (LIP) will be often compared with NSIP, thus will be categorized in the IIPs, but will be essentially categorized in the lymphoproliferative disorders.

Diagnosis of IIPs needs widely accepted surgical lung biopsy, including video-assisted thoracoscopic (VATS) biopsy and open-lung biopsy. Pathological diagnosis is most important for a definitive diagnosis of ILD. Surgical lung biopsy will be more informative for the evaluation of IIP than a small piece of material by TBLB. An ATS consensus statement recently recommended the diagnostic criteria for IPF without surgical lung biopsy (Table 1). TBLB will be done for the exclusion of other type of ILDs rather than for identifying IPF. If the patients with ILD meet all of the Major Criteria and at least three of the four items in Minor Criteria, we may clinically diagnose the patient with IPF.

Thus, we show you the "diagnostic flow chart" for the evaluation of IIPs (Fig. 1). Careful clinical evaluations lead to separating "possible IIP" and "not IIP". Patients presenting "possible IIP" will be further evaluated by high resolution computed tomography (HRCT), resulting in four groups. The group that can be confidently diagnosed with IPF will receive bronchoscopic examinations to exclude other IIPs. TBLB and/or BAL will give us valuable information in the consideration of a diagnosis. The patients who show pathological features to support any alternative diagnosis will need to receive surgical lung biopsy for further evaluation. If the feature of HRCT shows "atypical IPF", the patient will directly receive surgical lung biopsy. In the case of suspected or confidently diagnosed other diffuse parenchymal lung diseases (DPLDs), a lung biopsy will not always be necessary.

Table 1. Diagnostic criteria of IPF without surgical lung biopsy.

Major criteria (all items)
- Exclusion of other unknown causes of ILD
(drug toxicities, environmental exposures, CVDs, etc.)
- Abnormal pulmonary function studies
(VC$\downarrow$, FEV1/FVC$\uparrow$, $PaO_2\downarrow$, DLco$\downarrow$)
- HRCT abnormalities
(bibasilar reticular, minimal GGO)
- TBBs or BAL showing no features to support an alternative diagnosis
Minor criteria (at least three out of four items)
- Age > 50 years
- Insidious onset of otherwise unexplained dyspnea on exertion
- Duration of illness $\geqslant 3$ months
- Bibasilar, inspiratory crackles (dry or 'Velcro' type)

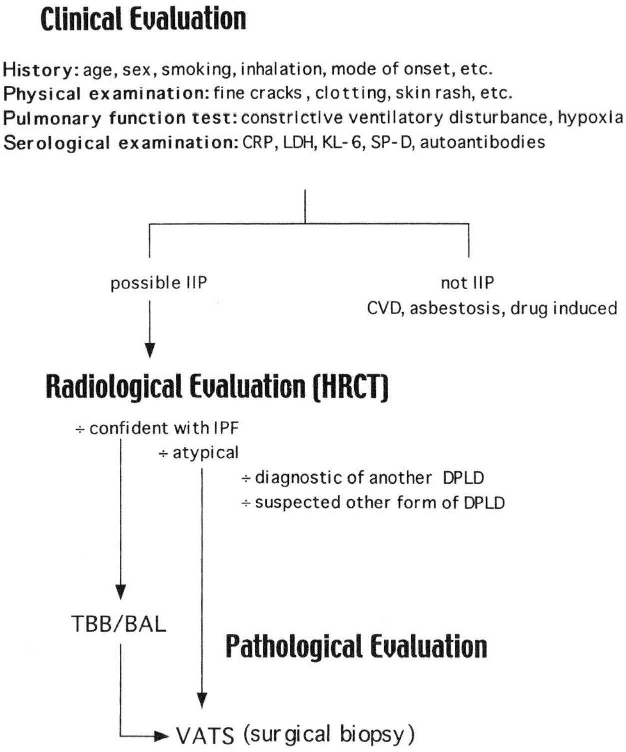

Fig. 1.

I would like to say that all pulmonary physicians work together with cooperation for achieving accurate diagnosis of patients with ILD. Therefore, we have to keep in mind that TBLB will give us a limited diagnostic value for ILD. I hope this paper will be offered to help pulmonary physicians with their assessment and care of patients.

References

1. Katzenstein AL, RF Fiorelli. Nonspecific interstitial pneumonia /fibrosis: histologic features and clinical significance. Am J Surg Pathol 1994;18:136–147.
2. Travis WD, Matsui K, Moss J, Ferrans VJ. Idiopathic nonspecific interstitial pneumonia: prognostic significance of cellular and fibrotic patterns: survival comparison with usual interstitial pneumonia and desquamative interstitial pneumonia. Am J Surg Pathol 2000;24:19–33.
3. King Jr TE, Costabel U, Cordier JF, DoPico GA, Du Bois RM, Lynch D, Lynch JP, Myers J, Panos R, Raguh G, Schwartz D, Smith CM. Idiopatic pulmonary fibrosis: diagnosis and treatment. International consensus statement. Crit Care Med 2000;161:646–664.

Bronchology and Bronchoesophagology: State of the Art.
H. Yoshimura et al., editors.

Bronchoscopy to diagnose infection

Robert P. Baughman
Department of Internal Medicine, University of Cincinnati Medical Center, Cincinnati, Ohio, USA

Abstract. Bronchoscopy is the most common procedure performed by pulmonologists in order to evaluate pneumonia. It allows one to visualize the airways and take samples for culture and pathologic examination. A wide variety of organisms can be detected by bronchoscopy, including viral, bacterial, fungal, and mycobacterial. It has proved particularly helpful in the evaluation of immunosuppressed patients. In patients with possible *Pneumocystis carinii (P. carinii)*, the bronchoalveolar lavage (BAL) has provided a diagnosis in most cases. However, it should not be linked to just one organism, since it has proved useful in diagnosing mycobacterial and fungal infections. Semiquantitative cultures of the protected brush or bronchoalveolar sample are useful in assessing possible bacterial infection.

Keywords: bronchoscopy, *Pneumocystis carinii*, pneumonia, tuberculosis.

Introduction

For many institutions, diagnosis of pneumonia is the most common reason for performing bronchoscopy [1]. Bronchoscopy itself provides several types of information regarding pneumonia, including visualization of the airway, bronchial wash and bronchoalveolar lavage (BAL) for culture, and biopsy of tissue to assess for invasion of lung parenchyma. All of these have a role in diagnosing infection [2].

In the immunosuppressed patient, bronchoscopy has proved useful [2]. This is in part because of the value of BAL in diagnosing certain infections, such as *P. carinii* [3]. Not all immunosuppressed patients are the same. Categorizing the type of immunosuppression will help identify which organisms to worry about [4]. For example, the patient with multiple myeloma or chronic lymphocytic leukemia has abnormal immunoglobulins. Therefore, they are at risk for encapsulated organisms such as *S. pneumoniae* and *H. influenzae*. The HIV-infected patient or solid organ transplant has a decreased number of T lymphocytes. They are at risk for infections controlled by cell-mediated immunity. These include *P. carinii*, *M. tuberculosis*, *Legionella*, and cytomegalovirus. In the non-immunocompromised host, bronchoscopy may provide useful information in some circumstances. These include the patient with possible tuberculosis or fungal infection. For the patient with ventilator associated pneumonia, bron-

Address for correspondence: Robert P. Baughman MD, University of Cincinnati Medical Center, P.O. Box 670564, Cincinnati, OH 45267-0564 USA. Tel.: +1-513-558-0347. Fax: +1513-558-0360.
E-mail: bob.baughman@uc.edu

choscopy with BAL or protected brush may be quite useful [5].

In evaluating a particular pathogen recovered from lung, it is useful to determine the invasiveness of the organism itself. If one finds *P. carinii* or *M. tuberculosis* in the sample, one is dealing with this as the cause of the pulmonary problem. On the other hand, some organisms can colonize the airways and lead to some confusion. For example, up to 5% of the healthy population is said to be colonized with *S. pneumoniae*. However, if a patient has a fever, purulent sputum, a lung infiltrate, and *S. pneumoniae* in his sputum, he is assumed to have pneumococcal pneumonia. Some other colonizers/pathogens are less obvious. These include herpes virus, especially cytomegalovirus. For *Aspergillus*, it may be necessary to prove that there is actual tissue invasion to assure that it is the cause of pulmonary disease. Finally, some organisms such as candida can colonize the airway and rarely cause pneumonia [6].

Pneumocystis carinii pneumonia

The identification of *P. carinii* by bronchoalveolar lavage led to the recognition of the use of BAL to evaluate immunocompromised patients [7]. In HIV-infected patients, *P. carinii* was a particular problem and BAL became widely used to diagnose this infection, since it was safer and usually as reliable as transbronchial biopsy [3]. In AIDS patients, it was noted that examination of sputum samples could identify the organism. While a successful strategy, even in the best centers it only diagnoses 60% of the cases of *P. carinii* pneumonia [8]. More importantly, other pathogens, including *M. tuberculosis* may be missed if sputum is the only specimen examined [3,8].

The utility of various stains enhances the diagnostic yield in less than adequate sample. For example, the immunofluorescent stain has a higher sensitivity than the silver stain or Wright-Giemsa stain in detecting *P. carinii*. However, this difference is only significant when examining sputum or bronchial wash. These differences in stain are not significant when one examines BAL, where a larger numbers of organisms are seen.

Another technical feature of lavage is to perform the lavage in the area of most infiltrate. Some authors found lavage exclusively in the middle lobe was associated with a yield as low as 60% in some groups of AIDS patients [9]. Others have found that lavage directed to the area of infiltrate enhanced the diagnostic yield [10]. We had developed a method for quantitating the amount of *P. carinii* recovered by BAL. This has proved useful in following patients while on therapy. It also found that *P. carinii* was more abundant in the upper lobes than lower lobes, whether or not the patients were on aerosol pentamidine [11]. Thus, the use of two lavages, with at least one to the infiltrate or into the upper lobe of patients with diffuse infiltrate has kept the yield for *P. carinii* above 95%.

Tuberculosis and fungal infections

Bronchoscopy has also proved useful in the evaluation of both tuberculosis and fungal infections [12]. This has proved true in both the AIDS and non-AIDS patients. In a study in our institution, we looked at the role of bronchoscopy in 50 patients with *M. tuberculosis* and another 41 with deep-seated fungal infections. Most of these patients were not infected with HIV, but underwent studies because the diagnosis was unclear. For *M. tuberculosis*, sputum smear was positive in 34% of cases tested and culture positive in 51% while bronchoscopy samples were smear positive in 68% and culture positive in 92%. For fungal infections, the sputum smear was never positive and only one patient had a positive culture while the bronchoscopy sample was smear positive in 34% and culture positive in 85%.

Others have found the bronchoscopy sample useful in identifying *M. tuberculosis* [13] and fungal infections. Some authors have felt that biopsy will enhance the yield and should be part of the routine evaluation [14]. However, biopsy does increase the risk of pneumothorax.

Among the uses of bronchoscopy is to identify airway lesions due to mycobacteria. *M. tuberculosis* is associated with airway lesions and can lead to airway stenosis [15,16]. Endobronchial lesions have also been seen with atypical mycobacterium [17].

Bacterial infections

The role of bronchoscopy to diagnose bacterial infection has relied on two procedures, the protected brush and BAL. Both require semiquantitative cultures to provide the clinician with the ability to separate between colonization and true infection [18]. For the ventilated patient, evidence-based analysis of the published literature has found no difference in the protected brush sample and the BAL-derived specimen [5].

Pneumonia due to bacteria remain a common cause in all groups of patients being evaluated for pneumonia. Therefore, the addition of samples for routine bacterial cultures should remain routine. In patients without pneumonia, bacteria at significant numbers are rarely cultured. In our original study, we found that none of our controls grew $>100{,}000$ colony-forming units (cfu) of bacteria/ml of BAL [18]. This means that a BAL sample can be handled similar to a urine culture.

Conclusion

Bronchoscopy has provided a large number of ways to examine the lung. In patients with possible pneumonia, it can be useful in a wide array of infections. Its value includes: what you see, what you send, and what you do with the information.

References

1. Baughman RP, Golden JA, Keith FM. Bronchoscopy, lung biopsy, and other diagnostic procedures. In: Murray JF, Nadel JA, Mason RJ et al. (eds) Textbook of Respiratory Medicine. Philadelphia: W.B. Saunders Company, 2000;725–780.
2. Baughman RP. Use of bronchoscopy in the diagnosis of infection in the immunocompromised host. Thorax 1994;49(1):3–7.
3. Baughman RP, Dohn MN, Frame PT. The continuing utility of bronchoalveolar lavage to diagnose opportunistic infection in AIDS patients. Am J Med 1994;97(6):515–522.
4. Baughman RP. The lung in the immunocompromised patient: infectious complications part 1. Respiration 1999;66:2–11.
5. Grossman RF, Fein A. Evidence-based assessment of diagnostic tests for the diagnosis of ventilator-associated pneumonia: executive summary. Chest 2000;117:177S–181S.
6. el Ebiary M, Torres A, Fabregas N et al. Significance of the isolation of *Candida* species from respiratory samples in critically ill, nonneutropenic patients. An immediate postmortem histologic study. Am J Respir Crit Care Med 1997;156(2 Pt 1):583–590.
7. Stover DE, Zaman MB, Hajdu SI et al. Role of bronchoalveolar lavage in the diagnosis of diffuse pulmonary infiltrates in the immunosuppressed host. Ann Intern Med 1984;101:1–7.
8. Huang L, Hecht FM, Stansell JD et al. Suspected Pneumocystis carinii pneumonia with a negative induced sputum examination. Is early bronchoscopy useful? Am J Respir Crit Care Med 1995;151(6):1866–1871.
9. Jules-Elysee KM, Stover DE, Zaman MB et al. Aerosolized pentamidine: effect on diagnosis and presentation of Pneumocystis carinii pneumonia. Ann Intern Med 1990;112:750–757.
10. Levine SJ, Kennedy D, Shelhamer JH et al. Diagnosis of *Pneumocystis carinii* pneumonia by multiple lobe, site-directed bronchoalveolar lavage with immunofluorescent monoclonal antibody staining in human immunodeficiency virus-infected patients receiving aerosolized pentamidine chemoprophylaxis. Am Rev Respir Dis 1992;146(4):838–843.
11. Baughman RP, Dohn MN, Shipley R et al. Increased *Pneumocystis carinii* recovery from the upper lobes in *Pneumocystis* pneumonia. The effect of aerosol pentamidine prophylaxis. Chest 1993;103(2):426–432.
12. Baughman RP, Dohn MN, Loudon RG et al. Bronchoscopy with bronchoalveolar lavage in tuberculosis and fungal infections. Chest 1991;99(1):92–97.
13. Chan HS, Sun AJ, Hoheisel GB. Bronchoscopic aspiration and bronchoalveolar lavage in the diagnosis of sputum smear-negative pulmonary tuberculosis. Lung 1990;168(4):215–220.
14. Salzman SH, Schindel ML, Aranda CP et al. The role of bronchoscopy in the diagnosis of pulmonary tuberculosis in patients at risk for HIV infection. Chest 1992;102(1):143–146.
15. Smith LS, Schillaci RF, Sarlin RF. Endobronchial tuberculosis: serial fiberoptic bronchoscopy and natural history. Chest 1987;91:644–647.
16. Lee JH, Park SS, Lee DH et al. Endobronchial tuberculosis. Clinical and bronchoscopic features in 121 cases. Chest 1992;102(4):990–994.
17. Connolly MG Jr, Baughman RP, Dohn MN. Mycobacterium kansasii presenting as an endobronchial lesion. Am Rev Respir Dis 1993;148(5):1405–1407.
18. Thorpe JE, Baughman RP, Frame PT et al. Bronchoalveolar lavage for diagnosing acute bacterial pneumonia. J Infect Dis 1987;155:855–861.

Bronchology and Bronchoesophagology: State of the Art.
H. Yoshimura et al., editors.

Significance of BAL fluid findings as a diagnostic tool in patients with interstitial lung disease

Sonoko Nagai, Takeshi Mikuniya, Masanori Kitaichi, Michio Shigematsu, Kunio Hamada, Taishi Nagao, Tadashi Mio, Yuma Hoshino, Hiroyuki Miki and Takateru Izumi

Department of Respiratory Medicine, Graduate School of Medicine, Kyoto University, Kyoto, Japan

Abstract. Based on our BAL panel of interstitial lung diseases (ILD) and current classification of interstitial pneumonia (IP), we tried to summarize whether bronchoalveolar lavage fluid cells (BALF) are a feasible diagnostic tool for differentiation, and whether the BALF cell findings predict prognosis. In an analysis of 400 healthy subjects and 151 patients with idiopathic IP (IIP) histologically diagnosed by surgical lung biopsy, we investigated how BALF cell findings were related with histology, disease severity, and prognosis. The BALF cell findings were found to be useful for differentiating between UIP and the non-UIP lesions, and also to be related to prognosis among the IIP subjects. However, the BALF cell findings were not useful for differentiating the IIP and predicting the prognosis in patients with IP-CVD.

Keywords: BAL fluid cell findings, collagen vascular disease, differential diagnosis, idiopathic interstitial pneumonia, prognosis.

Background

The definite diagnosis of interstitial pneumonia (IP) fundamentally requires a histological diagnosis from a surgical lung biopsy. It is important to obtain a histological diagnosis as differences in histology strongly relate to the prognosis. However, a surgical biopsy itself is an invasive approach for diagnosis. Since the cells obtained from a bronchoalveolar lavage (BAL) are collected from more widely dispersed lesion sites than the cells obtained from a surgical lung biopsy, the BAL method might constitute an alternative means for definite diagnosis. BAL was evaluated as a liquid-lung biopsy when this method was introduced to the fields of interstitial lung diseases (ILD).

We have accumulated BAL fluid cell findings in 400 healthy subjects and recognized that a smoking status drastically affects the findings (BALF healthy patterns: nonsmokers and smokers: Table 1) [1]. We have also accumulated BALF cell findings from about 1,600 cases with ILD [2,3]. Based on our experiences, we tried to classify the findings using three different BALF cell patterns (sarcoidosis-pattern, BOOP-pattern, and UIP-pattern) [1]. The patterns were

Address for correspondence: Sonoko Nagai MD, Department of Respiratory Medicine, Graduate School of Medicine, Kyoto University, Kawaharacho 54, Shogoin, Sakyoku, Kyoto 606-8507, Japan. Tel.: +81-75-751-3831. Fax: +81-75-751-4643. E-mail: nagai@kuhp.kyoto-u.ac.jp

Table 1. BALF cell findings in healthy subjects.

	Nonsmokers	Smokers
Fluid recovery (%)	63–83[a]	55–78
Cell recovery (1×10^5/ml)	0.3–1.1	0.7–3.9
Macrophage (%)	78–98	89–100
Lymphocyte (%)	1–20	0–9
Neutrophil (%)	0.0–1.5	0.0–1.4
Eosinophil (%)	0.0–1.6	0.0–0.7
CD 4/8 ratio	1.0–3.8	0.0–2.6

Nonsmokers (Never 177, Former 60); Smokers (180); [a](Mean – SD) – (Mean + SD).

defined according to the most common findings found in patients with sarcoidosis, idiopathic BOOP, and idiopathic UIP, respectively. BALF-sarcoidosis pattern is characterized by the presence of CD4-lymphocytosis, the BALF BOOP-pattern is characterized by the presence of CD8-lymphocytosis with or without an increase in granulocytes, and the BALF UIP-pattern is characterized by a frequent absence of lymphocytosis in spite of apparent increases in granulocytes. Given the strong relationship between the histology and prognosis in IIP patients [2,4], we tried to examine whether these BALF cell patterns could be used to predict histology in IIP.

Methods

First, we tried to classify 151 biopsy-proven idiopathic IP (IIP) using the respective BALF cell patterns. Next, we analyzed whether there were statistical differences among the IIP patients. Finally, we examined how the BALF cell patterns related to disease severity and prognosis.

Results

The BALF UIP-pattern strongly increases the likelihood that UIP lesions are present, and the BALF BOOP-pattern encompasses a variety of histologies, including those of BOOP, NSIP, UIP-CVD, and a subgroup of AIP (Table 2).

Table 2. IPs and BALF cell patterns (%) (n = 151).

	AIP	BOOP	cNSIP	fNSIP	RBILD	DIP	UIP
BOOP-p	45	85	87	53	17	13	7
UIP-p	55	8	7	29	0	75	66
Sar-p	0	0	0	7	0	0	0
Healthy-p	0	7	6	11	83	12	27

-p = -pattern; p value (overall) = 0.00001.

Table 3. BALF cell patterns and prognosis (%) (n = 151).

	BOOP-p	UIP-p	Sar-p	H-p
Improved	62.2	10.0	100	16.7
Unchanged	17.8	25.7	0	53.3
Worsened	2.2	4.3	0	3.3
Died	17.8	60.0	0	23.3

p value = 0.00001.

BALF cell patterns had a statistically significant correlation with prognosis overall (Table 3). However, since BALF lymphocytosis is present even in UIP lesions [5], BALF cell patterns could not predict the histology in patients with IP associated with collagen vascular diseases (IP-CVD) (Table 4).

Conclusion

BALF cell patterns are useful for differentiating UIP from other non-UIP lesions in patients with IIP. In particular, the BALF cell BOOP-pattern reflects a pathophysiological process in which increases in lymphocytes can be found in the lesion sites.

Table 4. BALF cell findings.

	Healthy control	IPF/UIP	UIP-SSc	UIP/CVD non-SSC
No. of patients	175	16	6	9
Fluid recovery (%)	73.2 ± 9.7	57.6 ± 18.5[a] (27.0–83.3)	53.5 ± 14.2 (33.2–70.3)	68.2 ± 10.3 (48.3–83.0)
Recovered cells (1×10^5/ml)	0.71 ± 0.5	1.62 ± 0.63 (0.55–2.93)	1.37 ± 0.96 (0.34–2.54)	1.44 ± 0.93 (0.55–3.30)
Macrophages (%)	88.8 ± 10.7	84.2 ± 20.6 (28.4–98.9)	92.5 ± 2.8 (88.7–96.5)	70.7 ± 21.3 (36.6–97.7)
Lymphocytes (%)	10.4 ± 10.3	7.8 ± 11.4 (1.0–47.1)	4.4 ± 3.7 (1.2–10.0)	27.7 ± 21.1[b] (2.0–62.8)
Neutrophils (%)	0.5 ± 1.0	6.0 ± 12.6 (0–47.9)	1.7 ± 1.4 (0.7–4.2)	0.8 ± 1.2 (0–3.3)
Eosinophils (%)	0.2 ± 0.6	2.2 ± 3.8 (0–11.4)	1.9 ± 1.7 (0–4.2)	0.5 ± 0.9 (0–2.8)
CD4+/CD8+	2.65 ± 1.58	2.12 ± 2.12 (0.49–9.02)	1.73 ± 1.41 (0.22–3.58)	2.23 ± 2.25 (0.05–6.95)

[a]Values are expressed as mean ± SD (with range of values); [b]significantly increased ($p < 0.05$) compared to IPF/UIP and UIP-SSc. SSc = systemic sclerosis; CVD = collagen vascular diseases.

References

1. Nagai S, Fujimura N, Hirata T, Izumi T. Differentiation between idiopathic pulmonary fibrosis and interstitial pneumonia associated with collagen vascular diseases by comparison of the ratio of OKT4+ cells and OKT8+ cells in BALF T lymphocytes. Eur J Respir Dis 1985;67:1–9.
2. Nagai S, Izumi T. Bronchoalveolar lavage. Still useful in diagnosing sarcoidosis. Clin Chest Med 1997;18:787–797.
3. Nagai S, Kitaichi M, Itoh H, Nishimura K, Izumi T, Colby TV. Idiopathic nonspecific interstitial pneumonia/fibrosis: comparison with idiopathic pulmonary fibrosis and BOOP. Eur J Respir Dis 1998;12:1010–1019.
4. Nagai S, Kitaichi M, Izumi T. Classification and recent advances in idiopathic interstitial pneumonia. Curr Opin Pul Med 1998;4:256–260.
5. Nagao T, Nagai S, Kitaichi M, Hayashi M, Shigematsu M, Tsutsumi T, Satake N, Izumi T. Usual interstitial pneumonia: idiopathic pulmonary fibrosis versus collagen vascular diseases. Respiration 2000 (In press).

Bronchology and Bronchoesophagology: State of the Art.
H. Yoshimura et al., editors.

Approach to the peripheral airway epithelial cells by an ultrathin bronchoscope

H. Takizawa[1], M. Tanaka[2], K. Takami[1], T. Ohtoshi[1], Y. Okada[3], F. Yamasawa[3] and A. Umeda[3]

[1]Department of Laboratory Medicine, Tokyo University; [2]WHO Collaborating Center, Tokyo Medical College; and [3]Department of Diagnostic Radiology, Keio University, Tokyo, Japan

Abstract. The inflammatory changes in small airways have been believed to be important in the pathogenesis of chronic obstructive pulmonary disease (COPD). We successfully harvested epithelial cells from sites in these small airways by using an ultrathin fiber optic bronchoscope BF2.7 (Chest 1994;106:1443). We first evaluated IL-8 (interleukin-8) and ICAM-1 expression in small airway epithelium, both being important in the recruitment and activation of inflammatory cells such as neutrophils. The IL-8 and ICAM-1 mRNA levels, corrected by β-actin transcripts, were significantly more increased in COPD patients and smokers than nonsmokers. Secondly, we studied the levels of TGFβ-1 expression, an important growth factor in tissue remodeling. Heavily smoking volunteers (> 1 pack/day), COPD patients and nonsmokers underwent bronchoscopic examination after an informed consent, and epithelial cells from small airways were harvested. Levels of TGFβ-1 mRNA/β-actin transcripts were significantly higher in smokers and COPD patients than in nonsmokers. The levels showed a positive correlation with daily cigarette consumption. Importantly, there was an inverse correlation between TGFβ-1 mRNA and V25 in flow-volume curves. In conclusion, small airway epithelium of smokers and COPD express higher levels of IL-8, ICAM-1 and TGFβ-1, which may be involved in neutrophil inflammation and irreversible airway obstruction found in small airways.

Keywords: COPD, ICAM-1, IL-8, small airway, smoker, TGFβ-1.

Introduction

Tobacco smoke has been implicated as one of the most important factors that can cause small airway disease, and following it COPD (chronic obstructive pulmonary disease) [1,2], but the molecular mechanisms by which small airway obstruction occurs remain unknown. Direct evaluation of inflammatory responses in these regions of humans remains extremely difficult to carry out, since it is presently impossible to see the mucosa using conventional bronchoscopy. Tanaka and his associates developed a number of ultrathin scopies, which enabled direct vision of small airways (inner diameter less than 2 mm) [3,4]. We harvested living epithelial cells by brushing the small airway mucosa under direct vision by using an ultrathin bronchofiberscope BF-2.7T (the outer diameter: 2.7

Address for correspondence: Dr H. Takizawa, Department of Laboratory Medicine, University of Tokyo, School of Medicine, 7-3-1 Hongo, Bunkyo-ku, Tokyo 113, Japan. Tel.: +81-3-3815-5411. Fax: +81-3-5689-0495. E-mail: TAKIZAWA-PHY@h.u-tokyo.ac.jp mm with a biopsy channel of 0.8 mm in diameter) [5,6]. To evaluate if this bronchoscopy helps in the assessment of inflammatory responses in small airways, we studied the mRNA levels of IL-8 (interleukin-8) and ICAM-1 in small airway epithelium from tobacco smokers by reverse transcription-polymerase chain reaction (RT-PCR) as the first project. Recent studies suggest some fibrogenic growth factors may be involved in the remodelling processes in the small airways [7]. One of the most potent and extensively studied growth factors is TGFβ-1, which induces fibroblast proliferation, increased production of collagen and other extracellular matrix proteins and decreased collagen degradation [8]. Therefore, TGFβ-1 mRNA levels in small airway epithelium from tobacco smokers and COPD patients were evaluated using the RT-PCR technique and the magnitudes of this fibrogenic factor expression were correlated with the small airway obstruction.

Materials and Methods

Subjects

In total, 23 healthy Japanese volunteers of whom 13 (9 males and 4 females, mean age 57.6) were current smokers and 10 nonsmokers (7 males and 3 females, mean age 54.2) were included in the study. The study was planned according to ethical guidelines, following the declaration of Helsinki, was given institutional approval and informed consent was obtained from each subject.

Bronchoscopy with an ultrathin scope

The subjects underwent a bronchofiberscopic examination with a BF-XT20 fiberscope (Olympus, Tokyo, Japan) in a standard fashion. Under fluorographic guidance, an ultrathin fiberscope (BF-2.7T) was inserted through a 2.8-mm diameter biopsy channel. A newly modified BC-0.7T brush was then inserted to collect cells by brushing the airway mucosal surfaces several times. Brushing of the mucosa was routinely performed at three or four different 9th to 10th lower lobe bronchioles. The cells were immediately collected by vortexing the brush in RPMI 1640 medium supplemented with 10% fetal-calf serum (FCS, heat-inactivated, GIBCO, Grand Island, New York). The cells were centrifuged for 5 min at 1000 rpm. The recovered cells were washed twice in Hanks' balanced salt solution without calcium and magnesium (HBSS, GIBCO). The number of cells was counted by a standard hemocytometer and the cell viability was assessed using the trypan blue dye exclusion technique [6].

RT-PCR for IL-8, ICAM-1 and TGFβ-1 mRNA in small airway epithelial cells

To assess the IL-8, ICAM-1 and TGFβ-1 mRNA levels in human small airway epithelial cells, a semiquantitative assay utilizing RT-PCR [6] was performed. We used the epithelial cell samples for RT-PCR, only if the samples contained less than 5% of nonepithelial cells as evaluated by Diff-Quik and keratin stainings. Total RNA was isolated from epithelial cell samples using the guanidinium thiocyanate-phenol-chloroform extraction method [6]. Extracted RNA was reverse transcribed to cDNA by using a Takara RNA-PCR kit according to the manufacturer's recommendation. The PCR cycle was determined by preliminary experiments showing a linear relationship between PCR cycles and the intensity of signals on ethidium-bromide stained agarose gels. The PCR product was run on a 1.0% agarose gel, and the intensity of ethidium-bromide fluorescence was evaluated by NIH Image version 1.61.

Statistics

The results were analyzed by nonparametric equivalents of analysis of variance (ANOVA) for multiple comparison, as reported [6]. Spearman's rank correlation test was used for correlation analysis between the two data.

Results

Cell harvest, viability, and morphology

The number of recovered cells ranged from 1.20×10^6 to 2.30×10^6 with a mean of 1.86×106. The cell viability ranged from 62.5 to 79.5% with a mean of 68.7%. More than 95% of the cells were positive to keratin staining. Approximately 70% of the viable cells were nonciliated round cells.

Small airway epithelial cells in smokers and COPD patients showed increased IL-8, ICAM-1, and TGFβ-1 mRNA as compared to those in nonsmokers by RT-PCR

The signals for IL-8, ICAM-1, TGFβ-1 and β-actin were detected in all cases, and the relative intensity of the 3 markers were statistically increased in smokers and patients with COPD compared to nonsmokers. The TGFβ-1 mRNA levels in COPD patients were significantly higher than those of healthy smokers.

Correlation between the levels of IL-8, ICAM-1 or TGFβ-1 mRNA and smoking history

Among current smokers without airway obstruction, IL-8, ICAM-1 and TGFβ-1 mRNA levels correlated positively with the extent of smoking history when the signals were normalized by β-actin transcripts. The magnitudes of TGFβ-1 expression in cases with COPD also showed a statistically significant correlation with smoking history ($r = 0.653$, $p < 0.001$).

Correlation between mRNA levels of TGFβ-1 and lung function tests

The mRNA levels of TGFβ-1 correlated significantly with %V25 and V50/V25 in smokers, but seemed to show no relationship to %V50, %FVC or FEV1.0%. Those of COPD patients showed significant correlation with %V50, as well as, %V25, but not with V50/V25, %FVC or FEV1.0%.

Discussion

In the present studies, we were able to successfully evaluate the expression levels of inflammatory markers in small airways by using the ultrathin bronchofiberscope. We found that IL-8 and ICAM-1 expression was significantly more increased in small airway epithelium from tobacco smokers than nonsmokers, which are believed to play important roles in the recruitment of inflammatory cells into local sites. There was a positive correlation between the consumption of cigarettes and IL-8 levels, but no correlation between these inflammatory markers and airway obstruction in small airways as assessed by V25. We found that the levels of TGFβ-1 mRNA were significantly increased in small airway epithelium in smokers and COPD patients. The magnitudes of TGFβ-1 signals, corrected by β-actin transcripts, showed a positive correlation with consumption of cigarettes. More importantly, TGFβ-1 gene expression levels correlated with the degrees of peripheral airway obstruction as assessed by the measurements of flow-volume curves.

It is well known that cigarette smoking causes inflammatory responses in small airways [1,2]. These changes include infiltration of inflammatory cells, such as neutrophils, macrophages and mast cells, and thickenings of the airway walls with increased collagen deposition, which is believed to be closely related to the obstruction of the small airways. Local migration of neutrophils may be induced by the direct effects of the contents of tobacco, however, additional data suggest that cigarette smoke stimulates airway epithelial cells to release chemotactic activities for neutrophils such as IL-8 [9]. TGFβ-1 has been hypothesized to be involved in airway remodelling found in chronic airway inflammatory disorders such as COPD and asthma. De Boer et al. [10] studied the expression of TGFβ-1 mRNA and proteins in resected lungs from smokers and COPD cases using immunostaining and in situ hybridization techniques. They showed that semiquantitative histological scores of TGFβ-1 mRNA and protein levels assessed by a visual analogue scoring system were significantly increased in bronchiolar and alveolar epithelium as well as endothelium from these subjects. Our results seem to support the contention that airway epithelium play a role in the tissue remodelling seen in tobacco smokers and those with COPD via expressing TGFβ-1.

In conclusion, we have demonstrated a clear upregulation of IL-8, ICAM-1 and TGFβ-1 mRNA in small airway epithelium from healthy smokers and patients with COPD. It has also been suggested that small airway epithelial cells are active members participating in the processes of airway inflammation and remodelling, and thus, in resultant obstructive changes in the small airways.

References

1. Wright JL, Cagle P, Churg A, Colby TV, Myers T. Diseases of the small airways. Am Rev Respir Dis 1992;146:240–262.
2. Kilburn KH, McKenzis W. Leukocyte recruitment to airways by cigarette smoke and particle phase in contrast to cytotoxicity of vapor. Science 1975;189:634–636.
3. Tanaka M, Satoh M, Kawanami O, Aihara K. A new bronchofiberscope for the study of diseases of very peripheral airways. Chest 1984;85:590–594.
4. Tanaka M, Kawanami O, Satoh M, Yamaguchi K, Okada Y, Yamasawa F. Endoscopic observation of peripheral airway lesions. Chest 1988;93:228–233.
5. Tanaka M, Takizawa H, Satoh M, Okada Y, Yamasawa F, Umeda A. Assessment of an ultrathin bronchoscope which allows cytodiagnosis of small airways. Chest 1994;106:1443–1447.
6. Takizawa H, Desaki M, Ohtoshi T, Kawasaki S, Kohyama T, Sato M, Tanaka M, Kasama T, Kobayashi K, Nakajima J, Ito K. Erythromycin modulates IL-8 expression in human bronchial epithelial cells: Studies with normal and inflamed airway epithelium. Am J Respir Crit Care Med 1997;156:266–271.
7. Jetten AM, Vollberg TM, Nervi C, George MD. Positive and negative regulation of proliferation and differentiation in tracheobronchial epithelial cells. Am Rev Respir Dis 1990;142:S36–S39.
8. Massague J. The transforming growth Factor-β family. Ann Rev Cell Biol 1990;6:597–641.
9. Mio T, Romberger DJ, Thompson AB, Robbins RA, Heires A, Rennard SI. Cigarette smoke induces interleukin-8 release from human bronchial epithelial cells. Am J Respir Crit Care Med 1997;155:1770–1776.
10. De Boer WI, Van Schadewijk A, Sont JK, Sharma HS, Stolk J, Hiemstra PS, Van Krieken JHJM. Transforming growth factor β1 and recruitment of macrophages and mast cells in airways in chronic obstructive pulmonary disease. Am J Respir Crit Care Med 1998;158:1951–1957.

Controversies in stenting

Bronchology and Bronchoesophagology: State of the Art.
H. Yoshimura et al., editors.

Multiple and combination stenting in tracheobronchial stenoses

Teruomi Miyazawa, Yasuo Iwamoto and Yuka Miyazu
Department of Pulmonary Medicine, Hiroshima City Hospital, Hiroshima, Japan

Abstract. During a therapeutic bronchoscopy, in some cases further implantation of the same stent and/or additional implantation of a different stent were needed. As a result, combination stenting procedures have been performed.

At Hiroshima City Hospital between July 1991 and April 2000, multiple and combination stenting (19 Dumon stents including six Dumon Y-stents, 47 Ultraflex stents, one Dynamic stent, and two Covered Wallstents) using a rigid bronchoscope were performed as emergency procedure in 23 patients with life-threatening tracheobronchial obstruction (11 cases of lung cancer, nine of esophageal cancer, one of colon cancer, one of relapsing polychondritis, and one of Von Recklinghausen's disease).

Symptomatic relief of dyspnea was achieved in 87% of the patients. Due to long bilateral stenosis of varying diameters, in one patient seven stents had to be implanted, six stents in one patient, five stents in one patient, four in two, three in one, and two in three.

Combination stenting should be considered in some cases. Certain complicated situations seem to point towards this approach to treatment, e.g., cases of long stenosis, bilateral bronchial stenoses and stenosis with fistula.

Keywords: dumon stents, ultraflex stents.

Background

We mainly use Dumon stents [1,2], but have recently started using Dumon Y-stents. The placement of 30 Dumon Y-stents was performed at our institution and the stents have proven to be safe and effective. Furthermore, in our experience of all the commercially available expandable metallic stents, the Ultraflex nitinol stent looks most promising due to its excellent flexibility and biocompatibility [3]. However, the ideal stent for all cases does not exist. Whilst we have used various stent types, we opted to use the stent best suited in a specific situation. In some cases, further implantation of the same stent and/or additional implantation of a different stent were needed during therapeutic bronchoscopy. Therefore, combination stenting has been quite frequently performed at our institution.

Address for correspondence: Teruomi Miyazawa MD, Department of Pulmonary Medicine, Hiroshima City Hospital 7-33, Moto-machi, Naka-ku, Hiroshima 730-8518, Japan. Tel.: +81-82-221-2291. Fax: +81-82-223-1447. E-mail: ikyoku@city-hosp.naka.hiroshima.jp

Methods

Between July 1991 and May 2000 at Hiroshima City Hospital, various airway stents were implanted in 142 patients with tracheobronchial stenoses: Dumon stents in 90 patients, Ultraflex stents in 30, Gianturco stents in 13, Montgomery T tubes in 10, Dynamic stents in five, and Covered Wallstents in three.

Combination stenting procedures (19 Dumon stents including six Dumon Y-stents, 47 Ultraflex stents, one Dynamic stent and two Covered Wallstents) using a rigid bronchoscope were performed as an emergency procedure in 23 patients with life-threatening tracheobronchial obstruction. The diseases were as follows: 11 cases of lung cancers, nine cases of esophageal cancers, one case of colon cancer, one case of relapsing polychondritis and one case of Von Recklinghausen's disease.

Results

Symptomatic relief of dyspnea was achieved in 87% of the patients. Due to the diffuse narrowing of the airway extending along the trachea into both mainstem bronchi and beyond, in one patient seven stents had to be implanted, six stents in one patient, five stents in one patient, and four in two. Due to long stenosis,

Table 1. Implantation of combination stents of several types for each patient.

Patient No. and diagnosis	Number and type of stents
1. Lung cancer (sq)	2 Dumon + 3 Ultraflex
2. Lung cancer (sq)	2 Ultraflex
3. Lung cancer (sq)	2 Ultraflex
4. Lung cancer (sq)	3 Ultraflex
5. Lung cancer (ad)	1 Dumon Y + 6 Ultraflex
6. Lung cancer (ad)	3 Ultraflex
7. Lung cancer (ad)	1 Wall + 1 Ultraflex
8. Lung cancer (ad)	1 Dumon + 2 Ultraflex
9. Lung cancer (ad)	2 Ultraflex
10. Lung cancer (ad)	2 Ultraflex
11. Lung cancer (ad)	1 Dumon Y + 1 Ultraflex
12. Lung cancer (ad)	1 Dumon + 1 Ultraflex
13. Colon cancer	1 Dumon Y + 1 Dumon
14. Esophageal carcinoma	1 Wall + 4 Ultraflex
15. Esophageal carcinoma	1 Dumon Y + 1 Ultraflex
16. Esophageal carcinoma	2 Ultraflex
17. Esophageal carcinoma (fistula)	2 Dumon + 2 Ultraflex
18. Esophageal carcinoma (fistula)	1 Dumon + 2 Ultraflex
19. Esophageal carcinoma (fistula)	1 Dynamic + 1 Dumon
20. Esophageal carcinoma (fistula)	1 Dumon Y + 1 Dumon
21. Esophageal carcinoma (fistula)	1 Dumon Y + 1 Dumon
22. Relapsing polychondritis	4 Ultraflex
23. Von Recklinghausen's disease	6 Ultraflex

in one patient five stents had to be implanted, three in two, and two in three. Due to bilateral bronchial stenosis, in three patients two stents had to be implanted. Due to stenosis with fistula, in one patient three stents had to be implanted, and two in four (Table 1).

Conclusion

Combination stenting should be considered in some cases. This therapy seems to be appropriate in certain complicated situations, e.g., cases of long stenosis, bilateral bronchial stenoses, and stenosis with fistula.

References

1. Dumon JF, Cavaliere S, Diaz-Jimenez JP et al. Seven-year experience with the Dumon prosthesis. J Bronchol 1996;3:6–10.
2. Miyazawa T, Arita K. Airway stenting in Japan. Respirology 1998;3:229–234.
3. Becker HD. Stenting of the central airways. J Bronchol 1995;2:98–106.

Diagnosis and treatment of early stage central type lung cancer

Bronchology and Bronchoesophagology: State of the Art.
H. Yoshimura et al., editors.

The role of PDT for bronchogenic carcinoma

Tetsuya Okunaka, Kinya Furukawa, Hidemitsu Tsutsui, Jitsuo Usuda, Junichi Nitadori, Yukari Kuroiwa, Chimori Konaka and Harubumi Kato

Department of Surgery, Intractable Disease Research, Tokyo Medical University, Nishishinjuku, Shinjuku-ku, Tokyo, Japan

Abstract. Photodynamic therapy (PDT) utilizing photofrin has proven to be an effective modality that can be used in the treatment of a wide variety of solid tumors and luminal cancers. Over the past decade, 285 patients (338 lesions) with central type lung cancers have been treated in our hospital. Overall, complete remission (CR) was obtained in 50.3% of the 170 lesions, significant remission in 48.9% and no remission was obtained in 0.8%. However, among 149 early-stage lesions CR was obtained in 128 (85.9%), and 48 cases were disease free over 2 to 228 months. We conclude that PDT is efficacious for the advanced bronchogenic carcinoma combined with surgery, as well as in the treatment of superficial lung cancer where complete remission may be achieved.

Keywords: excimer dye laser, lung cancer, photodynamic therapy.

Introduction

Photodynamic therapy (PDT) is a new cancer treatment modality that selectively destroys cancer cells by means of an interaction between absorbed light and a retained photosensitizer. The authors began the investigation of these techniques in collaboration with Dougherty (1978) and demonstrated their effectiveness in both diagnosis and treatment in canine lung cancer models, and applied these methods in clinical cases in 1980 [1,2]. Since then, 420 cases, including 285 lung cancer patients (338 lesions), have been treated with PDT in our institution. There were several cases of 5-year survival, including the first such case in the world treated by PDT alone [3]. In this paper, our experience of PDT, especially in terms of early-stage lung cancer, will be discussed.

Methods

Bronchoscopical PDT was performed with topical anesthesia approximately 48 h after the intravenous injection of 2.0 mg/kg body weight of Photofrin [4]. After the injection of Photofrin, the patients were instructed to avoid direct sunlight for at least 2 weeks. The laser beam (630 nm wavelength) was transmitted via a quartz fiber (400 mm) inserted through the instrumentation channel of a fiber-

Address for correspondence: Tetsuya Okunaka, Department of Surgery, Intractable Disease Research, Tokyo Medical University, 6-7-1 Nishishinjuku, Shinjuku-ku, Tokyo 160-0023, Japan. Tel.: +81-3-3342-6111. Fax: +81-3-3349-0326. E-mail: okunaka@tokyo-med.ac.jp optic bronchoscope. The fiber tip, 1 to 2 cm from a perpendicular target, yields a circular area of illumination of 4 to 8 mm^2. The power output at the fiber tip was adjusted to 100 to 400 mW/cm^2 in cases using the argon dye laser. Using the excimer dye laser, the frequency was 30 Hz and the energy was adjusted to 4 mJ/pulse. For surface irradiation of early-stage lung cancer, illumination time generally ranged from 10 to 40 min giving energy densities of 100 to 800 J/cm^2. However, in advanced obstructing lung cancer, interstitial irradiation is performed with the fiber tips inserted into the tissue [5]. After PDT procedure, bronchial toilet should be performed every 2 or 3 days for 1 week. The effectiveness of PDT was evaluated both bronchoscopically and histologically 2 to 4 weeks after the PDT. In preoperative PDT cases, the operation would be performed 2 to 9 weeks after the PDT.

Results

The total number of cases was 113, consisting of 149 lesions, with an age distribution ranging from 37- to 82-years-old. There were 111 males and 2 females. Histologically, all the cases were squamous cell carcinoma except for one case of adenocarcinoma. All patients were required to have histopathologically and cytologically proven superficial cancer of the lung. Each patient had a bidimensionally measurable lesion. Informed consent was obtained from all patients or their relatives. Reasons why PDT was conducted in the enrolled patients were the refusal of surgery, inoperability because of poor organic functions, serious concomitant disease, advanced age or the possibility of cure by this modality.

One month after treatment, the tumor response to PDT was evaluated endoscopically, roentgenographically, cytologically, and histologically. In surgically resected or autopsied cases, the treated areas were examined endoscopically and histologically.

Complete remission was obtained in 98 cases (128 lesions, 85.9%) out of 113 cases (149 lesions) and partial remission in 21 lesions. Surgical resection was undergone in 15 cases, and radiotherapy or some other modality was in four. Recurrence was recognized in a total of 19 cases (12.7%) which were then treated by surgery or PDT again.

The therapeutic effectiveness of PDT was analyzed according to both the longitudinal tumor size and the visibility of the distal tumor margin. The univariate analysis was based on 2×2 tables and differences were tested by the χ^2test. Of the 112 cancer lesions that had a longitudinal tumor extent of 1 cm or less, 105 (93.8%) obtained a CR after initial PDT, however, of the 37 carcinomas that had a longitudinal tumor extent of greater that 1 cm, 23 (62.2%) showed CR after PDT. There was a statistically very significant difference between the two groups ($p = 0.00001$). Of the 118 carcinomas with a clearly visible distal tumor margin, 110 (93.2%) had a CR after initial PDT. Of the 31 carcinomas without a clearly visible distal tumor margin, 18 (58.1%) had a CR after PDT. However, distal margin visibility was not significantly related to CR ($p = 0.09$).

Survival was calculated on the basis of the period from the start of treatment to death or last follow-up. The survival curve was calculated using the Kaplan and Meier method. The overall survival rate for the 82 patients was 57.6%.

Discussion

In the field of endobronchial malignancy, over 500 patients have been treated with PDT. The results of various investigations are remarkably consistent, with CR + PR rates ranging from 70% to 100% [4]. The best results were obtained with mucosal tumors or early (stage 0) lung cancers. Our data also suggest that PDT provides an alternative to surgical resection as the primary treatment of patients with early-stage central type lung cancer [6,7]. The overall CR rate for early superficial lesions was 66.7% (108/162), which indicates that PDT may be good substitution for surgery in these type of cases [5]. From our therapeutic results, we consider the indications for successful use of PDT in early stage lung cancer to be as follows: 1) the entire lesion should be visible endoscopically; 2) the tumor should be in a location where the laser beam can be delivered easily and sufficiently; 3) the lesion should be superficial and 1 cm or less in its greatest dimension; 4) the histological type should be squamous cell carcinoma; and 5) there should be no lymph node involvement.

We studied lung cancer cases, including early-stage cases, which did not show complete remission by examining them histologically on the basis of resected specimens. Complete remission was not obtained in lesions which were anatomically difficult to photoirradiate or in those located submucosally if photoradiation from an angle of 90° to the surface of the lesion was impossible, nor was it achieved in lesions located beyond the cartilage or in extensive lesions. To solve these problems, PDT using cylindrical quartz fibers with 360° delivery using increased laser power is recommended.

References

1. Dougherty TJ, Laurence G, Kaufman JH et al. A photoradiation in the treatment of recurrent breast carcinoma. J Natl Cancer Inst 1979;62:231–237.
2. Hayata Y, Kato H, Konaka C et al. Hematoporphyrin derivative and laser photoradiation in the treatment of lung cancer. Chest 1982;81:269–277.
3. Kato H, Konaka C, Ono J et al. Five-year disease-free survival of a lung cancer patient treated only by photodynamic therapy. Chest 1986;90:768–770.
4. Marcus SL, Dugan M. Global status of clinical photodynamic therapy: the registration process for a new therapy. Lasers Surg Med 1992;12:318-324.
5. Kato H, Okunaka T. Photodynamic therapy in early tumors. In: Hetzel M (eds) Minimally Invasive Techniques in Thoracic Medicine and Surgery. London: Chapman and Hall Medical, 1995;149–172.
6. Furuse K, Fukuoka M, Kato H et al. A prospective phase II study on photodynamic therapy with Photofrin II for centrally located early stage lung cancer. J Clin Oncol 1993;11:1852–1857.
7. Kato H, Horai T, Furuse K et al. Photodynamic therapy for cancers: a clinical trial of Porfimer sodium in Japan. Jpn J Cancer Res 1993;84:1209–1214.

Bronchology and Bronchoesophagology: State of the Art.
H. Yoshimura et al., editors.

Is brachytherapy for early-stage hilar cancers cost-effective?

G. Sutedja
Department of Pulmonology, Free University Academic Hospital, Amsterdam, The Netherlands

Abstract. Although endobronchial brachytherapy has been shown to be effective in treating early-stage hilar cancers in phase II studies, the relatively expensive facility, more complex logistics, the necessity of repeated fractions, radiation fibrosis because of nonselective damage, and the important fact that response rate of treating early-stage cancer is more related to tumor stage rather than treatment techniques, may lead brachytherapy to be less cost-effective than other, more competitive intraluminal treatment modalities such as cryotherapy and electrocautery.

Keywords: brachytherapy, cost-effectiveness, early-stage hilar cancer.

Introduction

Endobronchial brachytherapy is the use of tiny radioactive seeds to irradiate tumors in hollow organs using a catheter [1]. This afterloading technique makes local intraluminal irradiation less hazardous for health care personnel. Bronchoscopically, a catheter has to be accurately positioned in the target area, inside the tracheobronchial tree where the tumor is located. Transnasal positioning of the catheter is more secure for its fixation during treatment. After confirmation of the catheter's position with chest X-rays, dosimetry can be calculated and the dwell time and position of the radioactive seed preprogrammed. Remote control and an automatic stepper device motor are used to transport the radioactive seed into the catheter. The session can be started after fixing the catheter at the nasal orifice and connecting its proximal end to the remote afterloading device. High dose rate brachytherapy has been the most popular method, because treatment duration is ±10 min. Usually ±10 Gy is given at 1 cm from the source axis. In patients with a small intraluminal tumor, endobronchial ultrasound (EBUS) has been used to assess the tumor thickness [2]. This may allow more accurate assessment of tumor infiltration in the bronchial wall and enable more accurate dosimetric calculation.

In practice, several fractions are needed to minimize damage to normal tissue, e.g., radiation bronchitis and fibrosis [3]. Treatment requires several sessions, while the effect is clearly nonimmediate if compared to tissue damage caused by thermal lasers or electrocautery [4]. As brachytherapy is performed under local anesthesia, coughing and spontaneous breathing during the session may ulti-

Address for correspondence: Dr G. Sutedja MD, PhD, FCCP, Department of Pulmonology, Free University Academic Hospital, P.O. Box 7057, 1007 MB, Amsterdam, The Netherlands. Tel.: +31-20-444-4444. Fax: +31-20-444-4328. E-mail: tg.sutedja@azvu.nl mately affect the dosimetry. The bronchoscopist, however, is hampered by the afterloading principle. Thus, correction during treatment to accurately target tumor tissue is not possible. The multidisciplinary approach requires support from the radiation oncologist and laboratory technician in a specialized unit with radiation facility. Therefore, brachytherapy is relatively expensive and requires more cumbersome logistics when compared to some bronchoscopic modalities which can be performed in the standard endoscopy room. All these factors have to be taken into account in analyzing its cost-effectiveness.

Brachytherapy with curative intent

Of all the prognostic factors for non-small cell lung cancer, by far the most important one is the size of the primary tumor. To detect and treat lung cancer at the earliest stage is a valid approach and will be rewarding because of the improved outcome. Early detection of roentgenographicallly occult lung cancer (ROLC) is difficult [6,7]. But the cure rate of ROLC is in the range of 80–100%. One of the advantages of diagnosing ROLC at the earliest stage is the availability of several therapeutic options, even for patients with severe chronic obstructive pulmonary disease (COPD) [8], cardiac problems, or after previous resections. Bronchoscopic treatment with curative intent may provide an alternative to surgical resection [9]. Whether any bronchoscopic treatment will result in cure strongly depends on tumor size and the degree of tumor infiltration in the bronchial wall. The prime importance of tumor size and its relation to nodal disease cannot be overstated, and surgical data have supported this important oncological concept [10–12]. This concept has to be taken seriously when dealing with early-stage hilar cancer. We reported that high resolution computed tomography may be of value in helping to classify patients with ROLC [13]. Autofluorescence bronchoscopy (AFB) seems to improve the accuracy of staging even more, and the role of endobronchial ultrasonography is currently being explored [14–16].

Photodynamic therapy (PDT) has been the focus of attention for treating early-stage lung cancer [17]. As well as PDT and brachytherapy, laser and electrocautery are also potentially curative. Details of the many studies in this area, primarily in treating microinvasive squamous cell cancers, have been reviewed in detail [5]. There is a lack of consensus about brachytherapy as regards total dose, fractions, and margins of the target volume required, in treating ROLC with curative intent.

The curative potential of any intraluminal therapy is obvious, because microinvasive tumor and carcinoma in situ appear to consist of malignant cells of several layers thick only [18]. The ability to treat tumors in depth is therefore not the only argument to justify the use of brachytherapy or PDT for ROLC. Intraluminal tumors >3 mm deep and >1 cm^2 are not suitable for any intraluminal approach with curative intent, be it brachytherapy, PDT or electrocautery [5,9–12]. Especially when treating ROLC bronchoscopically as an alternative for surgical resection, one has to keep in mind the inaccuracy of staging [5,13]. It is likely that the relatively expensive facility, more complex logistics, the necessity of repeated fractions, radiation fibrosis because of nonselective damage, and the important fact that response rate of treating early-stage cancer is more related to tumor stage rather than techniques, may prevent brachytherapy from being a cost-effective procedure [5]. If ROLC is accurately staged, repetitive treatments are indeed more expensive, cumbersome and causing more morbidity to the patients than a single approach, e.g., extensive biopsy or electrocautery [19]. Further clinical studies in treating early-stage lung cancer are warranted due to the magnitude of the problem and the resurgence of interest in sputum cytology screening. We are now in the comfortable position of being able to treat intraluminal tumors at the earliest stage possible with any kind of bronchoscopic treatment modality, provided that accurate staging is possible. Tailoring our diagnostic and treatment ability to each individual patient in this screening era is most likely to be pursued in interventional bronchology.

References

1. Villanueva AG, Lo TC, Beamis JF. Endobrochial brachytherapy. Clinics Chest Med 1995;16: 445–454.
2. Ono R, Hirano H, Egawa S et al. Bronchoscopic ultrasonography and brachytherapy in roentgenologically occult bronchogenic carcinoma. J Bronchol 1994;1:281–287.
3. Speiser BL, Spratling L. Radiation bronchitis and stenosis secondary to high dose rate endobronchial irradiation. Int J Radiat Oncol Biol Physics 1993;25:589–597.
4. Sutedja G, Postmus PE. Review article. Bronchoscopic treatment of lung tumours. Lung Cancer 1994;11:1–17.
5. van Boxem TJ, Venmans BJ, Postmus PE, Sutedja G. Curative endobronchial therapy in early-stage non-small cell lung cancer. Rev J Bronchol 1999;6:198–206.
6. Kato H, Horai T. A colour atlas of endoscopic diagnosis in early-stage lung cancer. Aylesbury, England: Wolfe, 1992;35.
7. Sato M, Saito Y, Usuda K, Takahashi S, Sagawa M, Fujimura S. Occult lung cancer beyond bronchoscopic visibility in sputum cytology positive patients. Lung Cancer 1998;20:17–24.
8. Petty TL. Lung cancer and chronic obstructive pulmonary disease. Med Clin N Am 1996;80: 645–655.
9. Edell ES, Cortese DA. Photodynamic therapy in the management of early superficial squamous cell carcinoma as an alternative to surgical resection. Chest 1992;102:1319–1322.
10. Woolner LB, Fontana RS, Cortese DA. Roentgenographically occult lung cancer: pathologic findings and frequency of multicentricity during a 10-year period. Mayo Clin Proc 1984;59: 453–466.
11. Usuda K, Saito Y, Nagamoto N, Sato M, Sagawa M, Kanma K, Takahashi S, Endo C, Fujimura S. Relation between bronchoscopic findings and tumor size of roentgenographically occult bronchogenic squamous cell carcinoma. J Thorac Cardiovasc Surg 1993;106:1098–1103.
12. Nagamoto N, Saito Y, Ohta S, Sato M, Kanma K, Sagawa M, Takahashi S, Usuda K, Nakada T, Hashimoto K. Relationship of lymph node metastasis to primary tumor size and microscopic appearance of roentgenographically occult lung cancer. Am J Surg Pathol 1989;13:1009–1013.
13. Sutedja G, Golding RP, Postmus PE. High resolution computed tomography in patients referred for intraluminal bronchoscopic therapy with curative intent. Eur Respir J 1996;9:1020–1023.
14. Hung J, Lam S, LeRiche JC, Palcic B. Autofluorescence of normal and malignant bronchial tis-

sue. Lasers Surg Med 1991;11:99–105.

15. Lam S, MacAulay C, Hung J, LeRiche JC, Profio AE, Palcic B. Detection of dysplasia and carcinoma in situ with a lung imaging fluorescence endoscopy device. J Thorac Cardiovasc Surg 1993;105:1035–1040.
16. Kurimoto N, Murayama M, Yoshioka S, Nishisaka T, Inai K, Dohi K. Assessment of usefulness of endobronchial ultrasonography in determination of depth of tracheobronchial tumor invasion. Chest 1999;115:1500–1506.
17. Hayata Y, Kato H, Furuse K, Kusunoki Y, Suzuki S, Mimura S. Photodynamic therapy of 169 early-stage cancers of the lung and oesophagus: a Japanese multicentre study. Lasers Med Sci 1996;11:255–259.
18. Auerbach O, Stout AP, Hammond C, Garfinkel L. Changes in bronchial epithelium in relation to cigarette smoking and in relation to lung cancer. N Engl J Med 1961:265:253–268.
19. van Boxem TJ, Venmans BJ, Schramel FM, Mourik JC van, Golding RP, Postmus PE, Sutedja G. Radiographically occult lung cancer treated with fiberoptic bronchoscopic electrocautery: a pilot study of a simple and inexpensive technique. Eur Resp J 1998;11:169–172.

Bronchology and Bronchoesophagology: State of the Art.
H. Yoshimura et al., editors.

Optimizing autofluorescence bronchoscopy

Hubert van den Bergh
Institute of Environmental Engineering, Swiss Federal Institute of Technology, Lausanne, Switzerland

Abstract. Dual wavelength autofluorescence (AF) imaging bronchoscopy is optimized by studying the AF excitation-emission matrix over a wide spectral range. This study was carried out under endoscopic conditions in patients with various stages of malignancy as proven by biopsy. The results show major AF spectral differences between 1) healthy bronchial mucosa; 2) metaplasia or inflammation; and 3) dysplasia or carcinoma in situ. The optimal AF excitation wavelength at the applied conditions was found to be near 410 nm. It is suggested that red backscattered light may be a better reference for the disease-related decrease in green AF intensity than the red fluorescence itself. An imaging AF bronchoscope was constructed based on these findings which was tested on 50 patients. The AF results appear to be superior to those obtained by white light bronchoscopy. The combined use of both techniques leads to a much improved positive predictive value for the identification of early-stage central lung squamous cell malignancy as compared to each technique used by itself.

Introduction

Lung cancer is the most common cause of cancer-induced death worldwide, and may well remain so for many decades to come. The poor prognosis of this disease tends to be related to clinical presentation/diagnosis at a late stage of its development. Hence, there is a need for detecting lung cancer at much earlier stages, when treatment has a higher probability of being curative.

Autofluorescence bronchoscopy [1] is probably too expensive for the screening of early disease in all but the highest risk groups. Thus, it would seem reasonable to apply it, for instance, in patients who have undergone a lobectomy for invasive central lung cancer or who have had an invasive squamous cell carcinoma in the head and neck region. For the much larger group of heavy smokers ($\geqslant$ 30 pack years), the chance of finding a carcinoma in situ (CIS) or high grade dysplasia is sufficiently small so that the cost of using AF bronchoscopy as a screening/localization device would be generally unacceptable. Thus, large volume application of AF bronchoscopy will depend on the appearance of a cheap effective screening procedure for early-stage disease. Several approaches for this are currently under investigation.

Other reasons for developing an effective autofluorescence bronchoscope include using it in 1) the evaluation of new sputum tests; 2) in chemoprevention trials; and 3) in research into the pathogenesis of lung cancer. Thus, the primary

Address for correspondence: H.E. van den Bergh, Institute of Environmental Engineering, Swiss Federal Institute of Technology, EPFL-DGR/LPAS-1015 Lausanne, Switzerland. Tel.: +41-21-6933620. Fax: +41-21-6933626.

objective of the present study was to define optimal spectral conditions to detect precancerous and early cancerous lesions with a bronchoscope which images the tissue autofluorescence. This implies optimizing the sensitivity and specificity of the AF bronchoscopy until they are significantly higher than is the case in the "golden" standard white light reflectance bronchoscopy. If in the first instance we cannot attain this goal, using AF bronchoscopy as a stand-alone technique, it should at least be useful in complementing existing technology. Hence, we will search for the best AF-excitation wavelength, and the best AF-detection spectral domains, and use this information to design an AF-bronchoscope. Whereas two-wavelength fluorescence endoscopy was to a large extent pioneered by Profio et al., the early accents on the use of autofluorescence came mostly from Palcic and Lam et al. Most of the historical and instrumental aspects of these developments have been reviewed recently by Wagnières et al. [2].

Materials and Methods

50 patients were involved in this study, and 3578 AF emission spectra were measured at 82 sites. 47 of these sites were identified by biopsy as being healthy, 25 were identified as either inflammatory tissue or metaplasia, and 10 sites were identified as dysplasia or CIS. Ten spectra were taken per site for each excitation wavelength. The latter ranged from 350 to 495 nm in steps of 15 nm. The tissue samples were classified by a histopathologist and divided into 3 classes:

1. Normal mucosa (i.e., tissue without inflammation or metaplasia or hyperplasia) was classed as "HEALTHY".
2. Inflammation, metaplasia or hyperplasia was classed as "INFL./MET.".
3. Mild, moderate and severe dysplasia, as well as carcinoma in situ were classed as "DYS./CIS".

An optical fiber based spectrofluorometer [3] consists of a Xenon lamp and a monochromator for the excitation light, a special fiber bundle for transmitting the excitation light through the endoscope to the tissue, as well as the AF light from the tissue to the detector, and a detection system consisting of a spectrograph, a cooled CCD detector and a PC. The fiber bundle was passed through the biopsy channel of a flexible bronchoscope which was fitted at its distal end with a 3.5 mm spacer. The latter was used to ensure that all AF spectra were taken, with the fiber bundle tip at 3.5 mm, from the mucosa surface. This distance is important as it influences the spectral distortion, and it represents an approximate "average" observation distance in bronchoscopy.

Results and Discussion

Figure 1 represents the average autofluorescence emission spectra [4] of the human respiratory mucous membrane, measured mostly in the trachea (carena), the main bronchus, truncus intermedius, and the upper, middle and lower lobe bronchus [5]. It may be essential to specify this as the optical properties will

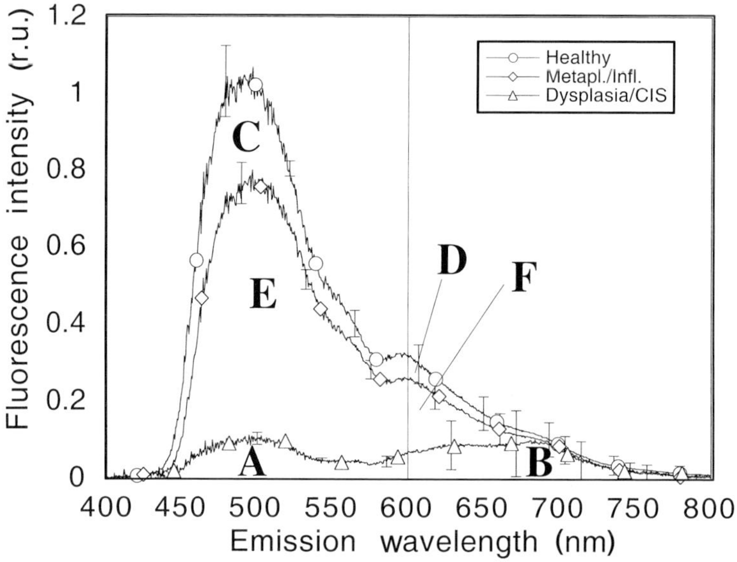

Fig. 1. Average AF emission spectra of the upper part of the tracheobronchial tree.

change when moving in the bronchopulmonary tree from the trachea via the segmental and subsegmental bronchus towards the alveoli [5]. The excitation wavelength was 405 nm. One should note the large reduction in "green" AF between 450 and 600 nm of about one order of magnitude between healthy (area C) and dysplastic tissue/CIS (area A). It is this nature-given factor of 10 difference between normal and neoplastic tissue that makes AF imaging so attractive. In the "red" AF spectra, between 600 and 700 nm, this decrease (area D as compared to area B) is much smaller. Also, note that the intermediate curve which corresponds to metaplasia/inflammatory tissue is quite close to the healthy tissue, which should in principle lead to a small number of false positives.

In the apparatus one measures C/A, i.e., (Healthy/Dysplasia or CIS) which is related to the sensitivity and E/A (metaplasia or inflammatory tissue/Dysplasia or CIS) which is related to specificity. These ratios must be corrected for the topography, i.e., the distance between the distal end of the endoscope and the fluorescing surface. This was at first done by dividing by the corresponding "red" AF, i.e., $\frac{C/A}{D/B}$ is the "sensitivity" corrected for distance, whereas $\frac{E/A}{F/B}$ is the "specificity" corrected for distance. As the surfaces D, F and B tend to be small, one may gain by using the reflected red light from the Xenon lamp source as a reference as there is more of this light, i.e., bigger signals. Also, the reflected red light does not show the small decrease in intensity that is typical of the red fluorescence (D/B) which partially reduces the contrast C/A in the distance-corrected $\frac{C/A}{D/B}$ quasi sensitivity. Furthermore, the use of crossed polarization between incident and returning light can be of interest both for the reflected light (limitation of specular reflectance) and the fluorescence. In future versions of such endoscopes, one may also want to use white light composed of multiple diode, multiple wavelengths, sources in order to be able to reduce the endoscope diameter.

The next problem was where optimally to chose the wavelength of the dichroic, i.e., where to separate between "red AF" and "green AF". Figure 2 shows the AF spectra of Fig. 1 normalized at the green maximum near 500 nm [4]. The difference spectrum between the normalized healthy and dysplasia/CIS is also shown with a maximum around 690 nm. Somewhat arbitrarily we now choose the position of the dichroic at half the peak height of the difference spectrum, i.e., near 600 nm to get an essentially optimal "specificity", "sensitivity" and light intensity compromise. When carrying out this procedure at many excitation wavelengths between 350 and 495 nm, we find that interestingly the optimal beam splitter separation wavelength, both for "sensitivity" and "specificity" is between 595 and 600 nm. This is shown in Fig. 3 [4]. It should be noted that without measurement of "negatives" these sensitivity and specificity values do not correspond directly to the real sensitivity and specificity.

Finally, Fig. 4 summarizes the values of

$$R = \frac{nomal\ tissue\ green\ AF/tumoral\ green\ AF}{normal\ red\ AF/tumoral\ red\ AF}$$

for different excitation wavelengths of the human respiratory mucous membrane in the upper part of the tracheobronchial tree as defined above [4]. It shows that optimal excitation is near 405 nm for the apparatus used, and that UV light contributes nothing positive toward R. The wavelengths above 410 nm are used in

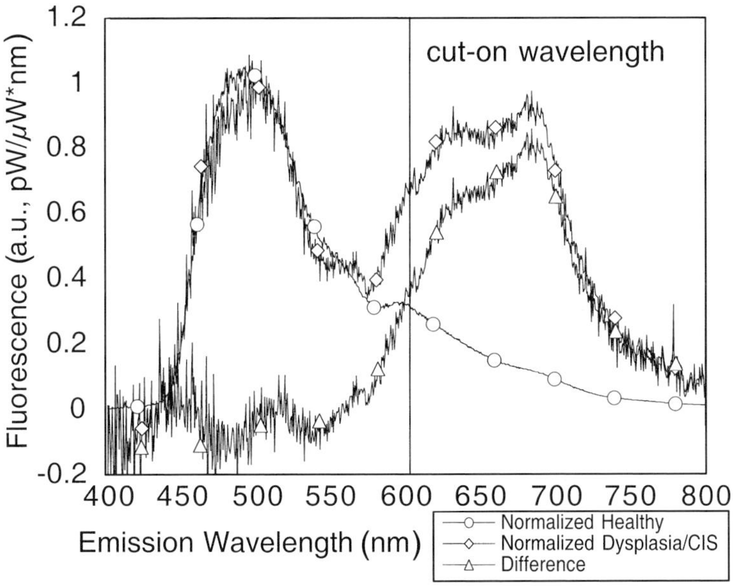

Fig. 2. Average AF emission spectra normalized at 500 nm and subtracted.

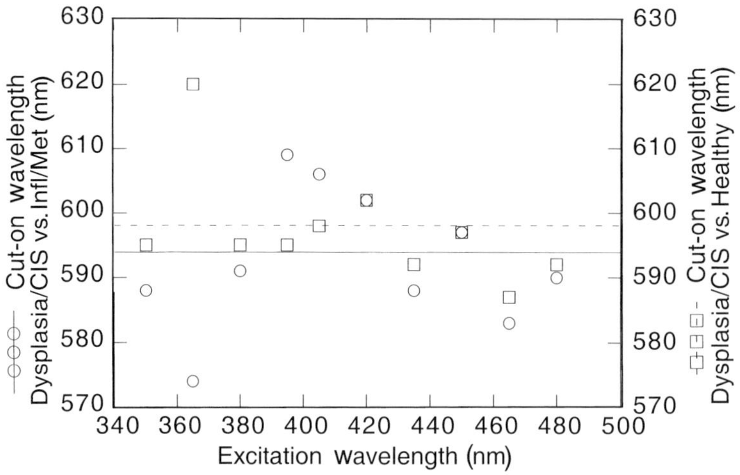

Fig. 3. Cut-on wavelength of the dichroic as a function of the AF excitation wavelength, as optimized for quasisensitivity and specificity.

order to acquire enough signal in the allotted time under the applied conditions.

Based on the results presented above, an AF imaging fluorescence bronchoscope was constructed which demonstrated, in a very preliminary investigation on 15 patients with 20 biopsies taken, that 1) the sensitivity of AF bronchoscopy

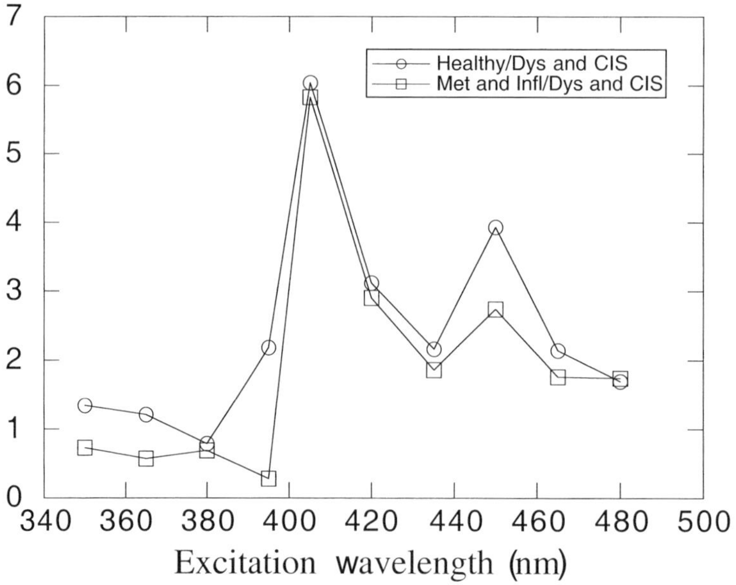

Fig. 4. The ratio R = (normal green/tumor green)/(normal red/tumor red) measured at different AF excitation wavelength.

was larger than that of white light bronchoscopy; and 2) that the positive predictive value defined as the ratio between true positives and the sum of true positives and false positives was larger for AF (75%) than for white light bronchoscopy (38%) [4]. It should of course be noted that in both types of endoscopy as well as in the histopathological analysis, there is room for observational error, and individual learning curves are hard to assess quantitatively at this point in time.

Conclusions

1. The excitation wavelength yielding the highest sensitivity and specificity is above 400 nm with a peak value near 405 nm.
2. The shapes of the AF spectra taken on healthy, inflammatory and metaplastic bronchial tissues are similar, so that the latter two conditions should to a large extent not generate false positives.
3. When the AF spectra are normalized at the maximum near 500 nm, the region of divergence between the tumor and normal tissue AF spectra is consistently situated above 600 nm.
4. The optimum transition wavelength between the green and red AF spectral regions is between 595 and 600 nm, independent of the excitation wavelength, under the applied conditions (excitation wavelength between 350 to 495 nm). This may hint at the fact that mainly one fluorochrome is responsible for the spectral shape changes. One might suggest that this is hemoglobin in the lamina propria.
5. In a more final form of this apparatus, a mathematical evaluation or other supplementary spectral analysis of the suspect area may lead to a true optical biopsy, i.e., a noninvasive staging of the tumor development.
6. The positive predictive value for the small sample of tumor dection endoscopies could be raised significantly (from 38% to 100%) by combining classical white light bronchoscopy with AF bronchoscopy.

Acknowledgements

The author acknowledges the contributions of M. Zellweger who did his PhD thesis on this subject. The other persons who have contributed significantly were D. Goujon, G. Wagnières, Ph. Monnier, and P. Grosjean. The latter were both at the ENT clinic of the CHUV Hospital in Lausanne.

References

1. Fujisawa T. Autofluorescence Bronchoscopy: Principles and Clinical Applications. Tokyo: Kanehara and Co., 1999.
2. Wagnières GA, Star WM, Wilson BC. In vivo fluorescence spectroscopy and imaging for oncological applications. Photochem Photobiol 1998;68:603–632.
3. Forrer M, Glanzmann T, Braichotte D et al. In vivo measurement of fluorescence bleaching of mTHPC in the esophagus and the oral cavity. Proc SPIE, 1995;2627:33–39.

4. Zellweger M, Goujon D, Monnier P, van den Bergh H, Wagnières G. In vivo autofluorescence spectroscopy of human bronchial tissue to optimize the detection and imaging of early cancers. Accepted for publication in J Biomed Optics.
5. Classification of lung cancer. The Japan Lung Cancer Society, 1st English edn. Tokyo: Kanehara and Co. Ltd, 2000.

Diagnosis and treatment of peripheral lesions and solitary pulmonary nodules

Bronchology and Bronchoesophagology: State of the Art.
H. Yoshimura et al., editors.

Transbronchial approaches for the diagnosis and treatment of small peripheral pulmonary lesions

Toshiaki Kobayashi
Endoscopy Division, National Cancer Center Hospital, Tokyo, Japan

Abstract. Patients with small peripheral lung cancers, which are mainly detected by computed tomography (CT) are deemed to survive longer and have better chances of cure when given standard treatment, i.e., lobectomy with lymph node dissection. CT detection of such small lesions is relatively easy. However, establishing a definitive diagnosis for indeterminate small peripheral lesions is difficult and often requires more invasive diagnostic procedures such as surgical resection.

While surgical resection of lung cancer can indeed offer the most reliable prognosis, it can be considered too invasive an approach for smaller lung cancers, particularly in elderly individuals. Managing these lesions with traditional bronchoscopy is difficult. However, combining CT with bronchoscopy offers new diagnostic and therapeutic options. We have studied the application of CT to bronchoscopy using a high-resolution spiral CT system with CT fluoroscopy that provides near real-time image visualization and is additionally equipped with a standard X-ray fluoroscopy system.

CT-guided bronchoscopic biopsy of small lesions allows definitive diagnosis of even fluoroscopically invisible lesions with high diagnostic accuracy and with few complications. In addition, the procedure has a high negative predictive value. It can preclude unnecessary and invasive surgical resections in patients with true benign lesions. To facilitate video-assisted thoracic surgery (VATS) resection of minute peripheral pulmonary lesions, a radio opaque marker (0.1–1.0 ml barium sulfate suspension) can be placed using the CT-guided bronchoscopy technique. This permits more accurate and less invasive VATS resection. CT-guided bronchoscopy also allows the performance of brachytherapy to small peripheral malignancies. As such, treatment becomes possible for patients who cannot tolerate even VATS.

The introduction of CT has extended the utility of bronchoscopy from mere diagnosis to actual treatment of small peripheral pulmonary lesions.

Introduction

Despite recent improvements in the treatment of lung cancer, patient survival

Address for correspondence: Endoscopy Division, National Cancer Center Hospital, 5-1-1 Tsukiji, Chuo-ku, Tokyo 104-0045, Japan. Tel.: +81-3-3542-2511. Fax: +81-3-3542-3815.

rates are not satisfactory, particularly in stages IIIA, IIIB, and IV disease. Earlier detection would seem to be one solution, however, several randomized controlled studies have failed to prove efficacy of screening using sputum cytology and chest radiography [1–4]. In addition, the 5-year survival rate of even stage I patients is approximately 70% or less which is not satisfactory [5], and new strategies to improve survival of lung cancer patients must be investigated.

When very early lung cancer detection occurs, a better survival rate is naturally expected as earlier treatment can begin. This situation is facilitated by the use of computed tomography (CT) which can be used for various purposes such as diagnosis of diffuse pulmonary diseases, detection of metastasis from other primary sites, and screening for lung cancer. CT in lung cancer screening yields a detection rate close to 0.5% of all subjects screened, and approximately 90% of cases detected by CT were in stage I [6,7].

There are various diagnostic options for these indeterminate peripheral pulmonary lesions including high-resolution CT which is the most common method of examinations in institutions in which the equipment is available. High-resolution CT has relatively good diagnostic accuracy particularly in typical well-differentiated adenocarcinoma cases, however, it yields poorer results with squamous cell carcinoma, small cell carcinoma, and poorly differentiated adenocarcinoma. In addition, image diagnosis cannot provide a definitive diagnosis. Therefore, highly accurate definitive diagnostic methods are required for these lesions.

Fluoroscopy-guided bronchoscopy is a standard approach to diagnosis of peripheral pulmonary lesions, however, small lesions are difficult [8–13] and fluoroscopically invisible lesions are almost impossible to diagnose. Transthoracic approaches under fluoroscopy and CT guidance are indicated in these lesions and have yielded good results [14–20]. Another option is video-assisted thoracic surgery (VATS) which has a diagnostic accuracy of close to 100% when lesions are properly resected [21–24]. When lesions are too small to be visualized through thoracoscopes and fluoroscopes, markers can be placed to show the lesion sites [25,26].

Although the transthoracic approaches have good diagnostic accuracy, they carry risks of complications such as pneumothorax and hemorrhage [16–20,27–29]. Pneumothorax is not a severe complication, however, the discomfort of a chest tube cannot be ignored. Hemorrhage is not usually severe, however, it sometimes can be fatal. In addition, implantation of malignant cells [30–33] and air-embolism [34] are rare, however, they can be catastrophic if they happen.

Patients with earlier lung cancers are considered to be cured or to survive longer following the standard treatment which at present is surgical resection. In particular, the 5-year survival of some lung cancer patients with certain histologic characteristics is close to 100% [35]. Considering the nature of minute and earlier peripheral lung cancers, diagnostic methods should be as minimally invasive as possible. In addition, even less invasive treatments might have to be applied in certain patients considering lung cancer characteristics as well as patient conditions such as advanced age and poor pulmonary function.

Bronchoscopic examination is considered to be a standard approach to the diagnosis of peripheral pulmonary diseases despite its difficulty in accessing lesions. This is attributed to the fact that it is a less complicated procedure and allows examinations to be performed even in an outpatient setting. If these small peripheral pulmonary lesions can be accessed transbronchially, bronchoscopy would be a standard approach even for these lesions. In addition, small, early lesions may be responsive to bronchoscopic treatments.

Because detection or confirmation of the existence of these lesions is done by CT, CT guidance is naturally expected to be applied even to bronchoscopy. Consequently, CT-guided bronchoscopy for small peripheral pulmonary lesions was developed [36]. CT-guided bronchoscopic techniques used at present are CT-guided bronchoscopic biopsy [36,37], CT-guided bronchoscopic barium marking for VATS [38], and CT-assisted transbronchial brachytherapy for small peripheral pulmonary malignancies [39].

CT-guided bronchoscopic biopsy

CT-guided bronchoscopic biopsy was initially applied to fluoroscopically invisible peripheral pulmonary lesions such as minute lesions, indistinct lesions, and those concealed by anatomical structures. Subsequently, the indications were extended to include fluoroscopically visible lesions 2 cm or less, as decided by the Ministry of Health and Welfare at the time of authorization of the technique as a highly advanced medical treatment. Because this category of medical treatment is not covered by national health insurance in Japan, the examination was mostly carried out in patients in whom extremely reliable diagnosis was required, yet in whom complications had to be avoided as much as possible.

The situations in which extremely reliable diagnoses were required were encountered in patients in whom diagnostic or therapeutic procedures would be highly invasive, considering their physical condition such as poor pulmonary function and minute lesions which would require lobectomy for definitive diagnosis. In addition, extremely reliable diagnosis was also required to avoid unnecessary surgical procedures for lesions in which nonmalignant diagnosis was strongly suspected. Representative complications which were avoided by applying CT-guided bronchoscopic biopsy were pneumothorax in lesions on or close to the pleura, and hemorrhage in lesions near larger blood vessels. These situations were extremely significant in patients with a poor physical condition.

The CT systems used are equipped with a CT-fluoroscopy mode which allows near real-time image visualization by reconstructing six images per second with a 0.67 s delay. In the first five cases, CT alone was used to guide the sampling instruments. In the following cases, a CT system with a c-arm fluoroscope system placed adjacent to the CT system was used. The present CT system is coupled to a biplane fluoroscope system which was specially designed for bronchoscopy equipped in a bronchoscopy room. Both CT and fluoroscopy systems have one table for patients which allows an easier transfer of the patients between CT and fluoroscopy systems.

We preferred thin video-bronchoscopes which have a 5.3 mm distal tip diameter and a 2.0 mm working channel, because video-bronchoscopes allow increased control since the examiner does not have to look into an eyepiece. Ultra-thin bronchoscopes were used only occasionally in the initial period, because of problems of maneuverability and obtained specimens which are small. Biopsy forceps are mainly used to obtain specimens for pathologic diagnosis because of easier manipulation, histologic specimens, and confirmation of exact biopsy sites on high-resolution CT.

The procedure is essentially similar to that of fluoroscope-guided bronchoscopic biopsy. The bronchoscope is inserted orally under topical anesthesia and the tracheobronchial tree is inspected. The sampling instruments for examination (forceps, brush, curette, and transbronchial aspiration needle) are inserted to the target bronchus and guided to a possible lesion site under fluoroscopic guidance. The possible lesion site on fluoroscopes is assessed by comparing the lesion site on CT taken before the procedure, and the anatomical structures such as the vertebrae which can be observed on fluoroscopy.

When the sampling instrument is considered to be close enough to the lesion fluoroscopically, the patient is moved to the CT scanner. First, the lesion is scanned with the sampling instrument by CT-fluoroscopy. When the sampling instrument is close enough to the lesion, the high-resolution CT scan measures three-dimensional distances between the lesion and the sampling instrument. The distances are adjusted under fluoroscopic guidance after moving the patient to the fluoroscopy system. This procedure is repeated until the sampling instrument reaches the lesion. Precise adjustment of the tip of the sampling instrument is made under CT-fluoroscopic guidance. The final biopsy site is confirmed by high-resolution CT and biopsy is performed under CT-fluoroscopic guidance.

Since 1995, more than 200 examinations have been performed at the National Cancer Center Hospital, and the diagnostic accuracy is now close to 100% [37]. In addition, when the sampling instruments are confirmed exactly inside the lesions on high-resolution CT and pathologic findings of the obtained specimens are compatible with image diagnosis, even a diagnosis of nonmalignancy is highly reliable, and consequently, the procedure can be used to avoid surgical resection of probably benign lesions.

The advantages of CT-guided bronchoscopic biopsy over CT-guided transthoracic needle biopsy are that there are much fewer complications like pneumothorax, hemorrhage, implantation, and air-embolism. Although pneumothorax is easily controlled by chest tube placement, the discomfort it causes and the hospitalization period are similar to those with VATS resection of the lesions. Since the other conditions can be fatal, utmost effort should be made to prevent them, which makes bronchoscopy a standard approach to peripheral pulmonary lesions.

The advantages of CT-guided bronchoscopy over standard fluoroscopy-guided bronchoscopy are the improved confirmation of biopsy sites and the avoidance of dangerous anatomical structures such as the pleura and blood vessels. The former can increase the reliability of a diagnosis of nonmalignancy in cases of truly benign lesions as well as that of malignancy in malignant lesions. The latter can reduce complications such as pneumothorax and massive hemorrhage. As a result of these advantages, CT-guided bronchoscopic biopsy can be adopted as a standard approach to small peripheral pulmonary lesions with improved accuracy and diminished risk.

One of the present limitations of CT-guided bronchoscopy is the difficulty in accessing minute lesions. Even if CT can visualize a lesion and a sampling instrument clearly, the bronchoscopic technique per se is not assisted by CT. Consequently, the decisive factor concerning accessibility to lesions is the bronchoscopic technique itself. This means that CT-guided bronchoscopic biopsy requires experienced bronchoscopists in order to achieve satisfactory results.

Another problem is the equipment needed for the procedure, i.e., CT systems. The system used for the procedure should consist of a CT which allows rapid image reconstruction, a fluoroscope, and a patient table. This type of CT system was initially developed for an interventional radiology CT (IVR-CT) system, and is mainly used for treatments of the liver [40]. At present, few IVR-CT systems are available, and it would be difficult to have such a system dedicated only to bronchoscopy.

CT alone without fluoroscopy can be used for CT-guided bronchoscopic biopsy, however, it may have some problems. Standard fluoroscopy-guided bronchoscopic biopsy can diagnose malignant lesions because even a single cancer cell is diagnostic for malignant lesions. If CT-guided bronchoscopic biopsy performed by CT alone as the first examination revealed no malignancy, the examination could be said to have failed because it was only by CT. The examination might have been successful if it had been done by fluoroscopic guidance, because CT alone cannot show the direction of a sampling instrument which makes the procedure very difficult. On the other hand, CT guidance should be used even for the first examination to confirm the benign nature of lesions in which benign pathologic conditions are highly suspected.

When a lesion is strongly suspected to be malignant, surgical resection of the lesion is the final diagnostic option even if all obtained specimens are nonmalignant. If the results of a nonsurgical examination do not affect future diagnostic plans, the nonsurgical examination should not be performed and surgical approaches such as VATS should be the first diagnostic option when informed consent is obtained. However, since surgical resection is highly invasive in some cases, nonsurgical diagnostic procedures should be aimed for as much as possible, to avoid unnecessary invasion. This situation is often experienced in lesions located close to the hilum and requiring lobectomy, and also in patients with less than ideal physical conditions. The latter case is particularly important because the number of older patients is set to increase.

Diagnostic methods for small peripheral pulmonary lesions should not only be accurate but also minimally invasive, and should be decided on after considering the lesion characteristics and patient conditions as well. In this respect, CT-guided bronchoscopic biopsy is a good standard approach for the diagnosis of small peripheral pulmonary lesions.

CT-guided bronchoscopic barium marking

In small peripheral pulmonary lesions in which malignancy cannot be denied, VATS resection is a good diagnostic option. However, even in VATS resection, the smaller the lesions are, the more minimal the invasiveness of the procedure should be. When lesions are so small as to potentially present problems thoracoscopically or fluoroscopically, markers such as coils and wires can be placed by transthoracic approaches under CT guidance to show lesion sites and/or resection lines in order to preserve as much residual lung function as possible [25,26].

However, the transthoracic approach carries risks of inherent complications. Pneumothorax and hemorrhage are common complications, however, they would compromise the marking procedures, and placing of the chest tube should be under local anesthesia prior to the induction of general anesthesia for VATS. Steps to prevent fatal complications must be taken to the greatest extent possible, even if such a probability is low. In addition, marker migration, dislodgement, and disappearance are common problems even if markers are placed properly without any complication. Furthermore, accurate histologic diagnosis is compromised because metallic markers cannot be cut for histologic examinations and they must be removed.

CT-guided bronchoscopic barium marking was developed using the CT-guided bronchoscopic biopsy technique to place a marker for VATS resection of fluoroscopically and thoracoscopically invisible peripheral pulmonary lesions [38]. Barium sulfate was used as a marker. The technique is basically similar to that of CT-guided bronchoscopic biopsy. Lesions are approached by a transbronchial aspiration cytology needle whose needle tip is removed, and 0.1–1.0 ml of 100 w/v% barium sulfate suspension, the same substance as used for barium swallow, is instilled into bronchi near the lesions under CT guidance.

In our series, more than 30 barium markers were placed and all were detected fluoroscopically enabling accurate indication of proper resection lines, and all lesions were resected without any residual lesions. There were no complications related to the barium marking and no marker problem. There was no lesion which could not be diagnosed pathologically due to the barium.

The barium marker is a stable substance. This has been shown by the inhalation of barium at the time of barium swallow proving not to be problematic, even if the inhalation is massive. The barium marker does not compromise histologic examinations even when placed adjacent to a lesion or even at a lesion. Complications are considered to be minimal because the procedure is performed through bronchi and no invasive procedures such as biopsy are performed. Consequently, barium markers can be placed regardless of the date of surgical resection, and there would be no problem even if the barium markers were not resected.

The barium markers can be placed near a lesion to indicate the lesion site, either in a bronchus leading to the lesion which is to be resected together with the lesion, or in a segment to be resected. When barium markers are placed immediately under the pleura, the markers can be visualized thoracoscopically through the pleura as whitish areas. As the marking procedure is done through bronchi, it causes much less damage than a transthoracic approach. Considering these facts, the barium markers are anatomically and oncologically appropriate.

In addition, multiple markers can be placed to clearly show resection lines, and this can be convenient in cases with relatively large lesions to resect, while at the same time preserving residual lung functions in patients with poor pulmonary functions. Barium markers can also be placed in cases with thickened pleura which prevents accurate palpation of small lesions even with open thoracotomy. Another application was employed for CT-assisted transbronchial brachytherapy to exactly reproduce the same radiation field at each of fractions even under fluoroscopic guidance.

CT-guided bronchoscopic barium marking is thus a versatile technique. Even in surgical resection of small peripheral pulmonary lesions, invasiveness should always be restricted to a minimum and patients should never be subjected to unnecessary invasion, e.g., lobectomy for a minute benign lesion immediately under the pleura. From this point of view, barium marking is considered to be one of the best marking techniques.

CT-assisted transbronchial brachytherapy for small peripheral pulmonary malignancies

When peripheral pulmonary malignancies are small or very early, they may not have to be resected. This situation is sometimes encountered in patients with less than ideal physical conditions such as poor pulmonary conditions which preclude even VATS resection. This will be increasingly important as the number of older patients increases in the near future. In addition, multicentricity of malignancies will make less invasive or compromise treatment more desirable.

Transthoracic approaches are not ideal for these small and earlier lesions because of their inherent invasiveness. If small peripheral pulmonary malignancies can be precisely accessed bronchoscopically under CT guidance, treatment may be performed if appropriate instruments can be brought to the lesions. We use a high dose rate (HDR) remote-afterloading system the efficacy of which has been proved for several types of malignancies.

A dummy source is inserted into an applicator from the HDR remote-afterloading system, and the applicator is guided to the small peripheral pulmonary malignancy under local anesthesia using the CT-guided bronchoscopic technique [39]. The dummy source is usually used to calculate an accurate radiation dose to be delivered. The applicator which penetrates the lesion is fixed at the pleura and to the mouthpiece. If no bronchus penetrates the lesion, it is also possible to have multiple applicators inserted around the lesion. The three-dimensional relationship of the lesion and the applicator(s) is confirmed on high-resolution CT. The treatment plan is calculated, a radioactive source (iridium-192) is inserted into the applicator using the HDR remote-afterloading system after removing the dummy source, and the planned radiation dose is delivered. When multiple-fractioned radiation is planned, a barium marker can be placed immediately under the pleura through a bronchus penetrating the lesion. When the tip of the applicator is confirmed fluoroscopically to reach the barium marker, the applicator must be in the same bronchus penetrating the lesion. This facilitates the procedure by allowing the same radiation field to be used, because the CT system is not necessary after the first procedure.

No complication has occurred in our series until now and reduction of tumor sizes could be observed on high-resolution CT, however, its efficacy is difficult to prove because the treatment is indicated in patients whose physical condition would not allow even VATS resection. There was one lesion, which was metastatic from colon cancer, in which resection was later performed and no residual cancer cells were detected histologically.

Because a radiation dose is delivered from inside lesions or from bronchi surrounding lesions, the damage to noncancerous tissues is minimal and limited to a small area in the vicinity of the lesion. Consequently, a sufficient radiation dose can be delivered without causing damage to noncancerous tissues, and even single fraction radiation is allowed. In addition, radiation is not compromised by movements caused by respiration and heartbeat, which solves one of the important problems of heavy particle radiation.

Conclusion

Bronchoscopic approaches to small peripheral pulmonary lesions have been considered to be difficult and the use of a CT scanner can overcome these problems. Once these lesions are reached, transbronchial approaches are sure to offer several new applications including the treatments. The field of transbronchial approaches to small peripheral lesions under CT guidance has just begun to develop, however, it holds great promise for new diagnostic and therapeutic strategies for pulmonary malignancies.

References

1. Melamed MR, Flehinger BJ. Screening for early lung cancer. Chest 1984;86:2–3.
2. Tockman MS. Survival and mortality from lung cancer in a screened population: the Johns Hopkins study. Chest 1986;89(Suppl):324–325.
3. Fontana RS, Sanderson DR, Woolner LB, Taylor WF, Miller WE, Muhm JR. Lung cancer screening: the Mayo Program. J Occ Med 1986;28:746–750.
4. Kubik A, Polak J. Lung cancer detection. Results of a randomized prospective study in Czechoslovakia. Cancer 1986;57:2427–2437.

5. Naruke T, Tsuchiya R, Kondo H, Asamura H, Nakayama H. Implications of staging in lung cancer. Chest 1999;112:242S–248S.
6. Kaneko M, Eguchi K, Ohmatsu H, Kakinuma R, Naruke T, Suemasu K, Moriyama N. Peripheral lung cancer: screening and detection with low-dose spiral CT versus radiography. Radiology 1996;201:798–802.
7. Sone S, Takashima S, Li F, Yang Z, Honda T, Maruyama Y et al. Mass screening for lung cancer with mobile spiral computed tomography scanner. Lancet 1998;351:1242–1245.
8. Swensen SJ, Jett JR, Payne WS, Viggiano RW, Pairolero PC, Trastek VF. An integrated approach to evaluation of the solitary pulmonary nodule. Mayo Clin Proc 1990;65.173–186.
9. Stringfield JT, Markowitz DJ, Bentz RR, Welch RH, Weg JG. The effect of tumor size and location on diagnosis by fiberoptic bronchoscopy. Chest 1977;72:474–476.
10. Cortese DA, Mcdougall JC. Biopsy and brushing of peripheral lung cancer with fluoroscopic guidance. Chest 1979;75:141–145.
11. Fletcher EC, Levin DC. Flexible fiberoptic bronchoscopy and fluoroscopically guided transbronchial biopsy in the management of solitary pulmonary nodules. West J Med 1982;136:477–483.
12. Shure D, Fedullo PF. Transbronchial needle aspiration of peripheral masses. Am Rev Respir Dis 1983;128:1090–1092.
13. Radlke JR, Conway WA, Eyler WR, Kvale PA. Diagnostic accuracy in peripheral lung lesions: factors predicting success with flexible fiberoptic bronchoscopy. Chest 1979;76:176–179.
14. Wallace JM, Deutsch AL. Flexible fiberoptic bronchoscopy and percutaneous needle lung aspiration for evaluating the solitary pulmonary nodule. Chest 1982;81:665–671.
15. Berquist TH, Bailey PB, Cortese DA et al. Transthoracic needle biopsy. Mayo Clin Proc 1980;55: 475–481.
16. Böcking A, Klose KC, Kyll HJ, Hauptmann S. Cytologic versus histologic evaluation of needle biopsy of the lung, hilum and mediastinum. Sensitivity, specificity and typing accuracy. Acta Cytol 1995;39:463–471.
17. Hartner LP, Moss AA, Goldberg HI, Gross BH. CT-guided fine needle aspiration for diagnosis of benign and malignant disease. AJR 1983;140:363–367.
18. van Sonnenberg E, Casola G, Ho M, Neff CC, Varney RR, Wittich GR et al. Difficult thoracic lesions: CT-guided biopsy experience in 150 patients. Radiology 1988;167:457–461.
19. Haramati LB. CT-guided automated needle biopsy of the chest. Am J Roent 1995;165:53–55.
20. Katada K, Kato R, Anno H, Ogura Y, Koga S, Koga S et al. Guidance with real-time CT fluoroscopy: early clinical experience. Radiology 1996;200:851–856.
21. Yim APC. The role of video-assisted thoracoscopic surgery in the management of polmonary tuberculosis. Chest 1996;110:829–832.
22. Allen MS, Deschamps C, Jones DM, Trastek VF, Pairolero PC. Video-assisted thoracic surgical procedures: the Mayo experience. Mayo Clin Proc 1996;71:351–359.
23. DeCamp MM Jr, Jaklitsch MT, Mentzer SJ, Harpole DH Jr, Sugarbaker DJ. The safety and versatility of video-thoracoscopy: a prospective analysis of 895 consecutive cases. J Am Coll Surg 1995;18:113–120.
24. Daniel TM, Kern JA, Tribble CG, Kron IL, Spotnitz WB, Rodgers BM. Thoracoscopic surgery for diseases of the lung and pleura. Effectiveness, changing indications, and limitations. Ann Surg 1993;217:566–574.
25. Kanazawa S, Ando A, Yasui K, Tanaka A, Hiraki Y. Localization of small pulmonary nodules for thoracoscopic resection: use of a newly developed hookwire system. Cardiovasc Intervent Radiol 1995;18:122–124.
26. Plunkett MB, Peterson MS, Landreneau RJ, Ferson PF, Posner MC. Peripheral pulmonary nodules: preoperative percutaneous needle localization with CT guidance. Radiology 1992; 185:274–276.
27. Miller KS, Fish GB, Stanley JH, Schabel SI. Prediction of pneumothorax rate in percutaneous needle aspiration of the lung. Chest 1988;93:742–745.

28. Wescott JL, Rao N, Colley DP. Transthoracic needle biopsy of small pulmonary nodules. Radiology 1997;202:97–103.
29. Kazerooni EA, Lim FT, Mikhail A, Martinez FJ. Risk of pneumothorax in CT-guided transthoracic needle aspiration biopsy of the lung. Radiology 1996;198:371–375.
30. Ferrucci JT, Wittenberg J, Margolies MN, Carey RW. Malignant seeding of the tract after thin-needle aspiration biopsy. Radiology 1979;130:345–346.
31. Muller NL, Bergin CJ, Miller RR, Ostrow DN. Seeding of malignant cells into the needle tract after lung and pleural biopsy. J Can Assoc Radiol 1986;37:192.
32. Seyfer AE, Walsh DS, Graeber GM, Nuno IN, Eliasson AH. Chest wall implantation of lung cancer after thin-needle aspiration biopsy. Ann Thorac Surg 1989;48:284.
33. Sinner WN, Zajicek J. Implantation metastasis after percutaneous transthoracic needle aspiration biopsy. Acta Radiol 1976;17:473–480.
34. Aberle DR, Gamsu G, Golden JA. Fatal systemic arterial air embolism following lung needle aspiration. Radiology 1987;165:351–353.
35. Noguchi M, Morikawa A, Kawasaki M et al. Small adenocarcinoma of the lung. Histologic characteristics and prognosis. Cancer 1995;75:2844–2852.
36. Kobayashi T, Shimamura K, Hanai M, Kaneko M. Computed tomography-guided bronchoscopy with an ultrathin fiberscope. Diagn Ther Endo 1996;2:229–232.
37. Kobayashi T. CT-guided bronchoscopy for minute peripheral lung cancer: from diagnosis to future therapeutic strategies. Rev Oncol 1999;1(Suppl 2):41–45.
38. Kobayashi T, Kaneko M, Kondo H et al. CT-guided bronchoscopic barium marking for resection of a fluoroscopically invisible peripheral pulmonary lesion. Jpn J Clin Oncol 1997;27: 204–205.
39. Kobayashi T, Kaneko M, Sumi M et al. CT-assisted transbronchial brachytherapy for small peripheral lung cancer. Jpn J Clin Oncol 2000;30:109–112.
40. Takayasu K, Muramatsu Y, Asai S, Muramatsu Y, Kobayashi T. CT Fluoroscopy-Assisted Needle puncture and ethanol injection for hepatocellular carcinoma: A preliminary study. AJR 1999;173:1219–1224.

Diagnostic thoracoscopy and its problems

Bronchology and Bronchoesophagology: State of the Art.
H. Yoshimura et al., editors.

Malignant pleural mesothelioma: role of thoracoscopy

Philippe Astoul[1,2] and Christian Boutin[2]
[1]*Department of Pulmonary Diseases, Hôpital Sainte-Marguerite; and* [2]*UPRES 2050, University of the Mediterranean, Marseille, France*

Abstract. Malignant pleural mesothelioma (MPM) is refractory to the standard therapeutic options since chemotherapy is only partially effective, radiation therapy simply provides palliation against pain, and surgery, even when performed at a relatively early stage, is controversial.

Pleuroscopy is an essential procedure for the management of MPM for several reasons:

- It has provided insight into the pathogenesis of this disease in showing carcinogenetic asbestos fibers accumulating in black anthracotic zones of the parietal pleura. Further study suggests that these zones could be the equivalent of the milky spots that have been observed in animals.
- It allows a clinical approach in the following aspects: i) diagnosis: the sensitivity and specificity of thoracoscopy is higher than any other method. In addition, thoracoscopic biopsy is considerably more cost-effective than surgical biopsy. ii) prognosis: thoracoscopy allows for the division of Stage I Butchart mesothelioma into two subgroups, Ia, which is an early stage with only parietal pleura involvement, and Ib, which is characterized by the invasion of visceral pleura. iii) therapy: in patients with early-stage disease, pleuroscopy allows the placement of an implantable port for local immunotherapy which is a reasonable therapeutic approach.

Keywords: asbestos, malignant effusion, mesothelioma, pleura, thoracoscopy.

Pleural mesothelioma is more frequent than peritoneal mesothelioma, possibly because inhalation is the usual route of the pathogenic fibers [1,2] and the incidence has risen in recent years [3] and is expected to peak sometime between 1990 and 2010 [4].

This disease is refractory to the standard therapeutic options since chemotherapy is only partially effective, radiation therapy simply provides palliation against pain, and surgery, even when performed at a relatively early stage, is controversial [3—5].

Perhaps because of this poor prognosis, early screening has not incited great interest. However, this pessimism belies the fact that certain forms have a better prognosis when diagnosed early [2,5—7]. To better ascertain prognostic factors, multifactorial studies using the Cox model have been performed [1,3,4,8—12]. The most favorable factors are being under 50 years of age, and having an epithelial histopathological type, a good general condition and stage I disease.

Pleuroscopy is an essential procedure for the management of malignant pleural mesothelioma (MPM) for several reasons:

Address for correspondence: Philippe Astoul, Hôpital Sainte-Marguerite, Department of Pulmonary Diseases, 270 Boulevard Sainte Marguerite, B.P.29, 13274 Marseille cedex 09, France.
E-mail: pastoul@ap-hm.fr

- It has provided insight into the pathogenesis of this disease in showing carcinogenetic asbestos fibers accumulating in black anthracotic zones of the parietal pleura [13]. Further study suggests that these zones could be the equivalent of the milky spots that have been observed in animals [14].
- It allows a clinical approach in the following aspects: i) diagnosis: the sensitivity and specificity of thoracoscopy is higher than any other method [5, 8,9,15,16]. In addition, thoracoscopic biopsy is considerably more cost-effective than surgical biopsy. ii) prognosis: thoracoscopy allows for the division of Stage I Butchart mesothelioma into two subgroups, Ia, which is an early stage with only parietal pleura involvement, and Ib, which is characterized by the invasion of visceral pleura. iii) therapy: in patients with early-stage disease, pleuroscopy allows the placement of an implantable port for local immunotherapy which is a reasonable therapeutic approach [17,18].

Since mesothelioma has no characteristic clinical manifestations, this diagnosis should always be considered in any patient with pleural symptoms, especially in towns, harbors and geographic areas where the asbestos industry formerly developed. Systematic screening allowed detection of 3% of the patients in Ruffie's series [10].

CT-scan images were variable. CT scans were more precise if the fluid was removed but were most useful for follow-ups. In our series, 20% of patients had lesions visible on CT scans, whereas 40% had fibrohyaline or calcified pleural plaques seen during thoracoscopy. Thoracoscopy allows excellent visualization and diagnosis of these plaques. A decrease in the diameter of the affected hemithorax is frequent with mesothelioma but this finding is also associated with infectious pleurisy. Mediastinal changes are more specific, the hemithorax becomes uneven, and nodular thickening of the mediastinal pleura, pericardium, hilus, and its lymph nodes occur. As will be discussed further on, mediastinal status is an important factor in staging the disease. Mediastinal changes develop at an advanced stage of mesothelioma and are a highly unfavorable prognostic feature.

Value of diagnostic thoracoscopy

Indications

The reported sensitivity of pleural fluid cytology ranges from 0 to 64%. Likewise, the sensitivity of needle biopsy varies from 6 to 38%. Herbert [19] claimed that the value of both these methods was limited and advocated surgical biopsy. Thoracoscopy results achieved are similar in comparison to the surgery and better than fluid cytology or Abrams biopsy (Table 1). Cope or Abrams needle biopsy under CT-scan control is of limited sensitivity since the sample volume is usually too small for histology and negative findings do not rule out mesothelioma.

Thoracoscopy is indicated in practically all cases of suspected mesothelioma.

Table 1. The sensitivity of different diagnostic methods for diffuse malignant mesothelioma.

Diagnostic methods	No. of cases of successful diagnoses	Successful diagnoses (%)
Fluid cytology	49/175	28
Abrams needle biopsy	33/135	24
Thoracoscopy	185/188	98
Surgery	9/9	100

In a series of 188 patients [20], the indications were chronic pleurisy in 88% of the cases, empyema in 2%, chronic spontaneous pneumothorax in 1%, and radiographically documented pleural nodules without effusion in 9%. Of these patients, 80% recalled previous exposure to asbestos. Thoracoscopic biopsy was positive in every case in which it was feasible.

Thoracoscopic findings

In 137 of the previous 188 patients, the pleural cavity was completely free or displayed only loose or fibrinous adhesions that did not impede thoracoscopic examination. In the other 51 patients, the procedure was hindered by adhesions, and electrocoagulation was required to severe adhesions and obtain a cavity of at least 10 cm^3. Although complete examination was not possible in these cases, biopsy samples were almost always obtained from malignant lesions on the parietal and, if necessary, visceral pleura.

The following lesions were observed in the parietal pleura or diaphragm:

- nodules or masses ranging from 5 mm to 10 cm in 92 patients (49%). In 25 patients (13%), a grape-like aspect [9] characteristic of mesothelioma was noted;
- thickening of the pleura in 21 patients (11%). This thickening was more or less regular with elevated, pale, hard, poorly vascularized tissue suggesting malignancy;
- malignant-looking pachypleuritis in association with nodules or masses in 63 patients (33.5%); and
- nonspecific inflammatory aspect with fine granulations (1 to 2 mm in diameter), lymphangitis, congestion, hypervascularization or local thickening of the pleura in 12 patients (6.5%).

The sensitivity of thoracoscopic biopsy was 98% (185 positive biopsies including "extended thoracoscopy" out of 188 patients). In the three failed cases, thick adhesions prevented specimen collection and the diagnosis was only mesothelial hyperplasia. Conclusive biopsy samples were obtained by Abrams needle biopsy (one patient), repeat thoracoscopy (one patient) and surgical biopsy (one patient). The histologic type of mesothelioma was epithelial in 135 cases (72%), mixed in 38 (20%), and fibrosarcomatous in 15 (8%).

In contrast with the almost perfect sensitivity of thoracoscopy, the cumulative sensitivity of fluid cytology and needle biopsy was only 38.2%. The sensitivity of these conventional procedures in our patients with previously negative results was not necessarily lower than in other series reporting initial, plus repeat results. However, Herbert and Gallagher [19] concluded that the overall sensitivity of these techniques was poor and most investigators prefer open surgical biopsy.

We prefer thoracoscopy to thoracotomy because it is far less painful and safer for the patient. Although Ratzer et al. [21] were unable to achieve diagnosis twice and Law et al. [22] were successful in only 13 of 23, thoracoscopy seems to be a highly reliable method. Martensson et al. [15] achieved diagnosis of mesothelioma in 23 out of 24 thoracoscopies, Hirsch et al. [23] in 9 out of 9 and Lewis et al. [24] in 28 out of 28.

Prognosis of mesothelioma

Prognosis depends on numerous factors which have been studied separately or in multiple correlation studies (Cox model). As previously stated, a good overall condition, no weight loss and a good P.S. are favorable prognostic factors. Common sense would warrant the same conclusions without complex calculations. The value and significance of age, sex, and symptom-to-diagnosis intervals have varied widely from one study to another. Treatment was cited as a favorable factor in 5 out of 7 series [1,2,11,25,26] but none of these studies was randomized, and no definite conclusions can be drawn, especially with regard to surgery [7].

Histological type

The histological type appears to be important. Epithelial or mixed forms have a better prognosis than fibrosarcomatous forms. The mean time of survival is 10 to 17 months for patients with epithelial or mixed forms and 4 to 7 months for the latter. In our series, fibrosarcomatous types had the most unfavorable prognosis, with a mean survival time of 5.25 months.

Disease stages

Disease staging is useful, not only to establish a prognosis but also to allow evaluation of the effectiveness of treatment. The most widely used and first classification is that of Butchart [6], which includes 4 stages (Table 2). Only patients in the first two stages are eligible for curative treatment. In stage II, the chest wall and/or mediastinum is involved with or without mediastinal lymph nodes. In all classification systems, mesothelioma at stage III or IV becomes fatal after a few weeks to 4 or 5 months.

Although cited as a good prognostic sign in four multivariate studies, stage I disease was a highly favorable factor in only two. In the previous series mean survival at stage I was 13.4 months. This was statistically different from the other stages but hardly exceeded overall average survival. These facts could mean either that the stage of disease is not an important prognostic factor or that the

Table 2. Survival in terms of the Butchart classification system.

	Butchart [6]		Antman [1]		Brenner [10]		Alberts [11]	
	Nb	Survival (months)	Nb	Survival (months)	Nb	Survival (months)	Nb	Survival (months)
Stage I: localized tumor in homolateral pleura	13	17	31	16	62	13	202	11
Stage II: involvement of mediastinal organs, the wall or the contralateral pleura	4	11	4	9	52	11	35	8
Stage III: subdiaphragmatic involvement	2	9	5	5	7	4	13	7
Stage IV: remote metastasis	0	–	2	4	0	–	12	2

Butchart system is inadequate. In this regard, it should be emphasized that the number of patients in stage I, which has ranged from 30% [11] to 77% [27], tends to be overestimated.

Thoracoscopy

Thoracoscopic features seem to allow more accurate staging. In 50% of cases, patients with the longest survival times had tumors with an inflammatory or non-specific lymphangitic appearance [28]. The mean survival for these patients (12 in our series) was 28.3 months. In the other 50% of these cases, small nodules (less than 5 mm in diameter), fine granulations or slight pleural thickening were observed. In this early stage of the disease, the mediastinum as well as the visceral pleura appear normal through the thoracoscope, as well as on CT scan. Unlike Canto [29], no lesions exclusively on the visceral pleura were noted and from this the conclusion can be drawn that in most cases mesothelioma develops from the parietal or diaphragmatic pleura and invades the visceral and mediastinal pleura later. This is consistent with the location of benign asbestos plaques only on the parietal or diaphragmatic pleura. As reported by Adams, in 19 out of his 20 patients [30], benign asbestos plaques were observed in an extent with less involvement of the visceral pleura than that of the parietal pleura or diaphragm. If the visceral pleura was involved to any extent, mesothelioma had a very unfavorable prognosis with a median time of survival of 10 months. Conversely, the median survival for 48 patients with a normal visceral pleura was 22.4 months.

Staging of mesothelioma is an important but difficult problem that must be solved so that effective treatment, when it becomes available, can be applied at the earliest stage of the disease. Rusch and Ginsberg [31] listed the following requirements for validation of a classification system:

- confirmation of diagnoses by a panel of pathologists,
- good prognostic value, and
- corroboration by a prospective study.

The Butchart system has been criticized because it overestimates the number of patients in stage I, and because assessment of tumor thickness by conventional X-ray and even CT scan is difficult in cases of ipsilateral effusion. This criticism is equally valid for all other classification systems. The Mattson system [32] differs from the Butchart system mainly with regard to pericardial involvement which is included in stage II rather than in stage I. The Dimitrov system [33] is based on the measurement of the largest diameter of the tumor by CT scan, which would be much easier by thoracoscopy.

The TNM system proposed by Chahinian [2] has the advantage of being based on an international system. A simpler TNM classification has been proposed by the UICC [30].

In fact, thoracoscopy shows that patients with parietal pleura involvement which often occurs at an early stage of the disease should be classified separately, while patients with involvement of visceral pleura, which has, in our series, the same prognostic significance as mediastinal involvement, should be classified in another group. Based on this finding we divided stage I into two subcategories:

Stage IA. The parietal and/or diaphragmatic pleura are involved, but the visceral pleura appears to be disease-free by both thoracoscopy and CT scan (26 patients in our series). The median time of survival of stage IA patients is 28 months.

Stage IB. The features are the same as stage IA, but also includes evident visceral pleura involvement (70 patients). The median time of survival is only 11 months at stage IB. Thus, as soon as the visceral pleura is invaded, the prognosis becomes much worse, whatever treatment is attempted. In stage II, where the mediastinum is involved, survival is only predicted to be 10 months, suggesting that mediastinal involvement may occur very soon after visceral pleura invasion, and in some cases may even be synchronous.

Recently, a group of investigators working under the direction of Rush agreed on a new TNM system that included stages IA and IB [34].

Therapeutic thoracoscopy

Talc poudrage pleurodesis

In most cases, the goal of treatment when dealing with mesothelioma is simply to prevent recurrent effusions and obtain the longest possible time of survival with the best quality of life. As previously seen, the efficacy of chemotherapy and/or radiotherapy is controversial, and surgery is generally noncurative.

Thoracoscopy permits effective palliation with less morbidity than surgery or even chemotherapy or radiation therapy. Permanent pleurodesis may be achieved at the end of the thoracoscopic examination by spraying 6 to 10 ml (3 to 5 g) of talcum powder into the pleural space. A chest tube is inserted and all air is aspirated from the chest cavity. A final roentgenogram is taken to assess the position of the tube and to confirm full re-expansion of the lung. Drainage or aspiration under negative pressure (50 to 100 mmHg) is maintained for 4 to 6 days.

Talc poudrage prevented fluid reaccumulation in 81% of cases, vs. 83% after surgery [35]. When effusions recurred despite poudrage, surgery was contraindicated by poor general condition. A second talc poudrage in two patients produced good results.

Complications included one case of empyema after poudrage, which was resolved after drainage and pleural lavage, and four deaths (3, 4, 7 and 10 days after talc poudrage) in patients in very poor general condition. Three perioperative deaths occurred, one 60 days after pleuropneumonectomy from a bronchial fistula and two 10 days after pleurectomy. The median time of survival in the three groups was 210 days after surgery, 330 days after talc poudrage, and 120 days when using supportive care alone.

The decreased survival observed in the untreated group was most likely due to the advanced stage of the tumors. Conversely, there was no significant difference between the surgery and talc poudrage groups. These groups, however, were not randomized.

The percentage of survivors at 1 year for these three groups was 47% after talc poudrage, 28% after surgery, and 13% for supportive care.

Surgery did not prevent subsequent distant metastases. Among patients surviving more than 3 months, metastases developed in eight out of 12 patients after surgery as compared to 12 out of 32 patients after talc poudrage (Table 3).

Role of thoracoscopy in intrapleural treatment

Talc pleurodesis is a purely palliative procedure that enhances the functional and general status of the patient by eliminating the need for repeated puncture. A more active therapy is available to some patients. It is intrapleural chemotherapy using either a sclerosing agent (Adriamycine) or an antimitotic agent (5FU, Thio-TEPA, Bleomycine). Tolerance is proportional to the sclerosing effect which itself

Table 3. Effectiveness of thoracoscopy and surgery in preventing fluid recurrence.

	Thoracoscopy	Surgery
No. of patients with pleural fluid	32	12[a]
Results:		
Good	26 (81%)	10 (83%)
Poor	6	2
Hospital mortality at 1 month	4	2

[a]Of patients who underwent surgery, only 12 had chronic pleural effusions.

depends on the cytotoxic effect. This is particularly true for Adriamycine [36].

Patients with minimal peritoneal or pleural disease (< 5 mm in depth) experience the best response rates to intracavitary chemotherapy [37]. The necessity of inserting a catheter or chest tube for the administration of intrapleural chemotherapy inevitably poses a high risk of infection. Markman et al. [38,39] treated eight patients with malignant mesothelioma with intrapleural cisplatin (100 μg/m^2 in 250 ml of saline). Only one patient exhibited a response, but these patients had more extensive disease which severely limited the diffusion of drug throughout the pleural cavity. Two out of seven patients treated intrapleurally with cisplatin combined with cytarabine demonstrated a response [40]. A "Lung Cancer Study Group" trial published by V. Rush et al. [41] included 46 patients. The overall response rate was 49%. The outcome of this trial was encouraging enough to warrant the subsequent trials for pleural mesothelioma.

The incidence of pleural adhesions and the heterogeneity of lesions in the pleural cavity led us to place the catheter near the lesions under visual control during endoscopy in order to obtain the best possible delivery of intrapleural chemotherapy. The incidence of pleural infection due to catheter handling led us to place a subcutaneous port-A-cath at the level of the 4th intercostal space in the anterior axillary region. The catheter is tunneled 6 to 8 cm under the skin and the tip is placed under visual control. Healing is usually occurs within 8 to 12 days and treatment can begin after 2 weeks. Limiting contact with ambient air has practically eliminated the problem of pleural infection. Our experience now includes 70 patients treated in the department, plus over 100 patients from a multicentric study. Using interferon-γ [36,37] and interleukine-2 [42,43] we have obtained an objective response with prolonged survival.

Another indication for thoracoscopy is assessment of tumor response. A follow-up can be accomplished using repeated pleural fluid cytology [40], but when there is no more liquid, cytology is not feasible. Others judge response on the decrease in the amount of fluid [39]. It appears that a second thoracoscopy is the most effective means of visualizing tumor response. In our patients we perform thoracoscopy and a CT scan, before treatment, to achieve diagnosis and staging. Then 15 to 30 days after treatment we perform a CT scan after fluid removal. If the CT scan shows that the lesions have stabilized or regressed, we repeat thoracoscopy to confirm response [42]. In eight cases [36] we observed complete regression with negative biopsies. Thus, thoracoscopy appears to be an excellent method for evaluating tumor response.

Conclusion

As thoracoscopy is a simple and safe procedure, we recommend that it be used liberally in the following diagnostic indications:

- Patients with a history of previous asbestos exposure presenting chest pain, recent and untreatable cough, unexplained loss of weight, pleural effusion, empyema, or spontaneous pneumothorax. Thoracoscopy should be undertaken early. In our experience several patients developed mesothelioma after false-negative cytology. In these patients thoracoscopy was performed only after the recurrence of fluid, and as a result diagnosis was delayed for several weeks or months.

- X-ray or CT scans documented changes in visible pleural plaques.
- Recent unexplainable pleurisy, particularly in patients from areas liable to asbestos exposure.

In all these cases manifestations are very minor and most physicians are reluctant to recommend a highly invasive procedure like exploratory thoracotomy. For malignant mesothelioma this reluctance is detrimental to survival, since we observed complete responses to cytokines only in patients in the earliest stage of disease.

To allow more widespread use, thoracoscopy should not be reserved to the surgeon, physicians should also be trained to perform this procedure for diagnostic purposes. More and more groups, even in the USA or Canada, where resistance to thoracoscopy has traditionally been strong, are starting to report their experiences [44–46].

References

1. Antman K, Shemin R, Ryan L et al. Malignant Mesothelioma: prognostic variables in a registry of 180 patients, the Dana-Farber Cancer Institute and Brigham and Women's Hospital experience over two decades, 1965–1985. J Clin Oncol 1988;6:147–153.
2. Chahinian AP, Pajak TF, Holland JF, Norton L, Ambinder RM, Mandel EM. Diffuse malignant mesothelioma (prospective evaluation of 69 patients). Ann Int Med 1982;96:746–755.
3. Mac Donald AD, Mac Donald JC. Epidemiology of malignant mesothelioma. In: Antman K, Aisner J (eds) Asbestos-Related Malignancy. Boston: Grune and Stratton Inc., 1986;31–35.
4. Nicholson WJ, Perkel G, Selikoff IJ. Occupational exposure to asbestos: population at risk and projected mortality -1980–2030. Am J Ind Med 1982;3:259–311.
5. Boutin C, Viallat JR, Aelony Y. Practical Thoracoscopy. Berlin-Heidelberg: Springer-Verlag, 1991.
6. Butchart EG, Ashcroft T, Barnsley WC, Holden MP. Pleuropneumonectomy in the management of diffuse malignant mesothelioma of the pleura (experience with 29 patients). Thorax 1976;31: 15–24.
7. Rusch VW, Piantadosi S, Holmes C. The role of extrapleural pneumonectomy in malignant pleural mesothelioma. J Thorac Cardiovasc Surg 1991;102:1–9.
8. Boutin C, Viallat JR, Cargnino P, Farisse P. Thoracoscopy in malignant pleural effusions. Am Rev Respir Dis 1981;124:588–592.
9. Boutin C. Thoracoscopy in malignant mesothelioma. Pneumologie 1989;43:61–65.
10. Brenner J, Sordillo PP, Magill GB, Golbey RB. Malignant Mesothelioma of the Pleura. Cancer 1982;49:2431–2435.
11. Alberts AS, Falkson G, Goedhals L, Vorobiof DA, van der Merwe CA. Malignant pleural mesothelioma: a disease unaffected by current therapeutic maneuvers. J Clin Oncol 1988;6: 527–535.
12. Delaria GA, Jensik R, Faber LP et al. Surgical management of malignant mesothelioma. Ann Thorac Surg 1978;26:375–382.
13. Boutin C, Dumortier P, Rey F, Viallat JR, de Vuyst P. Black spots concentrate oncogenic asbestos fibers in the parietal pleura, thoracoscopic and mineralogic study. Am J Respir Crit Care

Med 1996;153:444–445
14. Le Bouffant L, Bruyere S, Daniel H, Tichoux G. Etude experimentale de devenir des fibres d'amiante dans l'appareil respiratoire. Rev Fr Mal Resp 1979;7:707–716.
15. Martensson G. Thoracoscopy in the diagnosis of malignant mesothelioma. Poumon-Coeur 1981;37:249–251.
16. Martensson G, Hagmar B, Zettergren L. Diagnosis and prognosis in malignant pleural mesothelioma : a prospective study. Eur J Resp Dis 1984;65:169–178.
17. Boutin C, Viallat JR, Astoul Ph. Le traitement des mésothéliomes par interferon gamma et interleukine-2. Rev Pneumol Clin 1990;46:211–215.
18. Driesen P, Boutin C, Viallat JR, Astoul Ph, Vialette JP, Pasquier J. Implantable access system for prolonged intrapleural immunotherapy. Eur Respir J 1994;7:1889–1892.
19. Herbert A, Gaxllagher PJ. Pleural biopsy in the diagnosis of malignant mesothelioma. Thorax 1982;37:816–821.
20. Boutin C, Rey F. Thoracoscopy in pleural malignant mesothelioma: a prospective study of 188 patients. Part 1: diagnosis. Cancer 1993;72;389–393.
21. Ratzer E, Pool JL, Melamed MR. Pleural mesotheliomas: clinical experiences with thirty-seven patients. Am J Roentgenol 1967;99:863–880.
22. Law MR, Hodson ME, Turner-Warwick M. Malignant mesothelioma of the pleura: clinical aspects and symptomatic treatment. Eur J Respir Dis 1984;65:162–168.
23. Hirsch A, Brochard P, De Cremoux H et al. Features of asbestos-exposed and unexposed mesothelioma. Am J Ind Med 1982;3:413–422.
24. Lewis RJ, Sisler GE, Mackenzie JW. Diffuse, mixed malignant pleural mesothelioma. Ann Thorac Surg 1981;31:53–60.
25. Spirtas R, Connelly R, Tucker MA. Survival patterns for malignant mesothelioma: the seer experience. Int J Cancer 1988;41:525–530.
26. Calavrezos A, Koschel G, Hüsselmann H et al. Malignant mesothelioma of the pleura. Klin Wochen Schr 1988;66:607–613.
27. Mac Cornack P, Nagasaki F, Hilaris BS et al. Surgical treatment of pleural mesothelioma. J Thorac Cardiovasc Surg 1982;84:834–842.
28. Whitaker D, Henderson DW, Shikin KB. The concept of mesothelioma in situ: implications for diagnosis and histogenesis. Sem Diag Pathol 1992;9:151–161.
29. Canto A, Saumench J, Moya J. Points to consider when choosing a biopsy method in cases of pleuritis of unknown origin, with special reference to thoracoscopy. In: Deslauriers J, Lacquet LK (eds) Thoracic Surgery: Surgical Management of Pleural Diseases. Saint-Louis, Missouri: C.V. Mosby Company, 1990;49–53.
30. Adams VI, Unni KK, Muhm JR, Jett JR, Ilstrup DM, Bernatz PE. Diffuse malignant mesothelioma of pleura: diagnosis and survival in 92 cases. Cancer 1986;58:1540–1551.
31. Rusch VW, Ginsberg RJ. New concepts in the staging of mesothelioma. In: Deslauriers J, Lacquet LK (eds) Thoracic Surgery: Surgical Management of Pleural Diseases. Saint-Louis, Missouri: C.V. Mosby Company. 1990;336–343.
32. Mattson K. Natural History and Clinical Staging of Malignant Mesothelioma. Envir J Respir Dis 1982;63:124–187.
33. Dimitrov NV, Mac Mahon S. Presentation, diagnostic, methods, staging and natural history of malignant mesothelioma. In: Antman K, Aisner J (eds) Asbestos Related Malignancy. Boston: Grune and Stratton Inc., 1986;225–238.
34. International Mesothelioma Interest Group. A proposed new international TNM staging system for malignant pleural mesothelioma. Chest 1995;108:1122–1128.
35. Viallat JR, Rey F, Astoul Ph, Boutin C. Thoracoscopic talc poudrage pleurodesis for malignant effusions. Review of 360 cases. Chest 1996;110:1387–1393.
36. Boutin C, Viallat JR, van Zandwijk N et al. Activity of intrapleural recombinant gamma-interferon in malignant mesothelioma. Cancer 1991;67:2033–2037.
37. Boutin C, Nussbaum E, Monnet I, Bignon J, van der Schueren R, Guerin JC, Menard O,

Mignot P, Cabouis G, Douillard JY. Intrapleural treatment with recombinant gamma-interferon in early stage malignant pleural mesothelioma. Cancer 1994;74:2460–2467.
38. Markman M, Cleary S, Pfeifle C, Howell SB. Cisplatin administered by the intracavitary route as treatment for malignant mesothelioma. Cancer 1986;58:18.
39. Markman M, Howell SB, Green M. Combination intracavitary chemotherapy for malignant pleural disease. Cancer Drug Deliv 1984;1:333.
40. Rusch VW, Figlin R, Godwin D, Piantadosi S. Intrapleural cisplatin and cytarabine in the management of malignant pleural effusions: a lung cancer study group trial. J Clin Oncol 1991;9: 313–319.
41. Rusch VW. Intrapleural chemotherapy for malignant pleural effusion. In: Deslauriers J, Lacquet LK (eds) Thoracic Surgery: Surgical Management of Pleural Diseases. Saint-Louis, Missouri: C.V. Mosby Company, 1990;409–414.
42. Astoul Ph, Viallat JR, Laurent JC, Brandely M, Boutin C. Intrapleural recombinant IL-2 in passive immunotherapy for malignant pleural effusions. Chest 1993;103:209–213.
43. Astoul Ph, Picat-Joossen D, Viallat JR, Boutin C. Intrapleural administration of interleukin-2 for the treatment of patients with malignant pleural mesothelioma, a phase II study. Cancer 1998;15;83(10):2099–2104.
44. Elony Y, King R, Boutin C. Thoracoscopic talc poudrage pleurodesis for chronic recurrent pleural effusions. Ann Int Med 1991;115:778–782.
45. Menzies R, Charbonneau M. Thoracoscopy for the diagnosis of pleural disease. Ann Int Med 1991;114:271–276.
46. Mathur P, Martin WJ. Clinical utility of thoracoscopy. Chest 1992;102:3–4.

Bronchology and Bronchoesophagology: State of the Art.
H. Yoshimura et al., editors.

Utility of medical thoracoscopy in diagnosis and treatment of pleural diseases

Yoshiki Ishii and Takesi Fukuda
Department of Pulmonary Medicine and Clinical Immunology, Dokkyo University School of Medicine, Mibu, Tochigi, Japan

Abstract. We report on our recent practices of medical thoracoscopy performed under local anesthesia in 162 cases. Of 144 patients with pleural effusion, 56 had pleuritis carcinomatosa, 14 had pleuritis tuberculosa, and 10 had malignant mesothelioma. We evaluated the utility of thoracoscopic observation and pleural biopsy in these three diseases. Almost all of the patients with malignant pleural effusion, initially undiagnosed by the cytology of pleural effusion, were diagnosed by thoracoscopy. Thoracoscopy lead to accurate diagnosis especially in the case of malignant mesothelioma. Since medical thoracoscopy under local anesthesia is a rapid, easy, safe, and well tolerated procedure with an excellent diagnostic yield, it is recommended as a diagnostic procedure for cases with pleural effusion. Medical thoracoscopy is useful not only for diagnosis but also for treatment of pleural diseases. We performed thoracoscopic debridment for acute prulent pleuritis under local anesthesia. Early thoracoscopic breakage of loculation and complete drainage resulted in shortening the length of drainage and hospitalization period. No serious complications were observed in the thoracoscopic procedures.

Keywords: acute empyema, malignant mesothelioma, pleural effusion, pleuritis carcinomatosa, pleuritis tuberculosa.

Background

Medical thoracoscopy performed under local anesthesia is a useful agent for diagnosis and treatment of pleural diseases [1,2]. Medical thoracoscopy is defined as thoracoscopy performed under local anesthesia with sedation, usually in an endoscopy suite, by pulmonary physicians, and usually through a single port, for the diagnosis and treatment of pleural diseases. Pulmonologists can, therefore, perform this procedure easily, safely, quickly, and inexpensively. Usually, an indication for medical thoracoscopy is a patient with pleural effusion. We reviewed our recent experiences of medical thoracoscopy performed under local anesthesia in 162 cases and investigated the utility of medical thoracoscopy in the diagnosis for pleural effusions and in the therapy for acute empyema.

Address for correspondence: Yoshiki Ishii MD, Department of Pulmonary Medicine and Clinical Immunology, Dokkyo University School of Medicine, 880 Kitakobayashi, Mibu, Tochigi 321-0293, Japan. Tel.: +81-282-87-2151. Fax: +81-282-86-5080. E-mail: ishiiysk@dokkyomed.ac.jp

Methods

From 1994 to 2000, we performed medical thoracoscopy in a total of 162 cases. The resulting indications are shown in Table 1. Almost all of the indications were diagnoses of pleural effusion and treatment of acute empyema. Major causes of pleural effusion were metastatic malignant pleuritis, malignant mesothelioma, TB pleuritis, and empyema.

Under local anesthesia, a video-thoracoscope was inserted through the single port. We used a newly developed flexi-rigid thoracoscope, XLTF-240, or a video-bronchoscopy. After aspiration of pleural effusion through the suction channel, pleural biopsy was performed with forceps through the suction channel.

Results

The diagnostic sensitivities for three major pleural diseases, metastatic malignant pleuritis, malignant mesothelioma, and TB pleuritis, were 100, 100 and 58.3%, respectively. Seventy percent of metastatic pleural malignancy cases were diagnosed by cytological examination of pleural effusion. Almost all of the cases undiagnosed by thoracentesis were successfully diagnosed by thoracoscopic

Table 1. Indications of medical thoracoscopy under local anesthesia.

1. Pleural effusion	
Pleuritis carcinomatosa	56 cases
primary lung cancer	44
other organ cancer	12
Empyema	19
Tuberculosis	14
Parapneumonic	12
Malignant mesothelioma	10
Meigs syndrome	2
Lymphona	2
Cylothorax	2
Lupus pleuritis	1
Reumatoid arthritis	1
Pancreatitis	1
Lipoma of chest wall	1
Diaphragma herniation	1
Colio-pleural fistula	1
Rounded atelectasis	1
Etiology unknown	20
Subtotal	144 cases
2. Pneumothorax	14
3. Intrapulmonary cavitary lesions	4
Total	162 cases

pleural biopsy.

We found that some kinds of metastatic pleural malignancy showed hardly positive cytology. In our experience, only one out of 11 cases with pleural effusion due to renal cell carcinoma was positive for cytology. In such cases medical thoracoscopy is very useful.

Mesothelioma is one of the best indications for medical thoracoscopy. Of our 10 cases with malignant mesothelioma, only three were positive for cytology. Measurement of hyaluronic acid was of no use. Typical findings were nodular lesions, pleural thickenings and pleural plaques. With the thoracoscopic pleural biopsy, we were able to get sufficient specimens for histological and immunohistochemical examinations, so that diagnosis was made in all cases.

In TB pleuritis, positive rates of smear and culture for TB in pleural effusion are very low. In our case they were less than 10%. Sensitivity of PCR for TB was also poor. Lymphocyte dominance and high ADA levels in pleural effusion were good suggestive indicators of TB pleuritis. Pleural biopsy yielded 58.3% positive for granuloma or acid-fast stain. In our case, thoracoscopic findings and the positive rate of pleural biopsy varied depending on the period of time between the onset of disease and the thoracoscopic examination. When the thoracoscopy was performed within 40 days, 83% of cases showed small nodular lesions on the parietal pleura and biopsies of these lesions were positive. In contrast, when thoracoscopy was undertaken after 40 days, the pleura became thick and nodular lesions disappeared, and the positive rate of pleural biopsy decreased to 33%. These findings suggest that to perform thoracoscopy as early as possible is a very significant and important aspect of a precise diagnosis.

Medical thoracoscopy is useful not only for diagnosis but also for treatment of pleural diseases. In acute empyema, pleural space is rapidly loculated by deposition of fibrin, resulting in multiple compartment formation. In such a situation, drainage may not be successful. We performed medical thoracoscopy to break down the fibrin loculation and to achieve effective drainage. Indication of thoracoscopy is as follows: acute onset empyema, no response to antibiotics, and multiloculated moderate or much effusion. In cases of acute empyema, fibrin loculation, intrapleural abscess were seen. The fibrin septum was easily broken down by forceps. Sometimes localized abscesses appeared. In six cases, good drainage and sufficient lung expansion were obtained by thoracoscopic breakdown of fibrin loculations. However, in three cases, we failed to procure complete drainage because of hard adhesion or peel formation. Finally, these three cases required surgical procedures. In the improved six cases, thoracoscopic drainage was performed within 30 days of onset, whereas in the three failure cases thoracoscopy was performed after 30 days. In success cases the drainage period and hospital stay were significantly shorter than those in the failure cases.

Conclusions

We evaluated the utility of thoracoscopic observation and pleural biopsy in these three diseases. The majority of patients with malignant pleural effusion, initially undiagnosed by the cytology of pleural effusion, were successfully diagnosed by thoracoscopy. Especially in malignant mesothelioma, thoracoscopy allowed accurate diagnosis. Since medical thoracoscopy under local anesthesia is a rapid, easy, safe, and well tolerated procedure with an excellent diagnostic yield, it is recommended as a diagnostic procedure for cases of pleural effusion. We also applied medical thoracoscopy to the treatment of acute empyema. Early thoracoscopic breakage of loculation and complete drainage resulted in shortening the length of drainage and hospitalization time. Thus, medical thoracoscopy is useful not only for diagnosis but also for treatment of pleural diseases.

References

1. Boutin C, Viallat JR, Carginino P et al. Thoracoscopy in malignant effusions. Am Rev Respir Dis 1981;124:588–592.
2. Boutin C, Loddenkemper R, Astoul P. Diagnostic and therapeutic thoracoscopy pulmonary medicine: techniques and indications in pulmonary medicine. Tuber Lung Dis 1993;74: 225–239.

Bronchology and Bronchoesophagology: State of the Art.
H. Yoshimura et al., editors.

What we need to detect very early malignant mesothelioma by thoracoscopy

Kazuhiko Takabe[1], Hikaru Higashinakagawa[1], Kimitake Tsuchiya[1], Toshihiko Fukuoka[1], Yoshibumi Kodaira[1], Yoko Shinohara[1], Shinngo Usui[2], Masaharu Inagaki[2], Naoya Funakoshi[2], Keiko Suzuki[3], Hirotaro Miura[4], Hitomi Ishiwata[5], Hisamasa Akabane[5] and Naohiko Inase[6]

Departments of [1]Internal Medicine, [2]Thoracic Surgery, and [3]Pathology, Tsuchiura Kyodo Hospital, Ibaraki; Departments of [4]Internal Medicine and [5]Pathology, Yokosuka Kyosai Hospital, Kanagawa; [6]Department of Respiratory Medicine, Tokyo Medical & Dental University, Tokyo, Japan

Abstract. Recent reports have described the utility of thoracoscopy for the diagnosis and staging of mesothelioma. However, current therapeutic modalities are usually still incapable of curing even the earliest stage of mesothelioma. To improve the prognosis of mesothelioma, we may have to perform thoracoscopy for high-risk asbestos-exposed patients prophylactically in order to detect early mesothelioma. High asbestos content in pleural plaque and the presence of Simian virus 40 DNA sequences in peripheral blood cells may become useful markers to identify high-risk patients. Moreover, histological analyses of parietal pleura from autopsy cases suggest that premalignant lesions may arise in or near pleural plaque. These studies are likely to extend the role of thoracoscopy in the diagnosis of mesothelioma.

Keywords: asbestos body, mesothelial hyperplasia, pleural plaque, Simian virus 40.

Introduction

Recent reports have described the usefulness of thoracoscopy in the diagnosis and staging of mesothelioma [1,2]. However, even the earliest stage (stage 1a) [3] of mesothelioma can seldom be cured by current therapeutic modalities [4]. To improve the prognosis of mesothelioma, we may have to perform thoracoscopy for asymptomatic asbestos-exposed patients prophylactically in order to detect very early mesothelioma. Since a relatively small proportion of people exposed to asbestos go on to develop mesothelioma [5], it may be necessary to find effective tests to identify high-risk patients in asbestos-exposed populations for this purpose. Our studies suggest that the analyses of asbestos content in pleural plaque and Simian virus 40 (SV40) DNA sequences in peripheral blood cells (PBCs) may become useful markers in the selection of high-risk patients. Given the limited information we have about the morphological manifestation of early

Address for correspondence: Kazuhiko Takabe MD, Department of Internal Medicine, Tsuchiura Kyodo Hospital, 11-7, Manabeshin-machi, Tsuchiura-shi, Ibaraki 300-0053, Japan. Tel.: +81-298-23-3111. Fax: +81-298-23-1160. E-mail: kazu-tak@ka2.so-net.ne.jp mesothelioma and premalignant lesions [6,7], we may also have to establish morphological criteria for them.

Asbestos content in pleural plaque

Although the presence of asbestos bodies and fibers in pleural plaque has been confirmed by several reports [8,9], the asbestos content in pleural plaque of mesothelioma patients has rarely been investigated. In a comparison of the asbestos content (/g of wet tissue) in pleural plaques between seven mesothelioma patients and 14 control subjects matched by lung asbestos body counts, we found that the asbestos content of mesothelioma patients was higher than that of control subjects (asbestos bodies: 482 ± 460 vs. 19 ± 16, $p = 0.123$, uncoated fibers ($5\ \mu \leqslant$) ($\times 10^3$): 254 ± 95 vs. 80 ± 18, $p = 0.078$, Mann-Whitney U test), albeit not to a significant degree. The aspect ratio (length/diameter) of uncoated fibers ($5\ \mu \leqslant$) was significantly higher in mesothelioma patients than in control subjects, though there was no significant difference between the two groups in the aspect ratio of uncoated fibers in lung tissues (pleural plaque: 33.9 ± 3.3 vs. 15.1 ± 8.1, $p < 0.0001$, lung: 35.5 ± 5.3 vs. 35.0 ± 2.7, $p = 0.709$, Mann-Whitney U test). These results suggest that there may be distinct differences between mesothelioma and other asbestos-exposed patients in the number and type of asbestos fibers in the pleural plaque. Hence, the fiber analysis of pleural plaque samples may be useful for the determination of the risk of mesothelioma. When

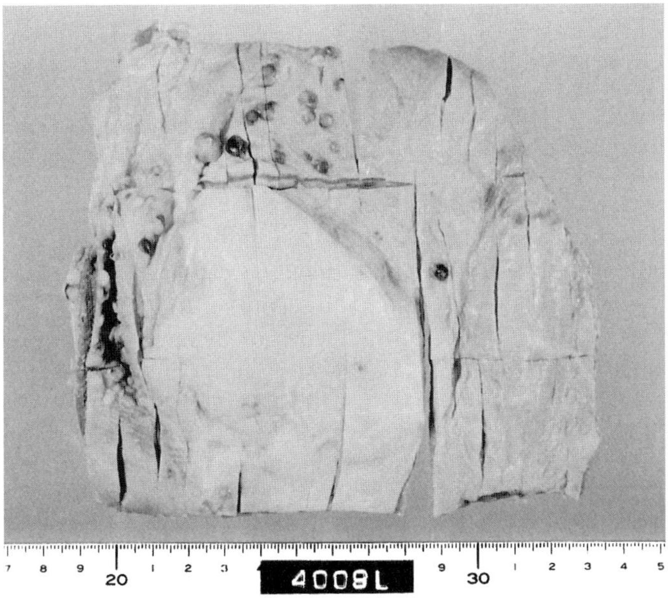

Fig. 1. Gross appearance of a diaphragm with pleural plaque. Pleura was serially sectioned into 10-mm strips and examined by routine light microscopy.

pleural plaque is not present, samples from pleural black spots, a foci of parietal anthracosis defined by Boutin et al. [10], can be obtained during thoracoscopy for fiber analyses.

SV40 DNA sequences in PBCs

Since Carbone et al. first reported the presence of SV40 DNA in mesothelioma in 1994 [11], SV40 DNA sequences have been found in 40 to 60% of mesothelioma patients in the US and several European countries [12,13]. We detected SV40 DNA sequences in 12 out of 18 (67%) Japanese patients with mesothelioma by PCR using primers as reported by Bergsagel et al. [14]. Furthermore, we have analyzed the presence of SV40 DNA sequences in PBCs and demonstrated that these sequences were contained in the PBCs of five out of six mesothelioma patients (83%), in contrast with only 13 out of 73 patients with other diseases (18%) ($p = 0.002$, Fisher's exact test). Although few samples have actually been obtained, SV40 DNA might be positive in the PBCs of mesothelioma patients. If this is the case, asbestos-exposed patients with positive SV40 DNA in the peripheral blood may have an increased risk of mesothelioma.

Establishing morphological criteria for early mesothelioma and premalignant lesions

We obtained the parietal pleural tissues from 48 autopsy cases with pleural plaques and examined them by routine light microscopy (Fig. 1). The features of the mesothelial hyperplasia could be classified into six categories (Fig. 2): cuboidal morphology, 47 cases (98%); multinucleated cells, 15 cases (31%); stratification, 25 cases (52%); papillary projection, 28 cases (58%); submesothelial infiltration into connective tissue, 15 cases (31%); and submesothelial infiltration into plaque, 20 cases (42%). We compared the frequency of each hyperplasia with lung and pleural asbestos content and the presence of pleural effusion. The cases with asbestos bodies in plaque demonstrated a significantly higher frequency of submesothelial infiltration into plaque than the cases without them (75 vs. 30%, $p = 0.008$, χ test), though asbestos bodies in the lung (>100/g of wet tissue) did not increase the frequency of any types of hyperplasia. It was also found that the frequency of submesothelial infiltration into connective tissue was significantly higher when pleural effusions (>100 ml) were present at the time of autopsy (42 vs. 14%, $p = 0.007$, χ test). These results suggest that submesothelial infiltration into plaque may relate to the pleural asbestos burden and the development of mesothelioma. Furthermore, some hyperplastic lesions (Figs. 3 and 4) can probably be differentiated from early mesothelioma or premalignant lesions by recent molecular biological techniques.

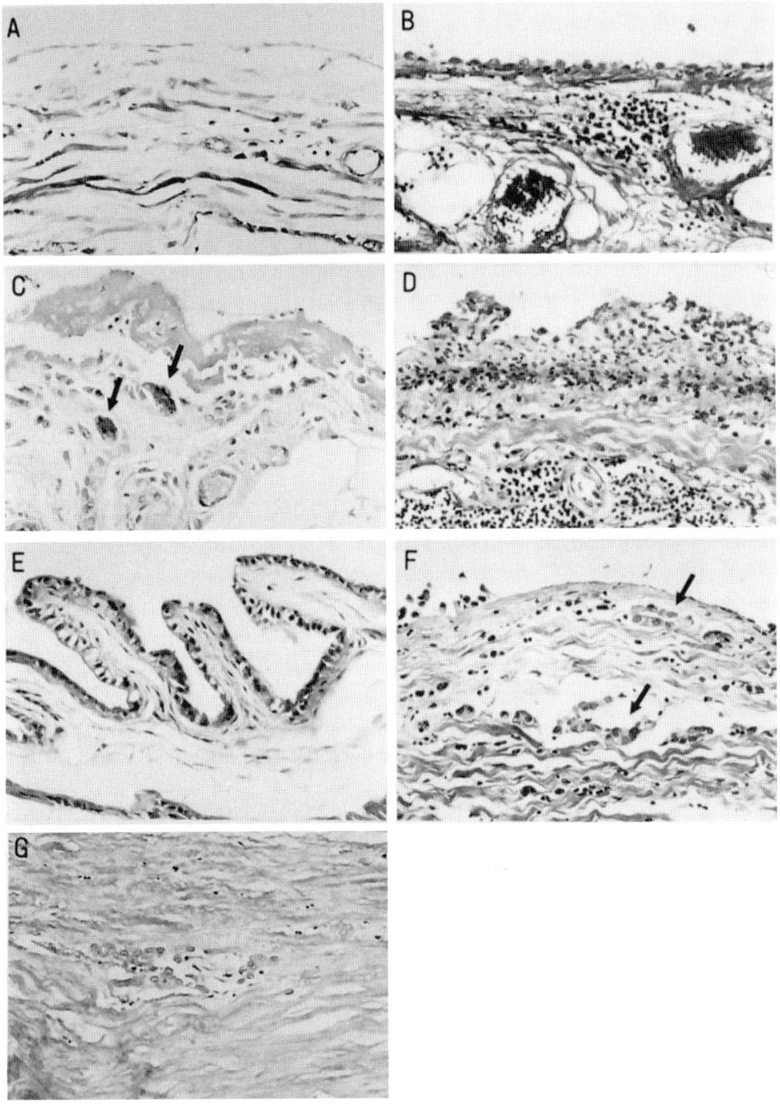

Fig. 2. Classification of mesothelial hyperplasia (H and E stain, × 200). **A:** Normal mesothelial cells. **B:** Cuboidal morphology. **C:** Multinucleated cells (arrows). **D:** Stratification. **E:** Papillary projections. **F:** Submesothelial infiltration into connective tissue (arrows). **G:** Submesothelial infiltration into plaque.

Conclusion

High asbestos content in pleural plaque and the presence of SV40 DNA sequences in PBCs may become useful markers to identify asbestos-exposed patients at a high risk of developing mesothelioma. Histological analyses of pari-

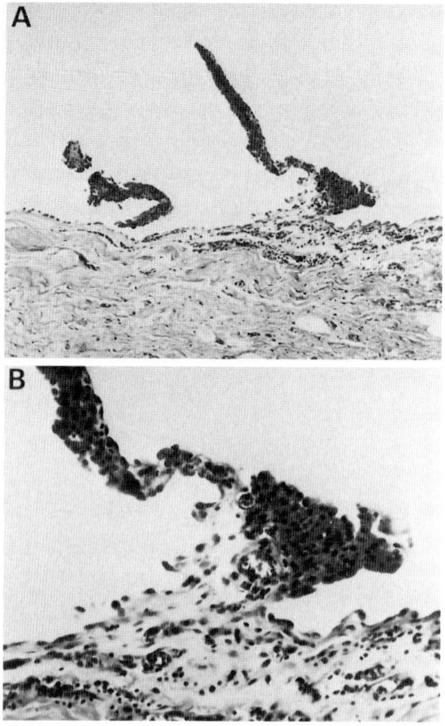

Fig. 3. A 79-year-old man. Died of pneumonia. Solid mesothelial cell proliferation is seen on a surface of the parietal pleura (H and E stain). **A:** × 200. **B:** × 400.

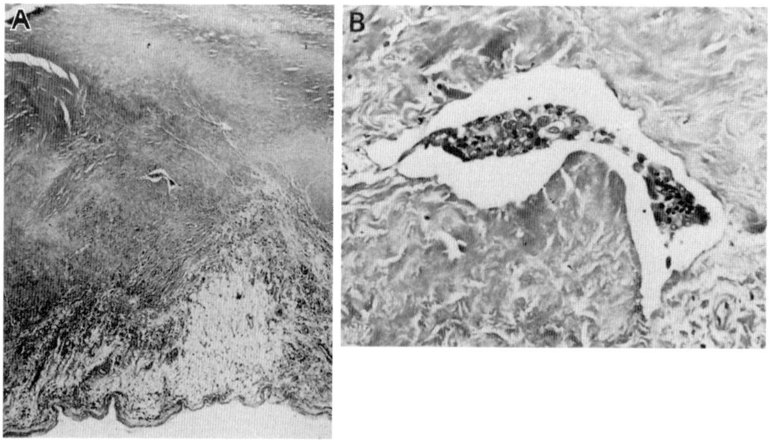

Fig. 4. An 85-year-old man. Occupation unknown. Died of pneumonia. Postoperative from bladder cancer; with no evidence of recurrence at the time of autopsy. A cluster of atypical mesothelial cells is seen in a plaque (H and E stain). Immunostaining for low molecular weight cytokeratins (CAM 5.2) showed immunoreactivity within some atypical cells (figure not shown). **A:** × 200. **B:** × 400.

etal pleura from autopsy cases suggest that premalignant lesions may arise in or near pleural plaque. These studies will extend the role of thoracoscopy in the diagnosis of mesothelioma in the future.

Acknowledgements

This work was partially supported by the 1993 Okinaka Research Fund and the 1998 Ibaraki Cancer Research Fund.

References

1. Page RD et al. Thoracoscopy: a review of 121 consecutive surgical procedures. Ann Thorac Surg 1989;48:66–68.
2. Boutin C et al. Thoracoscopy in pleural malignant mesothelioma: a prospective study of 188 consecutive patients. Part 1: diagnosis. Cancer 1993;72:389–393.
3. International mesothelioma interest group. A proposed new international TNM staging system for malignant pleural mesothelioma. Chest 1995;108:1122–1128.
4. Boutin C et al. Thoracoscopy in pleural malignant mesothelioma: a prospective study of 188 consecutive patients. Part 2: prognosis and staging. Cancer 1993;72:394–404.
5. Hillerdal G. Pleural plaque and risk for bronchial carcinoma and mesothelioma. Chest 1994;105:144–150.
6. Sheldon CD, Herbert A, Gallagher PJ. Reactive mesothelial proliferation. A necropsy study. Thorax 1981;36:901–905.
7. Whitaker D, Henderson DW, Shilkin KB. The concept of mesothelioma in situ: implications for diagnosis and histogenesis. Sem Diagn Pathol 1992;9:151–161.
8. Rosen P et al. Ferruginous bodies in benign fibrous pleural plaques. Am J Clin Pathol 1973;60: 608–617.
9. Dodson RF et al. Asbestos content of lung tissue, lymph nodes, and pleural plaques from former shipyard workers. Am Rev Respir Dis 1990;142:843–847.
10. Boutin C et al. Black spots concentrate oncogenic asbestos fibers in the parietal pleura. Thoracoscopic and mineralogic study. Am J Respir Crit Care Med 1996;153:444–449.
11. Carbone et al. Simian virus 40 like DNA sequences in human pleural mesothelioma. Oncogene 1994;9:1781–1790.
12. Pepper C et al. Simian virus 40 large T antigen (SV40LTAg) primer specific DNA amplification in human pleural mesothelioma. Thorax 1996;51:1074–1076.
13. Mayall FG et al. Mutations of p53 gene and SV40 sequences in asbestos associated and non-asbestos-associated mesotheliomas. J Clin Pathol 1999;52:291–293.
14. Bergsagel DJ et al. DNA sequences similar to those of Simian virus 40 in ependymomas and choroid plexus tumors of childhood. N Engl J Med 1992;326:988–993.

Dysphagia

Bronchology and Bronchoesophagology: State of the Art.
H. Yoshimura et al., editors.

Prevention of dysphagia after surgery for oral or oropharyngeal cancer in elderly patients

Yasushi Fujimoto, Yasuhisa Hasegawa, Bin Nakayama and Hidehiro Matsuura
Department of Head and Neck Surgery, Aichi Cancer Center, Nagoya, Japan

Abstract. *Background.* To prevent postsurgical dysphagia in oral or oropharyngeal cancer patients, crico-pharyngeal myotomy and laryngeal suspension are recommended, however, the criteria that determine this course of action remain controversial. We extended the criteria for crico-pharyngeal myotomy and laryngeal suspension for elderly patients (over 60-years-old), to also include those who received a hemiglossectomy (including tongue base) and extended resection of the oropharynx.

Patients and Methods. In order to verify the new indication and criteria, we examined two groups (group A, 15 cases, from June 1994 to September 1996; group B, eight cases, from October 1996 to November 1998) with both videofluorography and ability to sustain an oral diet. Upon determining the new criteria, group B patients received crico-pharyngeal myotomy and laryngeal suspension.

Results. In group A, two patients could not sustain an oral diet, but all the patients could in group B. In videofluorography, there was decreased aspiration in group B than in group A. We also noticed much residual bolus in the pyriform sinus in some patients in group A.

Conclusions. A crico-pharyngeal myotomy and a laryngeal suspension can contribute to the prevention of postsurgical dysphagia in elderly patients.

Keywords: crico-pharyngeal myotomy, laryngeal suspension, videofluorography.

Introduction

Dysphagia after surgical procedures carried out on advanced oral or oropharyngeal cancers not only hinders a patient's quality of life, but can also be a life-threatening problem. To prevent postsurgical aspiration pneumonia, a crico-pharyngeal myotomy and laryngeal suspension are recommended, however, the criteria that determine this course remain controversial [1,2].

Excluding surgery, aging is one of the most important factors in the onset of dysphagia [3]. The occurrence of this condition in elderly patients could indicate a muscle defect related to age or could be due to a neurogenic process. With aging, we can see reduced laryngeal movement, the lowering of the larynx in the neck, cervical arthritis, reduction in the strength of pharyngeal constriction, and pharyngeal delay. We can then deduce that elderly patients have a reduced swallowing ability reserve. Our earlier study showed a strong correlation between age and pharyngeal delay. The onset of upper esophageal sphincter opening was delayed in elderly patients after oral or oropharyngeal resection, thus suggesting

Address for correspondence: Yasushi Fujimoto, Department of Head and Neck Surgery, Aichi Cancer Center Hospital, 1-1 Kanokoden, Chikusa, Nagoya 464-8681, Japan. Tel.: +81-52-762-6111. E-mail: yasushif@land.linkclub.or.jp a higher risk of postoperative dysphagia [4].

Before 1996, we opted for crico-pharyngeal myotomy and laryngeal suspension when it was thought that patients would lose the mechanisms needed to elevate the larynx or to produce oropharyngeal pressure [5]. Because of concern about the effect of aging on swallowing ability, we extended the criteria for crico-pharyngeal myotomy and laryngeal suspension for elderly patients (over 60-years-old) in 1996. This paper will discuss our new set of criteria.

Patients and Methods

In this paper, we categorized a wide resection in which we recommended crico-pharyngeal myotomy and laryngeal suspension as type 1. This includes total or subtotal glossectomy with bilateral resection of suprahyoid muscles, or a wide resection of the oropharynx including tongue base. Resection larger than one-half of mobile tongue but smaller than a type 1 resection was categorized as type 2, in which case we were able to preserve the contralateral suprahyoid muscles. From June 1994 to November 1998, we operated on 23 elderly patients (over 60-years-old) with a type 2 resection. We categorized the patients from June 1994 to September 1996 as group A (15 cases), and the patients from October 1996 to November 1998 as group B (eight cases). Upon defining the new criteria, group B patients received crico-pharyngeal myotomy and laryngeal suspension. In order to verify the new indication, we examined both groups by videofluorography and the ability to sustain an oral diet. Videofluorography was carried out just after the wound had healed, using 5 ml of liquid barium. Severity of aspiration and residue in the pyriform sinus was compared between the two groups. Aspiration was defined as the entry of liquid into the trachea below the vocal folds. "Severe aspiration" was classified as more than one-half of the bolus flowing into the trachea. Residue in the pyriform sinus was classified as follows: "normal" meaning no stasis; stasis that can be cleaned up after a dry swallow as "slight stasis"; a little stasis after repetitive dry swallow as "moderate stasis"; and a lot of stasis after repetitive dry swallow as "severe stasis".

Results

Out of the patients in group A, 85% (11/13) of patients could successfully withstand an oral diet later, but only 13% (2/15) of patients could swallow without aspiration immediately following surgery, and 33% had moderate or severe aspiration (Fig. 1). However, all the patients in group B could sustain an oral diet, and no patients had severe aspiration. Figure 2 shows residue in the pyriform sinus. We could identify 87% (13/15) of the patients in group A with moderate or severe residue in the pyriform sinus after swallowing, whereas there were no patients with severe stasis in the pyriform sinus in group B.

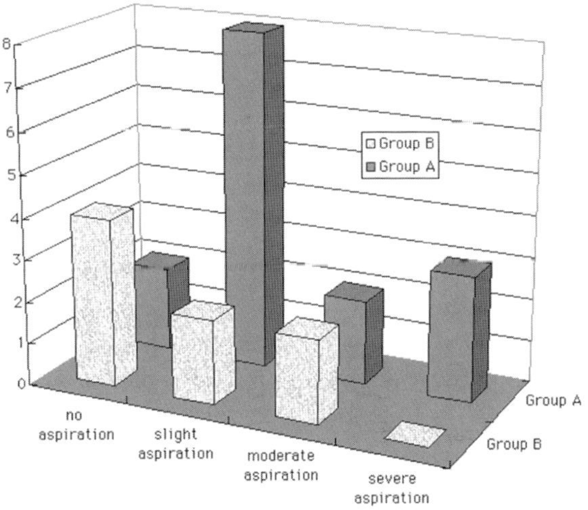

Fig. 1. Severity of aspiration.

Discussion

Residue in the pyriform sinus means that an inappropriate opening of the upper esophageal sphincter has reduced anterior laryngeal motion or reduced swallowing pressure of the oropharynx, both of which cause aspiration after swallowing. The length of laryngeal elevation and posterior movement of the tongue base was reduced after a tongue resection with neck dissection. Usually these difficulties are compensated by the contralateral side structures, but in elderly patients

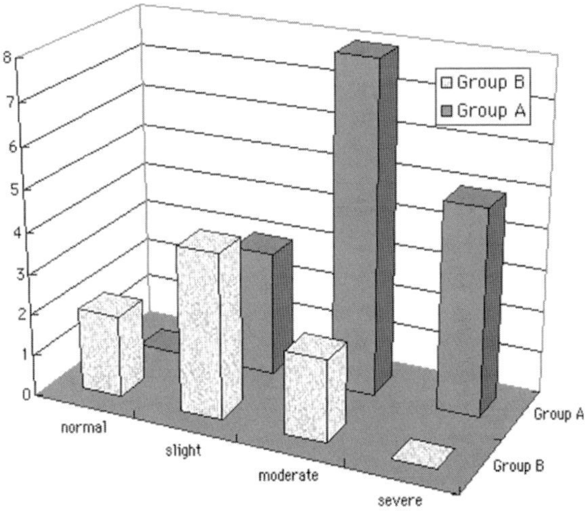

Fig. 2. Residue in the pyriform sinus.

this will sometimes take more time and effort. The laryngeal suspension method is added not only to support elevation of the larynx to close the airway, but also to contribute to the upper esophageal sphincter opening. With the crico-pharyngeal myotomy, we can make the upper esophageal sphincter open wider.

Thus, we changed our strategy after 1996. We opted for crico-pharyngeal myotomy and laryngeal suspension when we planned type 2 resection for patients over 60-years-old. Compared with our former criteria (group A), we were able to treat postoperative patients more safely and all patients could achieve an oral diet in group B. A crico-pharyngeal myotomy and a laryngeal suspension can contribute to the prevention of postsurgical dysphagia in elderly patients. The procedure allows for improved maintenance, safer rehabilitation, a reduced risk of pneumonia, and a shorter hospital stay for the patient.

References

1. Mladic RA, Horton CE, Adamson JE. Cricopharyngeal myotomy: application and technique in major oral-pharyngeal resections. Arch Surg 1971;102:1–5.
2. Tiwari RM. Total glossectomy: reconstruction and rehabilitation. J Laryngol Otol 1989;103: 917–921.
3. Kaneko I. A cinefuluorographic study of hyoid bone movement during deglutition. J Otolaryngol Jpn 1992;95:974–987.
4. Fujimoto Y, Hasegawa Y. Analysis of swallowing reflex after surgery for oral and oropharyngeal cancer. XVI World Congress of Otorhinolaryngology Head and Neck Surgery. 1997;239–243.
5. Fujimoto Y, Hasegawa Y. Usefulness and limitation of cricopharyngeal myotomy and laryngeal suspension after wide resection of the tongue or oropharynx. J Otolaryngol Jpn 1998;101: 307–311.

Bronchology and Bronchoesophagology: State of the Art.
H. Yoshimura et al., editors.

Treatment package of dysphagia in a semiconscious epileptic case

Leili Hayati
Department of Speech and Language Pathology, University of Rehabilitation Sc., Teharn, Iran

Abstract. A 16-year-old boy with a history of epilepsy lost consciousness 13 months back. He was discharged from hospital 6 months later, with near-normal internal conditions, in a semiconscious state, and feeding through a feeding tube.

The dysphagia treatment started 13 months after the epileptic attack, with the end goal of the treatment being the case's ability to sustain oral feeding. The treatment package included: A. Phase I – Sensory awareness: i) Touch, ii) Thermal; Phase II - Increase sensory input: i) More bolus flavors, ii) Type of bolus, iii) Volume of bolus, iv) Viscosity; B. Movement: i) Head position, ii) Chin position, iii) Reduce spasm in head and neck region.

The package outlined above helped us to increase the case's sensory awareness by manipulation of his sensation thresholds. Through the use of this package the range of his motion increased, including reflexes absent at the time of starting treatment which returned. Moreover, after 6 months of treatment the case could withstand oral food intake.

Keywords: bolus, sensory integration, swallowing.

Introduction

The normal human swallowing operation is comprised of a number of different actions which are used systemically in different contexts and which all result in moving food, liquid, saliva, etc., from the mouth to the stomach [1,2]. Swallow types differ in the strength of muscle activity and the range of motion of various neuromotor events comprising the swallow action. The exact sensory stimulus needed to trigger a pharyngeal swallow is not known. It is clear, however, that deeper proprioceptive receptors in the tongue, posterior oral cavity and pharynx are involved [3,4]. The different branches of the nine and 10 cranial nerves carry this sensory information to the nucleus tractus solitarius in the medulla and to the cortex. Tongue motion is also an important part of sensory input overall. When tongue motion is changed due to neural or structural damage, the patient will experience a delay in triggering the pharyngeal swallow, since the stimulation of the deeper proprioceptive receptors by tongue movement is altered and the pattern of sensory input to the cortex and brainstem will have changed. The nature of peripheral sensory stimuli is also important and to be considered.

Address for correspondence: Leili Hayati, Department of Speech and Language Pathology, University of Rehabilitation Sc., Avin Kodak yar St. PC. 19834, Teharn, Iran. Tel.: +98-21-6436203. Fax: +98-21-6436203. E-mail: ls.hayat@jamejam.net

Methods

A longitudinal study of a 16-year-old boy in a semiconscious state due to an epileptic attack which occurred 13 months back. He had lost many of his physical and mental system functions. When I started working with him he was using a feeding tube and was also suction-dependent. In the oral assessment we observed that: respiration was through the mouth only; the tongue was constantly pressed against the hard palate (this was visible in that damage to the soft tissue of hard palate could be seen); no chewing or biting was seen; spasmodic reflexes were observed, but no gag reflex was seen.

First in the process we worked at stimulating the tongue. By stimulating the tongue and facilitating head and neck movement through indirect swallowing therapy (by means of resistance and facilitation exercises), the range of motion of the lips, tongue and jaw increased. Other exercises were designed to increase sensory input. We used thermal therapy in which icing was applied to the face and the oral cavity. Tactile therapy included tapping on the face and faucial arch. We also gradually used more flavorful boluses (e.g., sour boluses). "Head back" and "chin down" postural techniques were used to eliminate aspiration or residue resulting from the swallowing disorder (Table 1).

Results

After 1 month the gag reflex was observed once more, and subsequently the use of suction for the removal of mucous in oral cavity was discontinued. An increase in the range of motion of the tongue, jaw and lips was observed, and control of extra movement and spasm was achieved (Figs. 1 and 2).

Discussion

Sensory integration (SI) as a theory has been in use for the last two decades. It is used for clients with neuromuscular dysfunction developmental delay and sensory impairment. SI is a form of information processing. In cases where neurodevelopmental lags occur, a programme that structures the environment and uses sensory input, motor output and sensory feedback techniques is believed to

Table 1. Successful postural techniques to eliminate aspiration or residue resulting from various swallowing disorders.

Disorder observed on fluoroscopy	Posture applied if aspiration occurs	Rational for postural technique effectiveness
1. Inefficient oral transit	- Head back position	- Utilizes gravity to clear oral cavity
2. Delay in triggering the pharyngeal swallow	- Chin down position	- Narrows air way entrance[a]

[a]Reproduced from [5].

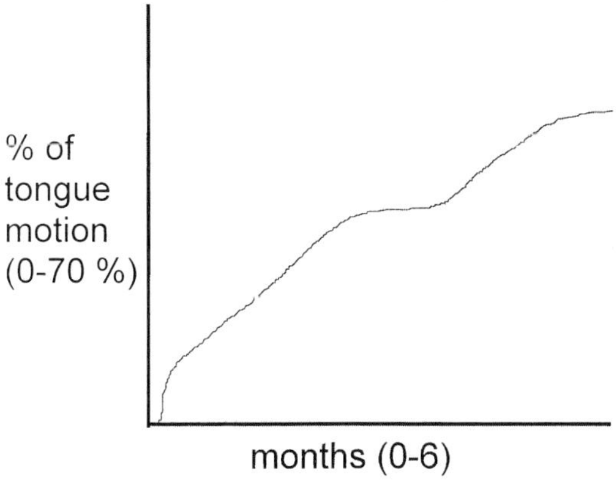

Fig. 1.

influence neural organization, and hence facilitate maturation [6]. Postural techniques are the first stage in the management of oropharyngeal dysphagia. In 50% of cases these techniques can effectively eliminate aspiration. If postural techniques do not promote the patient's swallowing action, increased sensory input may be utilized or in some cases these two techniques applied together will further ameliorate the client's condition. Increased sensory input is designed to alert the central nervous system prior to the swallowing action. This increased sensory input can take the form of the introduction of larger, more viscous or flavorful boluses, thermal/tactile stimulation, or a suck-swallow action prior to the placement of food in the mouth. Another technique employed is to rub a cold plastic tongue blade on the anterior faucial arch where both tactile and thermal receptors lie [7,8]. Swallowing therapy is designed to actually change the swallow physiology [9]. Swallow therapy is either carried out directly with food in the mouth, or indirectly with only saliva. Indirect swallowing techniques are utilized

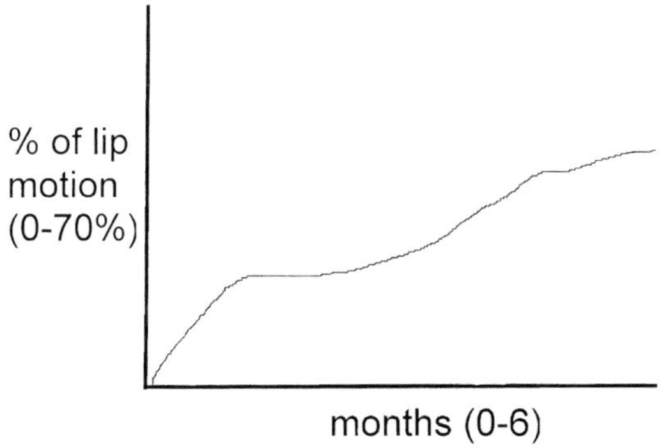

Fig. 2.

when the client is having difficulty with aspiration or significant residue. As for the gag reflex, in this case it was imperative to protect the pharynx from vomit.

Acknowledgements

I am indebted to my client and his family, especially his mother for her great help and assistance. The same goes to the University of Rehabilitation Sc., especially the Speech and Language Pathology Department and the IT section.

References

1. Logemann JA. A manual for video fluoroscopic evaluation of swallowing, 2nd edn. Austin: Pro-Ed, 1993.
2. Palmer JB, Rudin NJ, Lara G, Crompton AW. Coordination of mastication swallowing. Dysphagia 1992;7:187–200.
3. Larson CR. Neurophsiology of speech and swallowing. Sem Speech Lang 1985;6:275–291.
4. Miller AJ. The search for clarity. Dysphagia 1993;8:185–194.
5. Shanahan TK, Logemann JA, Rademaker AW, Pauloski BR, Kahrials PJ. Chin down posture effects on aspiration in dysphagic patients. Arch Phys Med Rehab 1993;74:736–739.
6. Ziviani J, Poulsen A, Obrien A. Effect of a sensory integration/neurodevelopmental programme on motor and academic performance of children with learning disabilities. Austr J Occup Ther 1982;29(910):27–33.
7. Doty RW. Neural organization of deglutition. In Code CF (ed) Handbook of physiology: alimentary canal. Washington: Am Physiol Soc, 1986;1861–1902.
8. Storey A. A functional analysis of sensory units innervating epiglottis and larynx. Exp Neurol 20;366–383.
9. Logemann JA. Evaluation and treatment of swallowing disorders. Austin: Pro-Ed, 1983.

Early cancer of the esophagus

Bronchology and Bronchoesophagology: State of the Art.
H. Yoshimura et al., editors.

Place of radiotherapy and chemoradiotherapy for superficial esophageal carcinoma

Satoshi Ishikura[1] and Atsushi Ohtsu[2]
[1]*Radiation Oncology Division and* [2]*Gastrointestinal Oncology/Gastroenterology Division, National Cancer Center Hospital East, Kashiwa, Japan*

Abstract. *Purpose.* In Japan, the number of patients discovered to have superficial carcinoma of the esophagus has been increasing, mainly due to the prevalence of endoscopic examinations with Lugol's iodine solution. Surgery has been a standard treatment, and endoscopic mucosal resection (EMR) has an established role for certain selected patients with superficial carcinoma confined to the mucosa. The purpose of this paper is to clarify the role of radiotherapy with or without concurrent chemotherapy.

Methods and Results. We reviewed literature reporting the nonsurgical approach to superficial carcinoma of the esophagus. There were only a few retrospective studies that reported the results of radiotherapy alone with 5-year disease-specific survival rates of more than 90% for tumors confined to the mucosa and around 70% for tumors invading the submucosa. Concurrent chemoradiotherapy has proven to be superior to radiotherapy alone in a recent clinical randomized trial. Some reports also suggest that the results of concurrent chemoradiotherapy are comparative in survival and superior in quality of life to surgery.

Conclusions. Radiotherapy alone may be the alternative to surgery but not to EMR. Concurrent chemoradiotherapy has potential to be the standard treatment for superficial carcinoma of the esophagus and it should be confirmed by prospective trial.

Keywords: combined modality therapy, endoscopic mucosal resection (EMR), organ-preserving therapy, surgery.

Introduction

Recent advances in the diagnosis of esophageal carcinoma by endoscopy with Lugol's iodine solution have led to early detection of the tumor. Endoscopic mucosal resection (EMR) has established a role for itself concerning selected patients with tumors confined to the mucosa [1], because these tumors have a low probability of lymphnode metastasis [2–6] and need local treatment only, and the 5-year overall survival rate is around 90% [1,2]. However, surgery is still a standard treatment for superficial tumors if EMR is not applicable. Surgery has 5-year overall survival rates of around 90% for tumors confined to the mucosa and around 50 to 60% for tumors invading the submucosa [3–6]. The purpose of this report is to clarify the role of radiotherapy and concurrent

Address for correspondence: Satoshi Ishikura MD, Radiation Oncology Division, National Cancer Center Hospital East, 6-5-1 Kashiwanoha, Kashiwa 277-8577, Japan. Tel.: +81-471-33-1111. Fax: +81-471-31-4724. E-mail: sishikur@east.ncc.go.jp chemoradiotherapy as an organ-preserving therapy in the treatment of superficial carcinoma of the esophagus.

Definitive radiotherapy without chemotherapy

We reviewed literature reporting the nonsurgical approach to superficial carcinoma of the esophagus. Definitive radiotherapy without chemotherapy has been used mainly for medically inoperable patients due to morbidity, senility, etc., and there are only a few retrospective reports with a limited number of patients. Okawa et al. [7] reported the results of a retrospective analysis with 105 cases of superficial carcinoma of the esophagus treated by definitive radiotherapy with or without intracavitary brachytherapy. The depth of tumor invasion was assessed mainly by endoscopy and barium swallow except for some cases where endoscopic ultrasonography was used. In 37 out of 105 patients, the precise depth of tumor invasion was unknown. They only included those who completed the planned radiotherapy, and the indication of intracavitary brachytherapy was not clearly mentioned. Nemoto et al. [8] reported the results of a retrospective analysis with 78 cases of superficial carcinoma of the esophagus, treated definitively by external beam radiotherapy alone. The depth of tumor invasion was determined more accurately by endoscopic ultrasonography in 34 patients, however, it was unknown in 44 of 78 patients. According to these reports, the 5-year disease-specific survival rate for tumors confined to the mucosa seems to be more than 90% and the 5-year overall and disease-specific survival rates for tumors invading the submucosa seem to be around 40% and 70% (Table 1).

These results suggest that definitive radiotherapy without chemotherapy may be an alternative to surgery as an organ-preserving therapy, however, less invasive EMR should be considered first, if applicable.

Table 1. Radiotherapy for superficial esophageal carcinoma.

Author	Depth of invasion	Number of patients	Radiotherapy dose (Gy)	5-year survival (%)	
				Disease-specific	Overall
Okawa et al.	m	15		100	NA
	sm	53		68.5	NA
	unknown	37			
	total	105	66 (mean)	71.0	38.7
Nemoto et al.	m	6		NA	100
	sm	28		NA	45
	unknown	44			
	total	78	65.5 (mean)	NA	45

m = mucosa; sm = submucosa; and NA = not available.

Table 2. Results of RTOG 85-01.

Treatment	Number of patients	Severe toxicity (%)	Survival		
			Median (months)	2-year (%)	5-year (%)
RT	62	28	9.3	10	0
CMT	61	64	14.1	36	26

CMT = combined modality therapy.

Concurrent chemoradiotherapy

In a recent clinical randomized trial of RTOG 85-01 [9], concurrent chemoradiotherapy was compared to radiotherapy alone. In this trial, patients with T1 through to T3 tumors, classified by the 1983 AJCC-TNM staging system, without evidence of distant metastasis were included. The combined modality therapy consisted of four courses of cisplatin and fluorouracil with concurrent radiation at 50 Gy in 25 fractions over 5 weeks. The radiotherapy alone, was delivered at 64 Gy in 32 fractions over 6.5 weeks. The results showed the superiority of chemoradiotherapy over radiotherapy alone (Table 2). There are some reports showing the effectiveness of concurrent chemoradiotherapy. Murakami et al. [10] also suggested that the results of concurrent chemoradiotherapy were comparative in survival and superior in quality of life to surgery, however, the advantage of chemoradiotherapy for superficial esophageal carcinoma has not been confirmed due to the limited number of patients.

Conclusions

Radiotherapy alone may be the alternative to surgery but not to EMR, for tumors confined to the mucosa. Concurrent chemoradiotherapy has potential to be the standard treatment of superficial carcinoma of the esophagus and it should be confirmed by prospective trials. In addition to this, further investigation concerning optimal combination of radiotherapy and chemotherapy including new cytotoxic agents is also necessary for further improvement of the outcome.

References

1. Kodama M, Kakegawa T. Treatment of superficial cancer of the esophagus: a summary of responses to a questionnaire on superficial cancer of the esophagus in Japan. Surgery 1998; 123:432–439.
2. Yoshida M et al. Endoscopic mucosal resection for radical treatment of esophageal cancer (in Japanese). Gan To Kagaku Ryoho 1995;22:847–854.
3. Ide H et al. Esophageal squamous cell carcinoma: pathology and prognosis. World J Surg 1994; 18:321–330.
4. Nishimaki T et al. Tumor spread in superficial esophageal cancer: histopathologic basis for

rational surgical treatment. World J Surg 1993;17:766–771.
5. Sugimachi K et al. Long-term results of esophagectomy for early esophageal carcinoma. Hepatogastroenterology 1993;40:203–206.
6. Kato H et al. Superficial esophageal carcinoma: surgical treatment and the results. Cancer 1990;66:2319–2323.
7. Okawa T et al. Superficial esophageal cancer: multicenter analysis of results of definitive radiation therapy in Japan. Radiology 1995;196:271–274.
8. Nemoto K et al. Treatment of superficial esophageal cancer by external radiation therapy alone: results of a multi-institutional experience. Int J Radiat Oncol Biol Phys 2000;46:921–925.
9. Cooper JS et al. Chemoradiotherapy of locally advanced esophageal cancer: long-term follow-up of a prospective randomized trial (RTOG 85-01). JAMA 1999;281:1623–1627.
10. Murakami M et al. Comparison between chemoradiation protocol intended for organ preservation and conventional surgery for clinical T1-T2 esophageal carcinoma. Int J Radiat Oncol Biol Phys 1999;45:277–284.

Bronchology and Bronchoesophagology: State of the Art.
H. Yoshimura et al., editors.

Differentiation of esophageal cancer of m3·sm1 from sm2·sm3 by EUS

Teruo Kouzu[1], Etsuo Hishikawa[1], Keitaro Nakao[2], Yasuo Suzuki[2] and Shinichi Miyazaki[2]
[1]Department of Endoscopic Diagnostics and Therapeutics and [2]Second Department of Surgery, Chiba University School of Medicine, Chuo-ku, Chiba, Japan

Abstract. It is mandatory to have a confident diagnosis for an extension of indication of endoscopic mucosal resection. From the standpoint of endoscopic ultrasonography (EUS) using a high-frequency ultrasound probe, it is important to scan as perpendicularly as possible in order to visualize the esophageal wall having at least nine layers. It is also important to confirm the deepest point of invasion by moving the probe over the whole area of the lesion of interest under endoscopic control. It is crucial to interpret subtle grayscale changes, visualized as a low-echoic areas. This is useful in order to be able to differentiate mass from cysts, esophageal glands, or blood vessels. It is especially necessary to recognize the lymph follicles, usually found in the lamina propria, in superficial esophageal carcinoma.

A tip to use, when trying to differentiate m3·sm1 from sm2·sm3, is to focus on the existence of the 3/9 layer of the muscularis mucosae during a high-frequency-probe EUS.

Keywords: endoscopic ultrasonography (EUS), muscularis mucosae, superficial esophageal carcinoma.

Introduction

As the interest in esophageal cancers has increased, efforts to detect superficial esophageal carcinoma, as a mucosal cancer, have been made, resulting in a rapid increase in cases. The main reason for this is the fact that there is no such lesion as esophageal cancer that has various degrees of invasiveness depending on surgical procedures to be applied. In other words, there are certain differences between the invasiveness of esophagectomy accompanied by lymphadenectomy in the third region and endoscopic mucosal resection (EMR), which has led to the prevalence of endoscopy and X-Ray diagnosis as the methods to detect cancers in their early stages.

The authors have been diagnosing esophageal carcinoma using endoscopic ultrasonography (EUS) since the beginning of the 1980s. The differentiation of sm1 from sm2·sm3 is a very important issue being discussed with regard to the expansion of indication of EMR. In this chapter we investigate the issue from the standpoint of EUS based on our experience. It is not necessary to mention the

Address for correspondence: Teruo Kouzu, Department of Endoscopic Diagnostics and Therapeutics, Chiba University School of Medicine, 1-8-1 Inohana, Chuo-ku, Chiba 260-8677, Japan. Tel.: +81-43-226-2331. Fax: +81-43-226-2368.

importance of both the detailed classification of esophageal carcinomas based on the extent of submucosal invasion and the analyses of the differences [1] between m and sm invasion in the frequencies of lymph node metastasis or infiltration into the vessels, since this should greatly influence the management of them.

EUS recognition of the layer structure visualized

It is most important, when using EUS, to be able to interpret the layer structure of the esophageal wall, visualized by the ultrasound waves. Our interpretation of the layer structures, visualized as having seven layers when using 7.5 MHz and having nine and 11 layers when using 20 MHz, are shown as schematics in Fig. 1. It is necessary to recognize that the layer structures visualized using 7.5 MHz are different from those visualized when using 20 MHz in the third layer towards the surface [2]. This same interpretation has been made by Kawano et al. [3]. We have proposed a common terminology or description. For the sake of easier understanding, we have been emphasizing that the layer structure visualized can be descibed as a fraction, with the total number of layers being the denominator and the numerator representing the layer in question [4].

Our interpretation of the layer structure visualized when using 20 MHz linear scanning is shown in Fig. 2. It is necessary to understand that there are boundary echoes sandwiching each layer. Based on our interpretation, we show typical images of m1 to m2, m3 to sm1, and sm2·sm3 invasion in Fig. 3. In case of m1·m2 invasion, the lesion is not visualized and there is usually no observed change in the layer structure. Whereas in case of sm2·sm3 invasion, the submucosal layer to be visualized as high echoic has a low-echoic infiltration.

Good image visualization in EUS

When using EUS, it is important to know how to obtain good images of the lesion of interest. It is essential to develop techniques how to retain water in the esophagus. In cases accompanied by hiatal hernias, it is useful to use a cardiac

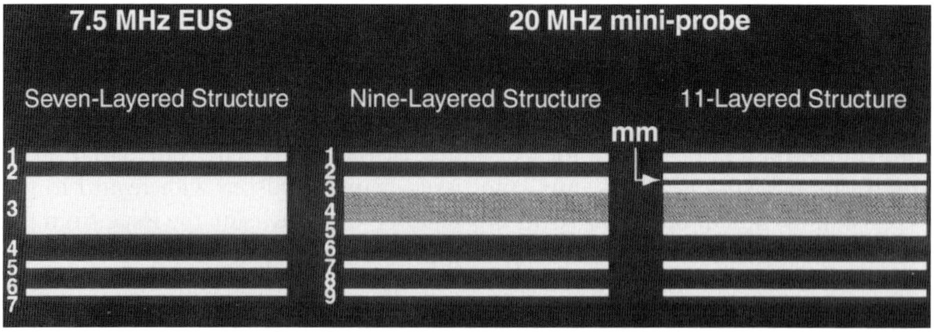

Fig. 1. The interpretation of an EUS image of the schematics of a normal esophageal wall.

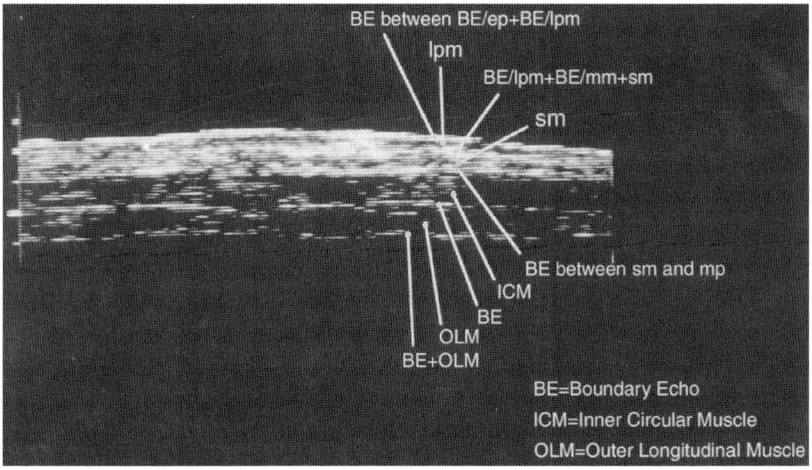

Fig. 2. The interpretation of a normal esophageal wall visualized by linear scanning using a high-frequency probe.

balloon to dam water at the cardia [5]. A two-channel endoscope and soft balloon have been used to retain water efficiently, and recently this multipurpose balloon

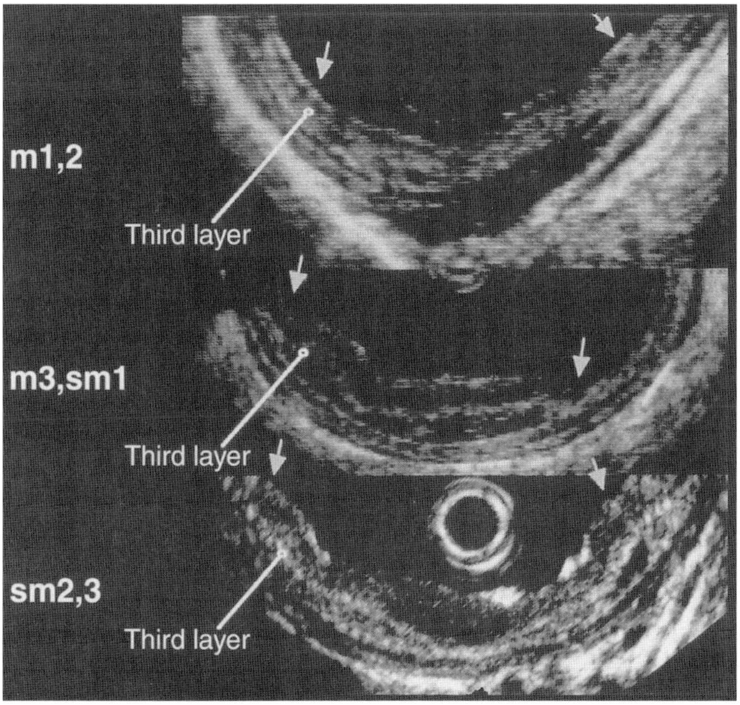

Fig. 3. EUS images visualizing various different invasion depths.

method has been used practically. As shown in Fig. 4, a panendoscope mounted with a multipurpose balloon is functionally converted into a two-channel scope. In case of difficulty in retaining water around the area of interest, it is recommendable to change in the posture of the patient from the left-lateral-supine position to the right one. Furthermore, it is important to select a suitable probe, which corresponds with the morphology of the lesion. Probes of 12, 15, 20 and 30 MHz are now commercially available. By and large, the authors have been using probes of 15 and 20 MHz for 0-I type lesions and flat 0-II type lesions, respectively.

Interpretations made based on our experiences of sm1, sm2 and sm3

In Japan, it has been suggested that the differentiation of m3 from sm1 is very difficult, even when making the most of precise X-Ray diagnosis [6], endoscopy [7], and pathology [8] at a time when the diagnostic consensus criterion for sm1 has been established to such a precise degree, i.e., the infiltration range 200 μmm from the muscularis mucosae. This means that the difference in infiltration between the two is pinpoint. We, therefore, decided to consider m3 and sm1 to be one group and instead investigated the depth invasion of sm1 and sm2·sm3. We selected five cases of well visualized lesions for the investigation of each invasion depth of m3·sm1 and sm2·sm3.

As described earlier, since the number of the layers visualized are different in each case, we have used the fraction description method to discuss the layer in question.

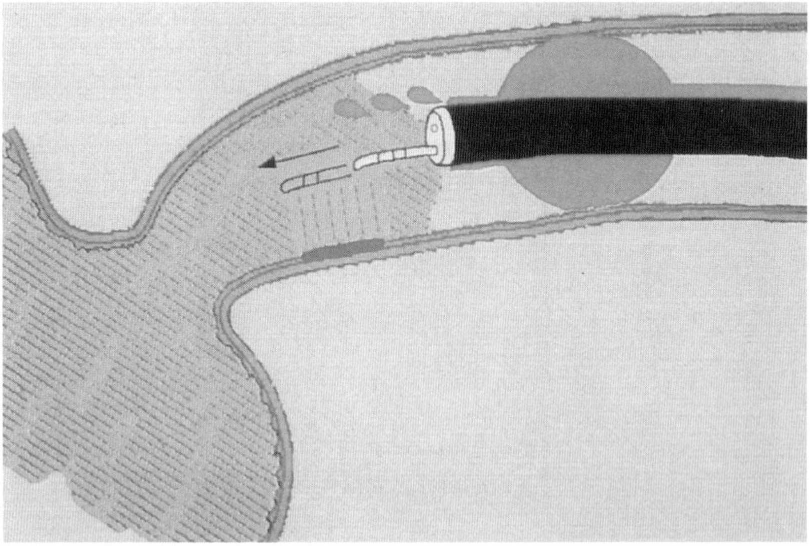

Fig. 4. A panendoscope loaded with a multipurpose balloon.

We were able to visualize 80% of layer 3/9, which included the muscularis mucosae layer. In the case of m3·sm1, a thickened area was observed toward the mucosa and in the case of sm2·sm3, a low-echoic area was observed beneath the 3/9 layer. Although low-echoic areas were observed beneath the 3/9 layer for two of the five m3·sm1 cases, because they are different from the low echoes of tumors, their echo levels could be judged as cystic lesions or blood vessels in the submucosa.

In a case with partial infiltration into the submucosa, a lot of lymph follicles were found in the lamina propria.

An actual interpretation of EUS findings

Case 1 (Fig. 5). This was a IIc lesion with a smooth depressed surface. The endoscopic finding was mucosal cancer. High-frequency-probe EUS visualized a low-echoic irregular area beneath the 3/9 layer. This echo-level change was much lower than that of the upper layer. It is very important to recognize that there are grayscale changes even in the same low-echo level. Histology revealed that the ectatic blood vessels in the submucosal layer were located beneath the m3 lesion, which was a reflection of the difference in echo levels.

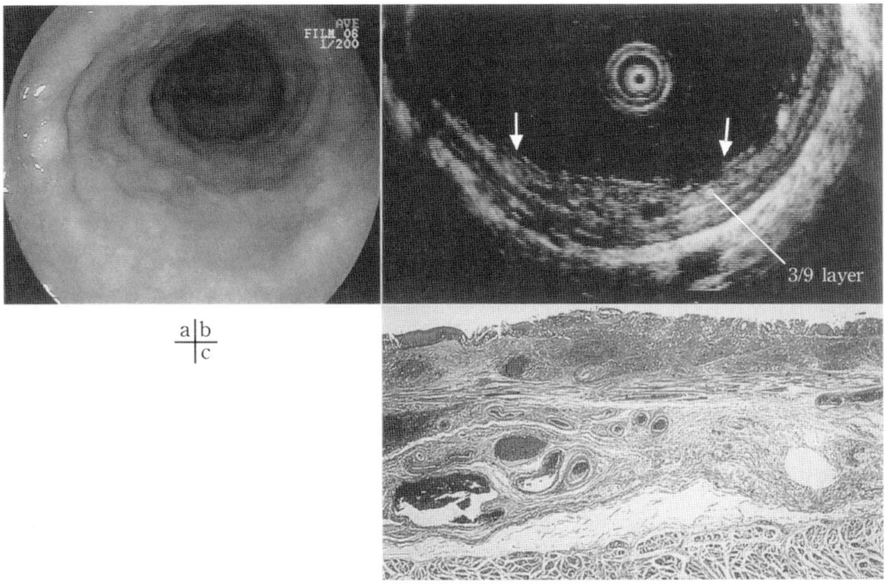

Fig. 5. **A:** A IIc lesion with a flatly depressed surface. **B:** The arrows depicts the mass. The low-echoic section can be observed in the submucosal layer. **C:** The depth of invasion was m3. Ectatic blood vessels can be observed.

%Differentiating m3·sm1 from sm2·sm3 in EUS

As pointed out earlier, it is crucial to visualize nine layers, at least, in high-frequency-probe EUS by placing the probe perpendicularly when a scanning is performed.

A whole lesion should be scanned by exploring the spread of the lesion under endoscopic control, in order to detect its deepest invasion.

It is also important to differentiate subtle changes in echo levels in areas which seemingly have a uniform echo level. This is useful when trying to differentiate between cystic lesions, esophageal glands or blood vessels. It is also important to be able to recognize lymph follicles in the lamina propria in higher frequencies, especially in superficial carcinomas.

In the case of high-frequency EUS, it is important to recognize the 3/9 layer by deliberate interpretation of the surrounding tissues visualized.

Conclusion

Today, the detection rate of esophageal mucosal carcinomas in the aged has rapidly increased. In compliance with this situation, an indication expansion of EMR, as the less invasive treatment, is under investigation in Japan.

Until now, m1·m2 invasion was always the indication of EMR. However, the expansion of this, to m3·sm1, is now mandatory in order to differentiate the latter from sm2·sm3 invasion. We investigated this issue from the standpoint of the importance of EUS images for confident diagnoses.

References

1. Kodama M, Kakegawa T. Summary report on questionnaires on treatment of superficial esophageal cancer - The 49th esophageal disease research meeting. J Soc Jap Surg 1996;97: 683–690.
2. Morikawa O, Kouzu T, Arima M et al. Radial scanning in the esophagus using the high-frequency ultrasound probe-investigation of the depth of invasion of superficial esophageal cancer. Abdom Imag Diagn 1994;604–614.
3. Kawano T, Nagai K, Inoue H et al. EUS in m3·sm1 esophageal cancer. Stomach and Intestine 1998;33:969–974.
4. Kouzu T, Arima M. EUS (invasion depth and lymph node metastasis). J Jap Bronchol 1999;50: 292–297.
5. Kouzu T. Basics of EUS in the esophagus. Stomach and Intestine 1997;32:191–194.
6. Yamaki G, Okura Y, Nagahama T et al. X-ray diagnosis of m3·sm1 esophageal cancer. Stomach and Intestine 1998;33:949–960.
7. Hoshihara Y, Yamamoto K, Hashimoto M. Endoscopy of m3·sm1 esophageal cancer. Stomach and Intestine 1998;949–960.
8. Okura Y, Nakajima H, Yamaki G et al. Pathology in m3·sm1 esophaeal cancer. Stomach and Intestine 1998;33:975–984.

Bronchology and Bronchoesophagology: State of the Art.
H. Yoshimura et al., editors.

Esophagectomy with extended lymphadenectomy for superficial esophageal cancer

Harushi Udagawa[1], Kenji Tsutsumi[1], Yoshihiro Kinoshita[1], Toyohide Nakamura[1], Masaki Ueno[1], Hiroshi Akiyama[1] and Masahiko Tsurumaru[2]
[1]Department of Surgery, Toranomon Hospital, Tokyo, Japan; [2]First Department of Surgery, Juntendo University, Tokyo, Japan

Abstract. *Background.* Advances in endoscopic mucosal resection (EMR) have made possible the local removal of superficial esophageal cancer. Therefore, the results of radical surgery should be reviewed in order to develop clear criteria for the appropriate selection of therapeutic measures in individual cases.

Methods. The clinical and pathological data on 168 patients who underwent esophagectomy with three-field lymphadenectomy (3FD-esophagectomy) at Toranomon Hospital from 1984 to 1999 were reviewed to identify the limits of EMR and the indications for extended radical esophagectomy in patients with superficial thoracic esophageal cancer.

Results. The hospital death rate after 3FD-esophagectomy was 3.0%. Factors indicating a poorer prognosis, i.e., nodal involvement, lymph vessel infiltration, blood vessel infiltration, and recurrence, were not detected in patients with lamina propria mucosae (lpm) or shallower tumors. Some of these factors were positive in more than 40% of patients with muscularis mucosae tumors, while the rate was 90% for cancers with massive submucosal invasion. The disease-specific 5-year survival rates in pTNM stages IVa and IVb were 83.3 ± 15.2% and 53.3 ± 17.6%, respectively.

Conclusion. EMR is a sufficiently curative procedure for lpm or shallower tumors. For deeper lesions, 3FD-esophagectomy should be the standard surgical procedure, and it achieves favorable results even in stage IV patients.

Keywords: endoscopic mucosal resection, recurrent laryngeal nerve, three-field lymphadenectomy.

Introduction

The development of endoscopic mucosal resection (EMR) has made it technically possible to completely remove superficial cancers of the esophagus without surgery as long as the lesion has not invaded the proper muscle layer. However, some superficial cancers do have lymph node metastasis, and local treatment is not sufficient for cure in such cases. The aim of this study was to review the results of our standard radical surgical procedure and develop a set of criteria to select appropriately between EMR and surgery in individual cases.

Address for correspondence: Harushi Udagawa MD, F.A.C.S., Chief of Gastroenterological Surgery, Toranomon Hospital 2-2-2, Toranomon, Minato-ku, Tokyo 105-8470, Japan. Tel.: +81-3-3588-1111. Fax: +81-3-3582-7068. E-mail: udagawah@tora.email.ne.jp

Materials and Methods

The subjects were 168 consecutive patients with superficial thoracic esophageal cancer who underwent esophagectomy with three-field lymphadenectomy (3FD-esophagectomy) at Toranomon Hospital between 1984 and 1999. The clinical features of the subjects are shown in Table 1. Patients with preoperative adjuvant therapy were excluded. More than 90% of the subjects had squamous cell carcinoma. Their clinical and histopathological data were investigated to clarify the limits of EMR in this group of patients, as well as to assess the short- and long-term results of 3FD-esophagectomy.

Results

In this series of 168 patients, the average number of dissected lymph nodes per patient was 114, with a range from 61 to 222. The average number of metastatic nodes was 0.9 and the maximum was 13. The hospital death rate after 3FD-esophagectomy was 3.0%. There were five hospital deaths, occurring between 2 and 188 days following the operation. Three of the deaths occurred in early patients treated before 1990. Two died because of severe tracheobronchial ischemia, which is avoided at present by preservation of the right bronchial artery, and the other hospital death before 1990 was caused by severe pneumonia. One of the two hospital deaths after 1990 was due to postoperative pulmonary thromboembolism, which is also effectively prevented at present by continuous pneumatic massage of the calves. The most recent hospital death was due to massive hemorrhage caused by sudden postoperative appearance of circulating anticoagulant factor.

The factors closely related to a poorer prognosis, i.e., nodal involvement, lymph vessel infiltration, blood vessel infiltration, and clinical recurrence, were investigated. The occurrence rates of these factors are listed in Table 2.

Table 1. Clinical features of the 168 subjects.

Histopathological dx.		Main tumor location		Depth of invasion		pTNM stage	
Dx.	No. of cases	Location	No. of cases	Depth	No. of cases	Stage	No. of cases
Squamous cell	155	Upper	31	ep	7	0	7
Adeno.	5	Middle	102	lpm	8	I	103
Adenosquamous	2	Lower	35	mm	23	IIb	39
Adenoid cystic	2			sm1	23	IVa	9
Basaloid	2			sm2	50	IVb	10
Mucoepidermoid	1			sm3	57		
Mal. melonoma	1						

ep: epithelium; lpm: lamina propria mucosae; mm: muscularis mucosae; sm1, sm2, sm3: Japanese subclassification of submucosal invasion (shown in [1]).

Table 2. Histopathological and clinical factors relating to a poor prognosis.

Depth of invasion	Histopathological and clinical factors (% of subjects)				
	n+	ly+	v+	rec+	any+
ep	0	0	0	0	0
lpm	0	0	0	0	0
mm	17	30	17	4	44
sm1	39	26	35	4	74
sm2	32	54	64	12	86
sm3	51	56	65	21	90

n+: positive lymph node metastasis; ly+: positive lymph vessel infiltration (from [1]); v+: positive blood vessel infiltration (from [1]); rec+: clinically identified recurrence; any+: one or more of these factors was positive.

Disease-specific survival curves stratified by tumor depth and pTNM-stage are shown in Figs. 1 and 2. The overall 5-year survival rate of the 168 subjects (including all causes of deaths) was 74.7 ± 3.8%, and the mean survival period was 10.5 ± 0.6 years.

The relationship between tumor location and lymph node metastasis is shown in Table 3. Metastasis in nodes along the thoracic duct occurred at a rate of 2.0% (three out of 153 patients with mm or deeper tumors).

Discussion

We started to use 3FD-esophagectomy as our routine surgical procedure for thoracic esophageal cancer in 1984. Although there were several problems, the

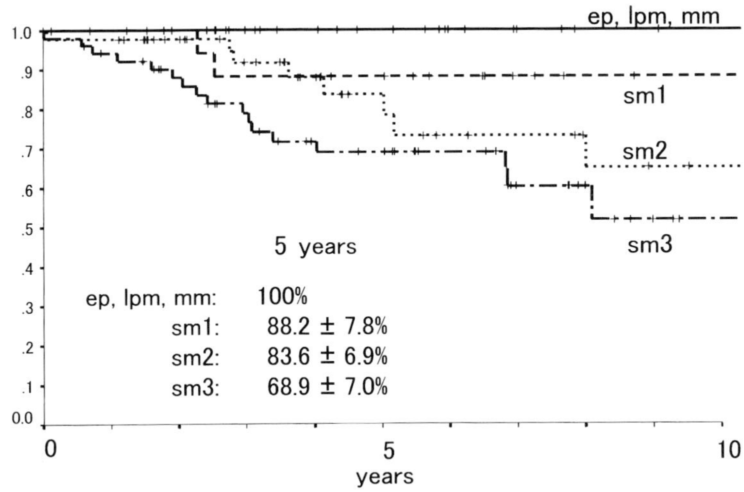

Fig. 1. Disease-specific survival curves stratified by tumor depth.

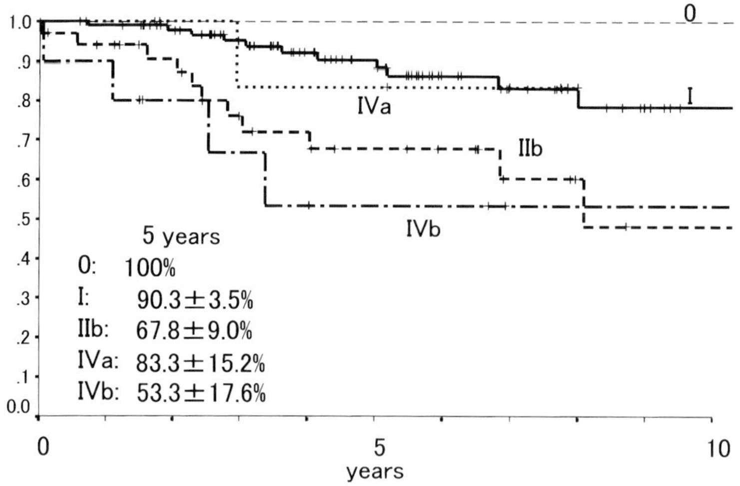

Fig. 2. Disease-specific survival curves stratified by pTNM stage.

short-term results obtained were satisfactory, and we now consider this operation to be an acceptable standard therapeutic measure. The most important part of this procedure is the thorough and meticulous clearance of lymph nodes in the superior mediastinum including the nodes along the bilateral recurrent laryngeal nerves [2,3].

The accumulated data on 3FD-esophagectomy provide us with detailed and reliable information on the pattern of tumor spread. According to our results, it is clear that EMR is sufficiently curative for lpm or shallower tumors. However, once a tumor invades beyond lpm, lymph node metastasis can occur, and the number of poor prognostic factors increases rapidly until it reaches 90% for cancers with massive submucosal invasion. It should be noted that 12.4% of our 153 sub-

Table 3. Tumor location and lymph node metastasis.

Site of metastasis	mm or deeper tumors limited to:		
	Upper esophagus	Middle esophagus	Lower esophagus
No. of cases	18	59	19
Cervical	4 (22%)	5 (8%)	0 (0%)
Upper mediastinal	4 (22%)	9 (15%)	1 (5%)
Middle thoracic	0 (0%)	1 (2%)	1 (5%)
Lower mediastinal	0 (0%)	1 (2%)	5 (26%)
Paragastric	1 (6%)	3 (5%)	7 (37)
Celiac[a]	0 (0%)	1 (2%)	0 (0%)

Tumors located in two or more esophageal regions are excluded. [a]Celiac: lymph nodes along the common hepatic artery and the proximal half of the splenic artery are included.

jects with mm or deeper tumors were classified as stage IV by the pTNM system.

The long-term result of 3FD-esophagectomy is favorable. The survival of pTNM stage IVa patients is no worse than that of stage IIb patients after this procedure, and even stage IVb patients have a 5-year survival rate higher than 50%.

Several small modifications can be made to the 3FD-esophagectomy procedure without decreasing its curability rate. The celiac nodes can be left alone when the tumor is located in the upper esophagus, and neck dissection can be safely omitted for a superficial tumor in the lower esophagus. A more significant modification is preservation of the thoracic duct. The thoracic duct is removed in our standard procedure, but lymph node metastasis along the duct is quite rare in patients with superficial cancer. Thoracic duct preservation makes the operation much safer because it prevents a dramatic postoperative decrease of the circulating plasma volume.

The long-term outcome following a 3FD-esophagectomy is favorable, but still requires improvement. We consider that postoperative adjuvant chemotherapy is effective [4], and the results shown here were obtained with very active postoperative adjuvant therapy for n-positive patients. However, we have to further clarify and define the criteria used in the selection of patients for adjuvant treatment, as well as for determining the mode and timing of adjuvant therapy. Reliable indicators for this purpose are needed, which we lack now.

There are many new options for the treatment of superficial esophageal cancer. Video-assisted surgery, sentinel node navigation surgery, and nonsurgical treatment with chemo-radiation are all under investigation for clinical application. These methods are attractive in terms of individualizing treatment and preserving a patient's quality of life, but many uncertainties need to be clarified and refined, and more technical advances are required before their indications can be precisely determined.

Superficial esophageal cancer is not identical to early cancer. Any tumors with mm or deeper invasion should be regarded as potentially advanced cancer with possible lymph node involvement. The most reliable treatment for these tumors is still some method of esophagectomy with extended lymphadenectomy, such as 3FD-esophagectomy.

References

1. Japanese Society for Esophageal Diseases. Guide Lines for the Clinical and Pathologic Studies on Carcinoma of the Esophagus, 9th edn. Tokyo: Kanehara, 1999.
2. Akiyama H. Surgery for Cancer of the Esophagus. Baltimore: Williams and Wilkins, 1990; 19–42.
3. Akiyama H, Udagawa H, Kirk RM. Oesophageal cancer. In: Kirk RM (ed) General Surgical Operations, 4th edn. London: Harcourtbrace (In press).
4. Udagawa H, Tsurumaru M, Ono Y, Kajiyamaaa Y, Matsuda M, Suzuki M, Watanabe G, Akiyama H. Evaluation of Adjuvant Therapy for Esophagectomy with Collo-Thoraco-Abdominal Lymph Node Dissection. In: Nabeya K, Hanaoka T, Nogami H (eds) Recent Advances in Diseases of the Esophagus. Tokyo: Springer-Verlag, 1992;884–890.

Gastroesophageal reflux

Bronchology and Bronchoesophagology: State of the Art.
H. Yoshimura et al., editors.

Gastroesophageal reflux disease and otolaryngologic manifestations: use of videofluorography

Eugenio Fiorentino[1], Giovanni Pantuso[1], Filippo Barbiera[2], Gianfranco Cupido[3], Riccardo Speciale[3] and Salvatore Restivo[3]
Departments of [1]Surgery, [2]Radiology, and [3]Otolaryngology, University School of Medicine, Palermo, Italy

Abstract. *Background.* The aim of this study is to evaluate the appropriateness of videofluorography (VFG) in otolaryngologic patients with symptoms of suspected gastroesophageal reflux-related (GER) origin.

Methods. 151 consecutive patients underwent esophageal VFG following a clinical ENT examination. These patients had pharyngo-laryngeal symptoms of uncertain etiology such as chronic cough, hoarseness, throat clearing, globus sensation and voice changes.

Results. There were anatomical and/or functional disorders of the esophagus and gastroesophageal junction such as sliding hiatal hernia (HH), episodes of barium reflux, and decreased esophageal clearing occurring in the vast majority of patients: HH 81%, GER 75%. Given certain necessary lifestyle changes in the patient, prolonged acid suppression with higher doses of proton pump inhibitors (PPI) and prokinetics agents was the pharmacologic treatment of choice. In 3 months 86% of the controlled patients showed a significant improvement of otolaryngologic symptoms thereby proving the causal relationship between reflux and symptoms.

Conclusions. In our opinion in all cases of chronic aspecific pharyngo-laryngitis VFG is the diagnostic test most favorably accepted by patients, and is even more useful in confirming the relationship between GERD and otolaryngologic symptoms if used in association with the so-called "PPI test".

Keywords: chronic cough, gastroesophageal reflux, hiatal hernia, hoarseness, videofluorography PPI test.

Introduction

Gastroesophageal reflux disease (GERD), which is the consequence of the retrograde flow of gastric contents into the esophagus with an abnormal acid exposure of the esophageal mucosa, can include typical symptoms of heartburn and acid regurgitation, as well as ear-nose-throat (ENT) symptoms such as chronic cough, hoarseness, throat clearing or dysphonia [1,2]. Currently, it is widely accepted that with the onset of otolaryngologic manifestations of GERD, proximal and distal esophageal 24 h pH monitoring [2,3] and endoscopic examination are reliable methods to first confirm the relationship between GER and symptoms, and to also diagnose hiatal hernia and/or esophagitis via the latter. Videofluorography can be used additionally in order to detect morphological and functional

Address for correspondence: Eugenio Fiorentino MD, University of Palermo - Policlinico Universitario, Via Biagio Petrocelli 12, 90142 Palermo, Italy. Tel.: +39-0339-378-3375.

alterations in GERD [4]. In our department it has been used as a first test, in conjunction with a therapeutic trial with proton pump inhibitors (PPI), when GERD was suspected. The aim of this study is to evaluate the pertinency of VFG in patients where GERD was suspected to be the cause of prevailing pharyngo-laryngeal symptoms and, with diagnosis relying mainly on this test, to evaluate the preliminary results after 12 weeks of a specific antireflux medical treatment with PPI in order to prove the causal connection between reflux and symptoms. The 1-year results will be available at the end of the study.

Materials and Methods

Patients

In order to test the hypothesis that some ENT disorders of uncertain etiology are associated with occult and/or intermittent GERD, 151 consecutive otolaryngologic patients with suspected GER-related pharyngo-laryngeal symptoms were evaluated over a 1-year period. All patients in the study were referred to the Unit for Diagnosis and Treatment of Esophageal Diseases for esophageal evaluation and then to the Department of Radiology for a VFG. The study sample was comprised of 151 patients (52% women and 48% men) with a mean age of 49.7 years (range from 18 to 84 years old).

History

All patients had been referred by otolaryngologists because of throat symptoms associated with no physical findings of specific chronic pharyngo-laryngitis, ranging from loss of the normal glistening appearance to redness, iperemia and edema of the pharyngeal and laryngeal mucosa and/or vocal cords. The presence of typical GER-related symptoms such as heartburn and/or acid regurgitation was also noted.

Videofluorography

All patients underwent barium esophageal VFG as the only diagnostic test. The VFG was carried out with patients standing and then lying recumbent with a bolster under the upper abdomen. No other provocative test or Trendelenburg position was used. Evaluations were made for reflux of barium from stomach into the esophagus, hiatal hernia and esophageal body motility abnormalities.

Treatment

The treatment of choice was a prolonged acid suppression therapy with PPI [5], constituting pantoprazole 40 mg twice a day for 8 weeks and then once daily for 4 weeks, along with prokinetics, such as cisapride, 10 mg twice a day before meals for 12 weeks. All patients were requested to alter certain lifestyle habits: to elevate the head of the bed, to remove fats, chocolate and excessive alcohol from the diet, to have three meals a day with no snacks in between and to have the last meal of the day several hours before sleep. After 2 weeks of therapy the patients were contacted by telephone to evaluate if the treatment suited them and then seen for the initial follow-up evaluation, by the same interviewers, after 12 weeks of treatment.

Follow-up

A follow-up evaluation after 3 months was carried out on 74% (112/151) of patients placed on antireflux treatment. Symptomatic improvement was considered as evidence of a response to antireflux therapy and was based on a nominal scale where: 4 = excellent, 3 = good, 2 = fair, 1 = no change and 0 = worsening of symptoms, as proposed by Schantz et al. [6] (Table 1).

Results

All patients had one or more of the otolaryngologic symptoms shown in Fig. 1. Globus pharingeus, referring to a foreign body or a lump sensation in the throat, was present in more than one-half of patients, and was the most frequent manifestation of pharyngoesophageal motor dysfunction. However, cervical dysphagia, referring to food sticking in the throat, had the lowest rate. Persistent chronic cough and chronic throat clearing, especially noted by patients when first getting up in the morning, were the most frequent symptoms of pharyngo-laryngeal mucosa inflammation, whereas throat burning and hoarseness had a lower rate. In 10% of cases nocturnal apnea prevailed as a symptom of pulmonary aspiration. Of the study sample, only 73% of patients had esophageal symptoms of acid regurgitation and/or heartburn, 27% had no esophageal symptoms and only throat symptoms as a manifestation of the disease. Acid regurgitation was more frequent than heartburn and this was more frequently seen than eructation. Eighteen percent of the patients complained about an exacerbation of symptoms when recumbent (Fig. 2).

Nineteen percent of patients had a completely normal VFG result. Hiatal hernia was seen in 81% of cases, reflux in 75% and dysmotility in 33% (Fig. 3).

Table 1.

Scale	Response	Definition
0	Worsening	Symptoms worse than before therapy
1	No change	Symptoms are the same as before therapy
2	Fair	Some improvement in symptoms but still a major complaint
3	Good	Symptoms are improved to the point of being tolerable but still noticeable
4	Excellent	Symptoms are totally resolved

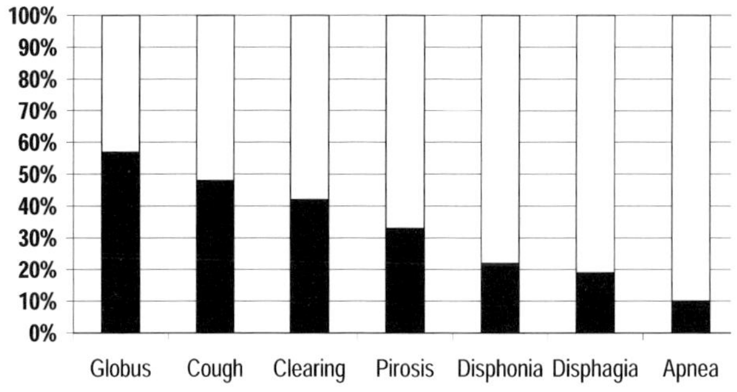

Fig. 1. ENT symptoms rate.

Nineteen patients had an endoscopy after VFG and in all the VFG finding was confirmed: 18 abnormalities (HH and/or reflux and/or esophagitis) and one completely normal. After 3 months 112 out of 151 patients (74%) were re-evaluated. Figure 4 summarizes the response to initial medical antireflux treatment: 85.5% (95/112) of patients showed a fair or good improvement, or a complete resolution of their symptoms, and 14.2% (17/112) of patients had worsening symptoms or exhibited no change. Among the patients with an improvement or resolution of symptoms, 86% (82/95) had hiatal hernia, 86% (82/95) had reflux, and 6% had no abnormalities at VFG (Fig. 5).

Discussion

Our data confirm that 73% of patients with otolaryngologic manifestations of GERD have esophageal symptoms, and in 27% of cases with no regurgitation and/or heartburn a high index of suspicion is essential to look for the relationship between GERD and throat symptoms. When GERD is very likely or suspected, prolonged esophageal pH monitoring with probes in the distal and

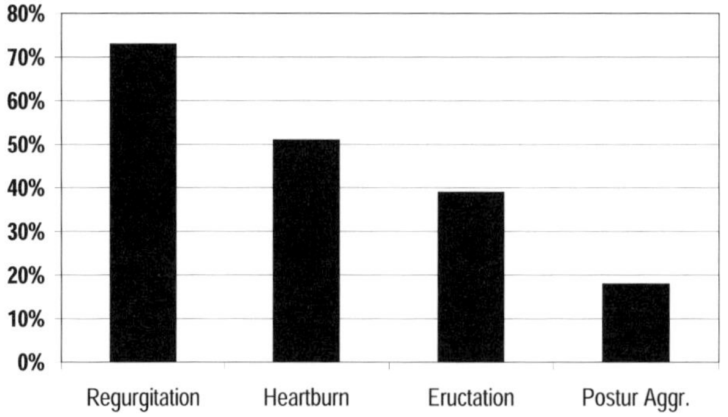

Fig. 2. GERD symptoms rate in ENT patients.

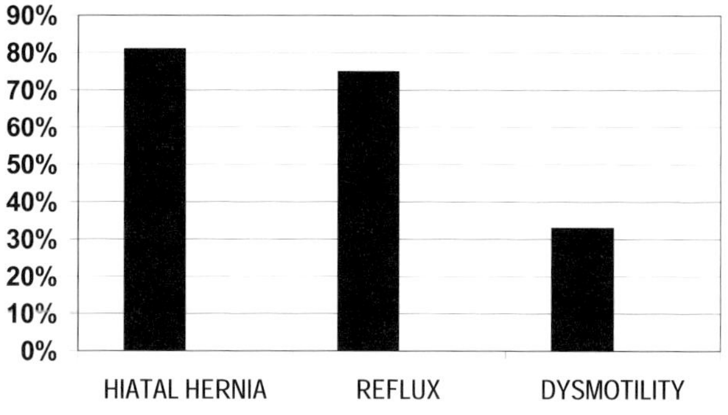

Fig. 3. HH and GER rate in ENT patients.

proximal esophagus, as well as an esophageal endoscopy should be indicated as the most helpful diagnostic tests. However, 24 h pH monitoring and endoscopy are unfavorably accepted by patients due to the invasiveness of these methods. We have subsequently used VFG in otolaryngologic patients with suspected GERD because it is not invasive and is much more widely available, hence much better received by patients. In our experience VFG proved to be a good diagnostic test in detecting the esophageal abnormality as HH (81%) and/or GER (75%) causing the abnormal acid exposure of the pharyngo-laryngeal mucosa. In the small group of patients having an endoscopy as well (19/151) the endoscopy results consistently confirmed the videofluorographic diagnosis thus demonstrating the satisfactory accuracy of this test. In our opinion the PPI therapeutic trial results with 85.8% (95/112) of improvement in symptoms or complete resolution along with the higher HH and/or GER rate in the same patients (86%: 82/95), proves the causal connection between HH and/or GER and throat symptoms. Regarding patients with no change in symptoms after 3 months therapy (12%), we think they need a longer period of treatment to show an improvement. We hope to confirm this at a 6-month follow-up evaluation.

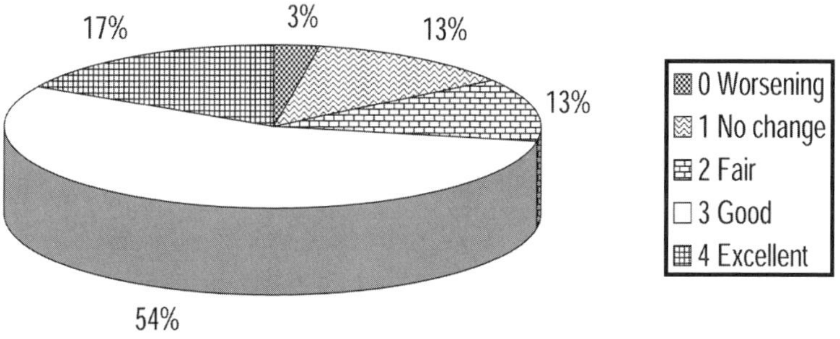

Fig. 4. Results after 3 months of IPP treatment.

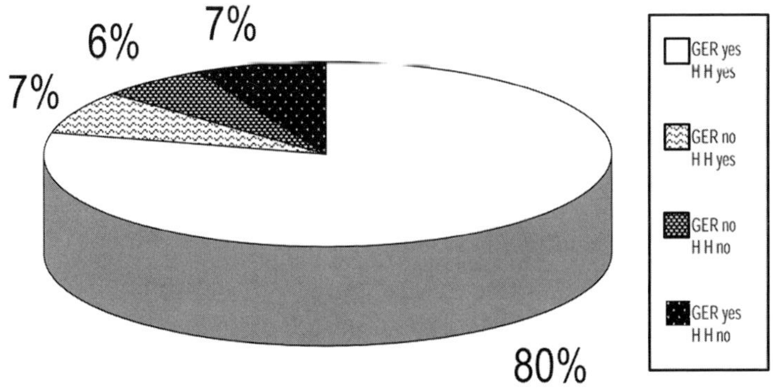

Fig. 5. HH and/or GER rate in patients improved with IPP.

Conclusions

Many of the throat symptoms of GERD are subtle and can be identified only by careful history monitoring and a high index of suspicion. VFG is a diagnostic test well-received by the patients, and it is accurate in showing GERD-related esophageal abnormalities, i.e., hiatal hernia and/or gastroesophageal reflux. In our opinion prolonged pH monitoring and esophageal endoscopy are indicated to confirm the disease in case of failure or when a complicated GERD is suspected. VFG is then useful in confirming the diagnosis of GERD in ENT patients especially if associated with an aggressive acid suppression regimen such as a proton-pump-inhibitor.

References

1. Koufman JA. The otolaryngologic manifestations of gastroesophageal reflux disease (GERD): a clinical investigation of 225 patients using ambulatory 24-hour pH monitoring and an experimental investigation of the role of acid and pepsin in the development of laryngeal injury. Laryngoscope 1991;101:1–64.
2. Gaynor EB. Otolaryngologic manifestations of gastroesophageal reflux. Am J Gastroenterol 1991;86:801–808.
3. Cote DN, Miller RH. The association of gastroesophageal reflux and otolaryngologic disorders. Compr Ther 1995;21:80–84.
4. Jamieson GG, Duranceau A. Gastroesophageal Reflux. Philadelphia: W.B. Saunders, 1976.
5. Richter JE. Extraesophageal presentations of gastroesophageal reflux disease : the case for aggressive diagnosis and treatment. Cleve Clin J Med 1997;64:37–45.
6. Schnatz PF, Castell JA, Castell DO. Pulmonary symptoms associated with gastroesophageal reflux: use of ambulatory pH monitoring to diagnose and to direct therapy. Am J Gastroenterol 1996;91:1715–1718.

Bronchology and Bronchoesophagology: State of the Art.
H. Yoshimura et al., editors.

A 24-h monitoring study of the upper esophagus in patients with gastroesophageal reflux disease

Kazuhiro Nakamura[1], Yusuke Watanabe[2], Ryoji Tokashiki[3], Hiroya Yamaguchi[1], Kohji Ohtsuka[3] and Hajime Hirose[4]
[1]Tokyo Senbai Hospital Otorhinolaryngology, Tokyo; [2]Osaka University Department of Otorhinolaryngology, Osaka; [3]Tokyo Medical University Department of Otorhinolaryngology, Tokyo; and [4]Kitasato University, School of Allied Health Sciences, Kanagawa, Japan

Keywords: diagnostic criteria, diagnostic standard, LPRD, pH monitoring.

Background

Several methods are available for the diagnosis of gastroesophageal reflux disease (GERD) and laryngo paryngeal reflux disease (LPRD), and a detailed history, laryngoscopy, esophagoscopy, pH monitoring, and radioisotope scintigraphy are some of them. Every method has its advantages and disadvantages.

Among the various different methods 24-h monitoring, which demonstrates gastric acid reflux into the esophagus, provides the most convenient and accurate method of diagnosis.

Methods

Thirty-two cases of GERD were subjected to 24-h pH monitoring. The 32 cases visited the ENT Clinic of Tokyo Senbai Hospital and Osaka Kousei-Nenkin Hospital with the chief complaint of abnormal sensation in the throat. They were diagnosed as having LPRD, based on their history and laryngeal findings.

Nineteen normal volunteers received pH monitoring and acted as the control group.

We used a type PH101-ZG pH monitor, manufactured by the Chemical Devices Company, and a Digitrapper MK III pH monitor, manufactured by the Synetics Medical Company. There were two sensor-input channels, and the two wires allowed intraesophageal pH monitoring to be performed at any site desired. Patients had to push the meal button, so that we could monitor the times when meals were consumed. After taking measurements for 24 h, we used special software to analyze the data.

The patients were hospitalized and the pH monitor was inserted for 24 h. They

Address for correspondence: Kazuhiro Nakamura, Tokyo Medical University, Department of Otorhinolaryngology, 6-7-1 Nishi-shinjuku, Shinjuku-ku, 160-0023 Tokyo, Japan. Tel.: +81-3-3342-6111, ext. 5788. Fax: +81-3-3346-9275. E-mail: eddy@tokyo-med.ac.jp were allowed to keep up daily habits such as smoking or drinking coffee. Light-out and sleeping times were also left to the patients' discretion.

After inserting the pH monitor electrode, we confirmed the position of the sensor with an X-ray. The electrodes were inserted transnasally under fluoroscopic guidance. The electrode was positioned behind the sternoclavicular joint, and intraesophageal pH was monitored continuously for 24 h.

Results

In this study we focused on two items: the total amount of time that the pH levels were lower than pH 4 and total amount of time that the pH levels were lower than pH 5, and assessed the data.

In view of the fact that the upper esophagus is influenced by saliva, which is alkaline, we conducted our assessment at pH < 5, as well as pH < 4, and measured the total amount time under pH 4 and under pH 5 per 24 h in the control and the patient groups.

In a similar manner, we measured the total amount of time that the pH levels were lower than pH 5 per 24 h in the control and the patient groups. Interestingly, although there were hardly any states where the pH levels were lower than pH 4 in the patient group, there was a large amount time between pH 4 and 5, and when we assessed the total amount of time that the pH levels were lower than pH 5, we found several patients with a very large amount of total reflux time. This phenomenon was not observed in the control group.

We statistically analyzed the total amount of time that the pH levels were lower than pH 4 per 24 h and the total amount of time that the pH levels were lower than pH 5 in the 19 subjects in the control group and the 32 patients in the patient group. We performed the Mann-Whitney test, using commercially available software. We obtained the median values as the representative values and ranges of the data as the minimal and maximal values. The median value for the total amount of time that the pH levels were lower than pH 4 was 38.5 min in the patient group, as opposed to only 4 min in the control group. This difference was found to be significant according to the Mann-Whitney test ($p = 0.0000226$). The median value for the total amount of time that the pH levels were lower than pH 5 was 112.5 min in the patient group, as opposed to only 11 min in the control group. This was also found to be significant according to the Mann-Whitney test ($p = 0.0000007$).

The influence of saliva must be taken into consideration during pH monitoring performed on the upper part of the esophagus. pH < 5 can be taken as a positive sign for diagnosis.

Conclusion

There was a significant difference in both the total time of pH < 4 and pH < 5, between controls and patients.

When we diagnose LPRD, the diagnostic standard of the upper esophageal pH monitoring is necessary. We propose considering pH values lower than 5 to be positive, because it may improve the rate of diagnosis of LPRD.

Bronchology and Bronchoesophagology: State of the Art.
H. Yoshimura et al., editors.

Proton-pump inhibitor (PPI) for laryngeal granulomas

Masaru Teraoka, Toshifumi Hasegawa, Miki Saito, Minoru Kinishi and Mutsuo Amatsu

Department of Otolaryngology - Head and Neck surgery, Kobe University School of Medicine, Kobe, Japan

Abstract. Laryngeal granuloma is a benign disease, usually located on the vocal process of the arytenoid cartilage. The causes of granuloma have been researched by many authors through the years. Major causal factors proposed have included intubation, voice abuse, and gastroesophageal reflux disease (GERD). A retrospective review of 30 patients with laryngeal granulomas who were examined between 1989 and 2000 at Kobe University School of Medicine, was carried out and analysed. Sixteen patients were treated with surgical removal, and after their operations nine patients had recurrence. Eleven patients were treated nonsurgically. In seven patients granulomas healed. Also, seven patients taking PPI medication were analyzed. Here, three patients were healed and three patients' granuloma decreased in size. With an esophagoscopy, it was revealed that only three patients of the five who had symptoms of GERD had reddened esophageal mucosa. In this study, PPI medication improved the symptoms of GERD, and indeed even the laryngeal granuloma of the patient who had no significant GERD findings from esophagoscopy.

Keywords: antireflux therapy, granuloma, larynx, reflux.

Introduction

Laryngeal granuloma is a benign disease, usually located on the vocal process of the arytenoid cartilage. Otolaryngologists have been mystified by granulomas' consistent tendency to recur. The causes of granuloma have been investigated by many authors through the years. Major proposed causal factors have included intubation, voice abuse, and gastroesophageal reflux disease (GERD). This report presents the clinical experiences, treatment and resulting condition of laryngeal granulomas at Kobe University School of Medicine.

Materials and Methods

A retrospective review of 30 patients with laryngeal granulomas, examined from 1989 to 2000 at Kobe University School of Medicine, was analyzed.

Address for correspondence: Masaru Teraoka MD, Kobe University School of Medicine 7-5-2, Kusunoki-cho, Chuo-ku, Kobe, 650-0017, Japan. Tel.: +81-78-382-5111. Fax: +81-78-382-6039. E-mail: teray@med.kobe-u.ac.jp

Table 1. Patients with granulomas (30 patients).

Causative factor	No. of patients
Postintubation	8 (27%)
Vocal abuse	6 (20%)
Idiopathic or GERD	16 (53%)

Results

The occurrence of granulomas was as follows: eight from intubation, six from vocal abuse, and 16 from idiopathic causes or GERD (Table 1). Sixteen patients were treated with surgical removal, and after their operations nine patients had recurrence. Eleven patients were treated nonsurgically. In seven patients granulomas healed, and in three patients they reduced in size. In one patient the granuloma remained (Table 2). Seven patients with PPI medication were analyzed. Three patients were cured, and three patients' granulomas reduced in size. One patient had no response to the PPI medication. With esophagoscopy, it was revealed that three patients out of five who had symptoms of GERD had reddened esophageal mucosa (Table 3).

Case reports

Case 1

The patient was a 58-year-old male. His primary complaint was globus sensation. The patient had seen an otolaryngologist due to the globus sensation and had his condition diagnosed as laryngeal granuloma. He underwent surgical removal twice and laser removal once, and experienced recurrence 3 times. He had had heartburn and regurgitation, and received PPI medication. The granuloma reduced after 4 weeks, and healed after 6 weeks medication.

The laryngeal granuloma was located on the left vocal process of the arytenoid cartilage prior to PPI medication (Fig. 1). The granuloma reduced after 4 weeks, and after 8 weeks PPI medication it healed.

Table 2. Patients with granulomas.

Treatment	No. of patients		
Surgical	16	– Healed:	7
		– Recurrence:	9
Nonsurgical	11	– Healed:	7
		– Reduction:	3
		– No response:	1

Table 3. Cases with PPI medication.

Response of granulomas	No. of cases	Symptoms of GERD		Esophagoscopy findings	
		+	–		
Healing	3	3	0	– Reddened esophageal mucosa	2
				– No examination	1
Reduction	3	2	1	– Reddened esophageal mucosa	1
				– No abnormal findings	1
				– No examination	1
No response	1	0	1	– No abnormal findings	1

Case 2

The patient was a 47-year-old male. Again his complaint was globus sensation. The patient had visited our hospital and also had been diagnosed with laryngeal granuloma. He underwent surgical removal where an operating microscope was used and experienced recurrence after 1 month. He had had heartburn and regurgitation, and was given PPI. The granuloma gradually reduced after medication.

The laryngeal granuloma was located on the left vocal process of the arytenoid cartilage before PPI medication (Fig. 2). The granuloma reduced after 4 weeks of PPI medication and further reduced after 8 weeks PPI medication.

Discussion

Gastroesophageal reflux (GER) has been defined as the retrograde flow of gastric contents into the esophagus. Patients with GERD exhibit classic symptoms of heartburn and regurgitation. Some patients display otolaryngologic manifestations of GERD which include globus sensation, chronic cough, sore throat,

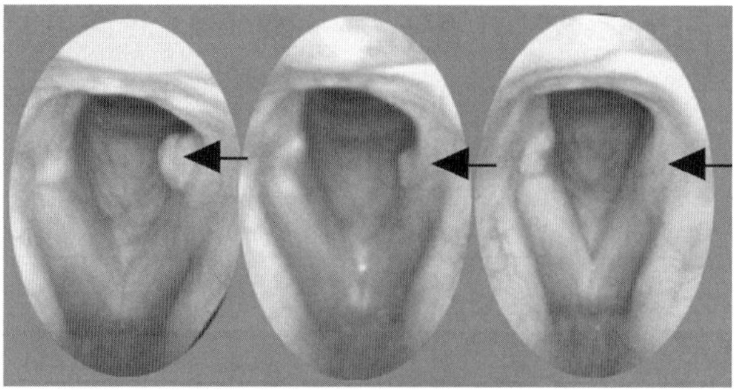

Fig. 1. Case 1: Laryngeal observations. The left was the finding before PPI medication, the center after 4 weeks, and the right after 8 weeks of PPI medication.

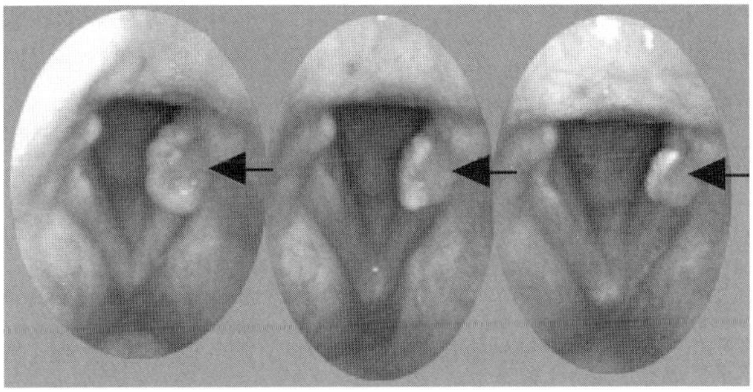

Fig. 2. Case 2: Laryngeal observations. The left was the finding before PPI medication, the center after 4 weeks, and the right after 8 weeks of PPI medication.

hoarseness, granuloma, and ulcers. It is possible that a clinical history may be monitored in order to identify symptoms of GERD. Pharyngolaryngoscopy, esophagoscopy, pH monitoring, and esophagography procedures were recommended to patients to identify GERD. Medical therapy included either protonpump inhibitor (PPI) or H2 blocker.

Several studies have proposed that GERD might be a contributory etiologic factor in granuloma formation. In 1968, Cherry and Delahunty reported that a causal effect might exist between GERD and the development of granuloma [1,2]. Goldberg, Ward and Feder supported the importance of the role of reflux and Feder believed that the effect of the acid content on the larynx and chronic forms of GERD-related trauma contributed to the formation of the granuloma [3–6]. Ohman and Tucher suggested that reflux mechanisms via vagus and recurring nerves may cause these symptoms and contribute to the appearance of granuloma [7,8]. Thomas reported that his assessment of 55 granulomas revealed an incidence of 42 patients (76%) with GERD where antireflux therapy was successful in achieving symptomatic resolution [9]. Paulo reported that his retrospective study of 66 patients, revealed 20 patients (30.3%) with GERD, and in 75% of the patients there was regression with clinical treatment [10]. Manish supposed that PPI medication is effective in the treatment of laryngeal granuloma, even in the absence of identifiable symptoms of GERD [11].

Conclusions

In our study, of seven patients with PPI medication, five patients showed symptoms of GERD. Three patients were cured, and three patients' granuloma reduced in size. In an esophagoscopy, it was revealed that only three patients of five who had symptoms of GERD had reddened esophageal mucosa. In this study, PPI medication improved the symptoms of GERD, and indeed even the laryngeal granuloma of a patient who had no significant GERD symptoms after esophagoscopy.

References

1. Cherry J, Margulies SI. Contact ulcer of the larynx. Laryngoscope 1968;78:1937–1940.
2. Delahunty JE, Cherry J. Experimentally produced vocal cord granulomas. Laryngoscope 1968; 78:1941–1947.
3. Goldberg M, Noyek AM. Laryngeal granuloma secondary to GER. J Otolaryngol 1978;7: 196–202.
4. Ward PH, Zwitman D. Contact ulcers and granulomas of the larynx. Otolaryngol Head Neck Surg 1980;88:262–269.
5. Feder RJ, Michell MJ. Hyperfunctional, hyperacidic and intubation granulomas. Arch Otolaryngol 1984;110:582–584.
6. Ward PH, Hanson DG. Reflux as an etiological factor of carcinoma of the laryngopharynx. Laryngoscope 1988;98:1195–1199.
7. Ohman L, Olofsson J. Esophageal dysfunction in patients with contact ulcer of the larynx. Ann Otol Rhinol Laryngol 1983;92:228–230.
8. Tucher et al. The larynx. New York: Thieme Medical, 1993;225–226.
9. Thomas E, Jocelyn P. A management strategy for vocal precess granulomas. Laryngoscope 1999;109:301–306.
10. Paulo A, Noemi G. Clinical evolution of laryngeal granulomas. Laryngoscope 1999;109: 289–294.
11. Manish K, Gayle E. Laryngeal contact granuloma. Laryngoscope 1999;109:1589–1593.

Bronchology and Bronchoesophagology: State of the Art.
H. Yoshimura et al., editors.

Otolaryngologic manifestations of gastroesophageal reflux in Japan

Yusuke Watanabe[1], Hiroshi Muta[2] and Takeshi Kubo[1]
[1]Department of Otolaryngology and Sensory Organ Surgery, Osaka University Graduate School of Medicine; and [2]National Osaka Hospital, Osaka, Japan

Abstract. The exact incidence of gastroesophageal reflux (GER) is unknown, although it is estimated that at least 25% of patients with GER have head and neck symptoms alone [1]. While there are many papers about Laryngo Paryngeal Reflux Disease (LPRD) in the USA and Europe, there are only a few in Japan. Our aim was to evaluate and treat LPRD patients in Japan. We evaluated and treated 80 patients (46 males and 34 females), who were seen in the Osaka Koseinenkin Hospital with complaints of heartburn, and who also had globus sensation, chronic coughs, dysphonia and/or pharyngeal pain. All the patients underwent an initial otolaryngologic examination. Twenty patients underwent 24-h esophageal pH monitoring. We used the so-called "Step-Down" therapy as treatment.

Concerning symptoms, 52 patients (65%) had globus sensation, 18 had a chronic cough, seven had dysphonia and three had pahryngeal pain. With regard to the 24-h pH monitoring study, the average number of reflux episodes observed in the lower probe was 156 and that of upper probe was 12. The results obtained between the upper and lower probes were significant in the total number of episodes of reflux events. We were unable to treat six of the patients (7.5%) without the use of PPIs.

Keywords: GERD, Japan, LPRD, symptoms.

Background

GERD/LPRD is a common disease in the USA and Europe, but there are few reports of it in Japan. Why are there so few Japanese GERD patients? Different eating habits and/or body weights could provide some explanation for this. We investigated Japanese LPRD patients' symptoms, laryngeal findings, etc., in order to explore this phenomenon.

Methods and Materials

Eighty patients visited ENT clinics of Osaka Koseinenkin Hospital. They were diagnosed as having LPRD based on their history, and laryngeal findings. There were 46 male cases and 34 female cases. Their ages ranged from 31 to 81 years. The average age was 56.7 years. The follow-up period varied from 12 to 96 weeks

Address for correspondence: Yusuke Watanabe, Department of Otolaryngology and Sensory Organ Surgery, Osaka University Graduate School of Medicine, 2-2 Yamadaoka, Suita, Osaka 565-0871, Japan. Tel.: +81-6-6879-3951. Fax: +81-6-6879-3959. E-mail: ywatanabe@ent.med.osaka-u.ac.jp (about 2 years). The mean follow-up period was 42.3 weeks. The following items were examined:

1. The symptoms of chief complaints, as described by Japanese LPRD patients.
2. The pH monitoring test, which had double electrodes (20 patients underwent this during hospitalization). The upper electrode was positioned around the hypopharynx, and lower electrode was 15 cm below. Their esophageal pH was monitored for 24 h.
3. Laryngeal findings of Japanese LPRD patients.
4. We used the so-called "step-down" therapy as treatment.

Results

Their symptoms

Globus sensation was present in 52 cases, amounting to 65% of all the patients. These cases included two laryngeal granulomas. Chronic coughs were present in 18 cases, and dysphonia is seven cases, which included three laryngeal granulomas.

In the dysphonia cases, all of the patients were male, and their ages ranged from 34 to 62 years. The average age was 45.8-years-old. The number of hospitals that patients had been to before they came to ours varied from one to four. The average number of hospitals, previously been to, was two. Treatment recieved at the other hospitals consisted of taking steroids, painkillers and resting the voice.

Three cases had sore throats. There was one male and two females and their ages ranged from 53 to 81 years. The average age was 67.4 years. The number of hospitals that these patients had been to before they came to ours varied from two to four hospitals. The average number of hospitals, previously been to, was three. The treatment recieved at the other hospitals consisted of taking painkillers, antibiotics and washing the mouth. (These are all total numbers.)

Case: An 81-year-old female. Her chief complaint was a sore throat after eating sweet things, such as cakes or chocolates. Her esophagitis was grade C in LA classification. She had hiatus sliding herniation. Her complaint disappeared after taking PPIs in dramatic amounts.

Some authors reported many symptoms in their papers, but in Japan there were no other symptoms of any kind.

24-h pH monitoring

Case: A 34-year-old female. Her chief complaint was globus sensation. Her esophageal motility was poor due to an operation on a hiatus herniation. Data collected from pH monitoring illustrated that even though many refluxes occurred at the lower electrode, fewer episodes occurred at the upper electrode.

We have abbreviated detailed data, however, from our results, we have determined that patients' symptoms can occur even though their reflux time is short or intermittent.

Laryngeal findings

Swelling, redness or arytenoid occurred in 63 cases. Interarytenoid pachyderm or edema was found in 58 cases. The pooling of saliva was complained of in 23 cases. Posterior laryngitis was present in 21 cases. Five cases had laryngeal granuloma, and seven cases had no specific findings.

Treatment

Step-down treatment was unsuccessful in six cases, consisting of four males and two female. Their ages ranged from 41 to 81 years. The mean follow-up period varied from 21 to 61 weeks. The average follow-up period was 32.3 weeks. The symptoms were two sore throats, two chronic coughs, one globus sensation and one dysphonia.

Discussion

The results from our study have made it clear that there are differences in GERD/LPRD pathology between Japan and other countries. In Japan we must consider the possibility of infection by Helicobacter pylori, because of high percentage of infection in over 50-year-olds. The presence of H. pylori infections can make gastric juice become hypoacidic, and the symptoms in Japan tend to be very mild. In this study we only encountered four symptoms (globus sensation, chronic coughs, dysphonia and sore throats), and never experienced any severe symptoms, such as otalgie, choking or dental caries, etc. Henderson et al. [2] noted that approximately 25% of patients with GER exhibit only head and neck manifestations.

We must pay great attention to the fact no LPRD patients ever have laryngeal findings (cherry spot arytenoid, interarytenoid edema, etc.). Therefore, it is a necessity to take down detailed histories from patients.

In many individuals, the occurrence of GER can be extremely difficult to document, even with further investigation.

References

1. Gainer EB. Otolaryngologic manifestations of gastroesophageal reflux. Am J Gastroenterol 1991;86(7):801–808.
2. Henderson RD, Woolf C, Marryatt G. Pharyngoesophageal dysphagia and gastroesophageal reflux Laryngoscope 1976;86:1531–1519.

Laryngeal cancer

Bronchology and Bronchoesophagology: State of the Art.
H. Yoshimura et al., editors.

The quality of life of laryngectomized patients

B. Krejovic, P. Stankovic, S. Krejovic and A. Trivic
Institute of Otorhinolaryngology and Maxillofacial Surgery, Clinical Center of Serbia, Belgrade, Yugoslavia

Abstract. The aim of this study is to define the frequency and distribution of factors affecting the quality of life of laryngectomized patients. During the 10-year period from 1989 to 1998, 3,615 patients were operated on for malignant tumors of the larynx at the Belgrade Institute of Otorhinolaryngology and Maxillofacial Surgery. Total laryngectomy was performed in 1,376 (38.06%) cases. The quality of life of laryngectomized patients can be affected by local factors, e.g., extent of surgical resection, postoperative complications, radiotherapeutic sequelae and tumor recurrence, as well as general factors, e.g., psychological condition, age, previous chronic diseases, hearing impairment, and social and familial surroundings of the patient.

Laryngectomies give rise to drastic changes in the patient's quality of life. The most prominently seen are psychological disorders as well as changes at matrimonial, professional, occupational and communication levels. Such frustrations are seen to be felt most intensively in females. Phoniatric rehabilitation is preferred by younger rather than older patients. Indeed, this rehabilitation is successful in over 83% of laryngectomees.

Restoration of verbal communication is only one of the aspects of rehabilitation. Significant enhancement in the quality of life of laryngectomized patients is achieved by phoniatric rehabilitation and through the societal contacts of laryngectomized patients.

Keywords: laryngectomy, quality of life, rehabilitation.

Introduction

Numerous questions have been raised regarding patients' quality of life following a total laryngectomy: quality and amenities of life, social contacts and communication in general. As Diedrich and Youngstrom [1] stressed, the laryngectomee becomes the patient when he starts talking, coughing, breathing, eating, crying, having a smelling sensation, having a bath or breaking into laughter.

The confrontation with a malignant disease, its unpredictability and uncertainty, according to Stankovic [2], is a difficult and traumatic experience for the patient's character. As Gilmore [3] stated, the notion and experience of being subjected to laryngectomy affects the patient in multiple psychodestructive ways. Many patients psychically experience laryngectomy in the form of castration, as emphasized by Stack [4]. The enteral alimentation through a nasogastric probe in the postoperative course fails to prevent the loss of muscle mass, namely, the catabolic phase of tissue proteins, as cited by Robe et al [5]. The major patho-

Address for correspondence: Prof Borivoje Krejovic MD, PhD, Institute of Otorhinolaryngology and Maxillofacial Surgery, Clinical Center of Serbia, 2 Pasterova St., 11000 Belgravia, Yugoslavia. Tel.: +381-11-643-694. Fax: +381-11-643-034.

physiological change is the enlarged pharyngeal resistance, as cited by Gould et al. [6].

As found by Traissac et al. [7], laryngectomy results in a reduction in the protecting function of upper airways, dysfunction of nasal reflexes, loss of function of respiratory muscle support, compromised deglutition, and the likelihood of bronchial aspiration. Frequently seen conditions in laryngectomized patients are the disordered function of lower esophageal sphincter, reflux esophagitis, severe changes in the cardiovascular system function, chronic and obstructive lung diseases, and sensorineural hearing impairment, as reported by Ross-Swain [8] and Robinette [9]. Following a laryngectomy, inspiratory air is not filtered, warmed or moistened. Le Huche et al. [10] reported on the conditions of prominently dry tracheal mucosa and bronchial hypersecretion. As stated by Krejovic et al. [11], the dissection of neck lymph nodes necessitates sacrificing the sensory branches of the superficial cervical plexus.

Materials and Methods

The prospective clinical study concerned laryngectomized patients, rehabilitated at the Department of Phoniatrics, Institute of Otorhinolaryngology and Maxillofacial Surgery, Clinical Center of Serbia, from 1989 to 1998. In this 10-year period, the frequency and distribution of factors affecting the quality of life of laryngectomized patients were investigated.

The following methods of investigation were used in the patients included in our study: 1) thorough anamnesis; 2) clinical otorhinolaryngological examination; 3) tonal liminal audiometry; 4) psychologic evaluation; 5) systematic sequence (through four designed rehabilitation phases); 6) group rehabilitation (groups defined by similar affinities in patients); 7) audiovisual comparison (VCR presentation of successfully rehabilitated patients may stimulate the motivation of patients beginning rehabilitation); 8) sociologic survey; and 9) statistical analysis.

Results

In the period from 1989 to 1998, 3,615 patients were surgically treated for malignant tumors of the larynx (Table 1). Due to locally expanded malignant tumors, 1,376 patients (38.06%) underwent total laryngectomies. Total laryngectomy was carried out most frequently, then pharyngolaryngectomy, and the resection of the base of tongue was carried out least frequently of the three (Table 2).

A neck dissection adversely affects the quality of life in laryngectomized patients, as it results in fibrosis and limited contractions of residual neck muscles, and for oncological reasons it often necessitates sacrificing some of cranial nerves or their branches. The dissection of neck was performed in almost every second laryngectomee, i.e., in 722 (52.47%) patients.

Out of 1,376 laryngectomized patients, 1,302 (94.62%) were male and only 74

Table 1. Surgical treatment of patients with laryngeal carcinomas with respect to year and type of surgery.

Type of surgery	Year of surgery (No. of cases)										
	1989	1990	1991	1992	1993	1994	1995	1996	1997	1998	Total
Conservative	66	58	57	63	63	100	78	92	94	93	764
Reconstructive	110	122	151	134	118	135	166	177	180	179	1472
Radical	94	92	121	141	124	142	163	164	170	168	1379
Total	270	272	329	338	305	377	407	433	444	440	3615

(5.38%) female. Our results revealed that the highest frequency of laryngectomized patients were aged between 50- and 70-years-old. The next most frequent group were patients aged from 41- to 50-years-old, and the least frequent was the group of patients under 40- and over 71-years-old.

Postoperative complications are inevitable in surgical treatment and have a considerable impact on the quality of life of laryngectomized patients. Postoperative complications were found in 210 (14.61%) laryngectomized cases. The most commonly occurring were as follows: pharyngocutaneous fistulas, postoperative hemorrhage, tracheostoma revision, and tracheal and esophageal stenosis.

While reviewing the laryngectomized patients, chronic diseases were diagnosed in 1,210 (87.93%) cases. Chronic respiratory disorders were significantly most frequent, while chronic digestive and neurological conditions were much less frequently occurring.

A hearing impairment was recorded in more than two-thirds of the laryngectomees, or in 930 (67.58%) cases. In 381 out of 930 (40.96%) laryngectomized patients, the hearing impairment interfered with social contacts. Perceptive hearing impairment was seen most frequently, while conductive or mixed hearing loss was significantly less common.

Table 2. Incidence of radical surgery based on resection extent.

Resection extent	No. of patients	
	Absolute	%
Total laryngectomy	1178	85.43
Pharyngo-laryngectomy	158	11.46
Pharyngo-laryngectomy with tongue base resection	43	3.11
Total	1379	100.00

Discussion

The total number of patients initially treated by surgery has been increasing significantly. The incidence of radical surgery in the treatment of patients with malignant laryngeal tumors, although somewhat less in comparison with former studies, is still very high. The reasons are the intolerable prolonging of "lost time" and the late presentation of patients for treatment.

Total laryngectomy was performed as the primary operation in the majority of patients. However, in 351 (25.51%) patients laryngectomy was carried out as secondary surgery following radiotherapy due to residue or recurring tumors. Postoperative radiotherapy after laryngectomy was applied in 422 (30.66%) patients. Due to primary localization of malignant tumors in the larynx, hyoid bone was concomitantly resected in 51.23% of the patients. The absence of hyoid is considered very important in reducing glossopharyngeal compression, relaxation and contraction of esophageal orifice having a direct effect on the site and quality of vibrations of pharyngo-esophageal junction. A high incidence of neck dissections is explicated by extremely expanded laryngeal tumors locally and advanced primary tumors of hypopharynx, base of tongue and supraglottis.

The fact that over three-quarters of laryngectomies, i.e., 926 (67.29%) cases, were carried out in patients of working age emphasizes the social as well as medical significance of laryngectomy, as well as the comfort and quality of life of these patients. For laryngectomized patients with particular occupations, a high degree of damage and disability to the patient can considerably reduce their working ability to a complete working inability. Phoniatric rehabilitation was preferred by younger patients rather than the older ones. As regards the patients' quality of life, postoperative complications are significant since they lead to modifications of already fairly altered anatomic relations, and from a psychological aspect to the reduction of motivation and general amenities. Given the age of laryngectomized patients and the fact they are commonly heavy smokers, the existing chronic respiratory, cardiovascular, digestive and neurological disorders are not surprising but are only additional problems. If indicated, hearing aids and concurrent audiological and phoniatric rehabilitation are applied in laryngectomized patients with hearing impairment.

The predominant psychological reaction in patients undergoing laryngectomy was fear of the surgery itself and of the sequelae of malignant disease. Resignation was observed in almost one-third of patients or 397 (28.85%) of them, while a defense mechanism, manifested with more intensive aggression was seen in 81 (5.88%) patients. Suicidal intentions, which must be taken seriously, were pronounced in 20 (1.45%) laryngectomees.

Conclusion

Restoration of verbal communication and vocal re-education is only one of the aspects of the quality of life of laryngectomized patients. Returning to family and society in general calls for planned and organized teamwork.

Laryngectomized patients can solve their numerous problems more easily by obtaining appropriate advice and support through the relevant societies, and this contributes to significantly improving their comfort and quality of life. Through these societies, both laryngectomized patients and their families are constantly and permanently educated in a new way of living and communication in general.

References

1. Diedrich WM, Youngstrom KA. Alaryngeal Speech. Springfield: Charles C. Thomas, 1966.
2. Stankovic P. Phoniatric Rehabilitation of Laryngectomized Patients by Establishing Oesophageal Voice and Speech using Modified Seemans Method. Belgrade: Doctoral Thesis. Medical Faculty of Belgrade, 1997.
3. Gilmore IS. The physical, social, occupational, and psychological concomitants of laryngectomy. J Speech Hear Res 1994;17:599–607.
4. Stack FM. The Feminine Viewpoint of Being a Laryngectomee. In: Keith RL, Darley FL (eds) Laryngectomee Rehabilitation. Austin, Texas: Pro-Ed Inc, 1994;515–521.
5. Robe Y, Moore P, Andrews HA, Holinger HP. A study of the role of certain factors in the development of speech after laryngectomy. Laryngoscope 1996;66:382–401.
6. Gould JW, Sataloff RT, Spiegel JR. Voice Surgery. St. Louis-Mosby, 1993.
7. Traissac L (ed) Réhabilitation de la Voix et de la Déglutition Après Chirurgie Partielle ou Totale du Larynx. Paris: Arnette, 1992.
8. Ross-Swain D. The Voice Advantage. London: Singular Publishing Group Inc, San Diego, 1991.
9. Robinette SM. Hearing problems associated with laryngectomy. J Speech Hear Res 1994;74: 80–85.
10. Le Huche F, Allali A, Miroux G. La Voix Sans Larynx, 4th edn. Paris: Maloine, 1987.
11. Krejovic B, Radulovic R, Stankovic P. One Thousand Laryngectomies in an Eleven-Year Period. In: Otorhinolaryngology, Head and Neck Surgery. Amsterdam: Kugler and Ghedini Publications, 1990;2413–2418.

Bronchology and Bronchoesophagology: State of the Art.
H. Yoshimura et al., editors.

Opening and closing mechanisms in the neoglottis in laryngectomees

Noriko Nishizawa[1], Yasushi Mesuda[1], Makoto Takahashi[2], Katsuhiko Tanaka[3], Noboru Sakai[4] and Yukio Inuyama[1]

[1]Department of Otolaryngology, Hokkaido University, School of Medicine; [2]Hokkaido University, School of Engineering; [3]National Sapporo Hospital; and [4]Health Science University of Hokkaido, Sapporo, Japan

Abstract. *Background.* In esophageal and tracheoesophageal speakers, the neoglottis acts not only as the orifice of the digestive tract but also as the airway and the voice source. An opening and closing mechanism is thought to be essential for these functions. Examinations were carried out in order to find out about the physical background of the opening and closing of the neoglottis.

Subjects and Methods. Subjects were volunteer esophageal and tracheoesophageal speakers. Neoglottal width, EMG of the inferior pharyngeal constrictor (IPC) and of the geniohyoid muscle (GH) were recorded simultaneously during swallowing, air intake, phonation and voicing distinction of stop consonants.

Results. The neoglottal closure was accompanied by activity of the IPC, which increased during phonation. During swallowing, the neoglottis was widely opened. Anterior traction of the anterior pharyngeal wall by the GH and reciprocal suppression of the IPC activity was thought to be the mechanism of the neoglottal opening in this case. Such simple reciprocity was not observed, however, during air intake or intervocalic voiceless consonant production, although transient opening of the neoglottis was commonly observed.

Conclusions. The GH and the IPC were found to open and close the neoglottis, respectively. Their activity was not always clearly reciprocal in the various functions of the neoglottis.

Keywords: alaryngeal speech, esophageal speech, laryngeal adjustment, neoglottal adjustment, tracheoesophageal speech, voicing distinction.

Introduction

In esophageal and tracheoesophageal speakers, the neoglottis acts as the orifice to the digestive tract and as the gateway for air intake before esophageal phonation, as well as being the voice source in esophageal and tracheoesophageal speech. The opening and closing mechanism is thought to be essential for these variously developed functions. It is not known, however, whether there is any active muscular control of neoglottal opening and closing.

We carried out a series of experiments to find out about the physical background of the opening and closing of the neoglottis [1]. Special attention was paid to the activities of the inferior pharyngeal constrictor and geniohyoid mus-

Address for correspondence: Noriko Nishizawa MD, Department of Otolaryngology, Hokkaido University, School of Medicine, Kita 15, Nishi 7, Kita-ku, 060-8638 Sapporo, Japan. Tel.: +81-11-716-1161 ext. 5959. Fax: +81-11-717-7566. E-mail: n-noriko@med.hokudai.ac.jp cles; the former is thought to be the constrictor of the neoglottis and the latter represents the combined activity of the suprahyoid muscles, which elicit anterior movement of the root of the tongue. In this paper, we review the findings of those experiments.

Subjects and Methods

Subjects were skilled esophageal and tracheoesophageal speakers. Behavior of the neoglottis was monitored during swallowing and air intake for esophageal speech and voiced/voiceless distinction of stop consonants. Parameters, recorded simultaneously along with the electromyographic activities of the inferior pharyngeal constrictor and the geniohyoid muscle, were as follows: 1) neoglottal width, monitored by photoglottography (PGG); and 2) intraoral air pressure and audio waveform.

Results

Experiment 1: Electrophysiologic examination of neoglottal opening during swallowing

The subjects were two esophageal speakers (subject 1 and 2). Figure 1 shows a typical course of the parameters during swallowing. The PGG waveform indicates that the neoglottis transiently opened during swallowing. The integrated EMG curve of the geniohyoid muscle shows prominent activity at the onset of neoglottal opening. Activity of the inferior pharyngeal constrictor, on the other hand, was suppressed during the opening of the neoglottis.

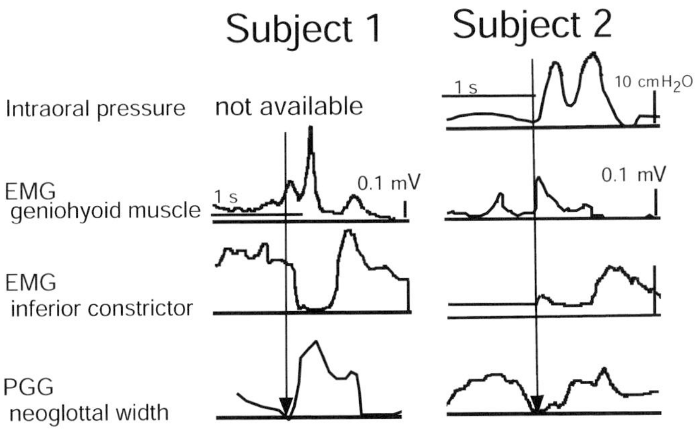

Fig. 1. Behavior of the neoglottis during swallowing. A typical course for two subjects is shown. The vertical arrow indicates the onset of the opening of the neoglottis. (Modified from Nishizawa et al. [1].)

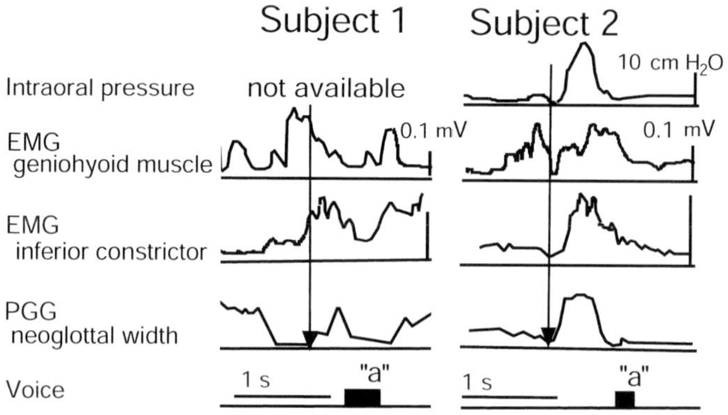

Fig. 2. Behavior of the neoglottis during the production of the vowel "a" by esophageal speech. A typical course for two subjects is shown. The vertical arrow indicates the onset of the opening of the neoglottis before phonation. (Modified from Nishizawa et al. [1].)

Experiment 2: Electrophysiologic examination of neoglottal opening during air intake

The subjects were the same as those in the first experiment. Figure 2 shows the behavior of the neoglottis during production of the vowel "a" using esophageal speech. It was shown that the neoglottis transiently opened at air intake, simultaneous with an increase in intraoral pressure. The EMG curve of the geniohyoid muscle shows increased activity at the onset of neoglottal opening, as it did during swallowing. The inferior pharyngeal constrictor, on the other hand, was continuously activated, and no significant suppression was observed during neoglottal opening.

Experiment 3: Electrophysiologic examination of neoglottal opening and closing during voicing distinction of stop consonants

The subjects were two tracheoesophageal (subject 3 and 4) and three esophageal speakers (subject 1, 2 and 5). Syllables containing contrasts of voiced/voiceless and double/single consonants between vowels were used in the test. The target of the test was the voicing distinction of these consonants. Each test word was repeated by each subject within the carrying sentence, "Hai —— desu, (Yes, it is——)". Activity of the inferior pharyngeal constrictor was surveyed in all subjects. Activity of the geniohyoid muscle was surveyed in only two of the subjects. Figure 3 shows a typical piece of behavior of the inferior pharyngeal constrictor and other parameters. Figure 4 shows a typical course of the parameters, including geniohyoid muscle activity.

Measurement of the duration of the silent period between the preceding and succeeding vowels confirmed that the voiced/voiceless and double/single consonant features could be successfully differentiated by all subjects. The average

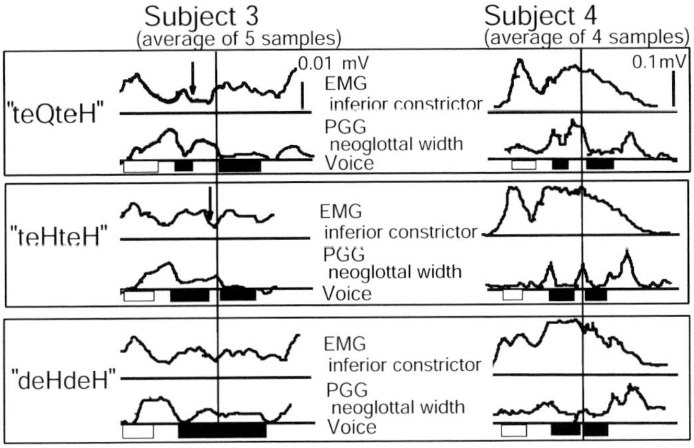

Fig. 3. Behavior of the neoglottis during voicing distinction. Activity of the geniohyoid muscle was not monitored in this test. The duration of voicing for vowels preceding and succeeding the consonants are shown by the black bars. The white bars indicate voicing of the leading word, "Hai". The vertical line indicates the timing of consonant release. The arrows indicate the suppression of the inferior pharyngeal constrictor. (Modified from Nishizawa et al. [1])

photoglottographic waveform, in all the subjects, indicated that there was a transient increase in neoglottal width during the production of voiceless consonants (Figs. 3 and 4). It was noted that the opening of the neoglottis during the production of voiceless consonants was accompanied by the suppression of EMG activity of the inferior pharyngeal constrictor in subject 3 (Fig. 3). However, in the other four subjects the inferior pharyngeal constrictor was continuously activated throughout the utterance, and no significant suppression was observed (Figs. 3

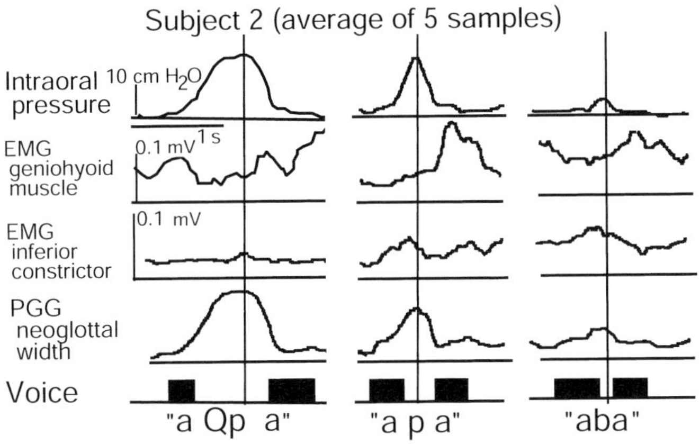

Fig.4. Behavior of the neoglottis during voicing distinction. Activity of the geniohyoid muscle was the target of this test. The duration of voicing for vowels preceding and succeeding the consonants are shown by the black bars. The vertical line indicates the timing of consonant release. (Modified from Nishizawa et al. [1].)

and 4). The average EMG curve of the geniohyoid muscle did not show any specific activity during neoglottal opening for voiceless consonant production in both subjects examined. Instead, both before and after the test syllables, the muscle showed normal articulatory activity in producing the "i" and "d" sounds in the carrying sentence that required the anterior movement of the tongue (Fig. 4).

Discussion

Identification of the opener and closer of the neoglottis

Fluorographic examination of swallowing in laryngectomees has shown it to be closely related to that of normal laryngeal subjects. At rest, the neoglottis is closed by the mucosal protrusion in the posterior pharyngeal wall. During swallowing, the mucosal protrusion in the posterior pharyngeal wall is partially flattened. At the same time, the anterior pharyngeal wall is pulled anteriorly by the root of the tongue, thus opening the neoglottis [1,2]. The activity of the geniohyoid muscle, observed in the present study, was thought to cause the anterior movement of the root of the tongue, which in turn pulls on the anterior pharyngeal wall. The suppression of the inferior pharyngeal constrictor was consistent with the flattening of the posterior mucosal protrusion during swallowing. Based on results of experiment 1, the geniohyoid muscle was identified as the opener of the neoglottis while the inferior pharyngeal constrictor was identified as the closer. Clear reciprocity between the two muscles was shown in opening the neoglottis during swallowing.

Such reciprocity between the opener and closer of the neoglottis was not observed, however, in neoglottal opening during air intake for esophageal speech. During air intake, neoglottal opening was caused mainly by the activity of the geniohyoid muscle and no reciprocal suppression of the activity of the inferior pharyngeal constrictor was observed. It must be taken into consideration, that the inferior pharyngeal constrictor may act, not only as the closer of the neoglottis, but as the tensor of the neoglottis as well. During air intake, the muscle was assumed to play a role in maintaining the tension of the neoglottis, which acts as the voice source in subsequent phonation.

Coordination of the opener and closer of the neoglottis during voicing distinction of consonants

The results of experiments on voicing distinction in laryngectomees showed a transient opening of the neoglottis, simulating normal laryngeal speech [3], to be associated with voiceless consonant production in all the subjects. Suppression of the inferior pharyngeal constrictor was associated with the opening of the neoglottis in only one of the subjects. This finding suggests that there is an active articulatory adjustment of the neoglottis itself during voiceless consonant production. It must be emphasized, however, that simple reciprocity between the opener and closer of the neoglottis cannot be assumed in voicing distinction in laryngectomees. In future experiments on voicing distinction in laryngectomees, we must be careful in our interpretation of neoglottal opening during voiceless consonant production. This mechanism might be an active articulatory adjustment or a passive movement reflecting adjustments occurring in other articulatory organs. It must also be kept in mind that the quite extraordinary adaptation that occurs in the substitution of the speech mechanism after total laryngectomy might not be uniform among patients.

Acknowledgements

We thank the subjects who voluntarily participated in our study. They are all members of the United Assembly of Japanese Laryngectomees. The outline of this review has already been published by the authors [1].

References

1. Nishizawa N, Mesuda Y. Neoglottal adjustments in tracheoesophageal and esophageal speech. Jap J Logoped Phoniatr 1998;39:468–476.
2. McIvor J, Evans PF, Perry A et al. Radiological assessment of post laryngectomy speech. Clin Radiol 1990;41:312–316.
3. Hirose H, Gay T. The activity of the intrinsic laryngeal muscles in voicing control – an electromyographic study. Phonetica 1972;25:140–164.

Bronchology and Bronchoesophagology: State of the Art.
H. Yoshimura et al., editors.

A comparison of various shunt methods for vocal rehabilitation

Hitoshi Saito, Shigeharu Fujieda, Toshio Ohtsubo, Takehisa Saito and Gota Tsuda
Department of Otolaryngology, Fukui Medical University, Matsuoka-cho, Yoshida-gun, Fukui, Japan

Abstract. Since 1975, we have been trying out various shunt method procedures on laryngectomized patients due to the malignancy of their airway/digestive tracts. A total of 87 cases of shunt method procedures were performed. These included 42 cases of the modified Komorn method (MK), 27 cases of the simple mucodermal method (SMD), 10 cases of the omohyoid loop method (OH), four cases of the tracheo-gastric shunt (T-G), and four cases of the tracheo-jejunal shunt (T-J). MK, SMD and OH belong to the tracheo-esophageal shunt (T-E). The technical ease, phonetic data, aspiration and success rate of these cases were evaluated.

The quality of voice obtained, using the esophageal mucosa, is significantly better than of that using the mucosa of digestive tract. This is due to the fact that the former forms a pseudo-glottic swelling on the mucosa. The success rates were 80% in MK, 81% in SMD, 90% in OH, 75% in T-G, and 100% in T-J 3 months after surgery. However, it is interesting that most of the success rates were close to 70% 1 year after the surgery.

Although the aspiration problem still remains to be solved, the shunt voice is very important in maitaining a higher quality of life for alaryngeal patients.

Keywords: aspiration, shunt voice, total laryngectomy, tracheoesophageal shunt, tracheogastric shunt, tracheojejunal shunt.

Background

Since 1975, we have been trying out various different shunt method procedures as a means of voice restoration for laryngectomized patients due to the malignancy of their airway/digestive tracts. Up untill now, we have tried out five different kinds of shunt method procedures, including the modified Komorn method (MK) [1], the simple mucodermal method (SMD) [2], the omohyoid loop method (OH), the tracheo-gastric shunt (T-G) [3], and the tracheo-jejunal shunt (T-J). MK, SMD and OH belong to the tracheo-esophageal shunt (T-E). The purpose of this paper is to evaluate and compare technical ease, phonetic data, aspiration and success rate among the different methods.

Address for correspondence: H. Saito MD, Department of Otolaryngology, Fukui Medical University, Shimoaizuki 23, Matsuoka-cho, Yoshida-gun, Fukui 910-1193, Japan. Tel.: +81-776-61-8404. Fax: +81-776-61-8118. E-mail: hisaito@fmsrsa.fukui-med.ac.jp

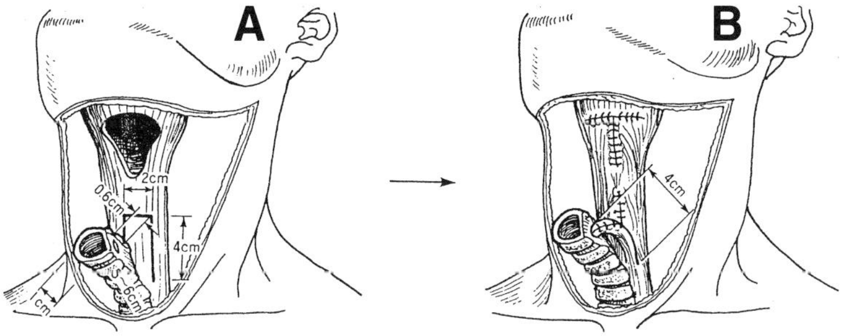

Fig. 1. The modified Komorn method. **A:** Surgical design after total laryngectomy. **B:** Completed T-E shunt procedure.

Patients and Methods

A total of 87 patients underwent shunt method procedures, and were subsequently analyzed. Of the 87 cases, 71 consisted of laryngeal cancer, 13 of hypopharyngeal cancer and three of mesopharyngeal cancer. Each of the five shunt method procedures mentioned are shown in Figs. 1 to 5.

Results

Data and results concerning the 42 patients who underwent the MK procedure are shown in Tables 1 and 2. The postoperative success rate at 3 months was 80%. The aspiration rate was noted to be 30%.

Data and results concerning the 27 patients who underwent the SMD procedure are shown in Tables 3 and 4. The postoperative success rate at 3 months was 81%. The aspiration rate was noted to be 56%.

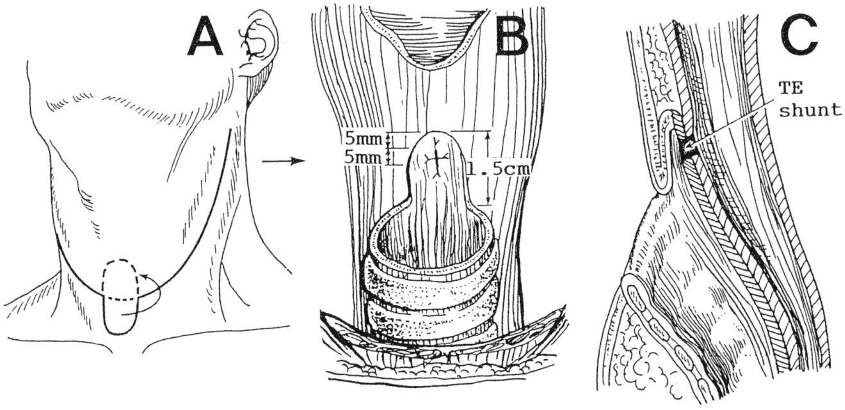

Fig. 2. The simple mucodermal method. **A:** Incision and skin flap. **B:** Mucosal design. **C:** Side view upon completion.

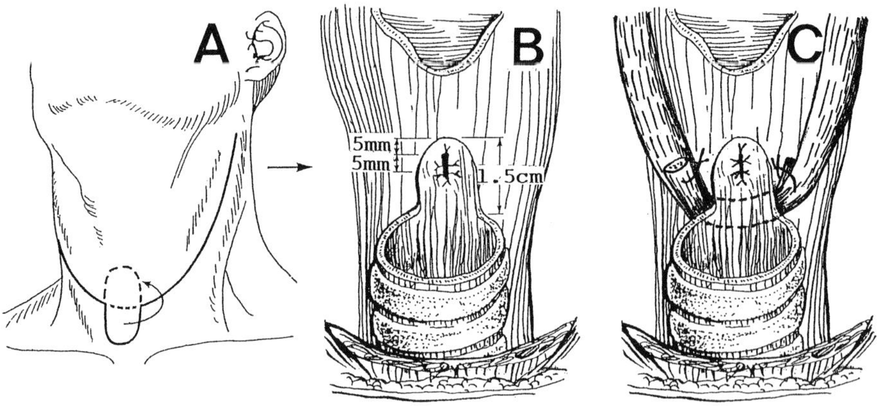

Fig. 3. The omohyoid loop method. **A:** Dermal incision. **B:** Mucosal design. **C:** Bilateral omohyoid loop.

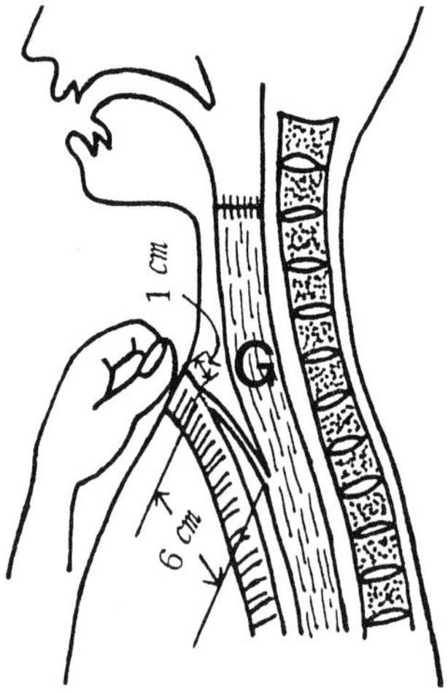

Fig. 4. Tracheogastric shunt. G = gastric tube.

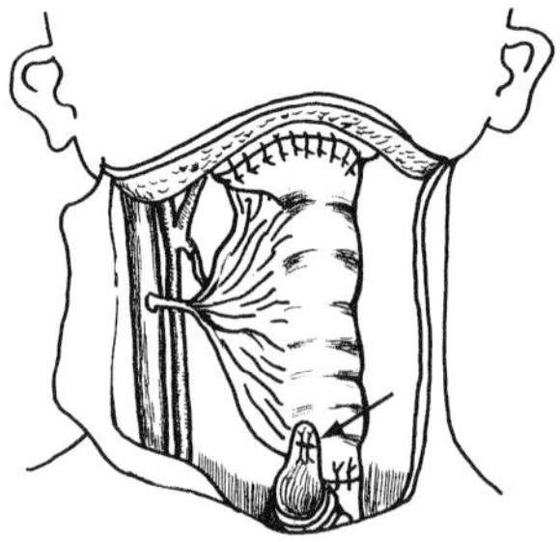

Fig. 5. Tracheojejunal shunt. The arrow indicates the T-J shunt with a horizontal incision.

Table 1. Cases that underwent the modified Komorn method procedure.

Laryngeal cancer	40
Primary	
Supraglottic	24
Glottic	13
Subglottic	1
Secondary	2
Hypopharyngeal cancer	2
Total	42

Age distribution: 44 to 73 years of age (mean age: 60.4 years).

Table 2. The results concerning the 42 patients who underwent the modified Komorn method procedure.

	3 months after surgery	1 year after surgery
Success	32 (80%)	28 (70%)
Failure	8 (20%)	
Stenosis or closure	4	
Surgical closure due to aspiration	2	
Voice prosthesis	2	
Excluded by death of other cause	2	
Total	42	

Mean first voice (n = 36): 31 POD. Aspiration: 30% (12/40).

Data and results concerning the 10 patients who underwent the OH procedure are shown in Table 5. The postoperative success rate at 3 months was 90%. The aspiration rate was noted to be 20%. However, when both omohyoid muscles were used, the success and aspiration rates were 100% and 10%, respectively.

A comparison of the three kinds of T-E shunt method procedures is shown in Table 6. The OH procedure is the most recommendable among these methods, at this point in time.

Table 3. Cases that underwent the simple mucodermal method procedure.

Laryngeal Cancer	24
Supraglottic	11
Glottic	12
Subglottic	1
Mesopharyngeal cancer	3
Total	27

Age distribution: 50 to 77 years of age (mean age: 62.4 years). Combined with radiation: 21/27 (78%).

Table 4. The results concerning the 27 patients who underwent the simple mucodermal method procedure.

	3 months after surgery	1 year after surgery
Success	22 (81%)	19 (70%)
Failure	5 (19%)	
Stenosis or closure	3	
Surgical closure due to aspiration	1	
Voice prosthesis	1	

Aspiration: 15 (56%). Mean first voice: 23 POD. Maximum phonation time: 17 s (N = 24). Maximum dB: 84 dB (N = 24).

Table 5. The results of patients that underwent a T-E Shunt using the omohyoid muscle (OM) loop procedure.

Patient No.	Age/sex	Primary condition	TNM	OM	Radiation	First voice (POD)	MPT (s)	Max. dB	Asp
1	62/M	SG	T4N0M0	Unilateral	+	14	14	67	+
2	65/M	Hypo	T3N2M0	Bilateral	+	14	18	75	–
3	46/M	G	rT2N0M0	Bilateral	–	35	20	78	–
4	64/M	Hypo	T3N0M0	Bilateral	+	19	18	88	–
5	58/M	SG	T2N0M0	Bilateral	+	—	—	—	–
6	60/M	Hypo	T3N2M0	Bilateral	+	57	30	75	–
7	66/M	SG	T3N0M0	Bilateral	–	33	15	94	–
8	50/M	G	T3N0M0	Bilateral	–	38	20	74	±
9	58/M	G	T3N0M0	Bilateral	+	21	18	80	–
10	59/M	G	T3N0M0	Bilateral	–	30	16	81	–
Mean	59				6	29	19	79	2 (20%)

Phonation after 3 months: 9/10 (90%); phonation after 1 year: 7/9 (78%); + = aspiration (asp) was prevented using a finger press; ± = asp was prevented using a neck extension; SG = supraglottic laryngeal cancer; Hypo = hypopharyngeal cancer; G = glottic laryngeal cancer.

Table 6. Comparison of the three different kinds of T-E shunt method procedures.

	MK	SMD	OH
No. of cases	42	27	10
Mean age (years)	60	62	59
Mean MPT (s)	18	17	19
Mean max. SPL (dB)	77	84	79
Operation time (min)	60	15	20
Aspiration rate (%)	30	56	20
Aspiration control	Stent tube	3 Steps	Neck extension
Success rate			
After 3 months (%)	80	81	90
After 1 year (%)	70	70	78

Table 7. Cases that underwent the tracheo-gastric (T-G) shunt procedure.

Patient No.	Age/sex	Primary	TNM	Method	MPT (s)	Max dB	Asp
1	53/M	Hypo-Cer	T2N0M0	primary tube	20	70	—
2	54/F	Hypo	T2N1M0	primary tube	7	65	—
3	60/M	Cer	T2N1M0	primary direct	?	?	?[a]
4	62/F	Hypo	T2N0M0	secondary direct	6	75	—
Mean	57.3				11	70	

[a]Died of renal failure. Hypo = hypopharynx; Cer = cervical esophagus; Asp = aspiration.

Table 8. Cases that underwent tracheo-jejunal (T-J) shunt procedures.

Patient No.	Age/sex	Primary condition	TNM	Method	MPT (s)	Max. dB	Asp
1	60/F	Hypo	T3N0M0	Secondary-voice pros	9	73	—
2	48/M	Hypo-Cer	T4N2M0	Secondary-voice pros	11	85	—
3	54/M	Hypo	T3N0M0	Primary-direct	4	75	—
4	67/M	Hypo	T3N1M0	Secondary-voice pros	8	82	—
Mean					8	78.8	

Data and results concerning the four patients who underwent the T-G procedure and those of the four patients who underwent the T-J procedure are shown in Tables 7 and 8. The success and aspiration rates in both methods were 100%, although there was a problem concerning the quality of voice obtained.

Comparisons of the maximum phonation times (MPT) and intensities (dB) between all the different methods are shown in Tables 9 and 10. The shunt voice of the digestive tract was shown to have a significantly shorter phonation time, and was of lower quality than the other T-E shunt voices. Among the T-E shunt voices, there were no significant differences in MPT and dB.

Table 9. Comparison of the maximum phonation times for each shunt method.

	N	Mean (s)	±SD	p (U-test)
T-G and T-J shunts	7	9.3	5.2	—
Mod. Komorn shunt	36	18.1	6.7	0.002
Mucodermal shunt	22	17.8	8.3	0.006
Omohyoid shunt	9	18.4	5.2	0.011

Table 10. Comparison of the maximum intensities (dB) for each shunt method.

	N	Mean (dB)	SD	p (U-test)
T-G and T-J shunt	7	75.0	6.8	0.006
Mod. Komorn shunt	33	77.1	6.1	
Mucodermal shunt	25	83.9	5.6	0.001
Omohyoid shunt	9	80.1	8.7	n.s.

Discussion

The quality of voice obtained, using gastric and jejunal mucosa, was revealed to be inferior to that of the T-E shunt voice. A fundamental difference in the way each method causes the formation of the neoglottis is believed to be the reason for this. In the case of the T-E shunt method, the neoglottis bulging from the posterior wall is formed by the stenotic portion due to thyropharyngeal muscle contraction [4]. On the other hand, such neoglottis is not formed in the cases of the T-G and T-J shunt methods, but peristalsis may contribute to voice formation.

Conclusion

The quality of voice obtained, using the esophageal mucosa, is substantially better than of that using the mucosa of digestive tract. This is due to the fact that the former forms a pseudo-glottis swelling on the posterior hypopharyngeal mucosa. The success rates were 80% in MK, 81% in SMD, 90% in OH, and 100% in T-G and T-J 3 months after surgery. However, it is interesting that most of the success rates were close to 70% 1 year after surgery.

Although the aspiration problem still remains to be solved, the shunt voice is very important in maintaining a higher quality of life for alaryngeal patients.

References

1. Saito H, Matsui M, Tachibana M et al. Experiences with tracheoesophageal shunt method for voice rehabilitation after total laryngectomy. Arch Otorhinolaryngol 1977;218:135–142.
2. Saito H, Yoshida S, Saito T et al. Simple mucodermal tracheoesophageal shunt method for voice restoration. Arch Otolaryngol Head Neck Surg 1989;115:494–496.
3. Saito H, Sato F, Saito A et al. Vocal rehabilitation by tracheogastric shunt method after pharyngolaryngoesophagectomy for malignancy. Arch Otorhinolaryngol 1984;240:35–41.
4. Omori K, Kojima H, Nonomura M et al. Mechanism of tracheoesophageal shunt phonation. Arch Otolaryngol Head Neck Surg 1994;120:648–652.

Bronchology and Bronchoesophagology: State of the Art.
H. Yoshimura et al., editors.

Indication of the supraglottic horizontal laryngectomy revisited

Hirohito Umeno, Kazunori Mori, Keiichi Chijiwa and Tadashi Nakashima
Department of Otolaryngology — Head and Neck Surgery, Kurume University, School of Medicine, Fukuoka, Japan

Abstract. *Background.* Recently, the number of patients who receive supraglottic horizontal partial laryngectomy (SHL) has decreased because of the improvements in the outcome of laser debulking surgery followed by radiotherapy [1,2]. In this paper the indication of SHL for the laryngeal cancer is revisited.

Methods. Sixty-eight cases (53 male and 15 female) who had undergone SHL in the Kurume University Hospital between 1971 and 1996 were analyzed.

Results. Almost all local recurrence was observed at the anterior commissure, ventricle or base of the tongue. A significant factor affecting the primary recurrence was invasion at the ventricle and the vocal fold. Invasion to the pre-epiglottic space or base of the tongue was not a significant factor. Age was deduced as being a significant factor affecting postoperative aspiration. The risk ratio is high for patients of 80-years-old and above in comparison with patients younger than 80 years of age.

Conclusion. Selected T3/T4 supraglottic carcinoma without invasion of the vocal fold or the ventricle can be an indication of SHL. However, patients 80-years-old or above are basically contraindications of SHL.

Keywords: aspiration, local recurrence, partial laryngectomy, radiotherapy, supraglottic cancer.

Introduction

From 1971 to 1997 supraglottic horizontal partial laryngectomy (SHL) was performed for sixty-eight cases at the Kurume University Hospital. However, after 1997, no patients underwent SHL. The decrease in the number of patients undergoing SHL in our hospital is due mainly to the improvement in the treatment outcome of laser debulking surgery followed by radiotherapy. The purpose of the present study is to revisit the indication of SHL.

Materials and Methods

Sixty-eight cases (53 males and 15 females) who had undergone SHL in the Kurume University Hospital between 1971 and 1996 were analyzed. Table 1 shows the number of SHL cases based on the 1987 UICC classification.

Based upon these subjects, the site of local recurrence following SHL and the

Address for correspondence: Hirohito Umeno MD, Department of Otolaryngology — Head and Neck Surgery, Kurume University, 67 Asahi-machi, Kurume 830-0011, Japan. Tel.: +81-942-31-7575. Fax: +81-942-37-1200. E-mail: umeno2@med.kurume-u.ac.jp

Table 1. No. of SHL cases.

T	Glottic	Supraglottic
T1	0	8
T2(rT2)	1(1)	36
T3(rT3)	0	13(1)
T4	0	10
Total	1	67

( ): recurrent case.

recurrence rate of patients with various invasion sites were analyzed. In addition, factors affecting postoperative aspiration were analyzed using multivariate logistic analysis due to the fact that aspiration is the most serious problem following SHL.

Results

Table 2 shows the sites of local recurrence following SHL. The most frequent sites of local recurrence were the anterior commissure and the ventricle and the base of the tongue.

Table 3 shows the recurrence rate in patients with various different invasion sites. Five patients had invasion of the vocal fold. Of these patients, three showed local recurrence after SHL. In this case, therefore, the recurrent rate of patients with vocal fold invasion was 60%. χ tests revealed that invasion of the vocal fold and ventricle alone were significant factors relating to local recurrence.

In total, severe aspiration appeared in seven patients after SHL. Table 4 shows the relationship between age and severe aspiration. Aspiration appeared in 50% of the patients over 80-years-old. Table 5 shows the relationship between postoperative radiation and severe aspiration. There was no significant relationship seen here. Table 6 shows the relationship between the extent of resection of the aryepiglottic fold and severe aspiration. Severe aspiration was more frequently observed in patients undergoing resection of the aryepiglottic fold than in

Table 2. Sites of local recurrence.

Site	T1	T2	T3	T4
Anterior commissure	1	3	0	0
Ventricle	0	2	0	0
Tongue base	0	1	0	1
Piriform sinus	0	0	1	0
Vocal fold	0	0	0	1
Total	1	6	1	2

Table 3. Recurrent rate of patients with various invasion sites.

Site	Invasion occurring	Invasion not occurring	p
Vocal fold	3/5 (60%)	8/63 (13%)	$p<0.01$
Ventricle	4/11 (36%)	7/57 (12%)	$p<0.05$
Tongue base	1/5 (20%)	10/63 (16%)	n.s.
Anterior commissure	2/4 (50%)	9/64 (14%)	n.s.
Preepiglottic space	5/16 (32%)	4/33 (12%)	n.s.
Arytenoid	1/6 (17%)	10/62 (16%)	n.s.
Aryepiglottic fold	3/27 (11%)	8/41 (20%)	n.s.
False fold	7/35 (20%)	4/33 (12%)	n.s.
Epiglottis lingualsurface	0/6 (0%)	11/62 (18%)	n.s.
Piriform sinus	0/6 (0%)	11/62 (18%)	n.s.

Table 4. Relationship between age and severe aspiration.

Age	Aspiration occurring	Aspiration not occurring
40–59	1 (5%)	18 (95%)
60–69	2 (9%)	20 (91%)
70–79	2 (9%)	21 (91%)
80–89	2 (50%)	2 (50%)
Total	7	61

Table 5. Relationship between irradiation and severe aspiration.

Irradiation	Aspiration	No aspiration
Occurring	1 (7%)	13 (93%)
Not occurring	6 (11%)	48 (89%)
Total	7	61

Table 6. Relationship between resection of the aryepiglottic fold and severe aspiration.

Resection	Aspiration	No aspiration
None	1 (4%)	24 (96%)
< bilateral 2/3	5 (14%)	32 (86%)
> bilateral 2/3	1 (17%)	5 (83%)
Total	7	61

Table 7. Relationship between neck dissection and severe aspiration.

Neck dissection	Aspiration	No aspiration
None	1 (4%)	22 (96%)
Ipsilateral	4 (11%)	32 (89%)
Bilateral	2 (22%)	7 (78%)
Total	7	61

patients with the aryepiglottic fold preserved. Table 7 shows the relationship between neck dissection and severe aspiration. Severe aspiration was more frequently observed in patients with neck dissections than in patients without neck dissection. A multivariate logistic analysis revealed that age alone was a significant factor affecting postoperative aspiration (Table 8). The risk ratio is 18.0 for patients 80-years-old or older in comparison with patients less than 80 years of age.

Discussion

One of the most frequent sites of local recurrence was the anterior commissure, and the recurrent rate of patients with anterior commissure invasion was 50%. Therefore, when the lesion invades the anterior commissure, a thin slice CT of the larynx should be employed. When carcinoma invades the anterior commissure, it can invade thyroid cartilage through the anterior commissure tendon [3].

When T3/T4 supraglottic carcinomas invade the base of the tongue, pre-epiglottic space or piriform sinus, local recurrence was not so frequent in this study. Therefore, they can be seen as indications of SHL.

Based upon these results, our conclusions are that selected T3/T4 supraglottic carcinoma without invasion of the vocal fold or the ventricle can be an indication of SHL. However, patients 80 years of age or older basically are a contra-indication of SHL.

Table 8. Results of multivariate analysis of factors affecting postoperative aspiration.

Factor	Variables	Risk ratio
Age	< 80	1
	$\geqslant 80$	18.0, $p = 0.04$
Neck dissection		Not determined
Aryepiglottic fold		Not determined
Irradiation		Not determined

References

1. Mori K, Mihoki H. Radiology after laser surgery for glottic T1 carcinoma conserving vocal function. Larynx Jpn 1997;9:145–149.
2. Mori K, Umeno H. Conservation for T1/T2 carcinoma of the larynx. Larynx Jpn 1999;11: 47–52.
3. Matsuoka H. A histopatholpgical investigation of glottic carcinoma A whole organ study. Otologia Fukuoka 1988;34:890–906.

Phonosurgery

Bronchology and Bronchoesophagology: State of the Art.
H. Yoshimura et al., editors.

Three-dimensional rigid endoscopic surgery of the larynx: initial experience

Masahiro Kawaida[1], Hiroyuki Fukuda[2] and Naoyuki Kohno[3]
[1]Department of Otolaryngology, Tokyo Metropolitan Ohtsuka Hospital, Tokyo; [2]Department of Otolaryngology-HNS, Keio University School of Medicine, Tokyo; and [3]Department of Otolaryngology, National Defense Medical College, Saitama, Japan

Abstract. The three-dimensional (3D) rigid endoscopic system has been developed to digitally process ordinary video signals. This 3D video system significantly improves visualization and enhances the ability of the surgeon to perform delicate endoscopic procedures. In this study we describe this system which displays the laryngeal cavity in three dimensions during endolaryngeal surgery. The system consists of the 3D converter, a 120 Hz display monitor, an active liquid crystal shutter panel, passive polarizing glasses, a high-bright light source, a light-guide cable, and a Karl Storz video-laryngoscope model II. The 3D video system enables endolaryngeal surgery to be performed with more accuracy, speed, and safety than with a conventional video system.

Keywords: 3D system, laryngeal cavity, phonosurgery.

Introduction

The video-laryngoscope which can be connected to a video camera has been developed to allow video images of the laryngeal cavity to be observed on a display monitor. However, the video images obtained during endolaryngeal surgery using the laryngoscope are flat two-dimensional (2D) ones, and the inability of the surgeon to obtain stereoscopic images is a problem. We attempted three-dimensional rigid endoscopic surgery of the larynx through a video-laryngoscope (3D surgery of the larynx) to remove laryngeal lesions. We used a three-dimensional video-assisted stereoendoscopic display system (3D display system) which can digitally process ordinary video signals. This 3D video system provides the surgeon with stereoendoscopic video images. In this study we describe this 3D surgical procedure and its underlying principles.

Methods and Techniques

To generate stereoscopic video images, two separate images of the observed objects have to be produced from different angles. Video images obtained with ordinary video signals captured with a conventional endoscope and CCD cam-

---

Address for correspondence: Masahiro Kawaida MD, Department of Otolaryngology, Tokyo Metropolitan Ohtsuka Hospital, 2-8-1 Minamiohtsuka, Toshima-ku, Tokyo 170-0005, Japan. Tel.: +81-3-3941-3211. Fax: +81-3-3941-9557. E-mail: kawaida-o@ohtsuka-hospital.toshima.tokyo.jp era are processed digitally with the 3D display system 3D-1A (Shinko Optical Company Ltd.) (Fig. 1). Video images obtained are shifted horizontally with the image memory inside the 3D converter, and so left and right images are reconstructed. These images are converted into digital image signals so that they can be displayed alternately at 120 Hz. The surgeon wears passive polarizing glasses (Fig. 2). Attached to the front of the display monitor is an active polarizing liquid crystal shutter panel. When the left and right images are made to enter the eyes alternately every 1/120 s, the left image into the surgeon's left eye and the right image into the right, lateral disparity can be obtained with the convergence angle and the other formed angle. As a result, the surgeon is able to successfully view stereoscopic images.

Results

The subjective impression from the surgeons is that a stereoendoscopic sensation and depth perception of the laryngeal cavity were successfully achieved, and that it was possible to confidently perform a resection of the lesions with forceps. Since the monitor was observed through both the shutter panel and polarizing glasses, the video images seemed somewhat dark. However, they were not too dark as to be an interruption or distraction in the procedure. The resolution of the image was also appropriate for the process.

Discussion

A video-laryngoscope incorporating a rigid endoscope has been developed

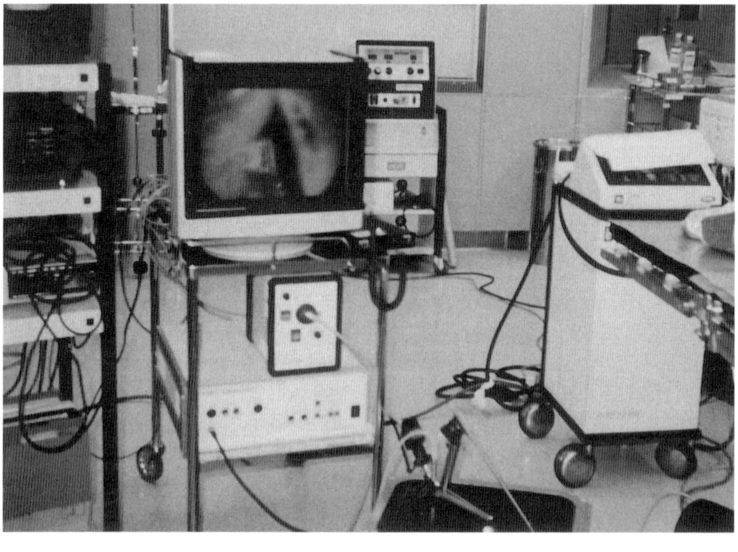

Fig. 1. A 3D display system 3D-1A manufactured by the Shinko Optical Co., Ltd.

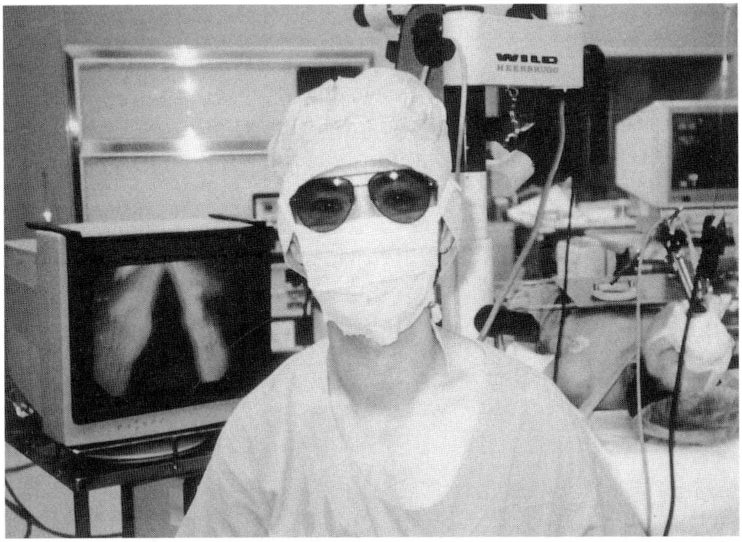

Fig. 2. The surgeon wears passive polarizing glasses.

through observing images displayed on a monitor [1,2]. The 3D display system connected to the video-laryngoscope offers a stereoscopic view and depth perception of the laryngeal cavity during 3D surgery of the larynx.

With most ordinary 3D display systems, the exclusive endoscope with two image guides connected to the exclusive CCD video camera captures individual left and right images which show different angles of the object/s being observed [3–5]. Consequently, the insertion portion of the endoscope is much thicker and the video camera is larger. For these reasons, it is not suitable for endolaryngeal surgery with a video-laryngoscope where there is a narrow lumen. However, the 3D display system used in this study could digitally process ordinary video signals and also the whole system was very compact. Accordingly, it was suitable for endolaryngeal surgery using a video-laryngoscope.

The main advantages of 3D surgery of the larynx apply to skilled operative endoscopy. Durrani et al. [5] report the advantages of the ability to perform endoscopic suturing accurately with the 3D display system. 3D surgery of the larynx appears to be useful in such procedures because the suturing technique is occasionally necessary in endolaryngeal surgery [6]. This 3D display system is superior with regards to its levels of depth perception, and it gave the surgeon a heightened feeling of confidence than a conventional 2D display system would. Therefore, 3D surgery with this 3D display system is also seen to be useful in video-assisted endoscopic endonasal sinus surgery.

Conclusion

Although 3D display systems are more expensive than conventional video systems, the increased stereoscopic sensation and depth perception generated by 3D display systems have been demonstrated to improve the performance of endolaryngeal surgical procedures. The enhanced depth perception allows improved visualization of the larynx, and may facilitate such complex procedures as endolaryngeal suturing. It is anticipated that the 3D display system will significantly improve the performance of current endolaryngeal surgical procedures.

Acknowledgements

The authors wish to thank Tsuneo Fukuyo (Shinko Optical Co. Ltd., Japan), Takanori Sekioka (Karl Storz Endoscopy Japan K.K.), and Takashi Ishii (MC Medical Inc., Japan) for their cooperation. This study has been supported by the JFE (the Japanese Foundation for Research and Promotion of Endoscopy) Grant, 1999.

References

1. Kantor EA, Berci G, Partlow E, Paz-Partlow M. A completely new approach to microlaryngeal surgery. Laryngoscope 1991;101:676–679.
2. Benjamin B. Thirty-five-millimeter photography using the Kantor-Berci video laryngoscope. Ann Otol Rhinol Laryngol 1998;107:775–778.
3. Satava RM. 3-D vision technology applied to advanced minimally invasive surgery systems. Surg Endosc 1993;7:429–431.
4. Birkett DH, Josephs LG, Este-McDonald A. New 3-D laparoscope in gastrointestinal surgery. Surg Endosc 1994;8:1448–1451.
5. Durrani AF, Preminger GM. Three-dimensional video imaging for endoscopic surgery. Comput Biol Med 1995;25:237–247.
6. Tsunoda K, Takanosawa M, Niimi S. Autologous transplantation of fascia into the vocal fold. A new phonosurgical technique for glottal incompetence. Laryngoscope 1999;109:504–508.

Bronchology and Bronchoesophagology: State of the Art.
H. Yoshimura et al., editors.

Outcome of functional videoendoscopic laryngeal surgery

Koichi Omori, Kaoru Shinohara and Nobuhiko Kazama
Department of Otolaryngology, Nishi-Kobe Medical Center, Kobe, Japan

Abstract. We present the outcomes of videoendoscope-assisted laryngeal surgery with office-based equipment, performed under local anesthesia. Laryngeal images are displayed by a flexible videoendoscope with a charge-coupled device. Specially designed fine-tipped forceps, scalpels and suction tubes are used. At each stage through surgery, the patient's voice and vocal folds are monitored and evaluated for functional control. Functional videoendoscopic laryngeal surgery was undertaken in 178 cases. Three patients were slightly intoxicated by local anesthesia but there were no other complications observed. Perioperative vocal function was reviewed by acoustic, aerodynamic, and perceptual analyses. In 55 polyp cases there was no recurrence and postoperative vocal function was improved. In 15 granuloma cases, three had recurrence. In five Reinke's edema cases, submucosal myxoid material was successfully removed and vocal function was improved. Functional videoendoscopic laryngeal surgery is a minimally invasive procedure as it monitors the patient's voice and provides clear visualization of the vocal folds during phonation.

Keywords: laryngeal surgery, office-based equipment, topical anesthesia, videoendoscope, vocal function.

Background

The procedure of laryngomicrosurgery with a suspension laryngoscope carried out under general anesthesia using an endotracheal tube has become a popular one [1]. It allows stability of the surgical field with no resulting gag reflex and enables identification of precise lesions. However, an endotracheal tube obstructs the surgical field and hence functional control cannot be achieved. Ideally, in phonosurgery the operator would be able to evaluate the patient's voice and observe the vocal fold vibration during phonation. Since 1991, Kojima et al. have been carrying out "fiberoptic laryngomicrosurgery with a stroboscope under local anesthesia" in a day surgery setting using office-based equipment [2]. The latest videoendoscope system employs a charge-coupled device chip built into the tip to offer larger images and deliver a higher level of resolution than a conventional fiberoptic endoscope [3]. Our previous study introduced videoendoscope-assisted laryngeal surgery with office-based equipment under local anesthesia [4]. This current study presents the outcome of functional videoendoscopic laryngeal surgery (FVLS) in a series of 178 patients. Vocal function was examined by well-attested aerodynamic, acoustic, and perceptual measures.

Address for correspondence: Koichi Omori MD, Department of Otolaryngology, Nishi-Kobe Medical Center, 5-7-1 Kouji-dai, Nishi-ku, Kobe 651-2273, Japan. Tel.: +81-78-997-2200. Fax: +81-78-993-3728. E-mail: koichi.omori@nifty.ne.jp

Materials and Methods

178 patients underwent FVLS under local anesthesia (Table 1). Surgical resection was undertaken in the patients with vocal fold polyp, vocal process granuloma, Reinke's edema, vocal fold nodule, laryngeal cyst, and laryngeal/pharyngeal benign lesions. A biopsy of the lesion was performed in the patients with laryngeal tuberculosis, epithelial hyperplasia, and laryngeal/pharyngeal cancer. A collagen injection in the vocal fold was carried out in the patients with vocal fold paralysis.

The videoendoscope system used in this study was the EVIS-200, a flexible videoendoscope ENF type 200, ENF type T200 (Olympus Optical Co. Ltd., Tokyo) and the EPM-1000, a flexible videoendoscope VNL-1330 (Asahi Optical Co. Ltd., Tokyo). Forceps with fine-tipped cups and scalpels with a fine-tipped blade were specially designed as described previously (Nagashima Co., Tokyo) [4].

The aerodynamic analysis of vocal function included measuring maximum phonation time (MPT), vocal intensity (VI), and mean flow rate (MFR), using a phonation analyzer PS-77 (Nagashima Co., Tokyo). The acoustic analysis involved recording pitch perturbation (jitter) and amplitude perturbation (shimmer), measured with a multidimensional voice analysis program CSL4300B (Kay Elemetrics Corp., Lincoln Park). Perceptual evaluations of the degrees of patients' roughness and breathiness of voice were determined by three experienced otolaryngologists. A score of 3 was given for a severely rough voice, a score of 2 for a moderately rough voice, a score of 1 for a slightly rough voice, and a score of 0 for no roughness of voice. The scores given by the three listeners were averaged and classified again into four categories: scores of 0, 1, 2, or 3. The degree of breathiness was also recorded as 0, 1, 2, or 3 in the same way.

Table 1. Functional videoendoscopic laryngeal surgery undertaken in 178 cases.

Condition	Surgery undertaken (No. of cases)	Surgery performed (No. of cases)
Lesions		
Vocal fold polyp	60	55
Vocal process granuloma	17	15
Reinke's edema	7	5
Vocal fold nodule	2	1
Laryngeal cyst	4	4
Laryngeal/pharyngeal benign lesion	16	16
Laryngeal tuberculosis	3	3
Epithelial hyperplasia	52	50
Laryngeal/pharyngeal cancer	15	14
Vocal fold paralysis	2	2
Total	178	165

Table 2. Preoperative and postoperative mean phonatory function in polyp, granuloma and Reinke's edema cases.

	MPT (s)	VI (dB)	MFR (ml/s)	Jitter (%)	Shimmer (%)
Polyp					
pre	14 (5)	75 (3)	215 (80)	2.6 (2.1)	6.3 (2.6)
post	21 (18)	78 (3)	170 (65)	0.9 (0.6)	2.6 (0.8)
Granuloma					
pre	28 (13)	77 (4)	184 (67)	2.0 (1.2)	4.1 (2.4)
post	31 (11)	79 (3)	169 (55)	0.8 (0.5)	2.3 (0.7)
Reinke's edema					
pre	11 (2)	75 (7)	245 (104)	5.4 (3.5)	8.8 (4.3)
post	19 (2)	79 (6)	185 (19)	1.7 (0.8)	3.4 (1.5)

Data: mean (SD).

Results

FVLS under local anesthesia was successfully performed in 165 out of 178 cases (93%), as shown in Table 1. In the remaining 13 cases FVLS could not be carried out because of patients' gag reflex. After surgery, three patients were intoxicated by the local anesthesia although they recovered 1 h later. There were no further complications seen, i.e., postoperative bleeding or aspiration of materials.

In 55 out of 60 cases operated on for vocal fold polyp, total resection of the polyp was achieved, and there has been no further recurrence in any of these 55 cases. Preoperative and postoperative vocal functions for the 40 cases of vocal fold polyp are summarized in Tables 2 and 3. Measures of MPT, VI, MFR, jitter and shimmer were seen to have significantly improved following this surgery (paired t test). In the perceptual evaluation analysis, scores for patients' roughness and breathiness of voice had also significantly improved after this surgery (Wilcoxon test).

Table 3. Preoperative and postoperative perceptual scores in polyp, granuloma and Reinke's edema cases.

	Voice roughness score (No. of cases)				Voice breathiness score (No. of cases)			
	3	2	1	0	3	2	1	0
Polyp								
pre	2	16	22	0	0	2	21	17
post	0	0	5	35	0	0	3	37
Granuloma								
pre	0	1	8	1	0	2	7	1
post	0	0	2	8	0	0	1	9
Reinke's edema								
pre	2	2	1	0	0	2	2	1
post	0	0	3	2	0	0	2	3

Total resection of the granuloma was successfully completed in 15 out of the 17 cases with vocal process granuloma. Following this surgery there has been recurrence seen in three of the 15 cases. Preoperative and postoperative vocal functions for the 10 cases with no recurrence are summarized in Tables 2 and 3. Vocal function for all measures was significantly improved post operation.

Submucosal myxoid material was successfully resected in five out of the seven cases with Reinke's edema, and there has been no apparent recurrence in any of these five cases. Preoperative and postoperative vocal functions for the five cases with successful resection are summarized in Tables 2 and 3. Again, vocal function for all measures was improved following the operation.

Conclusions

FVLS provides monitoring of the patient's voice and vocal folds during surgery which is reassuring for the surgeon as well as for the patient. This technique also allows good visibility of the lesion and hence permits precise manipulation. With these advantages, good vocal function can be obtained postoperatively. FVLS is a minimally invasive procedure for functional phonosurgery as opposed to conventional suspension laryngomicrosurgery.

Acknowledgements

This work was supported by a JFE (The Japanese Foundation for Research and Promotion of Endoscopy) Grant.

References

1. Scalo AN, Shipman WF, Tabb HG. Microscopic suspension laryngoscopy. Ann Otol Rhinol Laryngol 1960;69:1134–1138.
2. Kojima H, Honjo I. Fiberoptic laryngeal surgery with stroboscope. In: Isshiki N (ed) Syllabus of International Phonosurgery Workshop – Laryngeal Framework Surgery. Kyoto, Japan: Kyoto University, 1992;157–162.
3. Kawaida M, Fukuda H, Kohno N. Clinical experience with a new type of rhino larynx electronic endoscope Pentax VNL-1530. Diagn Ther Endo 1994;1:57–62.
4. Omori K, Shinohara K, Tsuji T, Kojima H. Videoendoscopic laryngeal surgery. Ann Otol Rhinol Laryngol 2000;109:149–155.

Bronchology and Bronchoesophagology: State of the Art.
H. Yoshimura et al., editors.

Surgical procedure concerning vocal cord cysts

Hiroya Yamaguchi[1], Kazuhiro Nakamura[1], Kiyoaki Tsukahara[1] and Hajime Hirose[2]

[1]*Department of Otorhinolaryngology, Tokyo Senbai Hospital, Tokyo; and* [2]*Kitasato University, Kanagawa, Japan*

Keywords: epidermoid cyst, laryngeal cyst, phono-surgery, retention cyst, surgical equipment.

Introduction

Vocal cord cysts are divided into two groups: acquired retention cysts and congenital epidermoid cysts [1].

Vocal cord cysts are usually located directly beneath the epithelial layer and can be easily ruptured during surgical excision. Once ruptured, the deflated vocal cord cyst, becomes extremely difficult to distinguish from the surrounding soft tissues.

If the vocal cord cyst is ruptured, the recurrence rate becomes higher. Excessive excision of the soft tissue of the normal vocal cord will result in undesirable postoperative deterioration of the quality of voice. Therefore, it is of extreme importance not to damage the cyst wall during surgical excision.

Different types of surgical methods for excision of vocal cord cyst have been reported, with emphasis on how to avoid rupturing the vocal cord cyst [2]. For this purpose, we developed special laryngo-micro surgical instruments and introduced a specific surgical method for the treatment of vocal cord cysts with promising surgical results.

Materials

During the past 2 years, 10 cases of vocal cord cysts were surgically treated at our institution. They consisted of four males and six females, and histopathological examination revealed seven epidermoid cysts, two retention cysts and one undiagnosed case.

The instruments that we developed are the laryngeal hook and the laryngeal dissector. They are ideal for the surgical excision of vocal cord cysts. Each instrument consists of two pieces, the shaft and removable handle. The laryngeal hook is a smooth and blunt probe-like instrument with the length of the hook portion being 3 mm, which is bent posterior at 60°. The laryngeal dissector is a spoon-

Address for correspondence: Hiroya Yamaguchi MD, Tokyo Senbai Hospital, 1-4-3 Mita, Minato-ku, Tokyo 108-0073, Japan. Tel.: +81-3-3451-8121. Fax: +81-3-3454-0067.

like shaped multipurpose instrument and has proved its use as a dissector, probe and elevator.

In addition, a sickle knife was also developed with a shallow curve for easy access and maneuverability for excision. The shafts of these instruments are black-finished, to minimize glare and to enable the use of them in laser surgery; thus, the surgical field can easily be observed. Furthermore, the shaft and handle combination make it easy for the surgeon to handle the length of the instrument depending on the distance to the surgical site or to change the angle of approach during surgery.

Surgical methods

The excision of vocal cord cysts commences by making an incision with the sickle knife, anterior to the midline of the cyst, followed by a posterior incision.

The laryngeal hook was inserted from the posterior position of the incision and the mucous membrane covering the cyst was undermined, exposing the superior surface of the cyst. The tip of the laryngeal hook is so smooth and blunt and the capsular margin of the cyst has enough flexibility, so that accidental rupture of the cyst can be prevented. Furthermore, since the mucous membrane is semi-transparent, the laryngeal hook can be observed during the surgical procedure. Therefore, damage to the mucous membrane was also prevented.

After undermining the mucous membrane of the superior potion of the cyst, anterior and posterior incisions were connected. Then the medial margin of the cyst was undermined. If the longitudinal axis of the vocal cord cyst is in the antero-posterior direction of the vocal cord, connective tissues, like the ducts of the cyst, are usually located at 12 o'clock. If the longitudinal axis is in right angle with the antero-posterior direction of the vocal cord, connective tissues, like ducts, can be usually found at 3 o'clock. If connective tissues, like ducts, are located at 3 o'clock, care must be taken during the undermining of the lateral margin of the cyst. At this stage of the surgery, most of anterior margin of the cyst was visible and freed from the soft tissues. Using the laryngeal dissector,the posterior margin and the inferior portion of the cyst were then undermined. The final step of the procedure was to grasp the anterior portion of the cyst and to cut it.

Results

Immediate postoperative observation revealed minute bleeding along the line of incision with minimal or no damage to the free margin of the cyst. In nine out of the 10 cases, regular and symmetrical wave patterns of the mucous membrane of the cyst were observed within 2 postoperative months, during stroboscopic examination. The remaining patient recovered after 3 months. Thus, satisfactory results were obtained in all the patients treated.

Conclusion

In the surgical treatment of vocal cord cysts, it is of extreme importance that the vocal cord cyst be excised without rupturing. Surgical damage to the free margin of the mucous membrane of the vocal cord must be avoided. The newly developed instruments, the laryngeal hook, laryngeal dissector and sickle knife, have proved to be outstanding and are extremely advantageous in the excision of vocal cord cysts without rupturing the cyst wall during surgery.

References

1. Milutinovic Z, Vasiljevic J. Contribution to the etiology of vocal fold cysts; a function and histrogic study. Laryngoscope 1992;102:568–571.
2. Hirano M, Yoshida Y, Hirade Y, Sanada T. Improved surgical technique for epidermoid cysts of the vocal fold. Ann Otol Rhinol Laryngol 1998;98:791–795.

Bronchology and Bronchoesophagology: State of the Art.
H. Yoshimura et al., editors.

Surgical management of microlesions of the vocal fold

Eiji Yumoto[1], Humihiro Katsura[1], Joji Kobayashi[2] and Tetsuji Sanuki[2]
[1]*Department of Otolaryngology Head and Neck Surgery, Kumamoto University, School of Medicine, Kumamoto; and* [2]*Department of Otolaryngology Head and Neck Surgery, Ehime University, School of Medicine, Shigenobu-cho, Onsen-gun, Ehime, Japan*

Abstract. The author performed microsurgery of the larynx on 23 patients who complained of hoarseness caused by lesions as small as, or smaller than, the size of a "typical" nodule. The patients included six men and 17 women. Nineteen of them had a history of vocal abuse. Their lesions were classified as "typical" bilateral nodules in three, "atypical" bilateral nodules in four, unilateral nodule and polyp in five, respectively, coexistence of nodule and polyp in three, cysts in two, and coexistence of polyp, nodule and polypoid change in the other. Lesions in five patients were complicated by microvascular pathologies. The mean airflow rate, in most patients, was distributed within the normal range and did not show a significant change after operation. On the contrary, the AC/DC ratio and acoustic measures (H/N ratio, jitter, and shimmer) showed a significant improvement after operation ($p < 0.05$). Detailed preoperative examination and meticulous manipulation during the operation is always required because these tiny lesions are usually atypical with more than two different kinds and because they often occur in professional vocalizers.

Keywords: examination of voice, microsurgery of the larynx, microvascular pathologies, nodule, polyp, professional vocalizer.

Introduction

Causes of hoarseness include inflammation, benign vocal fold masses such as polyps, nodules, polypoid degeneration and cysts, changes in stiffness of the mucosa, and various other causes. Of these benign vocal fold masses, polyps, polypoid degeneration and cysts are surgically managed, while voice therapy is the first choice in the treatment of nodules. Very often, tiny lesions of the vocal fold, often seen in people who use their voices frequently, are not clearly classified. Small polyps and nodules are especially difficult to differentiate based on laryngeal observation. Some nodules are atypical. In this study, we attempted to determine detailed diagnoses based on microscopic observation, operative procedures performed and perioperative vocal function in patients who complained of hoarseness caused by lesions as small as, or smaller than, the size of a "typical" nodules.

Address for correspondence: Eiji Yumoto MD, Department of Otolaryngology Head and Neck Surgery, Kumamoto University, School of Medicine, 1-1-1 Honjo, Kumamoto, Japan. Tel.: +81-96-373-5255. Fax: +81-96-373-5256. E-mail: yumoto@gpo.kumamoto-u.ac.jp

Patients and Methods

We have performed microsurgery of the larynx on 109 patients during the last 6 years in order to remove benign lesions of the vocal fold. Of these 109 patients, 23 had lesions as small as, or smaller than, the size of a "typical" nodule and were included in the study. Six were males and 17 were females. Their ages ranged from 22- to 74-years-old, with a mean age of 43-years-old. Only three had no apparent history of vocal abuse. Their occupations were teachers in 9 cases, karaoke or Japanese folk singers in 6, a saleswoman, a Buddhist monk and various other occupations.

Observation of the vocal fold was done under stroboscopic illumination in addition to continuous light. Laryngeal images were routinely observed on a monitor screen and recorded on a videotape. The vocal function test battery included aerodynamic and acoustic examinations.

Making the decision whether to proceed to surgical treatment or not depended on stroboscopic findings, the degree of dysphonia, and the need for vocal usage. The patients' understanding of pathological and functional changes of his or her own vocal fold was indispensable.

Tiny lesions were classified based on microscopic observation. Nodules, polyps and cysts were considered to be major lesions responsible for hoarseness, while minor lesions included edematous swellings reactive to polyps or cysts on the other side, microvascular lesions, nodules, mild polypoid change and inflammation. We surgically removed major lesions with cold instruments, not with lazer. A basic principle was to minimize the disruption of the mucosa and remove the least amount of tissue to preserve phonatory ability as much as possible. Reactive swellings and nodules which seemed to be minor lesions were not removed. Most microvascular lesions were cauterized with a low-powered KTP lazer. The sucking technique was utilized for polypoid change when the patient desired to raise their vocal pitch.

Results

Lesions of the vocal folds were classified into "typical" bilateral nodules in three cases, "atypical" bilateral nodules in four, unilateral nodules and polyps in five, respectively, coexistence of nodules and polyps in three, cysts in two, and coexistence of polyps, nodules and polypoid change in the other. Lesions in five of the patients were complicated by microvascular pathologies.

After placing a laryngoscope in the proper position, the lower surface of the vocal fold was always made visible by gently pressing the upper surface. Subsequently, major lesions were surgically managed. To emphasize the importance of the observation of the lower surface of the vocal fold, here is a description of a case involving a 63-year-old male. He experienced difficulty when trying to sing high tones and his voice became hoarse 4 years ago. Although stroboscopic examination revealed nodules and a slight polypoid change in the left vocal fold,

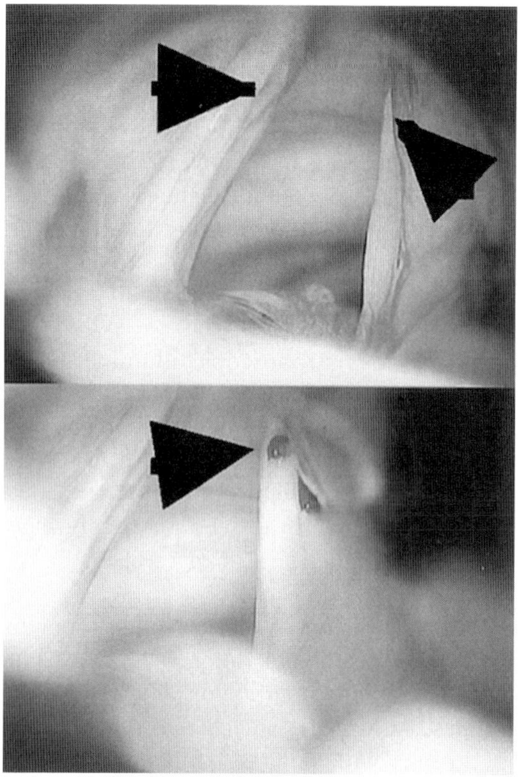

Fig. 1. A case involving a 63-year-old male. Upper half: conventional microlaryngoscopic view of the vocal fold. Triangles indicate nodules. Lower half: a small polyp (triangle) on the lower surface of the right vocal fold.

a tiny red polyp was found on the lower surface of the right vocal fold under direct microlaryngoscopy (Fig. 1). We resected this polyp and performed a sucking procedure on the left vocal fold to improve singing in high notes. The nodules were not removed. He recovered his singing voice postoperatively.

Figures 2 and 3 show pre- and postoperative aerodynamic and acoustic results during the sustained phonation of the vowel "a" with comfortable pitch and loudness, respectively. The ordinates in these figures represent the mean airflow rate (mL/s), vocal efficiency index (VEI, %), harmonics-to-noise ratio (HNR, dB), perturbations of pitch (jitter, %) and amplitude (shimmer, %). Airflow measurements were scattered in a wide range before and after the operation and no significant change was found. However, VEI increased postoperatively in all patients examined, except two, and this change was statistically significant ($p < 0.05$). HNR increased, and jitter and shimmer decreased postoperatively. These changes were also statistically significant ($p < 0.05$, $p < 0.01$ and $p < 0.001$, respectively).

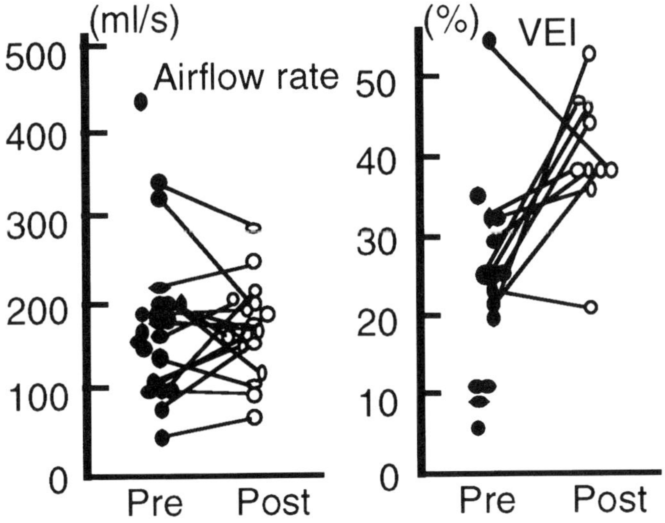

Fig. 2. Pre- and postoperative aerodynamic results. Left: mean airflow rate (mL/s). Right: vocal efficiency index (%). "Pre" and "Post" represent pre- and postoperative measurements, respectively.

Conclusions

1. Making the decision to proceed with the operation, or not, depends upon meticulous assessment of vocal fold vibration, the degree of dysphonia and the need for vocal usage. Patients' understanding of pathological and functional changes in his or her own vocal fold was indispensable.
2. Of 23 patients examined, 17 were women. All but three had a history of vocal abuse. Major lesions were labeled as nodules in 12 patients and only three of

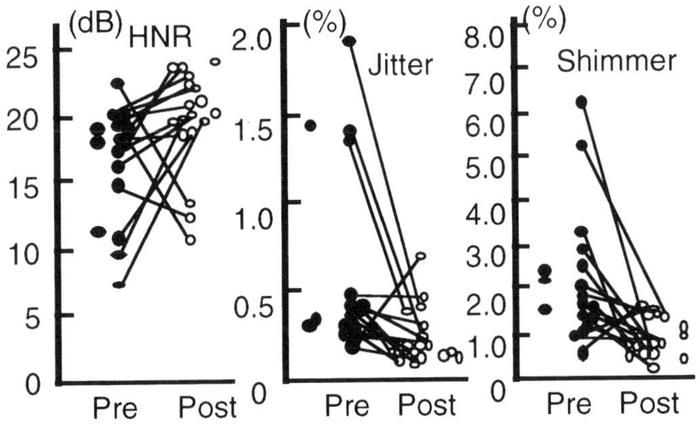

Fig. 3. Pre- and postoperative acoustic results. Left: harmonics-to-noise ratio (dB). Center: perturbation of pitch (%). Right: perturbation of amplitude (%).

them had "typical" nodules. Strategies on which pathological changes to remove should be tailored to individual patients. Acoustic analyses and VEI objectively assessed perioperative vocal functions, while airflow rate did not.

3. Management of microvascular lesions remains to be determined.

Tracheo-esophageal fistulae

Bronchology and Bronchoesophagology: State of the Art.
H. Yoshimura et al., editors.

Palliative treatment of esophagorespiratory fistulae with airway stenting or double stenting

Yasuo Iwamoto, Teruomi Miyazawa and Yuka Miyazu
Department of Pulmonary Medicine, Hiroshima City Hospital, Hiroshima, Japan

Abstract. The development of malignant esophagorespiratory fistulae are a life-threatening complication and can lead to a rapid deterioration in a patient's quality of life. Aspiration of esophageal content into the bronchial tree often causes severe pneumonia. Airway and esophageal stenting is the only way to seal the fistulae. We analyzed our experiences with single and double stenting in 13 cases of esophagorespiratory fistulae in patients.

Keywords: double stenting, esophagorespiratory fistulae.

Purpose, patients and methods

The purpose of this analysis is to evaluate the efficacy and problems of airway and double stenting in 13 patients with esophagorespiratory fistulae.

From September 1994 to December 1999, 13 patients with esophagorespiratory fistulae were inserted with single or double stents. The patients were all male with ages ranging from 51 to 73 years with a mean age of 60 years. Eleven patients had esophageal cancer and two had lung cancer.

All the data were collected from charts retrospectively.

Results

Table 1 shows the characteristics of the patients who were inserted with double stents. Out of these nine patients, four had fistulae located at the trachea, three at the left main bronchus, and two at the right main bronchus. For the fistulae located at the trachea we used one Dynamic stent, two Dumon Y stents and one Dumon stent. We used the Y-shaped stents because of the difficulty in fixing stents at the trachea. In one case, the fistula was too far from the carina to insert a Y-shaped stent and so a normal Dumon stent had to be used. The duration of patients' survival was counted from the insertion of the airway stents. The average survival period of these patients was 134 days.

Four patients were inserted with only airway stents. Three out of these four had fistulae located on the right side. In the third case, we had to insert a Covered

Address for correspondence: Dr Y Iwamoto, Department of Pulmonary Medicine, Hiroshima City Hospital, 7-33 Moto-machi, Naka-ku, Hiroshima 730-8518, Japan. Tel.: +81-82-221-2291. Fax: +81-82-223-1447.

Table 1. Characteristics of patients with double stenting.

Patient	Age	Etiology	Location	Esophagus stent	Airway stent	Survival (days)
1	60	EC	LMB	Wilson-cook	Dumon	53
2	73	LC	RMB	Covered ultraflex	Dumon	203
3	62	EC	RMB	Covered ultraflex	Dumon Y	7
4	63	EC	Trachea	Covered ultraflex	Dynamic	403[a]
5	68	EC	LMB	Covered ultraflex	Dumon Dy-	117
6	70	EC	Trachea	Covered ultraflex	namic	9
7	62	EC	Trachea	Covered ultraflex	Dumon Y	82
8	71	EC	LMB	Covered ultraflex	Dumon Y	103[a]
9	69	EC	Trachea	Covered ultraflex	Dumon	230

EC: esophageal cancer; LC: lung cancer; LMB: left main bronchus; RMB: right main bronchus; [a]patients still living.

Ultraflex stent because the tructus intermedius was too deformed for a Dumon stent to be used. The average survival period of these patients was 135 days.

Five of the nine patients who were inserted with double stents had airway stents inserted beforehand. In three of these five cases this was done to seal the fistulae and in the remaining two cases this was done to facilitate the insertion of the double stents and to maintain the airway.

The remaining four patients had esophageal stents inserted beforehand. In two cases, the airway stenosis was caused by compression of esophageal carcinoma after insertion of esophageal stents. In the other two cases the airway stents were inserted to seal the fistulae.

The functional results following stenting are as follows. After double stenting, five of the nine patients were able to swallow a solid diet without aspiration. Two patients could only swallow a liquid diet. The remaining two cases could not swallow either a liquid or solid diet. As regards the single stenting cases, two of the four patients were able to ingest a solid diet without aspiration but the remaining two cases could not swallow even a liquid diet.

The reasons for persisting dysphagia after double stenting are as follows. One patient could not even drink liquid because of recurrent laryngeal nerve palsy due to the invasion of esophageal cancer. In another case, the patient's general condition deteriorated rapidly after stenting, and died 8 days later.

We did not insert esophageal stents in some cases, in spite of persisting dysphagia. In one case we could not pass the guide wire through the esophagus because of tumor invasion. In another case it was impossible to seal the fistula because it was located between the right intermedius and the stomach. A major complication was airway stenosis caused by compression of esophageal stenting. A severe cough was seen in one case. We did not observe any migration of stents, hemoptysis or bronchial or esophageal necrosis following stenting.

In our study, seven patients died of pneumonia, three died of tumor progress and the remaining three patients are still alive.

Conclusion

We conclude that double stenting for esophagorespiratory fistulae improves patients' quality of life. We have found that when the fistulae are small, only airway stenting can be used to seal the fistulae sufficiently.

Bronchology and Bronchoesophagology: State of the Art.
H. Yoshimura et al., editors.

Comparison: tygon and polyflex stents for the palliation of esophageal obstructions and fistulas

István Kovács[1], Katalin Dévényi[2], Sándor Sz. Kiss[1] and Péter Sápy[1]
[1]*2nd Department of Surgery and* [2]*Department of Radiology, University of Debrecen, Medical and Health Science Center, School of Medicine, Debrecen, Hungary*

Abstract. *Background.* Patients with inoperable esophageal cancer have poor life expectancy without different types of palliation. The aim of this study was to compare stenting methods and investigate the complications and results.

Methods. The endoscopic intubation was introduced in 1992 and the Rüsch Polyflex stent became available from 1998. During this period 84+14 patients underwent palliation with Tygon and Polyflex prostheses. 53+10 patients had esophageal carcinoma, 21+2 had tumors of the cardia and 10+2 had pulmonary carcinoma. Among them 18+5 patients had fistula.

Results. The swallowing ability improved in all cases and the bronchoesophageal fistulas were occluded. Early complications: perforations 7, bleeding 3+1. Two patients (2%) died. Late complications: food impaction 7, tumor overgrowth 6+2, tube migration 4+1. We had no Polyflex stent-insertion related complication.

Conclusions. The risk of perforation during endoscopic intubation is high, especially in cases of tumors of the distal esophagus. Intubation with the Polyflex stent using fluoroscopic control is a safer procedure. Self-expanding stents have wider indications. The outcomes of treatments of fistulas are better when the placement of a Tygon tube is difficult or technically impossible. The improvement of the quality of life is as important a result as the improvement of the survival time due to better nutrition and prevention of aspiration.

Keywords: bronchoesophageal fistula, carcinoma, dysphagia, esophageal stents, esophagus.

Introduction

Surgical resection and esophageal reconstruction remains the dominant element in the surgeon's armamentarium for the management of esophageal carcinoma. The average resection rate reported is 40% despite major advances in surgical techniques, radiotherapy, use of cytotoxic drugs and the combination of these treatments [1]. Most of the patients have no real improvement in overall life expectancy because many display distant metastases and rather extensive tumor growth. Since life expectancy is short, the quality of life deteriorates in parallel with severe esophageal obstruction and communication between the respiratory system. The palliative treatment becomes very important in the management of these patients. Malignant tracheoesophageal fistula is a serious complication of

Address for correspondence: István Kovács, 2nd Department of Surgery, University of Debrecen, Medical and Health Science Center, School of Medicine, Móricz zs.krt.22., P.O. Box 13, 4004 Debrecen, Hungary. Tel.: +36-52-422-868. Fax: +36-52-422-868. E-mail: kovacs@jaguar.dote.hu cancer, usually arising in the esophagus, lung, or mediastinal metastases. Repeated aspiration and pneumonia lead to rapid deterioration and death. The prognosis is dismal and curative resections are controversial. Surgical bypass of the lesion has been performed but is associated with 25 to 60% mortality. Our treatment goal is to provide adequate palliation using the simplest available means and minimal amount of hospitalisation. The passage for food and saliva should be restored, and the tracheoesophageal fistula should be occluded to stop continued aspiration of food and saliva into the lungs [2]. These lesions can be adequately palliated by permanent esophageal intubation. The ability to swallow can be immediately restored, and the patient spared extensive operative procedures, as well as the physical and mental discomfort of external fistulas. Earlier, the pull-through technique was performed for relieving dysphagia when a Tygon prosthesis was inserted via laparotomy. The mortality rate of this method was up to 30%, and required long hospitalisation. With the introduction of the oral-pulsion technique, a Tygon prosthesis could be inserted over a fiber endoscope, under constant visual control using only local anaesthesia. The technique was then developed and many kinds of self-expanding endoprotheses are now available [3]. The major advantage of these stents are their small diameter in the compressed state, allowing easy insertion under continuous fluoroscopy control. The aim of this study was to summarise and compare our experiences with these techniques and analyse the related problems and complications.

Material and Methods

The palliative endoscopic intubation was introduced in 1992. Our procedure is a simplified version of the method described by Tytgat in 1986. The Rüsch Polyflex self-expanding stent has been available since 1998 in the 2nd Department of Surgery. During the last 8 years 84+14 (29+5 women, 55+9 men) consecutive patients underwent palliation with Tygon or Polyflex self-expanding prostheses. The mean age of patients was 68 years (range: 39 to 92 years) and the patients' average weight loss was 12.7 kg (0 to 26 kg). 53+10 (16+3 women, 37+7 men) patients had esophageal carcinoma, 21+2 (9+0 women, 12+2 men) had tumors of the cardia, and 10+2 (4+2 women, 6+0 men) had pulmonary carcinoma or malignant mediastinal masses. Among them, 18+5 (6+2 women, 12+3 man) patients had esophageobronchial fistula. Five cases had prosthesis insertion during operative exploration. One patient had tumor recurrence after esophagojejunostomy, three patients had previous B II. In three patients, a nonfunctioning Tygon prosthesis was removed endoscopically. After palliative treatment selected cases received intracavitary brachytherapy combined with chemotherapy.

Patients were selected with severe malignant upper intestinal obstruction and with bronchoesophageal fistulas irrespective of distant metastases. Other methods of surgery, chemotherapy and radiotherapy had already been exhausted. We excluded patients with a very limited life expectancy estimated at only a few weeks, unless there was a fistula, and in uncooperative or unmotivated cases.

The Tygon prosthesis was made from Polyvinyl tubing with an inside diameter of 12.5 mm and a wall thickncss of 1.6 mm. Length was measured individually varying from 8 to 19 cm in total length. The obstructed segment was measured endoscopically after dilatation, and about 3 to 4 cm were added to each end. The proximal end was converted into a funnel shape, the diameter of the flange measuring about 25 mm, to keep the tube from sliding distally. The distal end was cut obliquely which facilitates placement and enlarges the distal opening. Before introduction of the Tygon prosthesis, the obstructing lesion has to be properly dilated. Under local anaesthesia a guide wire was introduced well beyond the stricture, followed by gently passing in the Savary Miller dilator. Dilation is always possible if one succeeds in introducing the guide wire correctly. The tumor mass was then dilated to a diameter of 15 mm. A prosthesis was mounted over the endoscope together with a plastic pusher tube and positioned under continuous visual control. Assessment of the severity of the stenosis, the dilatation, and the positioning of the prosthesis itself is usually done during a single session. The next day, contrast X-rays were taken to confirm that no displacement had occurred and that the passage is adequate, at which point the patient is ready to eat a nearly normal diet, and can be discharged. When the prosthesis extends into the stomach the patient is routinely treated with H2 receptor blockers and advised to sleep elevating the head to avoid recumbency.

The Rüsch Polyflex self-expanding stent for the esophagus is a complete plastic stent which consists of a compound of a Polyester braid which is totally covered in silicone. It has an introducer set for easy insertion via the guide wire. The introducer system contains a sterile stent, which is available in a broad range of widths (16 to 21 mm) and lengths (9 to 15 cm), and a stent loader for loading the proper stent into the introducer sleeve. The insertion tube has a dilator tip for the atraumatic insertion after Savary Miller bougie dilatation. Following the introduction of the loaded Polyflex stent into the malignant stenosis we can release the stent from the introducer sleeve with the aid of a flexible positioner. The stent has different marks. Blue marks for visibility under endoscopic observation and black radio markers for fluoroscopic identification. Both kinds of marks are on either side of the stent and in the middle to provide orientation during the application. The funnel and protruding mesh surface, as well as the elasticity prevent migration of the stent. The thin wall and a smooth silicone inner surface impedes bolus impaction

Results

In general, after intubation there was a marked improvement in swallowing ability, usually lasting until death. The stents allowed the patients to eat a nearly normal diet. There were two failures of stent positioning, both occurring during our early experiences. The repositioning of the stent was performed under endoscopy. In three patients with very extensive tumor growth (involving the stomach up to the pyloric region where no lumen could be found with the guide wire) prosthesis insertion was carried out using the operative method. The length of hospital stay for uncomplicated intubation averaged 2 days. The results were the same in the Tygon and Rüsch Polyflex self-expanding groups.

The tracheoesophageal fistula is an absolute indication for intubation, as the tube seals of the fistula with consequent improvement in the quality of life, and in respiratory and nutritional status. There was good sealing of the fistulas in 11 (61%) cases, three incomplete sealings were achieved in the Tygon group. In three cases the traditional rigid tube placement did not provide adequate occlusion of the fistula, because they were located above or at the level of the funnel. The use of Polyflex self-expanding stents completely sealing the fistulas was verified by radiography. In all five cases with fistula, immediate relief of incessant coughing spells was obtained.

A minor, short-lasting rise in body temperature was commonly observed. Major bleeding, necessitating transfusion occurred in three and one cases.

Perforation occurred in the Tygon group in seven (8,3%) cases. Five cases had extensive cardia carcinoma with tortuous irregular lumen and two patients had long-narrow nonirradiated esophageal carcinoma, where no lumen could be found. After the successful insertion of a tube the patients were treated conservatively with adequate nasogastric aspiration, intravenous feeding and systemic antibiotics. Two patients with cardia tumors died due to mediastinal sepsis. There were no procedure-related perforations or deaths using the Polyflex stent.

Migration or dislocation occurred in four and one cases. The Tygon tube surface is smooth and if it is short in length, there is a greater chance of migration. The cause of failure using the Polyflex tube was due to the procedure itself, using a tube diameter that was too narrow. Both kinds of tubes needed to be removed and replaced by either a longer or wider self-expanding stent.

Obstruction occurred in seven cases due to food impaction in the Tygon group. Cleaning the tube can be performed with ambulatory endoscopy. Six and two cases had tumor growth above the funnel of the stent, necessitating the removal of the tube and replacement with a longer one with the pull-through method. If the stent could not be removed we placed a second self-expanding stent into the original one. We had no case with benign obstruction due to reflux esophagitis.

Pressure necrosis caused by the Tygon prosthesis funnel edge, usually of the tumor–invaded or irradiated esophageal wall, caused severe pain and mediastinal leaking in three cases. The chances of pressure necrosis occurring are greater when there is marked angulation between the esophagus and the prosthesis, leading to eccentric asymmetric pressure of the esophagus wall by the radial force of the self-expanding stent (one case). Pressure necrosis may ultimately lead to mediastinal contamination and even bleeding due to necrosis of the aorta.

Discussion

Despite extensive advances in diagnostic and treatment strategies, esophageal cancer remains largely an incurable disease. The insertion of a prosthesis ultimately appears to be the fastest and cheapest way of obtaining long-lasting palliation of dysphagia in the majority of the patients with malignacy of the esophagus and cardia. Esophageal endoprotheses, until recently, consisted of semirigid plastic stents being placed with the use of laparotomies and eventually being positioned using endoscopy. Although well established as an inexpensive, rapid and durable palliative procedure, placement of these semirigid endoprostheses has been associated with a high complication rate, including perforation, dislocation and obstruction. However, when successfully placed, the quality of swallowing is good and the patient can eat an almost normal diet. As a result, the self-expanding stent has provided a new and popular alternative to conventional plastic stents for palliation over the past 8 years [4]. The improvement in dysphagia using either tube was the same. Complications and malfunctioning of the stent were significantly higher in the plastic stent group. Recurrent dysphagia due to tumor overgrowth was the same in both groups. The malignant tracheoesophageal fistula is a serious complication of cancer usually arising in the esophagus, lung and mediastinum. Repeated aspiration and pneumonia lead to rapid deterioration and death. Complete sealing of the fistulas was verified by radiography in all patients receiving Rüsch Polyflex self-expanding stents. From a theoretical point of view, these stents have some obvious advantages over the plastic endoprostheses; namely a thin wall allowing for wider diameter and considerable flexibility. These stents also have a strong radial expansion force due to the mesh [5]. On the basis of our first experience with self-expanding silicon covered polyester mesh stents, we have greatly reduced the procedure-related morbidity and mortality, especially in advanced cases with a very long and torturous tumor, and in cases with tracheoesophageal fistula. The Rüsch self-expanding Polyflex stents may prove cost-effective because of decreased complication rates and shorter duration of hospitalisation in selected cases. The findings of the study suggest that the decision to use conventional semirigid plastic tubes or Polyflex stents should be chosen on an individual basis, taking such factors into account as tumor localisation, axis deviation and the presence of esophagorespiratory fistulas. The self-expanding stents have increased the indications and the outcomes of the procedure where the placement of a traditional tube is difficult or technically impossible [6]. With adequate palliation of these cases we may serve to improve quality of life and prolong survival.

References

1. Kovács I, Kiss S.Sz, Tóth P, Kiss Gy.G, Szluha K, Bágyi P, Sápy P. Malignus nyelõcsõ szûkületek palliatív endoscopos intubációja. Endoscopia 1999;2:7–9.
2. Schumacher B, Lubke H, Frieling T, Haussinger D, Niederau C. Palliative treatment of malignant esophageal stenosis: experience with plastic versus metal stents. Hepatogastroenterology 1998;45:755–760.
3. May A, Ell C. Palliative treatment of malignant esophagorespiratory fistulas with Gianturco-Z stents. A prospective clinical trial and review of the literature on covered metal stents. Am J Gastroenterol 1998;93:532–535.

4. Maier A, Pinter H, Friehs GB, Renner H, Smole-Juttner FM. Self-expandable coated stent after intraluminal treatment of esophageal cancer: a risky procedure? Ann Thorac Surg 1999;67: 781–784.
5. Olsen E, Thyregaard R, Kill J. Esophacoil expanding stent in the management of patients with nonresectable malignant esophageal or cardiac neoplasm: a prospective study. Endoscopy 1999;31:417–420.
6. Segalin A, Bonavina L, Carazzone A, Ceriani C, Peracchia A. Improving results of esophageal stenting: a study on 160 consecutive unselected patients. Endoscopy 1997;29:701–709.

Bronchology and Bronchoesophagology: State of the Art.
H. Yoshimura et al., editors.

Endoscopic diagnostics of esophageal-respiratory fistulas

Michael A. Rusakov and Ellyna A. Godjello

Department of Endoscopic Surgery of the National Research Centre of Surgery, Moscow, Russia

Abstract. X-ray has been used as the main method of diagnosing esophageal-respiratory fistulas. However, it does not give an exact diagnosis and can give false positive results. Traditional endoscopic methods are successful in identifying wide fistulas in patients, but less effective in the cases of thin fistulas. For this reason we have developed a combined esophagotracheobronchoscopy that delivers accurate diagnosis in patients and can also indicate an absence of fistula in some cases.

Introduction

X-ray is the main diagnostic method used for patients with esophageal-respiratory fistulas. If swallowed contrast agent is registered in lumens of both esophagus and tracheobronchial tree then the diagnosis is confirmed. However, the esophageal and respiratory orifices of a fistula are not precisely located with this technique and it can sometimes give a false positive result.

Endoscopical diagnostics are based on detection of the connection between both organs' lumens. It is easier to do this if the tracheo-esophageal fistula's diameter is large. In such a situation it is possible to see one organ's mucosa from the other organ's lumen (Fig. 1A). Indeed sometimes it is possible to pass an endoscope from the trachea into the esophagus or vice versa (Fig. 1B).

If the fistula's diameter is small the direct endoscopic diagnosis of esophageal-respiratory fistulas is impossible, especially in esophago-bronchial fistulas. We have therefore developed a method of combining esophagoscopy and tracheobronchoscopy under a general anesthesia. This procedure is especially useful in cases where endoscopic examination of the esophagus or respiratory passage shows a suspected hole on the fistula's orifice but on closer investigation there is none. First, in this procedure we insert two endoscopes into the esophagus and respiratory passage simultaneously (Fig. 2). Then, we insert a Teflon catheter into the suspicious hole and inject a solution of nontoxic paint in saline. The appearance of the paint in the lumen of the other organ is an accurate confirmation of the fistula. This method also allows us to precisely locate a position of the second fistula's orifice.

Address for correspondence: M.A. Rusakov, National Research Centre of Surgery, Abrikosovsky 2, Moscow 119874, Russia. Tel.: +7-95-248-11-42. Fax: +7-95-246-89-88.

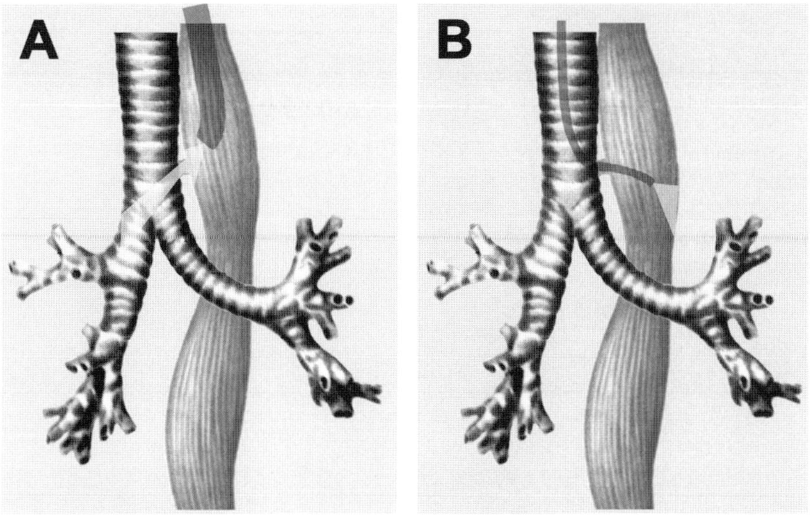

Fig. 1. **A:** An examination of tracheal mucosa from esophageal lumen. **B:** A bronchoscope is guided from trachea to esophagus.

Patients

From 1988 to 2000, 41 patients with suspected esophageal-respiratory fistulas were examined. In all of them X-ray had confirmed the diagnosis previously. Probable causes of fistulas are shown in Table 1.

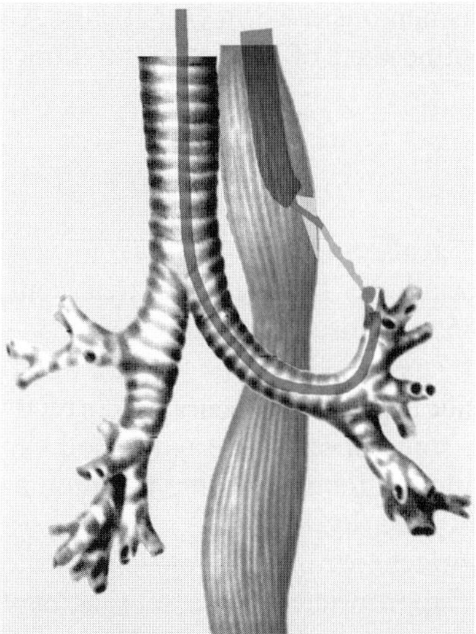

Fig. 2. An outline of the combined esophagotracheobronchoscopy.

Table 1. Probable causes of fistulas.

Etiology	No. of patients
Iatrogenic tracheal trauma	7
Bougienage of esophageal stricture	6
Esophageal diverticulum	5
Blunt chest trauma	5
Tumor destruction	5
Leakage of an esophageal anastomosis	3
Wall necrosis caused by stent	3
Congenital disease	3
Others	4
Total	41

Results

In 14 cases the fistula was diagnosed and both its orifices were found by esophagoscopy and tracheobronchoscopy, which were carried out separately. In these patients the diameter of a fistula was more than 5 mm and its respiratory mouth was in the trachea. In another 27 patients only one hole suspected on the fistula's orifice was revealed. These patients underwent the combined esophagoscopy and tracheobronchoscopy. In 17 patients small diameter fistulas were identified. In 10 patients the respiratory orifice was in the trachea and in 7 it was in segmental or smaller bronchus. In these cases the fistula location was only confirmed only due to the appearance of the paint in the lumen of bronchus.

Most significantly, the absence of fistulas was demonstrated in 10 patients. All these patients aspirated food and contrast agent because of the larynx's dysfunction.

Discussion

The accurate diagnosis of nontumor esophageal-respiratory fistulas is very important as regards their treatment and especially for their surgical treatment. Roentgenological (including CT) and traditional endoscopic methods can give good results only in patients where large fistulas are present. If the fistula's diameter is small then these methods cannot provide correct diagnoses or correctly determine both fistulas' orifices. Furthermore, sometimes the X-ray method can indicate signs of fistula present when there is in fact none. In such a situation as this, patients may be exposed to operation unnecessarily.

We believe that only the combined esophagotracheobronchoscopy can lead to exact diagnoses in these patients and to the appropriate choice of treatment methods for the individual patient.

Video, oral and poster presentations

Airway stenosis

Traumatic tracheal lesions in children: to stent or not to stent

S. Feijó, J. Rosal, I. Correia, M. Agarez and B. Almeida
Respiratory Endoscopy Unit, Department of Pulmonology, Hospital de Santa Maria, Lisbon, Portugal

Abstract. Central-airway traumatic lesions have multiple aetiologies. These lesions are a challenging problem for the bronchoscopist depending on the cause and localisation, on the symptomatology and on the degree of emergency. The decision to stent or not to stent is mainly dependent on the bronchoscopist's experience. We present three cases of tracheal traumatic lesions in children: first, a right main bronchus complete section caused by an accident with a tractor; second, an intubation trauma after a cardiac arrest caused by a car accident; and third, an accidental trauma with a knife.
The conclusion from these and other cases seems to be that stenting can play an important role in the treatment of these traumatic lesions. However, in some cases, to withhold this procedure may be appropriate.

Keywords: bronchoscopy, children, stent, tracheal stenosis, trauma.

Acquired laryngotracheal stenosis in children is more and more commonly seen, following the widespread adoption of prolonged endotracheal intubation for respiratory support, especially in cases with the respiratory distress syndrome or as a consequence of traumatic lesions due to domestic accidents or those involving vehicles.

Approximately 90% of infants and children with severe acquired laryngotracheal stenosis are tracheotomy-dependent and, therefore, impaired in their physical and speech development. In addition, tracheotomized infants can be damaged by the cannula due to crusting of secretions, dislocation, autoextubation and stomal collapse or stenosis secondary to the cannula, and in these cases early treatment is mandatory.

In some cases of unsuccessful intervention or in other cases in which intervention is not indicated or should be postponed, stenting is a therapeutical procedure which can play an important role in the management of these lesions. These lesions are a challenging problem for the bronchoscopist depending on the cause and localisation, on the symptomology and on the degree of emergency.

The decision of whether or not to stent is mainly dependent on the individual bronchoscopist's level of experience in this field.

Within the last 2 years, we have successfully treated three children with traumatic tracheal lesions:

Address for correspondence: S. Feijó, Unidade de Endoscopia Respiratória, Serviço de Pneumologia, Hospital de Santa Maria, Av. Prof. Egas Moniz, 1600 Lisboa, Portugal. Tel.: +351-21-7966739. Fax: +351-21-7966739.

First case:

- 11-ycar-old boy;
- Accident with a tractor;
- Endoscopy at 48 h: complete section of the right bronchial tree plus laceration of the distal third of the trachea;
- Right main bronchus reimplantation attempt plus tracheal "patch";
- Right pneumotomy plus thoracoplasty;
- Gastrectomy plus cervical esophogostomy.

Second case:

- 9-year-old boy;
- Car accident – 9 months;
- Severe cerebral damage, multiple episodes of mechanical ventilation after surgery and acute respiratory distress;
- Suprasternal depression with inspiratory collapse.

Third case:

- 5-year-old boy;
- Penetrating cervical wound with a knife;
- Severe subcutaneous emphysema;
- OT intubation with clinical stabilisation.

In the first case, we decided to insert a dynamic stent (Freitag) with right arm cut and closed with a thoracoscopy stapler. This gave excellent results with a successful weaning and tracheostomy closure within days. In the second case, a Dumon 12×30 mm stent was inserted with complete resolution of the clinical picture. There were no episodes of respiratory distress seen during 1 year of monitoring the postoperative condition. In the third case, we decided to wait and see. Four days later, the child was extubated without any complications.

Conclusion

- Decisive factors in treatment: time and experience.
- Silicone stents (easy to insert and easy to remove) are the best choice.
- More contributions on this matter are needed.

Bronchology and Bronchoesophagology: State of the Art.
H. Yoshimura et al., editors.

The examination of cicatricial stenosis of the larynx

Hirokazu Hattori, Tatsuya Sawada, Jun Mori, Yoshiaki Hayano, Makoto Murayama, Kenji Suzuki, Mikio Yagisawa and Tadao Nishimura
Department of Otolaryngology, Fujita Health University, The Second Affiliated Hospital, Nagoya, Japan

Abstract. We examined four patients with cicatricial stenosis of the larynx diagnosed and treated in our department over 4 years. We examined the literature concerning laryngeal stenosis published in Japan from 1990 to 1999. It appeared that treatment such as laryngomicrosurgery was useful for supraglottic stenosis, mild glottic stenosis and mild subglottic stenosis, and that laryngofissure was useful for severe glottic stenosis, subglottic stenosis and extensive stenosis. Concomitant use of a CO_2 laser was considered useful for inhibiting the formation of granulation tissue during the process of wound healing. A T-tube insertion period of 3 months or longer was considered necessary.

Keywords: laryngeal stenosis, laryngofissure, laryngomicrosurgery, T-tube.

Introduction

We occasionally come across the difficult case of treating cicatricial stenosis of the larynx resulting from a traffic injury or endotracheal intubation. We examined four patients with cicatricial stenosis of the larynx diagnosed and treated in our department over 4 years. We present here our results and a discussion of the relevant literature.

Cicatricial stenosis patients in our department

The details of the patients are summarized in Table 1. Patient 1 suffered from glottic stenosis after laryngomicrosurgery. The adhesion was eliminated by $C0_2$ laser under laryngomicrosurgery, and a silicon plate was inserted. This patient is currently doing well. Patient 2 also suffered from glottic stenosis due to a laryngeal injury. A laryngofissure was performed and granulation tissue was removed. Nevertheless, adhesion occurred after cricoarytenoid joint dislocation. There was an insufficient airway cavity, so a tracheal stoma retainer was inserted, however, the patient died of rectal cancer. Patients 3 and 4 are cases of subglottic stenosis following endotracheal intubation. In patient 3, cicatrices were removed by $C0_2$ laser via laryngofissure, and a T-tube insertion was carried out. In this case at present the tracheostoma is closed. In patient 4 tracheotomy was performed,

Address for correspondence: Dr Hirokazu Hattori, Fujita Health University, The Second Affiliated Hospital, 3-6-10 Otoubashi, Nakagawa-ku, Nagoya 454-8509, Japan. Tel.: +81-52-321-8171. Fax: +81-52-331-6843.

Table 1. Details of patients treated.

No.	Age	Sex	Cause of stenosis	Site	Chief symptoms	Method of treatment	Outcome
1	54	F	Laryngomicrosurgery	Glottic	Hoarseness, dyspnea	Tracheotomy, laryngomicro-surgery (CO_2 laser), silicon plate	Tracheostoma was closed 6 weeks later
2	47	M	Laryngeal injury	Glottic	Hoarseness, dyspnea	Tracheotomy, laryngofissure	Died of rectal cancer
3	74	M	Endotracheal intubation (2 weeks)	Subglottic	Dyspnea, wheeze	Laryngofissure (CO2 laser), T-tube	Tracheostoma was closed 4 weeks later
4	52	F	Endotracheal intubation (1 week)	Subglottic	Dyspnea, wheeze	Tracheotomy, T-tube	T-tube still inserted 2 years later

and a T-tube insertion was also undertaken. The T-tube is still inserted as the frame was extensively deformed over the tracheal cartilage.

Laryngeal stenosis in Japan (1990 to 1999)

We examined the literature concerning laryngeal stenosis published in Japan over 10 years from 1990 to 1999. We recruited laryngeal stenosis patients aged 16 years and older, and evaluated their condition.

There were 49 patients aged 17 to 80 years (average 49.3 years), and the ratio of males and females was 1:1.4 (Table 2). Traffic accidents were the most frequent cause of laryngeal stenosis cases (17 patients, 34.7%), followed by endotracheal intubation in seven patients (14.3%) and surgery in six patients (12.2%) (Table 3). Methods of approach to treatment at each site were classified into laryngo-microsurgery, laryngofissure and others. Laryngomicrosurgery was performed

Table 2. Distribution of the age and sex of patients.

Age	Male	Female	Unknown	Total
16–20	0	2	0	2
21–30	3	3	0	6
31–40	2	5	0	7
41–50	3	6	0	9
51–60	7	8	0	15
61–70	2	1	1	4
71+	3	3	0	6
Total	20	28	1	49

Table 3. Lesional site and cause of stenosis cases.

Cause	Supraglottic	Glottic	Subglottic	Two or more sites	Total
Traffic accident	5	2	4	6	17
Endotracheal intubation	0	3	4	0	7
Surgery	1	2	0	3	6
Tracheotomy	0	0	4	0	4
Percutaneous trachea needle puncture	0	0	1	0	1
Accident	0	2	1	2	5
Suicide	1	0	1	0	2
Others	0	1	4	2	7
Total	7	10	19	13	49

for supraglottic stenosis in five patients (71.4%). For treatment of glottic stenosis, laryngomicrosurgery was performed in three patients (30%) and laryngofissure in six patients (60%). For subglottic stenosis, laryngomicrosurgery was performed in five patients (26.3%) and laryngofissure in nine patients (47.4%). Laryngofissure was performed in 10 patients (76.9%) where stenosis was extensive in two or more sites (Table 4). A T-tube was applied in 15 (30.6%) of the patients, over a period of time ranging from 3 weeks to 3 years (9.5 months on average) (Table 5).

Discussion

Iatrogenic stenosis was observed in a total of 18 patients (36.7%), and was thus more frequently occurring than stenosis resulting from traffic accidents. Iatrogenic stenosis was observed in three of the four patients in our department. However, traffic accidents caused more extensive stenosis in a greater variety of sites than did other causes. Laryngomicrosurgery appeared to be an appropriate treatment due to the fact that in most cases stenosis could be controlled well by concomitant laser treatment. Laryngofissure was used more frequently than lar-

Table 4. Methods of approach and lesional site.

Method	Lesional site (No. of patients (%))				Total
	Supraglottic	Glottic	Subglottic	Two or more sites	
Laryngomicrosurgery	5 (71.4%)	3 (30.0%)	5 (26.3%)	2 (15.4%)	15 (30.6%)
Laryngofissure	1 (14.3%)	6 (60.0%)	9 (47.4%)	10 (76.9%)	26 (53.1%)
Others	1 (14.3%)	1 (10.0%)	5 (26.3%)	1 (7.7%)	8 (16.3%)
Total	7	10	19	13	49

Table 5. T-tube insertion period and lesional site distribution.

Insertion period	Lesional site (No. of patients)			Total
	Glottic	Subglottic	Two or more sites	
< 3 months	0	1	2	3
3–6 months	1	0	1	2
6–12 months	1	2	0	3
> 12 months	0	2	1	3
Unknown	0	4	0	4
Total	2	9	4	15

yngomicrosurgery for treating both glottic stenosis and subglottic stenosis. It appeared that when glottic stenosis and subglottic stenosis were mild, laryngomicrosurgery was a more useful treatment, and when they were more severe, laryngofissure was the more appropriate choice of treatment. Concomitant use of CO_2 laser appeared to be useful for inhibiting the formation of granulation tissue. Transplantation of the skin or membrane was considered necessary for certain conditions of the lumen, irrespective of site.

Sato et al. [1] reported that a T-tube insertion period of at least 3 months was required and that scar formation should be 3 months. When the T-tube was left for 2 months in patient 3, stenosis recurred, we therefore inserted the T-tube again for 4 months and obtained a good result. This finding suggests that the T-tube insertion period should be at least 3 months.

Conclusion

It appeared that laryngomicrosurgery treatment was useful for supraglottic stenosis, mild glottic stenosis and mild subglottic stenosis, and that laryngofissure was more successful for treating severe glottic stenosis, subglottic stenosis and extensive stenosis. Concomitant use of a CO_2 laser was considered effective for inhibiting the formation of granulation tissue during the process of wound healing. Transplantation of membrane was considered necessary for certain conditions of the lumen. Our results showed that a T-tube insertion period of at least 3 months would be considered necessary in most cases.

References

1. Sato K. Cicatricious stenosis of the larynx and trachea. Practica Otologica 1993:62;77–85.
2. Choi SS, Zalzal GH. Pediatric laryngotracheal reconstruction. Operat Tech Laryngol Head Neck Surg 1998:9;158–165.

Bronchology and Bronchoesophagology: State of the Art.
H. Yoshimura et al., editors.

Treatment of tracheal stenosis after surgery on a double aortic arch using a balloon-expandable metallic stent: a case report

Tivadar Márialigeti[1], Tamás Machay[2] and Kinga Jellinek[3]
[1]*Pediatric Department, County Pneumological Hospital, Törökbálint;* [2]*1st Pediatric Clinic, Semmelweis Medical University, Budapest; and* [3]*Jellinek and Partner Co. Anaesthesiologists, Martonvásár, Hungary*

Abstract. Due to a double aortic arch, a female newborn had to be operated. The operation was successful. The tracheal stenosis caused by the vascular ring was complicated by severe tracheobronchomalacia, stenosis, covering 95% of the left main bronchus, also causing — after extubation — hypercapnia, air trapping and ventril stenosis of the left lung. Permanent intubation was mandatory. At 6 weeks of age a balloon-expandable metallic stent was inserted into the lower part of the trachea. Her respiratory status improved dramatically after the insertion. Seven weeks postimplantation, severe respiratory distress occurred. Urgent stent removal was necessary due to an obstruction caused by granulation tissue, which could not be removed. During the removal, complete obstruction of the trachea occurred. After a successful reanimation, the patient's condition stabilised within 5 days. Six months later the tracheal and left main bronchus stenosis equalized at 60%, normal mucosa and no granulation was observed. Due to effort, on the part of the patient, only a mild case of stridor was present. The patient's physical and mental development was adequate. The insertion of stents is a very useful and less invasive method for the palliative treatment of airway stenoses.

Keywords: double aortic arch, stent removal, tracheobronchial stent, tracheomalacia.

Introduction

Following the surgical correction of the double aortic arch, a tracheal stenosis would generally be released to some extent [1]. However, because of the presence of some anatomical peculiarity, the extent of the release is limited.

In a follow-up study of the Pediatric Institute Svábhegy Budapest-Hungary, concerning the occurrence of different airway stenoses in childhood between 1971 and 1985, altogether 1,762 stenoses were found. Out of these, 49 were caused by vascular rings and 21 by double aortic arches [2]. In these 21 patients, the average degree of the stenoses was 80%, which decreased to 50% after surgery. Postoperative complications were observed in five babies, and one patient died.

If the tracheal stenosis is complicated by tracheomalacia, difficulties concerning extubation could emerge. This was the cause of the postoperative complications and death in the above follow-up study. We report the successfull treatment of tracheomalacia using a Tentaur 31.6LVM balloon-expandable metallic vascular stent in an infant, after surgery on a double aortic arch.

Address for correspondence: Dr Tivadar Márialigeti, Pediatric Department, County Pneumological Hospital, H-2045 Törökbálint, Munkácsy M.u.70., Hungary. Tel.: +36-23-338-022. Fax: +36-23-335-012. E-mail: tbti.@matavnet.hu

Case report

BB, a female newborn (born on 02.06.1999 at 38 weeks gestation; birth weight 2,900 g; from the fifth pregnancy as the first live baby, after in vitro fertilisation) suffered from serious stridor and apnoic attacks just after her delivery, which was normal. Her condition deteriorated rapidly, and artificial ventilation became necessary. On the 5th day of her life, 95% rigid tracheal and left main bronchus stenosis, softness of the cartilages and severe inflammation of the mucosa were diagnosed bronchoscopically. The suspected diagnosis of double aortic arch was confirmed by esophagography and angiography and she was operated on the 13th day after birth, without any complications.

During the 1st postoperative week she could not be extubated, because of hypercapnia, persistent air trapping and ventrilstenosis of the left lung. On the 7th postoperative day, a second bronchoscopy showed a 90% soft tracheal and left main bronchus stenosis. On the CT scan the tracheal stenosis was 13 mm long and a closed left main bronchus was detected. As extubation was unsuccessful, the implantation of a Tentaur 31.6LVM balloon-expandable metallic stent was indicated (KM Inc. 2360 Gyál, Hungary). Informed consent from the parents was obtained.

In placing the stent, we followed the method reported by Filler et al. [3]. The 20-mm long stent was inserted into the lower third of the trachea, just over the bifurcational carina, and expanded to 6 mm in diameter under general anaesthesia, using a rigid bronchoscope, sized 5 mm, under fluoroscopic control. The infant's respiratory status improved dramatically, and intubation was unnecessary. On the day of the implantation, it was possible to commence oral feeding and 2 days later the baby was sent home.

Four weeks passed by uneventfully. A control bronchoscopy showed epithelialisation and some granulation tissue. On the 7th week, severe respiratory distress occurred. Urgent bronchoscopy revealed a severe inflammatory reaction and obstructing granulation tissue, which could not be removed by scraping, and dilation of the stent also failed. Urgent stent removal was necessary. During the removal, complete obstruction of the trachea occurred. Successful reanimation lasted 8 min. The patient's condition stabilised within 5 days.

Three weeks after stent removal, bronchoscopy showed only 60% stenosis, some granulation and normal mucosa. Six months later the tracheal and left main bronchus stenosis was equally 60%, but normal mucosa and no granulation was seen. Due to effort, on the part of the patient, only mild stridor was present. The patient's physical and mental development was adequate. Long-term treatment consisted of the use of Budesonid spray, N-acetyl-cystein, ingested orally, and 0.9% NaCl inhalation.

Conclusions

The insertion of stents is a very useful and less invasive method for the palliative treatment of airway stenoses [3–5]. The major complication is the development of obstructing granulation tissue. Even small growths of granulation tissue have to be removed by frequent bronchoscopic manipulations. To reduce granulation the use of a covered stent is necessary [6]. Steroid inhalation seems to reduce granulation. Patients need very careful and continuous observation. During stent removal, major difficulties may emerge [3], as happened in our case, but they can be treated successfully.

References

1. Székely E, Farkas E. Pediatric bronchology, Akadémia Kiadó Budapest Hungary. University Park Press: Baltimore, 1978;300–305.
2. Márialigeti T, Székely E. Treatment and long term care of babies and infants suffering from airway stenosis. Eur Resp J 1988;1(Suppl 2):390.
3. Filler RM, Forte V et al. Tracheobronchial stenting for the treatment of airway obstruction. J Pediatr Surg 1998;33:304–311.
4. Filler RM. Current approaches in tracheal surgery. Pediatr Pulm 1999;S18:105–108.
5. Furman RH, Backer CL et al. The use of balloon-expandable metallic stents in the treatment of pediatric tracheomalacia and bronchomalacia. Arch Otolaryngol Head Neck Surg 1999;125: 203–207.
6. Sommer D, Forte V. Advances in the management of major airway collapse: the use of airway stents. Otolaryngol Clin North Am 2000;33:163–177.

Bronchology and Bronchoesophagology: State of the Art.
H. Yoshimura et al., editors.

Utilization of subtraction spiral computer tomography in evaluation of tracheobronchial stenosis

Kenwyn G. Nelson, David E. Griffith, Leslie A. Couch and David E. Finlay
University of Texas Health Center, Tyler, Texas, USA

For the last three decades computer tomography ("CAT SCANS") have been available for evaluation of tracheal lesions. These images have generally been taken in the transverse axis with 1.0 cm cuts. However, the trachea is a longitudinal structure best displayed in the coronal or sagittal planes. With the advent of spiral CT imaging it has been possible to display tracheal images in a longitudinal fashion. In addition, by subtraction of other organs (i.e., the heart and major vessels), it is now possible to obtain detailed studies of the trachea and major bronchi [1–3]. These studies are ordinarily done with breath-holding in both inspiration and expiration. However, when the patient is extremely compromised and cannot hold his breath, dynamic studies can be done with the patient breathing using an averaging technique [4–7].

An example of the first technique is a 72-year-old male admitted with recurrent respiratory failure. He was transferred intubated having had three recent previous intubations and extubations. Twenty-years previously he had suffered electrical shock, burns, smoke inhalation and had prolonged endotracheal intubation. Spiral CT with breath-holding in inspiration and expiration demonstrated a focal narrowing and buckling of the trachea that was worse on inspiration and was abnormal on both studies. Accurate measurements and location of the defect were made, and an appropriate stent was placed under fluoroscope control with immediate relief of symptoms. A grateful patient stated he had not breathed that well in 20-years.

In a second example, the patient was unable to hold his breath for the 30–45 s required for a spiral CT to be carried out. As a consequence, the study was averaged. This patient had severe tracheomalacia and bronchomalacia of unknown cause, suspected to be viral in origin. Collapse was so severe that it completely obstructed the trachea in expiration. Recurrent bouts of pneumonia had occurred due to inability to clear secretions. Measurements were taken and a stent was first placed in the left mainstem bronchus. Then the largest available tracheal stent (80 × 20 mm) was placed resting on the carina. Unfortunately with coughing the stent later displaced moving distally into the right bronchus and intermedius. This initially caused no difficulties, but as expected caused a late atelectasis of

Address for correspondence: Dr Kenwyn Nelson MD, University of Texas Health Center, 11937 US Highway 271, Tyler, Texas 75708-3154, USA. Tel.: +1-903-877-7460. Fax: +1-903-877-5548.

the right upper lobe and some changes in the left side.

The spiral CT showed that the upper trachea was essentially normal. As a consequence, the stent was brought up to this level by bronchoscopy with grasping forceps. Then, by limited retrosternal vertical tracheotomy at the fourth ring the stent was fixed by permanent sutures to the tracheal wall. Both stents have remained in place and have afforded the patient considerable relief of his symptoms. He is able to breathe quietly without oxygen support. He underwent bronchoscopy some 3 months after stent replacement and both stents were in appropriate position. Recent chest X-rays confirmed their unchanged position.

As illustrated by the above two cases, helical (spiral) CT scanning can be of considerable benefit in the treatment of tracheal disease by displaying the trachea in the long axis. Subtraction studies aid the accurate measurement of both longitudinal and transverse involvement. A number of terms have been used in describing these studies: 1) helical computed tomography; 2) spiral CT with multiplanar and three-dimensional reconstruction, and 3) virtual bronchoscopy. The only description I find fault with is 'virtual bronchoscopy' as the study is still a black, white and gray image and does not give the same information that a bronchoscopy, video or otherwise, gives.

These studies have been used in both adults and children, and in addition to tracheal stenosis and tracheomalacia, are also useful in tracheal tumors, and congenital variations, benign disease and in serial follow-up.

Conclusion

Spiral CT's with subtraction allow a highly accurate depiction of the tracheal anatomy and pathology, which can be used for accurate measurements for dilation, placement of stents or resection as indicated. Specific techniques should be adapted to the patient's condition and capabilities. Surgical intervention may be required to fix stent position in tracheal malacia.

References

1. Kozuka T, Minaguchi K, Yamaguchi R, Yamaguchi M, Taniguchi Y. Three-dimensional imaging of tracheobronchial system using spiral CT. Comput Meth Program Biomed 1998;57(102): 133–138.
2. Richenberg JL, Hansell DM. Image processing and spiral CT of the thorax. Br J Radiol 1998;71 (847):708–716.
3. Toki A, Todani T, Watanable Y, Sato Y, Yoshikawa M, Yamamoto S, Mitani M. Spiral computed tomography with three-dimensional reconstruction for the diagnosis of tracheobronchial stenosis. Pediatr Surg Int 1997;12(5–6):334–336.
4. Ferretti GR, Vining DJ, Knoplioch J, Coulomb M. Tracheobronchial tree: three-dimensional spiral CT with bronchoscopicemperspective. J Comput Assist Tomogr 1996;20(5):777–781.
5. LoCicero J 3rd, Costelo P, Campos CT, Francalancia N, Dushay KM, Silvestri RC, Zibrak JD. Spiral CT with multiplanar and three-dimensional reconstructions accurately predicts tracheobronchial pathology. Ann Thorac Surg 1996;62(3):811–817.
6. Remy-Jardin M, Remy J, Deschildre F, Artaud D, Ramon P, Edme JL. Obstructive lesions of the

central airways: evaluation by using spiral CT with multiplanar and three-dimensional reformations. Eur J Radiol 1996;6(6):807–816.

7. Whyte RI, Quint LE, Kazerooni EA, Cascade PN, Iannettoni MD, Orringer MB. Helical computed tomography for the evaluation of tracheal stenosis. Ann Thorac Surg 1995;60:27–33.

Asthma

Bronchology and Bronchoesophagology: State of the Art.
H. Yoshimura et al., editors.

Bronchial wall thickness in ovalbumin sensitized guinea-pig and asthmatic patients assessed by endoscopic ultrasonography

Hiroshi Tanaka, Satoshi Kaneko, Gen Yamada, Hiroki Takahashi, Toyohiro Saikai, Shin Teramoto and Shosaku Abe
Third Department of Internal Medicine, Sapporo Medical University School of Medicine, Sapporo, Japan

Abstract. To clarify the usefulness of endoscopic ultrasonography (EUS) in measuring airway wall thickness, we examined ovalbumin (OA) sensitized and control guinea-pigs, patients with chronic stable asthma and control subjects having lung cancer without abnormality in the bronchial tree. EUS was performed using an UM-S20-20R probe (1.7 mm diameter) with a 20-MHz transducer (Olympus Optical Co. Ltd), through a channel of video-imaged broncoscopy (type-P200, Olympus Optical Co. Ltd). Pathological-ultrasonographical correlation in OA sensitized guinea-pigs showed that five layers were observed in the wall of trachea, but these layers did not correlate with submucosal structures. Next, we used EUS to observe the right middle lobe bronchus and measured the length of bronchial wall. We evaluated seven EUS images in each patient. The mean thickness of bronchial wall in asthmatic patients increased in comparison with the control subjects. These results suggested that EUS could be used to measure the total bronchial wall thickness in patients with bronchial asthma, however, it could not identify each submucosal structure.

Keywords: airway remodelling, endobronchial ultrasonography.

Background

Thickening of the bronchial wall is one of the changes of the airway that can occur in chronic asthma. The assessment of bronchial wall thickness using an endoscopic ultrasonography (EUS) has been performed in bronchial tumor and adjacent large pulmonary vessels or lymph nodes, however, there has been no research done into evaluating bronchial wall thickness in asthmatic patients. This study aims to clarify the utility of EUS in measuring airway wall thickness.

Methods

We examined ovalbumin (OA) sensitized and control guinea-pigs, patients with chronic stable asthma (n = 2), and control subjects having lung cancer without abnormality in the bronchial tree (n = 2). EUS was performed using an UM-S20-20R probe (1.7 mm diameter) with a 20 MHz transducer (Olympus Optical Co. Ltd), through a channel of video-imaged broncoscopy (type-P200, Olympus

Address for correspondence: Dr Hiroshi Tanaka, Third Dept of Internal Medicine, Sapporo Medical University School of Medicine, South-1 West-16, Chuo-ku, Sapporo 060-8543, Japan. Tel.: +81-11-611-2111 ext. 3239. Fax: +81-11-613-1543. E-mail: tanakah@sapmed.ac.jp

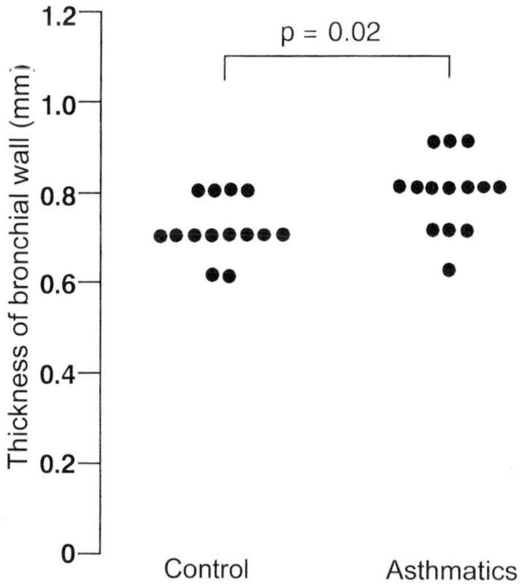

Fig. 1. Thickness of bronchial wall.

Optical Co. Ltd).

Results

Pathological-ultrasonographical correlation in OA sensitized guinea-pigs showed that five layers were observed in the wall of trachea, but these layers did not correlate with submucosal structures. We then observed the right middle lobe bronchus using EUS and measured the length of bronchial wall. We evaluated seven EUS views in each patient. The mean thickness of bronchial wall in asthmatic patients was significantly higher ($p = 0.02$) compared with the control subjects (Fig. 1).

Conclusion

EUS could measure total bronchial wall thickness in patients with bronchial asthma, however, it could not identify each submucosal structure.

Brachytherapy

Bronchology and Bronchoesophagology: State of the Art.
H. Yoshimura et al., editors.

Early experiences with HDR brachytherapy for lung cancer using a microselectron

Masahiro Imamura[1], Keizo Harima[1], Toshiko Shiga[1], Shuuji Kariya[2], Tomokuni Shiraishi[2], Satoshi Sawada[3], Yukihito Saitoh[4], Kazuyuki Yamaguchi[5] and Akiharu Okamura[6]

[1]Department of Radiology, Kansai Medical University Kohri Hospital, Neyagawa City; [2]Department of Radiology, Ishikiri Seiki Hospital, Higashi Osaka City; [3]Department of Radiology, [4]Department of Thoracic Surgery, [5]The First Department of Internal Medicine, and [6]Department of Surgical Pathology, Kansai Medical University, Moriguchi City, Japan

Abstract. High-dose-rate (HDR) brachytherapy using a microselectron, with ^{192}Ir serving as the source, was performed on 17 cases of lung cancer. The problems and values associated with this therapy were evaluated. In this paper we also present our device for HDR brachytherapy applied to lung cancer which has invaded the chest wall. Brachytherapy was undertaken by percutaneous insertion, with CT guidance, for palliation of pain, as one treatment, in multimodal therapy, achieving good pain relief.

Keywords: endobronchial HDR brachytherapy, MS-type applicator, percutaneous HDR brachytherapy.

Introduction

HDR brachytherapy is a recent development, enabling stable irradiation over a short period of time. As a result, locally concentrated irradiation, which could not be achieved with the conventional external beam irradiation procedure, is now possible [1]. We have been applying HDR brachytherapy since 1994 in order to stabilize the airway, restore patency, and secure more accurate local control of lung cancer.

Patients and Methods

Endobronchial HDR brachytherapy was performed on 17 cases (Table 1). Brachytherapy was performed using a microselectron HDR (Nucletron International B.V., The Netherlands) with a high-activity iridium-192 source (initial activity was 10 Ci, changed approximately every 3 months to 4.3 Ci). A flexible fiberoptic bronchoscope was inserted into the bronchus by way of the nose. During preparation and irradiation, patients were continually monitored in terms of

Address for correspondence: Dr Masahiro Imamura, Department of Radiology, Kansai Medical University Kohri Hospital, 8-45 Kohri Hondouri-cho, Neyagawa-shi, Osaka 572-8511, Japan. Tel.: +81-72-832-5321. Fax: +81-72-832-7336. E-mail: imamuram@takii.kmu.ac.jp

Table 1. Details of 17 cases undergoing endobronchial HDR brachytherapy.

Mean age	65.1 years (range: 42- to 85-years-old).
Sex	15 males; 2 females.
Tissue form	Squamous cell carcinoma: 14 cases; adenocarcinoma: 2 cases; small cell carcinoma: 1 case.
Clinical stage	IA: 3 cases; IB: 3 cases; IIIA: 6 cases; IIIB: 4 cases; IV: 1 case.
T factor	T1: 3 cases; T2: 6 cases; T3: 4 cases; T4: 4 cases.
Pretreatment	Surgical resection: 5 cases; chemotherapy: 6 cases (BAI: 2 cases).

pulse, blood pressure and pulse oxymetry. Continous oxygen, 3 to 4 l/min, was provided via an oxygen mask (Fig. 1).

We used an MS-type applicator (Create Medic Co., Ltd., Japan) to hold the catheter in a central location in the airway to avoid localized hot spots on the bronchial mucosa. The applicator was inserted using a 6 French catheter with dummy seeds. External beam radiation therapy was applied to the area encompassing the primary lesion hilus and mediastinum at a dose of 40 to 70 Gy in 20 to 35 fractions, followed by endobronchial HDR brachytherapy. Patients were treated with HDR brachytherapy in 4 fractions of 7 Gy at 1 cm. Figure 2 shows the range of irradiation, the area on the film represented by a solid line. The range was determined based on comprehensive findings of CTand bronchoscopy [2].

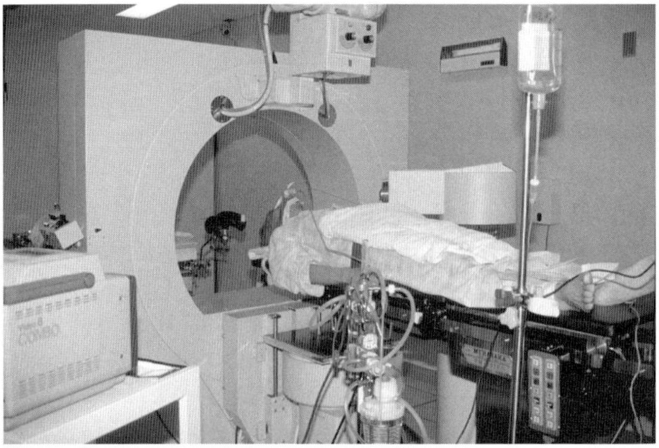

Fig. 1. An overall view of endobronchial HDR brachytherapy.

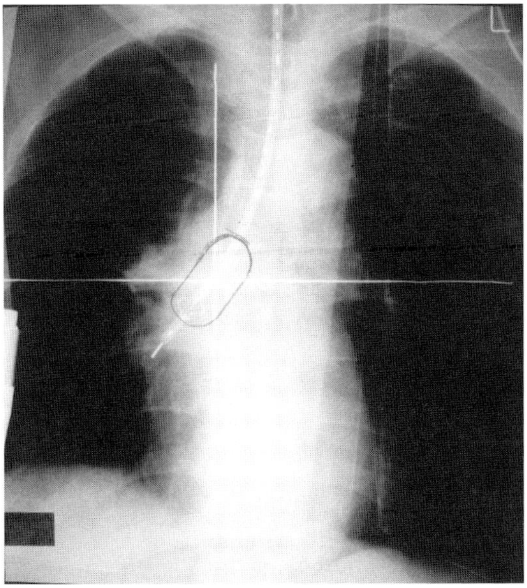

Fig. 2. The determination of the range of irradiation.

Results

Six of the 17 patients died due to systemic exacerbation. However, good local control has been maintained in the remaining patients (longest observation period: 22 months). Fatal hemoptysis, serious radiation bronchitis and fistulae are known to be complications in endobronchial HDR brachytherapy, but none developed in any of the patients.

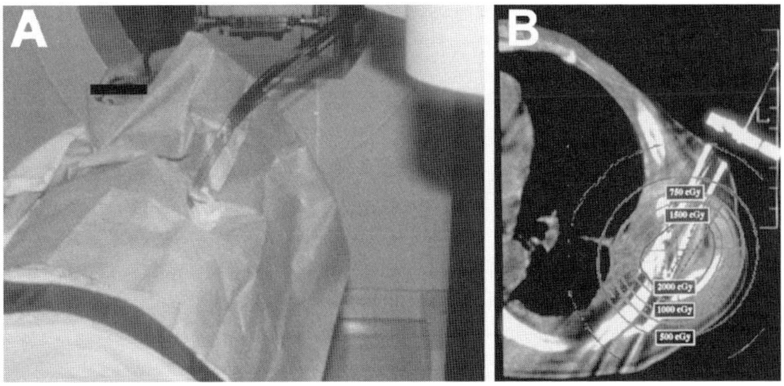

Fig. 3. Percutaneous HDR brachytherapy. **A:** Connection of each selectron needle to the main body of the microselectron apparatus. **B:** Dose distribution.

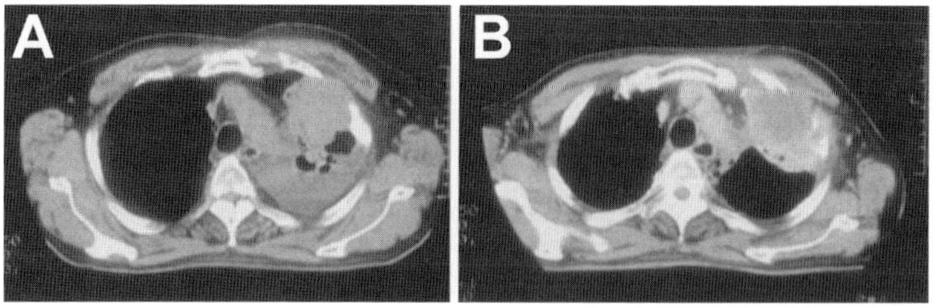

Fig. 4. Changes in CT image with percutaneous HDR brachytherapy. **A:** Before treatment. **B:** One month after treatment. The inside of mass which had infiltrated into the chest wall of the left upper lobe disclosed a low-density area showing central necrosis.

Discussion

There are two key issues necessitating future investigation. The first one is dose determination. Changing the dose in response to the changing caliber of the tracheobronchial tree is one method of securing a constant dose on the mucosal of the airway. The second one is fixation of the applicator. It was observed that sometimes the applicator failed to open completely, due to severe bronchial stenosis. It is necessary for the existing MS-type applicators to be improved to ensure, amongst other things, that the wing is strengthened. Wing size is changed in proportion to the internal diameter of the airway, and the number of wings is increased. To this end we have commenced our own research to develop a better applicator, with the intention to expand the adaptation of the microselectron HDR to enable us to improve the QOL of the patient, not only in curable cases but also for palliative benefits (Fig. 3). The subjects were three male patients aged between 38 to 64 years, suffering from lung cancer which had invaded the chest wall. Alleviation of spontaneous pain occurred in all three of the patients within 7 days after the completion of percutaneous HDR brachytherapy, and the pain-scoring scale for RTOG decreased to 1 within 2 weeks after completion. After hospital discharge, the pain-scoring scale remained in the range of 1 to 4 (Fig. 4).

References

1. Mehta MP, Speiser BL, Macha HN. High dose rate brachytherapy for lung cancer. In: Nag S (eds) High Dose Rate Brachytherapy: A Text Book. Armonk, New York: Futura Publishing Company Inc., 1994;295–319.
2. Imamura M, Murata M, Nagata K, Kimura H, Aoki Y, Harima Y, Uda M, Tanaka Y, Yonezu S, Umemoto M, Saitoh Y. Percutaneous and endobronchial high dose rate brachytherapy for lung cancer. Oncol Reports 1996;3:997–1002.

Bronchology and Bronchoesophagology: State of the Art.
H. Yoshimura et al., editors.

Intraluminal brachytherapy and external beam radiotherapy for early endobronchial cancer

Mari Saito[1], Takayoshi Uematsu[1], Akira Yokoyama[2], Hiroko Tsukada[2] and Yuzo Kurita[2]
Departments of [1]Radiology and [2]Internal medicine, Niigata Cancer Center Hospital, Niigata City, Japan

Keywords: high dose rate, intraluminal brachytherapy, low dose rate, roentgenographically occult endobronchial carcinoma.

Introduction

We have been carrying out this research since July 1991 to evaluate the efficacy and safety of the combination of external beam radiotherapy (EBRT) and Intraluminal brachytherapy (ILB) with ^{192}Ir for roentgenographically occult endobronchial carcinoma (ROEC).

Methods and Materials

The patients enrolled in this study had roentgenographically occult but endoscopically identifiable endobronchial squamous cell carcinoma, and were those for whom surgery had not been indicated due to various circumstances, e.g., decreased respiratory function, other serious complications, advanced age, refusal of operation, or at their own request. All patients gave informed consent prior to treatment.

Radiotherapy is in principle a combination of EBRT and ILB. In EBRT, a radiation field localized to the primary lesion is delivered by anterior and posterior parallel-opposed fields. Either a 6 or a 10 MV photon beam was used with a dose of 2 Gy/fraction, 5 times per week. With ILB, from July 1991, we started brachytherapy with four low dose rate (LDR) ^{192}Ir thin wires, and since 1996, we have also used a high dose rate (HDR) remote after-loading system, called Microselectron HDR. The radiation dose shown in Fig. 1 was given as our standard dose. If the residual tumor was observed at the final scheduled brachytherapy, we gave brachytherapy one or two more times. Because the diameters of the trachea and the bronchus differ by location, we chose the dose-prescribed point as Fig. 2 shows. We used applicators with wings for both LDR and HDR

Address for correspondence: Mari Saito, Department of Radiology, Niigata Cancer Center Hospital, Kawagishi-cho 2-15-3, Niigata-shi, Nigata 951-8566, Japan. Tel.: +81-25-266-5111. Fax: +81-25-233-3849. E-mail: m-saito@niigata-cc.niigata.niigata.jp

EBRT dose	**40 Gy/20 fr./4 weeks**
	+
ILB dose	
low dose rate (LDR)	**25 Gy/5 fr./2.5-5 weeks**
	or
high dose rate (HDR) 1	**20 Gy/5 fr./2.5-5 weeks**
	or
high dose rate (HDR) 2	**18 Gy/3 fr./3 weeks**

Fig. 1. Radiation dose.

brachytherapy.

A total of 98 lesions (in 88 cases) were examined from July 1991 to December 1999 (Fig. 3). As of December 1999, all enrolled patients but one were eligible for review of the treatment results. The one patient was still being treated at this time.

Results

The scheduled treatment was carried out for all but two patients. The follow-up period from the beginning of treatment for the 87 patients ranged from 3 to 100 months, with a median of 47 months.

After completion of radiotherapy, follow-up bronchoscopy with blushing cytology of the treated bronchus was performed. Stenosis and obstruction of the bronchi were observed, and Fig. 4 shows the resulting outcomes of the standard dose treated lesions.

Radiation pneumonitis, and subsequent radiation fibrosis in all but seven lesions were identified on chest X-ray and chest CT. As classified by NCI-CTC,

	LDR	HDR 1	HDR 2
Trachea	**9**	**10**	**10** (Trachea and Main bronchus)
Main bronchus	**7**	**7**	
Lobar and segmental bronchus	**5**	**5**	**5** (Lobar and segmental; Subsegmental and more peripheral)
Subsegmental and more peripheral small bronchus	**3**	**3**	

Fig. 2. Dose prescribed point from the source axis (mm).

Total enrolled	**88 patients 98 lesions**
Total eligible	**87 patients 97 lesions**
Sex	**All male**
Age	**55–83 (median 69)**
Clinical stage	**Tis-T2 N0 M0 (UICC)**
Indications	
Reduced respiratory function (patients)	**21**
Multiple lung cancer	**17**
Advanced age	**6**
Other complications	**5**
Requested by patients	**39**

Fig. 3. Patients enrolled in this study (from July 1991 to December 1999).

'Grade 2' radiation pneumonitis occurred in four lesions, all of which were treated with glucocorticoid and prophylactic antibiotics with subsequent improvement. Eighty-six lesions were classified as 'Grade 1' radiation pneumonitis.

Respiratory function tests were performed before treatment and once every year following treatment. For VC and FEV 1, we evaluated the reduction of each year's value as compared with the corresponding pretreatment value. The results of our standard dose treated patients are shown in Fig. 5. Prolonged symptoms, i.e., cough, sputum, dyspnea, or fatal toxicity, were observed in only two of all enrolled patients.

Thirteen patients developed recurrence. After recurrence, four of the seven patients who underwent surgery, and one of the four patients treated with EBRT,

Time from initiation of treatment (months)	3	6	12	18	24	36	60	over 60
Evaluated lesions	77	61	66	49	56	42	19	6
No change	54	36	34	22	20	19	4	2
Stenosis								
Lobar bronchus	0	0	0	0	2	0	0	0
Segmental bronchus	13	15	20	12	14	11	6	2
Subsegmental bronchus	6	5	3	2	4	0	1	0
Obstruction								
Lobar bronchus	0	0	0	0	0	0	0	0
Segmental bronchus	1	2	5	6	9	8	7	2
Subsegmental bronchus	3	3	4	7	8	4	1	0

Fig. 4. Bronchial stenosis and obstruction (pt. treated with our standard dose).

Time from initiation of treatment (Years)	Evaluated patients	%VC Decrease to >75-90% of pre-Tx value	%VC Decrease to >50-75% of pre-Tx value	FEV1.0 Decrease to >75-90% of pre-Tx value	FEV1.0 Decrease to >50-75% of pre-Tx value
1	41	4	1	5	1
2	33	1	0	3	1
3	25	2	1	5	3
4	16	1	1	3	2
5	18	1	1	3	3
6	4	0	0	2	0

Fig. 5. Respiratory function test (pt. treated with our standard dose).

were treated successfully. We were unsuccessful in the treatment of seven patients and they subsequently died. Fig. 6 shows the overall survival, cause-specific survival and disease-free survival rates for the 87 patients (97 lesions).

Conclusion

Our findings suggest that the combination of EBRT and ILB is an effective low-toxicity treatment for ROEC.

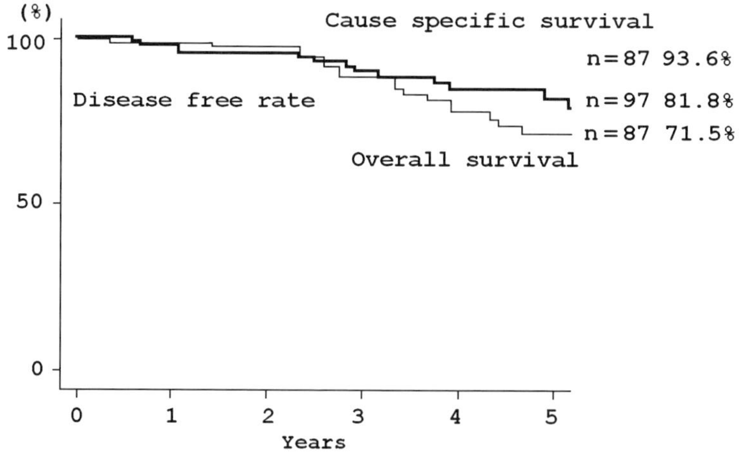

Fig. 6. Survival, cause-specific survival and disease-free rates.

Bronchology and Bronchoesophagology: State of the Art.
H. Yoshimura et al., editors.

Comparison of survival of high dose rate with low dose rate brachytherapy in endobronchial malignant lesions

Irena Spasova[1], Jiri Petera[2] and Miloslav Marel[3]
Departments of [1]Pulmonary Medicine and [2]Radiology and Clinical Oncology, University Hospital, Hradec Kralove; and [3]Department of Pulmonary Medicine, University Hospital Motol, Prague, Czech Republic

Abstract. *Background.* Endobronchial brachytherapy allows the delivery of higher radiation doses directly to tumor tissue, possibly leading to improved locoregional tumor control and subsequent prolonged survival in patients. In our study, we compare the long-term survival times of patients (pts) with malignant airway tumors treated by high dose rate (HDR), with those treated by low dose rate (LDR) endobronchial brachytherapy.

Methods. 122 pts with advanced inoperable malignant airway tumors were divided into two groups. Group A of 67 pts underwent 194 sessions of HDR ^{192}Iridium brachytherapy. The doses of between 500 and 1,000 cGy (median dose 750) were used in 1–5 fractions (median 3). Group B of 55 patients underwent 70 sessions of LDR ^{137}Cesium brachytherapy. The doses of between 300 and 1,000 cGy (median dose 1,000) were applied in 1–3 fractions (median 1). Pts were followed up for 6 to 120 months after treatment. The time of diagnosis, date of the first brachytherapy session and duration of survival were determined in May 1999. Kaplan-Meier curves of survival from the time of diagnosis and the first brachytherapy session were computed, and a log-rank test was used to compare the two groups.

Results. In Group A, the median survival time counted from the first diagnosis was 276 days, and in Group B 498 days. The median survival time from the first brachytherapy treatment was 167 days in Group A and 218 days in Group B. The duration of survival from time of diagnosis was significantly longer in Group B ($p = 0.027$). There was no statistical difference found between the two group's survival times from the first brachytherapy session.

Conclusions. Pts treated by LDR endobronchial brachytherapy in our study survived longer from time of diagnosis than those treated with HDR brachytherapy. However, there were similar effects of HDR and LDR brachytherapy on the survival time counted.

Keywords: bronchoscopy, lung cancer, radiotherapy.

Introduction

Brachytherapy allows the transmission of higher radiation doses directly to tumor tissue, possibly leading to improved locoregional tumor control and subsequent prolonged survival. In our study, we compare the duration of survival in patients (pts) with malignant airway tumors palliatively treated by high dose rate (HDR), with those treated by low dose rate (LDR) endobronchial brachytherapy.

Address for correspondence: Irena Spasova CSc, Department of Pulmonary Medicine, University Hospital, Pospisilova 365, 500 05 Hradec Kralove, Czech Republic. Tel.: +420-49-583-6341. Fax: +420-49-583-6226. E-mail: spasova@fnhk.cz

Methods and Patients

122 pts with advanced inoperable malignant airway tumors were divided into two groups. Group A (prospective) of 67 pts have undergone 194 sessions of HDR ^{192}Iridium intrabronchial brachytherapy. Using a Gammamed afterloading device the doses of between 500 and 1,000 cGy (median dose 750) were used in 1–5 fractions (median 3). The application time for these doses ranged from 7 to 15 mins. Group B (retrospective) of 55 patients had 70 sessions of LDR ^{137}Cesium intrabronchial brachytherapy. Either Microselectron (55 cases) or Selectron (15 cases) were used. The doses of between 300 and 1,000 cGy (median dose 1,000) were applied in 1–3 fractions (median 1). The total application time taken to deliver the planned treatment doses ranged from 0.3 to 20 h. Pts were followed up for 6 to 120 months after treatment. The time since first diagnosis and since the first brachytherapy session as well as the duration of survival, were determined in May 1999. Kaplan-Meier curves were computed for the survival time from the first diagnosis and from the first brachytherapy session. A log-rank test was used to compare the outcomes of the patients in the two groups.

Results

The median survival time from original diagnosis in Group A was 276 days and in Group B 498 days. In Group A, the median survival time from the first brachytherapy treatment was 167 days and 218 days in Group B. The survival time from first diagnosis was significantly longer in Group B ($p = 0.027$). No statistical difference was found in survival from the first brachytherapy. We found that pts in our study who received LDR endobronchial brachytherapy survived longer from the time of diagnosis compared with those treated with HDR brachytherapy. The effects of HDR and LDR brachytherapy were comparable regarding survival from the first brachytherapy treatment.

Discussion

Since the 1980s, different isotopes and dose rates for endobronchial brachytherapy have been used. HDR brachytherapy using ^{192}Iridium is clearly preferable, as this radiation treatment requires only a few mins time and is a more comfortable process for the patient. However, from a radiobiological point of view, LDR has been presented as an alternative method because it results in better irradiation of the tumor volume and has a lower incidence of complications, although there have been no randomized prospective study data results as yet to confirm this theory.

The only randomized study comparing survival times in patients receiving external irradiation alone with those receiving external irradiation plus additional brachytherapy, found slightly longer survival times in the brachytherapy group than in those with squamous cell carcinoma, but no overall advantageous survival rate when looking at the whole group of those with lung tumors. The brachytherapy group also displayed better local tumor control [1].

In his retrospective study, Shea proved a significantly longer survival time in patients with squamous cell carcinoma treated with endobronchial Nd-YAG laser therapy plus brachytherapy, compared with laser therapy alone [2].

In our study we found a significantly longer survival time counted from first diagnosis in pts treated with LDR brachytherapy, compared to HDR brachytherapy, and no difference in survival time from the date of the patients' first brachytherapy treatment. The endobronchial brachytherapy treatment used for pts in our study was only part of a multimodal treatment for the malignant lesions. The effects of brachytherapy should be confirmed in a large prospective randomized study in order to confirm its influence and significance on the duration of survival in patients.

References

1. Huber RM, Fischer R, Hautmann H, Pöllinger B, Häußinger K, Wendt T. Does additional brachytherapy improve the effect of external irradiation? A prospective randomized study in central lung tumors. Int J Radiation Oncol Biol Phys 1997;38:533–540.
2. Shea JM, Allen RP, Tharratt RS, Chan AL, Siefkin AD. Survival of patients undergoing Nd:YAG laser therapy compared with Nd:YAG laser therapy and brachytherapy for malignant airway disease. Chest 1993;103:1028–1031.

Bronchology and Bronchoesophagology: State of the Art.
H. Yoshimura et al., editors.

Combination therapy of preoperative endobronchial radiation therapy (EBRT) and surgery for malignant tracheo-bronchial stenosis in lung cancer

Toshiya Tokui[1], Masanori Kaneda[1], Katsumoto Hatanaka[1], Kazuhiro Tani[1], Tamotsu Morimoto[1], Kazuo Miyamura[2], Takashi Sakai[1] and Yoshihito Nomoto[3]

[1]Department of Thoracic and Cardiovascular Surgery and [2]Department of Anesthesiology, National Mie Chuo Hospital, Hisai; and [3]Department of Radiology, Mie University, School of Medicine, Tsu, Japan

Abstract. We have successfully treated two patients with malignant tracheo-bronchial stenosis using the combination of preoperative external and endobronchial radiation therapy (EBRT), and surgery. Our new applicator contributed to the improvement of the treatment results and reduction of the side effects caused by excessive irradiation. Thus, EBRT is effective therapy as preoperative adjuvant irradiation for patients with malignant tracheo-bronchial stenosis.

Keywords: endobronchial radiation therapy, malignant tracheo-bronchial stenosis, preoperative adjuvant irradiation, treatment.

Introduction

Radiation therapy has been used in the treatment of intrathoracic malignancies for approximately 80 years. Recently, endobronchial radiation therapy (EBRT) has been used with an Ir-192 high-dose-rate remote afterloading machine. EBRT has been carried out as a treatment for lung cancer. However, complications related to the EBRT, such as radiation bronchitis, stenosis and fatal hemoptysis have been indicated [1—3]. Thus, the primary objective of this treatment for patients with lung cancer was the treatment for major airway occlusion by inoperable carcinoma of the bronchus. We devised a new applicator [4], which improved treatment results and reduced the side effects caused by excessive irradiation, and have undertaken EBRT as the induction therapy for surgery. In this paper, we described two successful cases with malignant tracheo-bronchial stenosis, which was treated using the combination therapy of preoperative EBRT and surgery.

Address for correspondence: Toshiya Tokui MD, Department of Thoracic and Cardiovascular Surgery, National Mie Chuo Hospital, 2158-5 Myojincho, Hisai, Mie 514-1101, Japan. Tel.: +81-59-259-1211. Fax: +81-59-256-2651. E-mail: tokuit@miechuo-m.hosp.go.jp

EBRT Methods

The new applicator, which has two wings, can position the source in the center of the bronchial lumen. We placed the applicator at the treatment site and attempted to set up reference points according to bronchial diameter, for optimal dose distribution, as described previously [4]. Treatment consisted of external beam radiotherapy (70 Gy in case 1, 40 Gy in case 2) and EBRT in three fractions of 6 Gy each, separated by 1-week intervals. The patients were treated using a high-dose-rate afterloading device (microselectron HDR) with an Ir-192 source.

Case reports

Case 1

A 45-year-old woman began suffering from dyspnea during inspiration, 5 months prior to diagnosis. After unsuccessful treatment for bronchial asthma at another hospital, she transferred to our hospital for further evaluation. Physical examination revealed only inspiratory wheezing. Laboratory studies, including a variety of tumor markers, were all within the normal range. Chest radiography showed no abnormal shadow. Chest CT showed an endotracheal tumor, but no pneumonia or peripheral lung atelectasis. Bronchoscopy showed the tumor obstructing

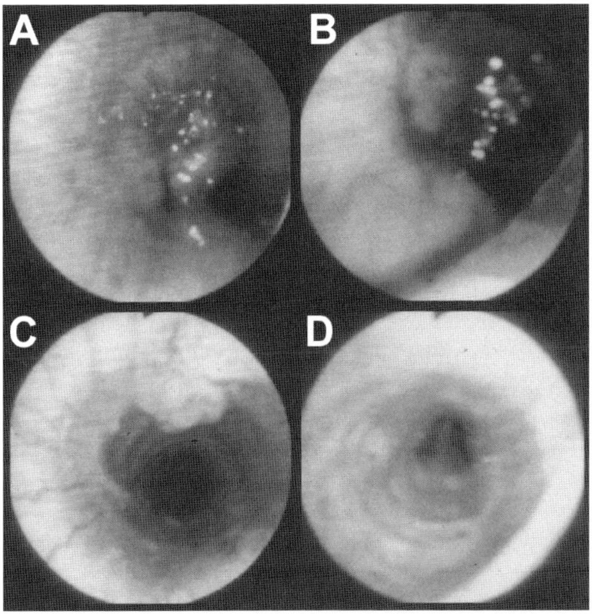

Fig. 1. Bronchoscopic findings. **A:** pretreatment; **B:** postlasertherapy; **C:** postirradiationtherapy; **D:** postoperation.

90% of the tracheal lumen and invading the tracheal wall (Fig. 1A). Biopsy of the endotracheal tumor indicated adenoid cystic carcinoma. Systemic examination revealed no distant metastasis, and the lung cancer was diagnosed as T4N0M0. For the palliation of airway obstruction, she was treated using an Nd-YAG laser. The laser provided good palliation for obstruction (Fig. 1B). After the relief of the dyspnea, she received EBRT in three fractions of 6 Gy each with external beam irradiation of 70 Gy (pre: 50 Gy, post: 20 Gy). A posttreatment bronchoscopy confirmed that the tumor had remarkably decreased in size (2 mm) (Fig. 1C). After 1 month of irradiation and five tracheal cartilages, resection and end-to-end anastomosis was performed under selective ventilation. The effectiveness of the Ef. 1 and Br (–) was hisologically confirmed, and so curative resection was done. The patient's postoperative course was uneventful and she is now doing well without cancer recurrence 49 months after surgery (Fig. 1D).

Case 2

A 54-year-old man complained of dry cough for 2 months. He saw his local physician and presented an abnormal shadow in the right hilus on a chest radiogram. He transferred to our hospital for further evaluation. He had no particular physical findings. Laboratory studies, including a variety of tumor markers, were all within the normal range. Chest radiography showed the swelling of right hilus. Chest CT showed that the tumor occluded the intermediate bronchus and also invaded the second carina (Fig. 2A). Bronchoscopy showed the tumor existed in

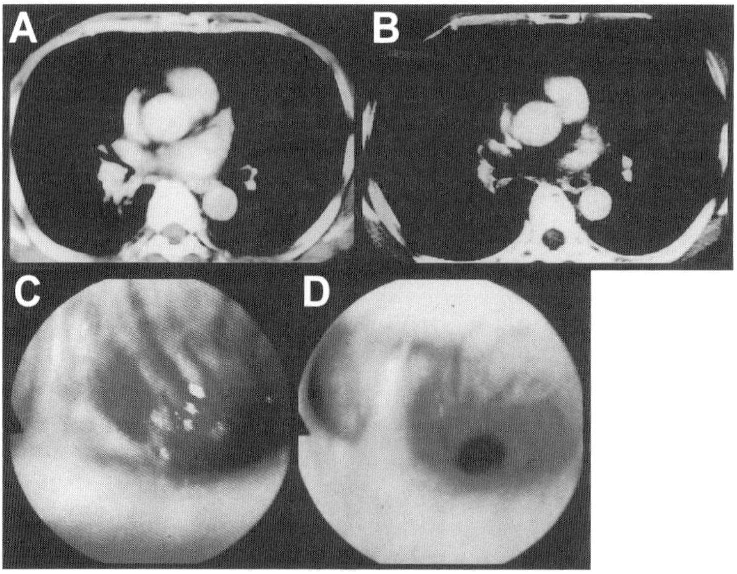

Fig. 2. CT findings; **A:** pretreatment, **B:** postirradiationtherapy. Bronchoscopic findings; **C:** pretreatment, **D:** postirradiationtherapy.

the right lower bronchus, and extended to bifurcation of upper bronchus and truncus intermedius (Fig. 2C). Biopsy of the tumor indicated squamous cell carcinoma. Systemic examination revealed no distant metastasis, and the lung cancer was diagnosed as T2N1M0. He received EBRT in three fractions of 6 Gy each after external beam irradiation of 40 Gy. A post treatment chest CT confirmed that the tumor remarkably decreased in size (Fig. 2B). A post treatment bronchoscopy confirmed almost complete remission of the tumor (Fig. 2D). After 1 month of irradiation, middle and lower lobectomy and bronchial wedge resection of the second carina was performed under selective ventilation by a double lumen endotracheal tube. The effectiveness of the Ef. 2 and Br (–) was hisologically confirmed, and so curative resection was done. The patient's post-operative course was uneventful and he is now doing well without cancer recurrence 84 months after surgery.

Comments

Thirty percent of lung cancers cause obstructions of the trachea and main bronchi with consequent respiratory distress, bleeding and infection [5], and result in the patient seeking medical assistance. Management of airway problems in lung cancer patients is a frustrating task because no definitive treatment exists. External beam radiotherapy can provide some relief but is limited both in the treatment area and total dose that can be given. Chemotherapy is also limited by a poor response rate and the low tolerance of normal tissues. Recently, EBRT has been carried out as a treatment for lung cancer. In 1921, Yankauer first reported EBRT as a possible treatment for lung cancer [6]. However, it was not in common use until the development of flexible bronchoscopes and an Ir-192 high-dose-rate remote afterloading machine. The complications related to EBRT, such as radiation bronchitis, stenosis and fatal hemoptysis have been indicated [1–3]. Thus, EBRT for patients with lung cancer has primarily been used in cases of local progression or recurrence. We devised a new applicator, which contributed to improved treatment results and reduction of the side effects caused by excessive irradiation. We conclude that this procedure is safe, useful and an easy method for the treatment of lung cancer patients [4]. Based on our experience, we have undertaken EBRT as a preoperative adjuvant irradiation for the treatment of lung cancer. When using irradiation therapy as a preoperative adjuvant therapy for a patient with malignant tracheo-bronchial stenosis, the most important point is the side effects to normal tissue included in the treatment area. In some cases, results could include poor healing and bronchopleural fistula after surgery. External beam radiotherapy has high risk factor concerning these problems. Due to the theoretic advantage that EBRT provides – improved localization to such an extent that the area containing the tumor receives the highest dose of radiation, while sparing normal tissue only a few centimeters away – it can be said to be more safe, more effective and a less complicative preoperative adjuvant therapy than external beam radiotherapy. In this paper, we treated two patients with malignant tracheo-bronchial stenosis using external beam radiotherapy and EBRT without technical difficulty or complications. After irradiation, we could perform curative resection safely. The patients gained a good postoperative course and a long time of survival. We conclude that EBRT is an effective preoperative adjuvant irradiation therapy for patients with malignant tracheo-bronchial stenosis.

Acknowledgements

We thank B. Tishkoff for critically reading the manuscript.

References

1. Gollins JM, Ryder WDJ, Burt PA, Barber PV, Stout R. Massive hemoptysis death and other morbidity associated with high dose rate intraluminal radiotherapy for carcinoma of the bronchus. Radiother Oncol 1996;39:105–116.
2. Khanavkar B, Stern P, Alberti W, Nakhosteen JA. Complications associated with brachytherapy alone or with laser in lung cancer. Chest 1991;99:1062–1065.
3. Speiser BL, Spartling L. Radiation bronchitis and stenosis secondary to high dose rate endobronchial irradiation. Int J Radiat Oncol Biol Phys 1993;25:589–597.
4. Nomoto Y, Shouji K, Toyota S, Sasaoka M, Murashima S, Ooi M, Takeda K, Nakagawa T. High dose rate endobronchial brachytherapy using a new applicator. Radiother Oncol 1997;45: 33–37.
5. Minna JD, Higgins GA, Glaistein EJ. Cancer of the lung. In: DeVita VT, Hellman S, Rosemberg SA, (eds) Cancer Principles and Practice of Oncology. Philadelphia: JB Lippincott, 1989; 591–705.
6. Yankauer S. Two cases of lung tumor treated bronchoscopically. NY Med J 1922;115:741–742.

Bronchial circulation

Bronchology and Bronchoesophagology: State of the Art.
H. Yoshimura et al., editors.

The diagnostic value of bronchial arteriography for hemoptysis

Toshio Sugane, Noriaki Takahashi, Hiroshi Akusawa, Chiharu Omori, Yoshiaki Koya, Tsuneto Akashiba and Takashi Horie
First Department of Internal Medicine, Nihon University School of Medicine, Tokyo, Japan

Abstract. *Purpose.* The purpose of this study was to evaluate the diagnostic value of bronchial arteriography for the determination of the bleeding sites in patients with hemoptysis.

Methods. Forty-five patients (29 men and 16 women) with hemoptysis were examined using bronchofiberscopy and bronchial arteriography. All the patients underwent bronchofiberscopy within 48 h of active bleeding in order to determine the bleeding sites. Bronchial arteriography was also carried out on all patients. Bronchiectasis, tuberculosis, aspergillosis and lung cancer were the causes hemoptysis in these patients. The correlation between those findings and the bleeding sites was evaluated.

Results. The angiographic signs were extravasation (11.1%), hypervascularization (97.7%), broncho-pulmonary shunts (51.1%), and aneurysms (11.1%), which tended to occur in upper bronchus. The sites of these signs were similar to the bleeding sites determined by bronchofiberscopy.

Conclusion. We suggested that bronchial arteriography was valuable for the determination of the bleeding sites of patients with hemoptysis.

Keywords: bronchial arteriography (BAG), bronchofiberscopy, hemoptysis.

Introduction

Hemoptysis is a symptom and sign commonly evaluated by chest clinicians. Despite considerable emphasis upon the approaches to this problem and its diverse presentations, the etiology of hemoptysis and the bleeding site are frequently elusive [1—3]. The purpose of this study is to evaluate the diagnostic value of bronchial arteriography as a means of determination of the bleeding sites in patients with hemoptysis.

Patients and Study design

121 patients with complaints of hemoptysis underwent bronchofiberscopy from 1997 to 1999 in our department.

Only 49 of those patients (30 men and 19 women, ranging in age from 28 to 85 years, the mean age being 68-years-old) had their bleeding site determined by bronchoscopy. Chest radiographs, chest CT scans and bronchial arteriography (BAG) were also performed on these 49 patients. All patients underwent bron-

Address for correspondence: Toshio Sugane, 1st Department of Internal Medicine, Nihon University School of Medicine, 30-1 Oyaguchi-kamimachi, Itabashi-ku, Tokyo 173-8610, Japan. Tel.: +81-3-3972-811. Fax: +81-3-3972-2893.

chofiberscopy within 48 h of active bleeding in order to determine the bleeding sites. Transfemoral bronchial arteriography was performed using the standard Seldinger technique, using 5.0 to 6.5 Fr catheters, and digital subtraction arteriography was performed on all patients.

In this study, we evaluated the correlation between bleeding sites and bronchioarteriographic findings.

Results

Underlying diseases

The underlying diseases were bronchiectasis (36 cases), mycobacterial infection (3 cases), lung cancer (3 cases), bacterial pneumonia (1 case), fungus infection (3 cases), racemose hemangioma (2 cases), and idiopathy (1 case).

Chest radiographic findings

In 14 cases, chest radiographs were interpreted as normal. CT scans were also revealed to be normal in two cases and bronchiectasis was revealed in the other 12. In five cases, nonspecific findings were shown, such as calcification, pleural thickness, and old lesions. Twelve cases who underwent chest radiographs were interpreted to have bronchial abnormalities, all of them were diagnosed to be bronchiectasis. Chest radiographs were interpreted as infiltrations in another 12 cases. Two of these cases were pneumonia and tuberculosis, another 10 cases were blood aspiration. In three cases, chest radiographs were interpreted as mass or cavities.

Bleeding sites

Although all 121 patients with hemoptysis underwent bronchofiberscopy within 48 h of active bleeding, hemorrhages were proved to occur in 49 cases (40%),

Table 1. Bleeding sites.

Site	No. of cases
Carina	1
Right main bronchus	1
Right upper lobe	25
Right middle lobe	4
Right lower lobe	5
Left upper lobe	8
Left lower lobe	5
Total	49

using bronchoscopy. Hemorrhages in right upper lobe were observed more often than in any other lobe (Table 1).

BAG findings

BAG was performed in all 49 cases. Forty-seven cases (96%) had abnormal BAG findings, such as hypervascularity (96%), enlargement of artery (14%), stain (29%), bronchopulmonary shunt (47%), pseudo aneurysm (10%), and extravasation (4%). These abnormal BAG findings tended to be obtained in upper branches.

BAG - Bronchoscopic correlations

In cases of single branch abnormality (Table 2), the site of BAG signs were similar to the bleeding sites determined by bronchoscopy. In cases of multiple branch

Table 2. Single branch abnormalities.

Patient No.	Bleeding site	BA site	BAG findings	correlation
1	Right upper	Left upper	H	–
2	Right lower	Right lower	H,ST	+
3	Right lower	Right lower	H,ST	+
4	Left upper	Left upper	H	+
5	Right upper	Right upper	H,SH	+
6	Left lower	Left lower	H,E,ST,SH	+
7	Right middle	Right upper	H,ST,SH	+
8	Left lower	Left lower	H,E	+
9	Left upper	Left upper	H,EX	+
10	Left lower	None	Intact	–
11	Right upper	Right upper	H,ST	+
12	Right upper	Right upper	H,ST	+
13	Carina	Right upper	H	+
14	Right upper	Right upper	H,SH	+
15	Right upper	Right upper	H,SH	+
16	Right upper	Right upper	H,SH	+
17	Right upper	Right upper	H,SH	+
18	Right upper	Right upper	H,ST	+
19	Right upper	None	Intact	–
20	Right upper	Right upper	H.ST,SH	+
21	Left upper	Left upper	H,SH	+
22	Right upper	Right upper	H,ST	+
23	Left lower	Left lower	H,E,SH	+
24	Left upper	Left upper	H,A	+
25	Right upper	Right upper	H	+
26	Right upper	Right upper	H,ST,SH	+
27	Right upper	Right upper	H,ST,SH	+
28	Right lower	Right lower	H,ST,SH	+

abnormalities (Table 3), at least one of these sites was similar to the bleeding site determined by bronchoscopy.

Discussion

Chest radiography, CT scans, and bronchofiberscopy might demonstrate some clues as to the source of bleeding, but are unreliable [4]. The positive diagnosis rate for bronchoscopic examination is not high [5]. Therefore, BAG plays an important role in localizing the bleeding site. According to our experience, extravasation is uncommon and only appeared in two patients with massive hemoptysis. In contrast, the indirect angiographic signs, such as hypervascularity, stains and bronchopulmonary shunt, are common indicators of the site of bleeding.

In cases of single branch abnormalities, the site of BAG signs were similar to the bleeding sites determined by bronchoscopy. Otherwise, in cases of multiple branch abnormalities, at least one of these sites was similar to the bleeding site determined by bronchoscopy. These results suggested that BAG was valuable in determining the bleeding sites of patients with hemoptysis.

Since abnormal BAG findings were also obtained in nonbleeding sites by broncoscopy, we were also able to speculate that these findings were valuable in pointing out another potential origin of hemoptysis.

Table. 3. Multiple branch abnormalities.

No.	Bleeding site	BAG findings			Cor.
1	Right upper	Right upper H, ST, SH	Right lower H, E, SH		+
2	Right upper	Right upper H, ST	Right lower H, ST		±
3	Right upper	Right upper H, ST	Left lower H, ST, SH		–
4	Right upper	Right upper H, ST	Right lower H		+
5	Right lower	Right upper H	Right lower H, ST		+
6	Right upper	Right upper H	Right lower H		±
7	Right upper	Right upper H, ST	Right lower H		+
8	Right main	Right upper H, ST, SH, A	Left lower H		+
9	Right upper	Right upper H, ST	Right lower H, ST		±
10	Left lower	Right lower H, SH, A	Left lower H, SH, A	Left lower H, ST, SH, A	+
11	Left upper	Right upper H, ST	Left upper H, A		–
12	Left upper	Right upper H, ST, SH	Left lower H, ST, SH		±
13	Left upper	Right upper H, ST	Left upper H, ST	Left lower H	±
14	Right middle	Right lower H, E, SH, A	Left lower H, E, A		+
15	Left upper	Right upper H, SH	Left upper H, E, SH		+
16	Left lower	Right lower H	Left lower H, SH		+
17	Right upper	Right upper H, SH	Right lower H, SH	Left lower H	±
18	Right middle	Right upper H, ST	Right lower H, ST	Left upper H	±
19	Right upper	Right upper H	Left lower H		±
20	Right lower	Right lower H, E, SH	Left lower H, SH		+
21	Right upper	Right upper H, ST	Left upper H, ST, EX		–

References

1. Poe RH, Israel RH, Marin MG, Ortiz CR, Dale RC, Wahl GW, Kallay MC, Greenblatt DG. Utility of fiberoptic bronchoscopy in patients with hemoptysis and a nonlocalizing chest roentgenogram. Chest 1988;93(1):70–75.
2. Adelman M, Haponik EF, Bleecker ER, Britt EJ. Cryptogenic hemoptysis. Clinical features, bronchoscopic findings, and natural history in 67 patients. Ann Intern Med 1985;102(6): 829–834.
3. Haponik EF, Chin R. Hemoptysis: clinicians' perspectives. Chest 1990;97(2):469–475.
4. Zhang JS, Cui ZP, Wang MQ, Yang L. Bronchial arteriography and transcatheter embolization in the management of hemoptysis. Cardiovasc Intervent Radiol 1994;17(5):276–279.
5. Saumench J, Escarrabill J, Padro L, Montana J, Clariana A, Canto A. Value of fiberoptic bronchoscopy and angiography for diagnosis of the bleeding site in hemoptysis. Ann Thorac Surg 1989;48(2):272–274.

Bronchial lavage

Bronchology and Bronchoesophagology: State of the Art.
H. Yoshimura et al., editors.

Bronchoscopic microsample probe assessment of pulmonary biochemical markers

Akitoshi Ishizaka[1], Masazumi Watanabe[2], Koichi Kobayashi[2] and Koji Kikuchi[3]
[1]*Tokyo Electric Power Company Hospital, Tokyo;* [2]*Keio University School of Medicine, Tokyo; and* [3]*Saitama Medical Center, Saitama, Japan*

Abstract. We have developed a noninvasive bronchoscopic microsampling (BMS) probe to be used to assess biochemical markers in epithelial lining fluid (ELF). In this study, we have compared the validity of the MS method to the bronchoalveolar lavage (BAL) method in control subjects. We have also employed the probe in subjects with acute lung injury/acute respiratory distress syndrome (ALI/ARDS) to test its clinical utility with such inflammatory pulmonary diseases. Two groups were studied: the control group (n = 7), and the ALI/ARDS group (n = 4). In the control group, BAL was also carried out following BMS treatment. Concentrations of albumin, LDH and interleukin-6 in ELF recovered by BMS were within the same range as those obtained by BAL in the control group. In the ALI/ARDS group, the albumin, LDH and IL-6 concentrations found in the ELF were significantly higher ($p < 0.0001$) than those of the control group. Basic-FGF (fibroblast growth factor) and neutrophil elastase were detected only in the ALI/ARDS group. These results suggest that the BMS probe is a useful tool in assessing pulmonary biochemical events in ALI/ARDS.

Keywords: ARDS, BAL, bronchoscopy, epithelial lining fluid, inflammation.

BMS procedure

Following routine premedication, a flexible fiberoptic bronchoscope (BF-XT40, Olympus, Tokyo, Japan) was inserted into the lungs. The fiberscope was wedged in a segmental bronchus of the right middle lobe. The BMS probe, which we developed in conjunction with Olympus Co. (Tokyo, Japan), was inserted into the lungs through a channel of the fiberoptic bronchoscope after flushing the channel with 10 ml of air to minimize contamination of samples. The probe consisted of an outer polyethylene sheath of diameter 2.0 mm, and an inner 1.2 mm cotton probe attached to a stainless steel guide wire (Fig. 1). After the sheath was wedged in place, the inner probe was advanced slowly into the distal airway and BMS was carried out for 5–7 s. The inner probe was then withdrawn into the outer tube and together they were pulled out. The inner probe was cut at 3 cm distal from the apex and placed in a preweighed tube. After weighing, the wet probe was kept in a -80°C freezer until further use.

Address for correspondence: A. Ishizaka, Tokyo Electric Power Company Hospital, 9-2 Shinanomachi, Shinjuku-ku, Tokyo 160-0016, Japan. Tel.: +81-3-3341-7121. Fax: +81-3-3341-9787.

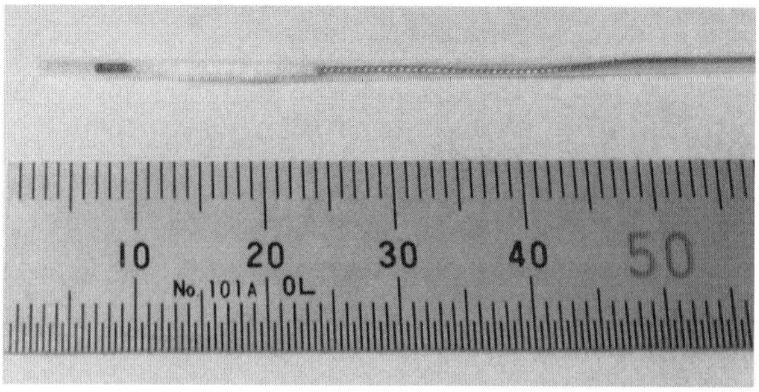

Fig. 1.

Results

Concentrations of albumin, LDH and interleukin-6 in ELF recovered by BMS were within the same range as those obtained by BAL in the control group. In the ALI/ARDS group, the albumin, LDH and IL-6 concentrations in ELF were significantly higher ($p<0.0001$, $p<0.0001$, $p<0.0001$, respectively) than those of the control group. Basic-FGF (fibroblast growth factor) and neutrophil elastase were detected only in the ALI/ARDS group.

Serial BMS was performed safely during a course of ALI/ARDS, and correlation between the biochemical events and clinical findings was noted. These results suggest that the BMS probe is a useful tool in assessing pulmonary biochemical events in ALI/ARDS.

Conclusion

Our results suggest that this microsampling method might be useful in contributing valuable information to the understanding of the pathophysiology of ALI/ARDS, and for evaluating disease activities, as well as the efficacy of treatments. Furthermore, application of the MS method to other kinds of pulmonary diseases may be possible.

Bronchology and Bronchoesophagology: State of the Art.
H. Yoshimura et al., editors.

The soluble form of Fas and Fas ligand in bronchoalveolar lavage fluid from patients with pulmonary fibrosis and bronchiolitis obliterans organizing pneumonia

Kazuyoshi Kuwano[1], Masayuki Kawasaki[1], Takashige Maeyama[1], Naoki Hagimoto[1], Norio Nakamura[2], Kamon Shirakawa[2] and Nobuyuki Hara[1]
[1]Research Institute for Diseases of the Chest, Graduate School of Medical Sciences, Kyushu University, Fukuoka; and [2]Bioscience Laboratory Research Center, Mochida Pharmaceutical Co., LTD. Tokyo, Japan

Abstract. *Background.* The Fas-Fas ligand (FasL) pathway is a representative system of apoptosis-signaling receptor molecules. We have previously described that this pathway may play an important role in the pathogenesis of fibrosing lung diseases. In this study, we hypothesized that the soluble form of Fas (sFas) and FasL (sFasL) may also be associated with this disorder.

Methods and Results. We measured sFas and sFasL levels in bronchoalveolar lavage fluid (BALF) from patients with idiopathic pulmonary fibrosis (IPF), interstitial pneumonia associated with collagen vascular diseases (CVD-IP), and bronchiolitis obliterans organizing pneumonia (BOOP), using enzyme linked immunosorbent assays (ELISA). BALF was obtained from all patients before prednisolone therapy. Soluble FasL levels were relatively increased in IPF ($p = 0.084$) and significantly increased in CVD-IP ($p < 0.05$) and BOOP ($p < 0.05$) compared with the controls. IPF or CVD-IP subgroups, with indications for prednisolone therapy, had elevated BALF sFasL levels, compared with those without indications for therapy. The BALF sFasL level in IPF was correlated with the total number of cells and lymphocytes. The BALF sFasL level in BOOP was relatively or significantly correlated with the total number of cells or lymphocytes, respectively. BALF sFas levels were significantly increased in BOOP, but not in IPF or CVD-IP.

Conclusions. We conclude that BALF sFasL levels may be associated with the accumulation of inflammatory cells and reflect the degree of lymphocyte alveolitis in IPF. The elevation of sFasL levels may be associated with the deterioration of IPF and CVD-IP. The elevation of BALF sFas levels may abrogate the cytotoxicity of FasL in BOOP, which may be associated with better prognosis of BOOP, compared with IPF or CVD-IP.

Keywords: alveolitis, collagen vascular disease, prednisolone.

Introduction

The Fas-FasL system is the representative system of apoptosis-signaling receptor molecules. We have previously demonstrated that the expression of Fas was upregulated in bronchiolar and alveolar epithelial cells and that Fas-Fas ligand (FasL) protein was upregulated mainly in infiltrating T lymphocytes in lung tissues from patients with idiopathic pulmonary fibrosis (IPF) [1]. Therefore, we

Address for correspondence: Kazuyoshi Kuwano MD, Research Institute for Diseases of the Chest, Faculty of Medicine, Kyushu University, 3-1-1 Maidashi, Higashiku, Fukuoka, 812 Japan. Tel.: +81-92-642-5378. Fax: +81-92-642-5389. E-mail: kkuwano@kokyu.med.kyushu-u.ac.jp hypothesized that the Fas-FasL pathway may be involved in the pathogenesis of IPF. Since the soluble forms of Fas (sFas) and FasL (sFasL) have not been studied in IPF, interstitial pneumonia associated with collagen vascular diseases (CVD-IP), and bronchiolitis obliterans organizing pneumonia (BOOP), we examined bronchoalveolar lavage fluid (BALF) levels of sFas and sFasL in these disorders.

Materials and Methods

BALF, used in enzyme linked immunosorbent assays (ELISA), was obtained before treatment. Patients with "acute exacerbation" were treated with prednisolone. In 10 out of 33 patients with IPF, diagnosis of IPF was confirmed by thoracoscopic lung biopsy. Out of nine cases of BOOP, 2 cases had histological findings of bronchiolitis obliterans organizing pneumonia, and 7 cases had organizing pneumonia with mononuclear cell infiltration of the interstitium. Out of 21 cases of CVD-IP, there were 12 cases of rheumatoid arthritis (RA), six cases of polymyositis/dermatomyositis (PM/DM), two cases of Sjögren syndrome, and 1 case of progressive systemic sclerosis (PSS).

Results

BALF sFas levels (mean±SD) were 21±54 pg/ml in the controls. BOOP exhibited significantly higher levels of sFas (215±215 pg/ml) as compared with the controls ($p < 0.05$). There was no significant difference in BALF sFas levels between IPF or CVD-IP and the controls. There was also no significant difference in BALF sFas levels between IPF or CVD-IP subgroups with or without indication for therapy. BALF sFasL levels (mean±SD) were 4.7±6.0 pg/ml in the controls. CVD-IP and BOOP exhibited significantly higher levels of sFasL, 32.9±42.5 ($p < 0.05$), and, 47.0±49.2 pg/ml ($p < 0.05$), respectively, as compared with the controls. BALF sFasL levels were relatively higher in IPF (40.1±69.1 pg/ml, $p = 0.084$) than in the controls. There was a significant difference in BALF sFasL levels between IPF ($p < 0.05$) or CVD-IP subgroups ($p < 0.01$) with or without clinical indication for prednisolone therapy. There was a significant correlation between the total number of BAL cells and BALF sFasL levels in IPF ($r = 0.45$, $p < 0.05$). BALF sFasL levels in IPF were also significantly correlated with the number ($r = 0.57$, $p < 0.005$) and percentage ($r = 0.64$, $p < 0.001$) of lymphocytes in BALF. BALF sFasL levels in BOOP were significantly correlated with the number of lymphocytes in BALF ($r = 0.74$, $p < 0.05$).

Discussion

We first demonstrated the sFas and sFasL levels in BALF obtained from patients with IPF, CVD-IP, and BOOP. The increased levels of BALF sFasL may reflect the accumulation of inflammatory cells and the exacerbation of the disease in

IPF. The transformation of mFasL to sFasL and the production of sFas may have an important role in the protection of epithelial cells from the cytotoxicity of FasL. Although the relationships between soluble and membrane-bound Fas and FasL appear to be complex, sFas and sFasL may have an important role in the pathophysiology of fibrosing lung diseases.

Reference

1. Kuwano K, Miyazaki H, Hagimoto N, Kawasaki M, Fujita M, Kunitake R, Kaneko Y, Hara N. The involvement of Fas-Fas ligand pathway in fibrosing lung diseases. Am J Respir Cell Mol Biol 1999;20:53–60.

Bronchology and Bronchoesophagology: State of the Art.
H. Yoshimura et al., editors.

KL-6, SP-A and SP-D in BALF and serum in patients with interstitial lung disorders

Takashi Mouri, Kohei Yamauchi, Toshiki Shikanai, Koko Yoshida, Harumasa Ito and Hiroshi Inoue
Third Department of Internal Medicine, School of Medicine, Iwate Medical University, Morioka, Japan

Abstract. *Background.* KL-6, SP-A and SP-D are newly developed markers for interstitial lung disorders. We compared these markers in bronchoalveolar lavage fluid (BALF) and serum to investigate whether these markers reflect the disease activity of pulmonary sarcoidosis and hypersensitivity pneumonitis.

Patients and methods. KL-6, SP-A and SP-D were measured using enzyme-linked immunosorbent assay (ELISA). Subjects presented with sarcoidosis (Sa) and hypersensitivity pneumonitis. The sarcoidosis group were divided into Sa-I (without interstitial change in lung fields) and Sa-II (with interstitial changes). The hypersensitivity pneumonitis group was composed of those presenting acute farmer's lung (a-fl), chronic farmer's lung (c-fl), serum precipitin positive asymptomatic dairy farmers (s-p) and exposed control (s-n).

Results. KL-6 in BALF was significantly higher in the Sa-II group (610±159 U/ml), compared with Sa-I (261±45) and the normal nonsmoking control group (NC) (222±21). KL-6 in serum was also significantly higher in the Sa-II (694±177) group compared with Sa-I (241±26) and NC (225±18). There was no significant difference in SP-A levels in BALF and serum in the Sa-II, Sa-I and NC groups. SP-D in BALF was significantly higher in Sa-II (1126±279 ng/ml) than NC (471±52). Regarding sarcoidosis, KL-6 in BALF showed significant positive correlation with the percentage of lymphocyte in BALF. KL-6 in BALF of a-fl (452±94) was significantly higher than NC. Some of the c-fl and s-p groups showed higher KL-6 levels in BALF (491±153 and 404±108, respectively).

It was suggested that KL-6 and SP-D levels reflect the stage of pulmonary involvement in sarcoidosis. In the farmer's lung and related patients, KL-6 and SP-D levels in BALF may not reflect the deterioration manifested in a chest roentgenogram.

Keywords: bronchoalveolar lavage fluid, farmer's lung, sarcoidosis.

Introduction

KL-6, SP-A and SP-D are newly developed markers for interstitial lung disorders and are considered to reflect the total disease activity present [1,2]. We compared these markers in BALF and serum to investigate whether these markers show a correlation with the disease activity of pulmonary sarcoidosis and hypersensitivity pneumonitis.

Address for correspondence: Prof Hiroshi Inoue, Third Department of Internal Medicine, School of Medicine, Iwate Medical University, 19-1, Uchimaru, Morioka, Iwate 020-8505, Japan. Tel.: +81-19-651-5111. Fax: +81-19-626-8040.

Patients and Methods

KL-6, SP-A and SP-D were measured with enzyme-linked immunosorbent assay (ELISA). Patients presented with sarcoidosis and hypersensitivity pneumonitis. Patients with histologically confirmed sarcoidosis (Sa) were divided into Sa-I (having lymphadenopathy without interstitial change in lung fields on chest roentgenogram), and Sa-II (having lymphadenopathy with interstitial changes in lung fields on chest roentgenogram). The hypersensitivity pneumonitis group was composed of those patients with acute and chronic farmer's lung (a-fl and c-fl, respectively), serum precipitin positive asymptomatic dairy farmers (s-p) and exposed control (s-n). They were diagnosed and grouped according to the following criteria: clinical manifestation in the environment, serum precipitin chest roentgenogram, and histopathology of the lung. These markers were compared with those in the normal nonsmoking control (NC) group.

Results

We performed statistical analysis using the Mann-Whitney test, with results shown in Table 1. KL-6 in BALF was significantly higher in the Sa-II group compared with Sa-I and NC. KL-6 in serum was also significantly higher in the Sa-II group compared with Sa-I and NC. There was no significant difference in SP-A levels in BALF and serum in the Sa-II, Sa-I and NC groups. SP-D in BALF and serum were significantly higher in Sa-II compared with Sa-I and NC. KL-6 levels in serum showed a significant positive correlation with those in BALF (y = (0.36)x + 265.69, p = 0.037, r = 0.5814). Furthermore, KL-6 levels

Table 1. Concentration of KL-6, SP-A and SP-D in serum and BALF in sarcoidosis and hypersensitivity pneumonitis group.

	Sa-II	Sa-I	c-fl	a-fl	s-p	s-n	NC
KL-6 (BALF)	610±159[a]	261±45	491±153	452±94[b]	404±108	200	222±21
KL-6 (serum)	694±177[a]	241±26	n.t.	n.t.	n.t.	n.t.	225±18
SP-A (BALF)	4160±873	4545±1072	2890±922	2047±779	3691±548	3250±580	3082±811
SP-A (serum)	31±17	45±9	n.t.	n.t.	n.t.	n.t.	47±20
SP-D (BALF)	1126±279[b]	654±116	651±175	929±139	644±87	357±87	471±52
SP-D (serum)	143±27[b]	81±10	n.t.	n.t.	n.t.	n.t.	56±14

[a]$p < 0.05$ compared with Sa-I and NC groups; [b]$p < 0.05$ compared with NC group; KL-6: U/ml; SP-A and SP-D: ng/ml; data results: mean±SEM.

in BALF showed a significant positive correlation with the percentage of lymphocyte in BALF ($y = (9.47)x + 84.07$, $p < 0.038$, $r - 0.454$).

KL-6 in BALF of the a-fl group (452±94) was significantly higher than NC. Some of the c-fl and s-p groups showed elevated KL-6 levels in BALF.

Discussion

KL-6 levels were found to be higher in the BALF and serum of those patients presenting interstitial lung disorders, including sarcoidosis and hypersensitivity pneumonitis [1]. SP-A and SP-D were seen as being useful markers for idiopathic pulmonary fibrosis and interstitial pneumonia with collagen vascular diseases [2]. In our study, significant high levels of KL-6 and SP-D concentration were shown in Sa-II and a-fl patients. Previous studies have shown that the s-p group present with bronchoalveolar lymphocytosis [3,4]. It is also interesting that some of this s-p group showed elevated KL-6 concentration in BALF.

Conclusion

As regards sarcoidosis, these results suggest that KL-6 and SP-D levels did reflect the stage of pulmonary involvement of sarcoidosis in patients. With the farmer's lung group, it was suggested that the KL-6 concentration in BALF may not reflect the deterioration manifested in the chest roentgenogram.

References

1. Kohno N, Awaya Y, Oyama T, Yamakido M, Akiyama M, Inoue Y, Yokoyama A, Hamada H, Fujioka S, Hiwada K. KL-6, a mucin-like glycoprotein, in bronchoalveolar lavage fluid from patients with interstitial lung disease. Am Rev Respir Dis 1993;148(3):637–642.
2. Kuroki Y, Takahashi H, Chiba H, Akino T. Surfactant proteins A and D: disease markers. Biochem Biophys Acta 1998;1408(2–3):334–345.
3. Cormier Y, Belanger J, Laviolette M. Persistent bronchoalveolar lymphocytosis in asymptomatic farmers. Am Rev Respir Dis 1986;133(5):843–847.
4. Mouri T. Cellular analysis of bronchoalveolar lavage fluid in patients with farmer's lung and serum precipitin positive asymptomatic dairy farmers. (Japanese) Kikanshigaku (The Journal of The Japan Society for Bronchology) 1987;9(2):103–114.

Bronchology and Bronchoesophagology: State of the Art.
H. Yoshimura et al., editors.

Factor XIII in bronchoalveolar lavage fluid from children with chronic lung disorders

Béla Nagy[1], Éva Katona[2], János Kappelmayer[3], György Baktai[4], Lajos Kovács[4], Tivadar Márialigeti[5] and László Muszbek[3]

[1]Department of Pediatrics, [2]Institute of Pathophysiology, and [3]Department of Clinical Biochemistry and Molecular Pathology, University of Debrecen, Health and Medical Science Center, Debrecen; [4]Children's Hospital for Pulmonology "Svábhegy", Budapest; and [5]County Hospital for Pulmonology, Department of Pediatrics, Törökbálint, Hungary

Abstract. *Background.* Bronchoalveolar lavage (BAL) is increasingly used in the assessment of different chronic bronchopulmonary diseases in children. In many cases, however, cellularity in BAL fluid samples or noncellular constituents are not enough for the evaluation of the severity of the disease process and of the treatment response. The presence of the alveolar macrophage (AM)-derived subunit A (A_2) and plasma-derived tetramer form (A_2B_2) of factor XIII (FXIII) in BAL fluid seems to be suitable for these purposes.

Methods. The cellularity and levels of A_2, as well as the presence of A_2B_2 of FXIII in BAL fluid samples obtained from 28 children with recurrent bronchitis and five children with fibrosing alveolitis were studied. Sixteen children were considered as a control group without inflammatory findings. The intracellular form (A_2) of FXIII in the AMs was detected by flow cytometry. A_2 and A_2B_2 concentrations of FXIII in BAL fluids were measured by ELISA.

Results. A_2 of FXIII was only detected in the cytoplasm of AMs, but was absent in other cell types of the recovered cell populations. In contrast to the control values, relative concentrations of FXIII A_2 in BAL fluid samples from bronchitics were elevated, and a weak correlation was seen with the number of injured AMs (r = 0.291). Low albumin related levels of cellular FXIII were measured in control subjects and the plasma FXIII (A_2B_2) was not detected at all in samples of BAL fluid. The presence of complex FXIII A_2B_2 in lavage samples from patients with bronchitis and alveolitis indicates plasma leakage without bronchoscopically observed bleeding.

Conclusions. The severity of inflammation on the bronchoalveolar surface can be assessed not only by the detection of cellularity and concentration of albumin, but the presence of FXIII A_2, as well as complex FXIII in BAL fluid samples may also be diagnostic in this relation.

Keywords: alveolar macrophages, bronchoalveolar lavage, chronic bronchitis, factor XIII, fibrosing alveolitis.

Introduction

Bronchoalveolar lavage (BAL) has frequently been used as a diagnostic tool in different inflammatory and granulomatous diseases of the respiratory tract. At the current time, however, not enough convincing BAL cellular or noncellular data have been shown to be predictive enough in determining the severity and

Address for correspondence: Béla Nagy MD, PhD, Department of Pediatrics, University of Debrecen, Health and Medical Science Center, H-4012 Debrecen, P.O. Box 32, Hungary. Tel.: +36-52-414-992. Fax: +36-52-414-992.

prognosis of the disease process or making therapeutic decisions [1,2].

The active form of factor XIII (FXIII) is a transglutaminase that can form crosslinks between two polypeptide chains stabilizing the fibrin clot [3]. It is also active in cell adhesion and migration, the healing of injured tissues, and it reduces endothelial permeability [4]. The presence of FXIII, its macrophage-derived cellular form (A_2) and plasma origin complex (A_2B_2) in BAL fluid, seems to be suitable for the detection of conditions of permeability on the bronchoalveolar surface as well as disease activity.

Patients and Methods

To determine the diagnostic value of FXIII subunits in bronchopulmonary disorders, we measured the lavage levels of subunit A and the presence of factor complex (A_2B_2) in BAL fluid samples in 49 children; 28 children with recurrent bronchitis (22 boys, six girls) aged 1- to 15-years-old and five children with fibrosing alveolitis (7 BAL procedures) (four boys, one girl) aged 2- to 14-years-old. The control group consisted of 16 children aged 2- to 17-years-old with suspicious histories of foreign body aspiration but it was not confirmed by bronchoscopy and no signs of bronchial inflammation were seen.

Bronchoscopy was performed in patients with recurrent bronchitis, and chronic bronchial mucosal inflammation was detected. In patients with alveolitis (three children with extrinsic allergic alveolitis, two children with idiopathic pulmonary fibrosis), the diagnosis was based on clinical symptoms, chest X-ray films, pulmonary function tests, dynamic inhalative lung scans and open lung biopsies.

BAL cell populations were labelled by a FITC-tagged anti-FXIII A monoclonal antibody or an irrelevant FITC-labelled IgG and by a Phycoerythrein (PE)-labelled anti-CD14 monoclonal antibody or an irrelevant PE-labelled IgG. Samples were analyzed on a BD FacScan flow cytometer within 8 h of staining.

The complex plasma FXIII concentrations of BAL fluids were measured by a one-step sandwich enzyme-linked immunosorbent assay (ELISA) [5]. FXIII subunit A concentrations were measured by another sandwich ELISA assay using two monoclonal antibodies specific to different antigenic determinants of FXIII A.

Results

Total cell counts were significantly higher in children with chronic bronchitis and fibrosing alveolitis than in control subjects. Besides predominance of alveolar macrophages, accumulation of neutrophils in bronchitics and of lymphocytes in patients with alveolitis were observed in BAL fluid samples.

FXIII A_2 was only detected in the cytoplasm of AMs by flow cytometry, but it was absent in other cell types of the recovered cell populations. Low albumin related levels of cellular FXIII (FXIII A_2) were measured in control subjects and the plasma FXIII (FXIII A_2B_2) was not detected at all in samples of BAL fluid (Fig. 1). Concentrations of FXIII A_2 correlated well with cell counts of injured macrophages ($r = 0.692$). In contrast to the control values, relative concentrations of FXIII A_2 in BAL fluid samples from bronchitics were elevated, and a weak correlation was seen with the number of injured AMs ($r = 0.291$).

In the case of alveolitis there was no significant difference in the mean relative concentration of BAL FXIII A_2 compared with the control group. No correlation was found between numbers of injured AMs and the relative concentrations of BAL FXIII A_2.

Discussion

Data from control subjects suggest the dominance of intact macrophages in the lavage cell populations and normal permeability without leakage from plasma into the bronchoalveolar surface. A low correlation between injured AMs and relative FXIII A_2 levels in bronchitis and alveolitis groups could be derived from other inflammatory factors, such as leakage. Presumably, extremely high lavage albumin levels altered the elevated FXIII A_2 levels in these groups of patients. The presence of complex FXIII (A_2B_2) in lavage samples from patients with bronchitis and alveolitis indicates plasma leakage without bronchoscopically observed bleeding.

The severity of inflammation on the bronchoalveolar surface can be assessed not only by the detection of cellularity and concentration of albumin, but the presence of FXIII A_2, as well as complex FXIII in BAL fluid samples may also be diagnostic in this relation.

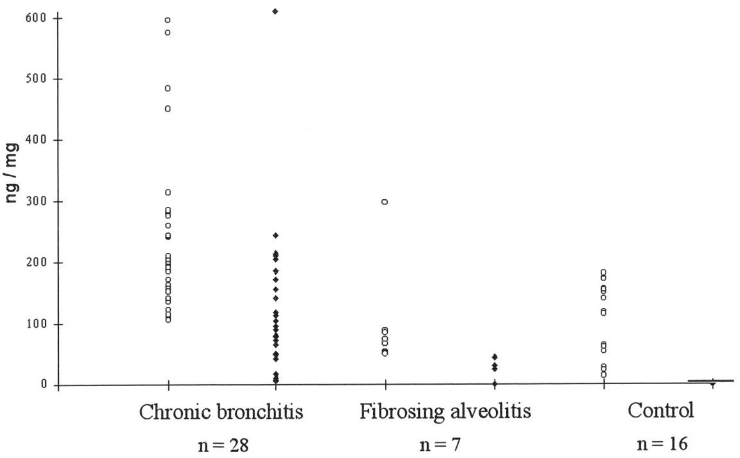

Fig. 1. Relative, albumin related concentrations of cellular FXIII A_2 (○) and complex FXIII A_2B_2 (◆) in BAL fluid samples from children with chronic bronchitis and fibrosing alveolitis compared to the control group. In contrast to the control values, relative concentrations of FXIII A_2 in BAL fluid samples from bronchitics were elevated and plasma FXIII (FXIII A_2B_2) was not detected at all.

References

1. de Blic J et al. Bronchoalveolar lavage in children. ERS Task Force on bronchoalveolar lavage in children. Eur Respir J 2000;15:217–231.
2. Nagy B et al. Fibronectin in bronchoalveolar lavage fluid and plasma from children with chronic inflammation of lungs. Acta Paediatr Scand 1988;77:727–733.
3. Muszbek L, Yee VC, Hevessy Zs. Blood coagulation factor XIII: Structure and function. Thromb Res 1999;94:271–305.
4. Noll T et al. Effect of factor XIII on endothelial barrier function. J Exp Med 1999;189: 1373–1382.
5. Katona et al. A simple, quick one-step ELISA assay for the determination of complex plasma factor XIII (A2B2). Thromb Haemost 2000;83:268–273.

Bronchoscopy

Bronchology and Bronchoesophagology: State of the Art.
H. Yoshimura et al., editors.

Bronchological aspects of pediatric lung and mediastinal tumors

A. Bánfi, G. Baktai, L. Kovács, E. Péterffy and L. Kádár
Pediatric Institute, "Svábhegy", Budapest, Hungary

Abstract. *Introduction.* In pediatric bronchological practice, there tends to be a low occurrence of benign tumors and their malignant counterparts. However, these alterations cause frequently significant airway compression and/or obstruction resulting in a severe condition.

Methods. Between 1989 and 1999, 12,280 chronic chest patients underwent bronchoscopic examination in our institution, with an occurrence of 31 tumors (0.25% of patients). Data were obtained from the retrospective analysis of the patients' files.

Results. There were 12 female and 19 male patients undergoing bronchoscopy, with a mean age of 7 years 8 months (age range from 2 months to 18 years) at the time of the procedure. The diagnosed tumors were as follows: hemangioma in six, neurogen tumors in four, thymoma in four, Hodgkin's disease in four, lymphangio-hemangioma in three and inflammatory pseudotumors in three cases. We diagnosed one case of each of the following conditions: adenoma, papillomatosis of epiglottis, hemangio-sarcoma, carcinoid, histiocytoma, leiomyoma. In one patient metastases was the subject of bronchology and retinoblastoma.

Conclusions. We have shown that bronchological examination reveals the exact endobronchial situation and airway stenosis caused by the tumor. The specimen gained may have an important role in establishing the diagnosis. Bronchograms map the dislocation of the bronchi and possible bronchiectasis. Furthermore, bronchoscopy is seen to be essential in managing the therapy and the follow-up of the patient.

Keywords: bronchological examinations, pediatric, tumor.

Introduction

Benign tumors and their malignant counterparts are rarely seen in pediatric bronchological practice. However, these alterations may cause significant airway compression and obstruction resulting in a severe condition. [1,3]

Materials and Methods

Patients with some form of tumor underwent bronchological examinations as an unavoidable part of the differential diagnosis. Data were obtained from the retrospective analysis of the patients' files. 12,280 rigid bronchoscopies were performed between 1989 and 1999 in our institute. Tumors were diagnosed in 31 cases, a 0.25% incidence. These were 12 females and 19 males, with a mean age of 7 years and 8 months at the time of their first bronchoscopy, ages ranging from 2 months to 18 years.

Address for correspondence: Dr Andrea Bánfi, Pediatric Institute "Svábhegy", Budapest, H-1535 Budapest Pf. 939, Hungary. Tel.: +36-1-3954922. Fax: +36-1-3957649.

Results

The 31 cases were categorised into four groups according to the localization of the tumors. Laryngotracheobronchial, parenchymal, mediastinal localizations, and chest wall tumors which spread to the airways appeared in six, 10, 12 and three cases, respectively.

Laryngotracheobronchial tumors

Tumors developing in the larynx and/or trachea may cause stridor and wheeze [1].

We could see a cauliflower-like alteration of the epiglottis which by histological examination proved to be papillomatosis. Considerably vascularized protrusion could be seen in the subglottical area, and hemangioma was diagnosed. This observed alteration led to diagnosis in two cases.

Tumors which narrowed or closed the bronchi were found in cases of cough and therapy-resistant pneumonias. These tumors occurring in large bronchi caused atelectasis. Smooth, shining, round tumors could be seen by bronchoscopy in three cases. On the basis of histology, these were found to be carcinoid, adenoma and histiocytoma, respectively [3]. Every tumor observed was situated in the right side.

Parenchymal tumors

Parenchymal tumors may be discovered by chance, as in three children in our study. There were varying symptoms in patients, e.g., recurrent bronchitis, fever and chest pain.

These tumors presented in two types of characteristic X-rays, solider pulmonale nodules were found in four, and irregular shadows found in six cases. Bronchoscopic pictures showed dilated vessels in the case of intrapulmonary hemangioma, occlusion of the left upper lobe bronchus in the patients suffering from hemangiosarcoma, and inflammation in the case of leiomyoma. Inflammatory pseudotumors were diagnosed in four patients. In these cases the bronchi were seriously compressed.

Mediastinal tumors

Mediastinal lesions result in direct pressure of the respiratory tract. Consequently, there are occurrences of dry cough, wheeze, pneumonia and fever [4]. In the X-ray pictures the mediastinal shadow was widened. Bronchoscopy revealed the compression of the trachea in a thymoma and a neuroblastoma.

There were two cases in which Hodgkin's disease caused stenosis and two in which it remained bronchoscopically asymptomatic.

Chest wall tumors

Three patients had chest wall tumors, i.e., lymphangio-hemangiomatosis. These spread onto the airways and caused hemoptysis and coughing [2]. We could see the opacity on the upper part of the chest X-ray. In the bronchoscopic picture the wall of the trachea was infiltrated by the tumor, this was the origin of the bleeding.

Other bronchological examinations

Bronchography was carried out in 17 patients. Tumors caused three types of alterations. Dislocation was revealed by mediastinal tumors in two cases. We experienced occlusion in the case of hemangiosarcoma. Bronchiectasis was diagnosed in the case of bronchial adenoma and histiocytoma. All these types of alterations were caused by pseudotumors [1].

Biopsies were performed in some bronchial tumors under bronchoscopy. Histological pictures of a histiocytoma and a carcinoid tumor were seen. Biopsy provided the exact tumor diagnosis in these cases [2].

Twenty follow-up bronchoscopies were performed in 10 patients. Recurrence of tumor was excluded in the case of carcinoid and histiocytoma, and was verified in the case of leiomyoma after being removed. Progression of the tumor was found in five children and subglottical hemangiomatosis showed a spontaneous regression in two cases.

Discussion

On the basis of our study we concluded that permanent chest X-ray shadow indicates bronchological examination. Bronchological examination describes the exact endobronchial situation of the tumors. Bronchograms map the dislocation and occlusion of the bronchi and the possible bronchiectasis. The specimen acquired may have an important role in establishing the diagnosis. Bronchoscopy is essential in managing the therapy and in the follow-up of the patient.

References

1. Székely E, Farkas E. Pediatric Bronchology. Baltimore and Akadémiai kiadó Budapest: University Park Press, 1978;116–131.
2. PS Harleston. M. D. Spencer's Pathology of the Lung, 5th edn, 1996.
3. PD Phelan, LI Landau, A Olinsky. Respiratory Illness of Children 3rd edn, 1990.
4. Kendig. Disorders of the Respiratory Tract 6th edn, 1998.

Bronchology and Bronchoesophagology: State of the Art.
H. Yoshimura et al., editors.

Bronchoscopy for difficult and special intubation

József Kas[1], Lajos Baranyai[1], Dorottya Kiss[2] and Veronika Simon[2]
[1]Department of Surgery and [2]Intensive Care Unit, Buda MÁV Hospital, Budapest, Hungary

Abstract. *Background.* The role of bronchoscopy was evaluated in difficult tracheal and special (endobronchial, double lumen tube, tracheostomy cannula and tracheal stent in place) intubation.
Methods. Both rigid (as an "optical stylet", dilator or ventilating tube) and flexible bronchoscopes were used for difficult and special intubation, except for the double lumen tube (Carlens) positioning.
Results. From 1978 to 1999 intubation, guided by bronchoscopy, was carried out on 142 patients for general, thoracic, and cardiovascular surgery, in both the operating room and the intensive care unit. Indications were as follows: tracheal compression caused by mediastinal disorders, benign or malignant tracheal stenosis, and failed conventional tracheal and planned endobronchial intubation.
Conclusion. Compared to other intubation methods and techniques, rigid and flexible bronchoscopy is an acceptable and useful but expensive procedure for difficult and special intubation.

Keywords: difficult tracheal, endobronchial intubation, rigid and flexible bronchoscopy.

Introduction

Tracheal intubation is a frequently used, safe and usually simple procedure in anesthesiology. All anesthesiologists, however, have to face difficulties in intubating from time to time. The concept of difficult intubation was not unequivocally clarified until the ASA (1993) [1] defined it as follows: the "proper insertion of the tracheal tube with conventional laryngoscopy requires more than 1) three attempts; or 2) 10 min." Its occurrence is about 0.5 to 14%, and is more frequent in women approaching labor than in other surgical patients. Although difficult intubation can be predicted by the careful examination of patients, it occurs unexpectedly in about 10%. Unsuccessful intubation occurs in 0.03 to 0.5%. The importance of the problem is underlined by the complications of death, brain and heart damage and airway injury. Difficult intubation may be due to various causes, such as anatomical variations, tumors, cysts, acute inflammation, congenital anomalies, scarred tissues, trauma, arthritis, spondylitis ankylopoetica, allergic edema, endocrine diseases and technical difficulties [2,3]. The majority of authors in international literature deal principally with the intubation difficulties of the upper airway. The present work is concerned primarily with difficult intubation due to complications in the lower airway and there is also a lot of attention given to some of the special intubation procedures (endobronchial intubation, the placement of a double lumen tube, the insertion of a tracheostomy cannula and intubation with a tracheal stent in place).

Address for correspondence: József Kas MD, Department of Surgery, Buda MÁV Hospital, Szanatórium u. 2/a., 1528 Budapest, Hungary. Tel.: +36-1-275-3535. Fax: +36-1-275-2529.

Methods

There are several different methods and instruments available in anesthesiology in order to solve the problem of difficult intubation. The rigid bronchoscope and the fiberoscope are among them. We made use of the rigid bronchoscope in three different ways, most frequently the "optical stylet" method as described by Katz and Berci [4]. In cases of major cicatrized tracheal stenosis, the bronchoscope was dilated before intubation with a series of 6- to 13-mm tubes and intubation with optical control was done thereafter. On rare occasions the rigid bronchoscope itself was left in the trachea during surgical intervention and respiration was carried out through it. The "optical stylet" method was suitable for both tracheal (translaryngeal and transstomal) and bronchial (main bronchi) intubation. The fiberoscope was first reported to be a useful instrument in the intubation of the trachea and main bronchi by Murphy [5] and later by Taylor and Towey [6]. We preferred transoral insertion to the nasal route. When intubation proved to be unexpectedly difficult and was unsuccessful by the conventional method, the tube was guided downwards with the use of fiberoscopy, on sleeping and spontaneously breathing patients. In those cases it was always necessary to pull the tongue forward and to lift the root of the tongue/epiglottis using the laryngoscope.

The bronchological assistance of a double lumen tube is extensively discussed in the literature [7]. The Carlens tube has been used at our institute for separate ventilation during pulmonary operations for about 30 years. A bronchoscope cannot be introduced into its narrow channel, thus, we have no experience with this technique. Tracheal intubation may be difficult in patients bearing an implanted stent of tracheal stenosis. In such cases where a laryngeal mask could not be used, the tube was introduced to the stent using optical control, and a ventilation bronchoscope was placed into the stent or at its opening. Finally, the stent may temporarily be removed to prevent hindering intubation.

Results

Rigid and flexible bronchoscopes were used in 142 cases between 1978 and 1999 for tracheal and bronchial intubation. The bulk of the interventions were done in our own institute, while in 12 cases they were performed in consultation with other institutes. 125 procedures were performed in the operating room, and the remaining 17 were done in ICU. The majority of the patients awaited either general, thoracic or vascular surgery, while a small number of them expected heart surgery. Indications are given in Table 1. Rigid bronchoscopes and fiberoscopes were used in 86 and 56 cases, respectively. Intubations that were unsuccessful using conventional techniques were solved by using the fiberoscope. In two cases, however, even this method was inefficient, surgery was postponed and the following fiberoscopic intubation was performed on the conscious patient.

Table 1. Indications for bronchoscpy guided intubation (1978 to 1999).

Condition	No. of cases
Tracheal compression (struma, mediastinal tumor)	12
Tracheal stenosis (postintubation, posttracheostomy, tumor)	26
Laryngeal stenosis	4
Failed tracheal intubation	30
Endobronchial intubation	59
Miscellaneous	11

Conclusions

Difficult and special intubation have been made much easier with the use of both rigid and flexible bronchoscopes in our experience, acquired over 22 years of practice. The advantages of bronchoscopic intubation are that there is safer execution assured by visual control, and the possibility of simultaneous bronchological intervention (dilation, excision, aimed suction). Disadvantages are the special experience and expensive instrumentation which are required.

References

1. ASA Task Force on Management of the Difficult Airway: Practice guidelines for management of the difficult airway. Anesthesiology 1993;78:597–602.
2. King TA, Adams AP. Failed tracheal intubation. Br J Anaesth 1990;65:400–414.
3. Ovassapian A. Fiberoptic airway endoscopy in anesthesia and critical care. New York: Raven Press, 1990.
4. Katz RL, Berci G. The optical stylet - a new intubation technique for adults and children with specific reference to teaching. Anesthesiology 1979;51:251–254.
5. Murphy P. A fibre-optic endoscope used for nasal intubation. Anaesthesia 1967;22:489–491.
6. Taylor PA, Towey RM. The bronchofiberoscope as an aid to endotracheal intubation. Br J Anaesth 1972;44:611–612.
7. Benumof JL et al. Margin of safety in positioning modern double-lumen endotracheal tubes. Anesthesiology 1987;67:729–738.

Bronchology and Bronchoesophagology: State of the Art.
H. Yoshimura et al., editors.

Bronchial brushing does not improve the diagnostic yield of biopsy and washing in bronchoscopically visible bronchial carcinomas

Bing Lam[1], Wah-Kit Lam[1], James C. M. Ho[1], Kenneth W. Tsang[1] and Gaik C. Ooi[2]
University Departments of [1]Medicine and [2]Diagnostic Radiology, Queen Mary Hospital, The University of Hong Kong, Hong Kong SAR, China

Abstract. *Background.* The diagnostic yield of fiberoptic bronchoscopy (FOB) can depend on the location and extent of a bronchial carcinoma. Although biopsy (BX) represents the gold standard in diagnosis of lung cancer, brushing (BR) and bronchial washing (BW) are frequently used complementary techniques.

Methods. We performed a prospective study to evaluate the diagnostic yield of BR and BW in addition to BX in patients with bronchoscopically visible tumors. For all patients, the sequence of procedure was BW ($>$ 50 ml), BX (four samples), and then BR whenever possible.

Results. Fifty-nine untreated patients with bronchoscopically visible tumors, subsequently proven to be bronchial carcinoma, were recruited. Forty-seven patients (80%) had BX confirmed bronchial carcinoma. For the 12 BX negative patients, BW and BR were positive in 10 (83%) and six (86%) of the patients, respectively ($p > 0.05$). All BR positive patients were also BW positive.

Conclusions. Our results suggest that BW is a useful complementary technique to BX in the diagnosis of bronchoscopically visible tumor, and BR provides no additional diagnostic benefit onto a combination of BX and BW.

Keywords: bronchial carcinoma, bronchoscopy, diagnosis.

Introduction

Bronchial carcinoma is one of the commonest malignant disorders and presents late in most affected patients [1]. Fiberoptic bronchoscopy is a standard procedure in the investigation of patients with suspected bronchial carcinoma, and is important in tumor staging and pathological typing. In bronchoscopy, various sampling techniques including forceps biopsy (BX) [2], bronchial washing (BW) and brushing (BR) are routinely employed [3,4]. While recent studies suggest that a combination of these techniques might increase the diagnostic yield of malignant cells [5–7], it is sometimes not always possible to perform all of these in the same patient. The costs of employing many sampling techniques in one routine investigation also need to be justified. However, only very limited data

Address for correspondence: Dr Kenneth Tsang MD (Hons), FRCP, FCCP, FCP, Associate Professor and Honorary Consultant Physician, University Department of Medicine, The University of Hong Kong, Queen Mary Hospital, Pok Fu Lam Road, Hong Kong SAR, China. Tel.: +852-2855-4775. Fax: +852-2872-5828. E-mail: kwttsang@hkucc.hku.hk are available comparing the relative yield of BAL, BW, and BR in the diagnosis of bronchial carcinoma [8–11]. We have, therefore, performed this prospective study to evaluate the diagnostic yield of these bronchoscopic sampling techniques (i.e., BAL, BW, and BR) in the diagnosis of bronchoscopically visible bronchial carcinoma.

Materials and Methods

Patients without prior cytological or histological evidence of bronchial carcinoma underwent bronchoscopy by the same bronchoscopist (K. Tsang) and were subsequently followed up at the Respiratory Clinic of the University of Hong Kong. Data were obtained for further analysis from those patients who had subsequently proven bronchial carcinoma. Inclusion criteria included written consent to undergo bronchoscopy for investigation of suspected bronchial carcinoma, and the presence of abnormal chest radiograph or thoracic computed tomography (CT). A diagnosis of bronchial carcinoma was established by BW or BR cytological results; compatible BX histological results; compatible clinical or radiological metastatic lesions with or without cytological or histological evidence; and absence of other malignancies or diseases that would otherwise explain the overall clinical picture. Bronchoscopy was performed using standard methods. BW (> 50 ml saline), followed by BX (⩾ four biopsies) and then BR (six smeared slides) were performed sequentially unless there was significant procedure induced bleeding, patient desaturation, or loss of patient cooperation.

Results

Between January 1996 and December 1997, 59 consecutive patients (18F, mean age 62, SD 13, age range 35- to 80-years-old) underwent bronchoscopy and were subsequently confirmed to have bronchial carcinoma. The diagnosis in two patients was based solely on clinical and imaging findings (mass lesions on chest radiograph and contrast thoracic CT scan, and metastatic lesions on brain CT scan) without histological or cytological confirmation. Stepwise performance of BW, BX and then BR in bronchoscopically visible lesions provided a diagnostic yield of 97% of cases who had subsequently proven bronchial carcinoma. Forty-seven (80%) patients had BX confirmed bronchial carcinoma. For the 12 BX negative patients, BW and BR were positive in 10 (83%: malignant cell in seven, suspicious cell in one, and atypical cell in two) and six (86%: malignant cell in four, and atypical cell in two) of the patients, respectively. All BR positive patients were also BW positive for malignant cells.

Discussion

The results of this study showed that bronchial carcinoma can be diagnosed efficiently by using fiberoptic bronchoscopy and its associated sampling techniques.

Stepwise performance of BW, BX and then BR in bronchoscopically visible lesions provided a diagnostic yield of 97% of cases who had subsequently proven bronchial carcinoma. BW was a useful complementary technique to BX in the diagnosis of bronchoscopically visible tumor, however, BR provided no additional diagnostic benefit to a combination of BX and BW. As our findings could have significant impact on the bronchoscopic diagnosis of bronchial carcinoma, i.e., physician's practice, costing, procedure time, and patient comfort, further studies should be performed in other centers to confirm our results.

References

1. Wingo PA, Bolden S, Tong T et al. Cancer statistics, 1996. CA Cancer J Clin 1996;46:5–27.
2. Zavala DC. Diagnostic fiberoptic bronchoscopy: techniques and results of biopsy in 600 patients. Chest 1975;68:12–19.
3. Linder J, Radio SJ, Robbins RA et al. Bronchoalveolar lavage in the cytologic diagnosis of carcinoma of the lung. Acta Cytol 1987;31:796–801.
4. Rennard SI. Bronchoalveolar lavage in the diagnosis of cancer. Lung 1990:168(Suppl): 1035–1040.
5. Saltzstein SL, Harrell JH, Cameron T. Brushings, washings, or biopsy? Obtaining maximum value from flexible fiberoptic bronchoscopy in the diagnosis of cancer. Chest 1977;71:630–632.
6. Popp W, Rauscher H, Ritschka L et al. Diagnostic sensitivity of different techniques in the diagnosis of lung tumour with the flexible fiberoptic bronchoscope: comparison of brush biopsy, imprint cytology of forceps biopsy, and histology of forceps biopsy. Cancer 1991;67:72–75.
7. Lachman MF, Schofield K, Cellura K et al. Bronchoscopic diagnosis of malignancy in the lower airway: a cytological review. Acta Cytol 1995;39:1148–1151.
8. Bedrossian CW, Rybka DL. Bronchial brushing during fiberoptic bronchoscopy for the cytodiagnosis of lung cancer: comparison with sputum and bronchial washings. Acta Cytol 1976; 20:446–453.
9. Jay SJ, Wehr K, Nicholson DP et al. Diagnostic sensitivity and specificity of pulmonary cytology: comparison of techniques used in conjunction with flexible fiberoptic bronchoscopy. Acta Cytol 1980;24:304–312.
10. Kvale PA, Bode FR, Kini S. Diagnostic accuracy in lung cancer: comparison of techniques used in association with flexible fiberoptic bronchoscopy. Chest 1976;69:752–757.
11. Lundgren R, Bergman F, Angstrom T. Comparison of transbronchial fine needle aspiration biopsy, aspiration of bronchial secretion, bronchial washing, brush biopsy and forceps biopsy in the diagnosis of lung cancer. Eur J Respir Dis 1983;64:378–385.

Bronchology and Bronchoesophagology: State of the Art.
H. Yoshimura et al., editors.

Flexible bronchoscopy in the diagnosis of tracheobronchial foreign bodies in children

Sang-Chul Lim and Jae-Shik Cho
Department of Otolaryngology, Chonnam National University Medical School, Gwangju, Korea

Abstract. The diagnosis of foreign body aspiration in children has not been satisfactory, although many methods have included history, physical examination, chest radiography, CT, MRI and lung scan. Therefore, a simple and definitive method is needed and we have studied the utility of flexible bronchoscopy in the diagnosis of tracheobronchial foreign bodies in children. A retrospective review of 67 cases referred with suspicion of foreign body aspiration was undertaken. The age of the patients ranged from 3 to 192 months. A flexible bronchoscopy was performed in 38 cases with topical-local anesthesia because the evidence of a tracheobronchial foreign body was not conclusive. We found foreign bodies in 27 cases (71%) and secretion suggesting foreign bodies in seven cases (18%). 34 children underwent rigid ventilating bronchoscopy and 32 had foreign bodies. Four of 38 children who had normal flexible bronchoscopic examination were discharged after improvement by medical treatment. There were no complications associated with the flexible bronchoscopy procedure. We suggest that diagnostic use of the pediatric flexible bronchoscopy is a safe, reliable and cost-effective method for the identification of tracheobronchial foreign bodies in patients.

Keywords: pediatric flexible bronchoscopy, tracheobronchial foreign body.

Introduction

There are various methods used in the diagnosis of tracheobronchial foreign bodies in children and in particular, if there is no definite history of a foreign body, a doctor's suspicion is essential. Diagnosis methods include history, physical examination, chest radiography, computed tomography and magnetic resonance imaging [1–5], but rigid bronchoscopy is the most accurate and definitive method although general anesthesia is needed. Since Wood [6] first described the application of flexible bronchoscopy in children for this purpose, many studies on its usefulness and safety had been performed [7–11]. We have carried out this study to evaluate the diagnostic value and usefulness of flexible bronchoscopy in diagnosing tracheobronchial foreign bodies in children.

Patients and Methods

Between January 1989 and May 1999, 67 children admitted to the Chonnam National University Hospital in Gwangju, Korea, for equivocal foreign body

Address for correspondence: Sang-Chul Lim, Department of Otolaryngology, Chonnam National University Medical School, 8 Hak-dong, Dong-gu, Gwangju 501-190, Korea. Tel.: +82-62-220-6773. Fax: +82-62-228-7743. E-mail: limsc@chonnam.ac.kr aspiration were recruited in this study. The age of patients ranged from 3 months to 15 years and there were 37 males and 30 females examined. Twenty-nine cases having a definite history of foreign body aspiration underwent immediate rigid bronchoscopy, and 38 cases with unclear history underwent flexible bronchoscopy under local anesthesia. The outcomes of bronchoscopy were presented.

We used a flexible bronchoscopy with an outer diameter of 3.6 mm, and topical anesthesia with 4% lidocaine and sedation with midazolam (0.1 mg/kg) was carried out. Equipment and medication for resuscitation were available and oxygen saturation was monitored. Patients were in a restrained sitting position (Fig. 1). The flexible bronchoscopy was inserted into one nostril and was passed carefully through the vocal cords so as not to cause a reflex cough and/or laryngospasm. The bronchoscope reached the orifice of the bronchiole and the foreign body could be inspected. Because any reflex cough of the patient caused movement of the larynx and interfered with detailed examination, sufficient topical anesthesia was required. In cases where the flexible bronchoscopy showed a foreign body or secretion indicating a foreign body, immediate rigid bronchoscopy was performed under general anesthesia, and appropriate treatment was planned.

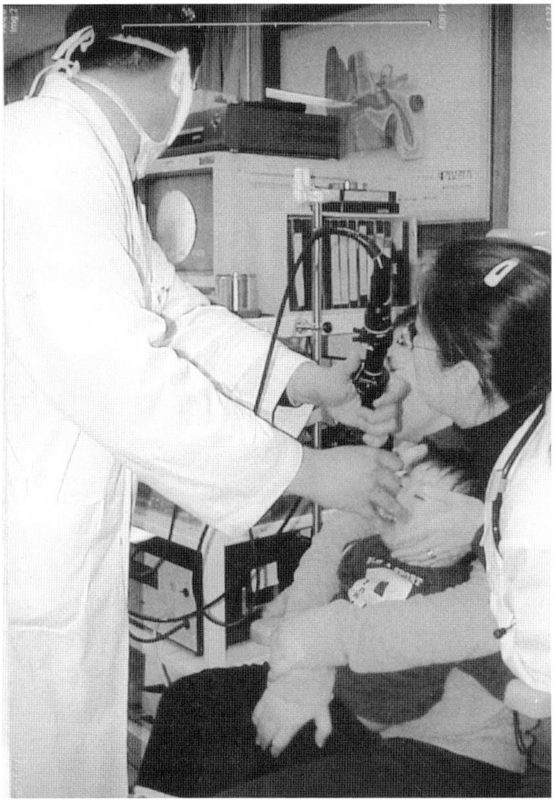

Fig. 1. Photography showing the patient in a restrained sitting position.

Results

Symptoms and signs of tracheobronchial foreign bodies were as follows: asphyxia (17 cases, 28%), respiratory difficulty (35 cases, 57%), cyanosis (15 cases, 25%), coughing (42 cases, 69%), decreased breathing sound of unilateral lung upon auscultation (33 cases, 54%) and stridor (15 cases, 25%). Chest radiological findings included emphysema (29 cases, 48%), pneumonia or atelectasis (13 cases, 21%) and metallic density (7 cases, 11%).

Twenty-nine cases who had a definite history of, e.g., choking underwent immediate rigid bronchoscopy, and here foreign bodies were found and extracted in 28 out of 29 cases. In 38 cases with an unclear history of foreign body aspiration, flexible bronchoscopy was performed first. Here, foreign bodies were found in 27 cases, seven had secretion suggesting a foreign body and the remaining four were negative. In 34 cases with positive findings of a foreign body with flexible bronchoscopy, rigid bronchoscopy was performed immediately. In 32 cases a foreign body was found and removed. Another four cases with negative findings recovered without rigid bronchoscopy (Fig. 2). There were no serious complications, except transient respiratory discomfort, seen in our study.

Locations of foreign bodies found is shown in Table 1. The most common found was a peanut (26 cases), and others included metal (8 cases), corn, a piece of plastic, seed of fruit, fish bone, etc.

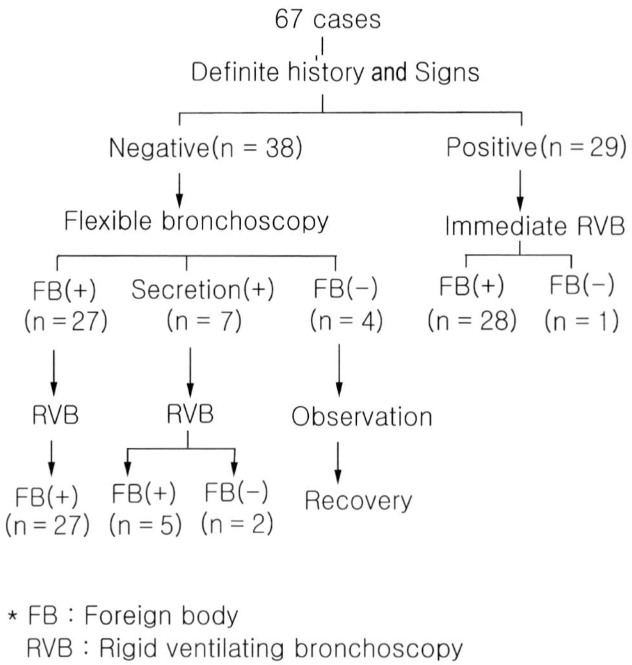

Fig. 2. Diagnostic approach for equivocal tracheobronchial foreign bodies.

Table 1. Location of foreign bodies.

Site	No. of cases (n = 60)
Left main bronchus	26
Right main bronchus	23
Above carina	7
Not determined	4

Discussion

Tracheobronchial foreign bodies are most common in children, especially those younger than 3-years-old [12,13]. Diagnostic methods for an equivocal tracheobronchial foreign body include history, physical examination, chest radiography, CT, MRI, lung scan, etc. [1–5]. History and physical examination of a tracheobronchial foreign body are asphyxia, cough, cyanosis, abnormal findings on auscultation [1,2], and radiological findings are emphysema, mediastinal shift, atelectasis, and pneumonia [12–14]. However, these conditions are not always present and not necessarily pathognomonic in the diagnosis of a tracheobronchial foreign body. Of the various possible methods, rigid bronchoscopy is the diagnostic and therapeutic method of choice, but needs general anesthesia and has a negative exploration rate of 26% [1].

In our opinion, one of the most helpful clues in examining a possible tracheobronchial foreign body situation is the patient's choking history. If there is a definite history of choking in the recent past then immediate rigid bronchoscopy is recommended. However, if the history is not definite and the duration of symptoms displayed is too long, then care has to be taken because rigid bronchoscopy has the possibility of negative exploration. Wood [6] first introduced the application of flexible bronchoscopy in the diagnosis of a tracheobronchial foreign body in children. The indication, diagnostic usefulness and safety of flexible bronchoscopies has subsequently been studied [7–11]. Indications of diagnostic flexible bronchoscopy in pediatric airway are stridor, persistent atelectasis, wheezing, recurrent/persistent pulmonary infiltrate, lung lesion of unknown etiology, chronic cough, hemoptysis, selective bronchography, equivocal tracheobronchial foreign body, assessment of injury from toxic inhalation or aspiration, sample collection of lower airway secretion and/or cells by bronchoalveolar lavage, brush biopsy and transbronchial biopsy [10,11,15]. Before the procedure, sedative and topical anesthesia are applied. Vital signs, skin color, position of head and oxygen saturation are checked, and equipment and medication for resuscitation should be prepared. Pediatric flexible bronchoscopy is carried out under local anesthesia, the advantages being the avoidance of the morbidity of general anesthesia and saving cost.

Complications associated with pediatric flexible bronchoscopy are: hypoxemia, laryngospasm or bradycardia due to inadequate topical anesthesia, respiratory depression due to the sedative, infection from instrument used, nasal bleeding, pneumothorax and hemoptysis [10]. From our experience, we believe that these complications should rarely occur if sufficient premedication with sedative and topical anesthesia are carried out, and if the procedure is performed carefully.

Because pediatric diagnostic flexible bronchoscopy is reliable and safe, we recommend flexible bronchoscopy first when physical examination and radiological findings are not conclusive. Our indications of diagnostic flexible bronchoscopy are: history of choking and unexplained respiratory problem unresponsive to conservative treatment, and contraindications are hypoxemia ($PaO_2 < 60$ mmHg), bleeding tendency, abnormal heart rate and poor general condition. Martinot et al. [8] propose that rigid bronchoscopy should be performed first in cases of asphyxia, a radiopaque foreign body, or association of unilaterally decreased breathing sounds and obstructive emphysema. They showed that the detection rate in flexible bronchoscopy was 30% (17 out of 55 cases), and that rigid bronchoscopy was not necessary in the remaining 38 cases. Our higher detection rate using flexible bronchoscopy (84%) and immediate rigid bronchoscopy (96%) may be attributable to stricter indication in this study.

Conclusion

We suggest that pediatric diagnostic flexible bronchoscopy is a reliable, safe and cost-effective method in detecting tracheobronchial foreign bodies in children.

References

1. Hoeve LJ, Rombout J, Pot DJ. Foreign body aspiration in children. The diagnostic value of signs, symptoms and preoperative examination. Clin Otolaryngol 1993;18:55–57.
2. Svedstrom E, Puhakka H, Kero P. How accurate is chest radiography in the diagnosis of tracheobronchial foreign bodies in children? Pediatr Radiol 1989;19:520–522.
3. Berger PE, Kuhn JP, Kuhns LR. Computed tomography and the occult tracheobronchial foreign body. Radiology 1980;134:133–135.
4. O'Unchi T, Tokumaru A, Mikami I, Yamasoba T, Kikuchi S. Value of MR imaging in detecting a peanut causing bronchial obstruction. AJR 1992;159:481–482.
5. Abramson AL, Rudavsky AZ. Use of lung scanning for the detection of endobronchial foreign bodies. Ann Otol 1972;81:832–839.
6. Wood RE, Fink RJ. Applications of flexible fiberoptic bronchoscopes in infants and children. Chest 1978;73:737–740.
7. Nussbaum E, Beach L. Flexible fiberoptic bronchoscopy and laryngoscopy in infants and children. Laryngoscope 1983;93:1073–1075.
8. Martinot A, Closset M, Marquette CH, Hue V, Deschildre A, Ramon P et al. Indications for flexible versus rigid bronchoscopy in children with suspected foreign-body aspiration. Am J Respir Crit Care Med 1997;155:1676–1679.
9. Wood RE, Gauderer M. Flexible fiberoptic bronchoscopy in the management of tracheobronchial foreign bodies in children: the value of a combined approach with open tube bronchoscopy. J Pediatr Surg 1984;19:693–698.
10. Green CG, Eisenberg J, Leong A, Nathanson I, Schnape BM, Wood RE. Flexible endoscopy of the pediatric airway. Am Rev Respir Dis 1992;145:233–235.
11. Godfrey S, Avital A, Maayan C, Rotschild M, Springer C. Yield from flexible bronchoscopy in

children. Pediatr Pulm 1997;23:261–269.
12. McGuirt WF, Holmes KD, Feehs R, Browne J. Tracheobronchial foreign bodies. Laryngoscope 1988;98:615–618.
13. Mu L, He P, Sun D. Inhalation of foreign bodies in Chinese children: a review of 400 cases. Laryngoscope 1991;101:657–660.
14. Mu L, Sun DQ, He P. Radiological diagnosis of aspirated foreign bodies in children: review of 343 cases. J Laryngol Otol 1990;104:778–782.
15. Wood RE, Sherman JM. Pediatric flexible bronchoscopy. Ann Otol 1980;89:414–416.

Bronchology and Bronchoesophagology: State of the Art.
H. Yoshimura et al., editors.

Assessment of bronchoscopic examination made by patient and physician

F. Salajka
Department of Respiratory Diseases, Masaryk University Hospital, Brno, Czech Republic

Introduction

In bronchology, as in other instrumental examinations, very little attention is paid to patients' subjective experience during the procedure or to his/her fears and feelings. The aim of our study was to evaluate bronchoscopic examination from a patient's point of view and to compare his assessment with that made by a physician.

Methods

In a group of 49 patients examined bronchoscopically for the first time, due to suspicion of pulmonary fibrosis, bronchoscopy and bronchoalveolar lavage were performed by the same bronchposcopist after routine premedication (midazolam, atropin) and local anesthesia (lidocain). An introductory explanation concerning the nature and course of the examination was given to all patients before starting the procedure. Using our own questionnaire, the level of discomfort and anxiety experienced by the patient, as well as the course of the bronchoscopy, were evaluated separately by the patients and by the physician immediately after finishing the procedure.

Results

Concerning the course of bronchoscopy (quiet/harsh), an agreement between patients' and the physician's evaluations was achieved in 32 cases (65%) (Table 1). The physician was able to determine correctly the grade of discomfort experienced by the patient in 25 cases (51%), but mostly underestimated the inconvenience (in 17 cases, 35%) (Table 2). The correlation between patients' and physician's evaluations of patients' anxiety was poor – the evaluation only reached agreement in 21 cases (43%) and, again, the physician's underestimation occurred frequently (in 24 cases, 49%) (Table 3). In all cases, the introductory

Address for correspondence: F. Salajka, Department of Respiratory Diseases, Masaryk University Hospital, Jihlavská 20, 639 00 Brno, Czech Republic.

Table 1. The evaluation of the course of the bronchoscopy.

		Physician' assessment		
		I	II	III
Patients' assessments	I	28	2	0
	II	8	4	3
	III	0	4	0

I = quiet; III = harsh.

explanation of the nature of bronchoscopic examination and the behavior of the bronchoscopic staff were assessed as very helpful and fully satisfactory.

Discussion

Most medical examinations represent a certain amount of stress for the patient. Due to many factors, bronchoscopy must be considered as one of the most stressful examinations. The fear the patient feels influences his experience during the examination considerably and can sometimes become an obstacle, making the procedure impossible to perform, or resulting in its turbulent course or premature end.

Surprisingly, only a little attention is given to this problem, generally. Sedation of the patient is routinely recommended and is considered a sufficient remedy. The use of diazepam (or midazolam) during the premedication of the patient is assessed as a standard method to quiet down the patient and to prevent undesirable manifestations of his anxiety. Very unusual, is the effort to increase the patient's comfort using various methods, such as listening to the music, etc.

In our study, it was not only the presence of the patient's anxiety and fear that was confirmed. At least some of the patients are unable to assess their behavior during the examination objectively when compared to the assessment made by the physician. On the other hand, in many cases the physician is unable to assess the patient's feelings, and his/her anxiety and experience during the examination. It is extremely important that the patient's unsuppressible stress be taken into consideration, and the physician should endeavor to take all possible measures

Table 2. The evaluation of the discomfort during the bronchoscopy.

		Physician's assessment		
		I	II	III
Patient's assessment	I	13	4	1
	II	12	11	2
	III	2	3	1

I = minor inconvenience; III = very unpleasant.

Table 3. The evaluation of the patient's anxiety during the bronchoscopy.

		Physician's assessment		
		I	II	III
Patient's assessment	I	13	3	0
	II	10	5	1
	III	6	8	3

I = low; III = high.

(not only medication) to minimize the adverse impacts of the stress on the patient. The need for close cooperation between the patient and the physician should be emphasized, especially in such stressful medical procedures as bronchoscopy.

Conclusion

Our results show that, even for an experienced bronchoscopist, it is difficult to recognize what the patient is experiencing during the procedure, and that the grade of stress is underestimated in most cases.

Bronchology and Bronchoesophagology: State of the Art.
H. Yoshimura et al., editors.

Fiberoptic bronchoscopic practice in Turkey

M. Sener and C. Ozturk
Department of Pulmonary Diseases, Faculty of Medicine, Gazi University, Ankara, Turkey

Purpose

The purpose of this study is to examine the facilities of medical centers in Turkey and the different personal approaches to the fiberoptic bronchoscopy (FOB) procedure.

Methods

This study was carried out by postal survey. Questionnaires containing a total of 59 questions were posted to hospitals. The first section of the questionnaire, concerning the facilities of the center, was required to be answered by one doctor, and the second section, covering individual approaches, was required to be responded to by all the physicians actively performing FOB in that medical center.

Results

The response rate of the survey was 77% (45 clinics). Eighty-six percent of the university hospitals and 100% of all the governmental hospitals specializing in respiratory diseases were examined. A total of 283 bronchoscopists (35 chest surgeons and 248 chest physicians) participated in the study.

Facilities

The number of fiberoptic bronchoscopes available in the medical centers ranged from one to four. The total number of FOB procedures performed during training was 60 to 100 in 30% of the clinics, and this training began within the first 3 months in 29% of the clinics. In 33% of the clinics, nurses and assistant doctors support the FOB procedure, whilst nurses alone assist the bronchoscopist in 29% of the clinics. The facilities of the medical centers are summarized in Table 1.

Address for correspondence: M. Sener, Gazi University Faculty of Medicine, Bagoat Caddesi Egemen Sokak, No:712 81030 Istanbul, Turkey. Tel.: +90-5325-022812. Fax: +90-2122-665995.

Table 1. FOB facilities in the medical centers.

Facility	No. of clinics (%)
Oxygen tube	45 (100.0)
Adrenalin	43 (95.6)
Laryngoscope	38 (84.4)
EKG monitor	28 (62.2)
Special room for post-FOB observation	27 (60.0)
Opiat antagonist	25 (55.6)
Pulse oxymeter	23 (51.1)
Videobronchoscopy	18 (40.0)
Defibrilator	17 (37.8)
Fluoroscopy	15 (33.3)
Blood pressure monitor	13 (28.9)
Balloon catheter	10 (22.2)
Endobronchial stent	5 (1.1)
Brachitherapy	4 (0.8)
Electrocother	1 (0.2)
Laser	1 (0.2)

Preparation for FOB

The patient's starvation time preceding FOB is accepted to be between 4 and 8 h by 52% of the doctors, while 2.9% of them allow less than 4 h. A chest radiograph is routinely carried out by 99.3%, EKG by 91.5%, respiratory function test by 44.2%, prothrombin time by 32.5%, blood count by 82%, Hbs Ag by 50.2%, HCV by 20.1%, HIV by 13.8%, and computerized tomography by 28.6% of the doctors.

Premedication and sedation

It was found that 6.7% of the responding doctors do not carry out any premedication. Regarding premedication, 91.9% of the doctors prefer atropine and 68.6% of them prescribe medication 30–45 min before FOB. Five percent of the doctors do not use sedatives, 85% use sedatives before FOB, and for 91.8% diazepam is the preferred sedative used.

Local anesthesia

Regarding anesthetic methods used, 89% of the doctors use lidocaine routinely and of these, most (47%) via a combination of the following techniques: nebulizer, bronchoscopic injection, and oral/nasal spray forms.

Table 2. Routine personal approaches for certain situations in FOB.

Procedure	Routine usage (% of doctors)
Sedation	76.7
Chest PA after TBB	75.7
Hospitalization after TBB	58.9
FOB via oral way	44.5
Oxygen therapy	41.6
Pulse oximeter usage	23.3
EKG monitorization	17.7
FOB in immunodeficiency	12.7
Videobronchoscopy	12.5
Mediastinal node aspiration	12.0
Midazolam usage	8.3
Protected brush	6.8
Fluoroscopy for TBB	2.9

Routine: used in more than 85% of cases; TBB: transbronchial biopsy.

Indications

The most common indications of FOB were seen to be hemoptysis (90.3%), tumor (87.5%) and foreign bodies (55.2%). Other less common indications were unresolved pneumonias (22.2%), atelectasis and pneumonia in ICU (21.9%) and tuberculosis diagnosis in smear negative patients (17.6%).

Personal approaches

The techniques that doctors would most like to be able to carry out in their clinics were: stent therapy (65.2%), photodynamic therapy (54.3%) and brachitherapy (52.8%). Other personal approaches are summarized in Table 2.

Conclusion

Several technical deficiencies limit the optimal performance of FOB in our country. In order to overcome economical problems, doctors should begin the approach to FOB by carrying out careful examination in order to choose the patient with the right indication, and by taking the cost into consideration.

Bronchology and Bronchoesophagology: State of the Art.
H. Yoshimura et al., editors.

Bronchoscopy without sedatives during premedication in 550 patients

Ageliki Sotiri and Maria Mattheou
Department of Pulmonary Medicine, General Hospital of Ioannina "G. Hadjicosta", Athens, Greece

Abstract. *Background.* The aim of the study was to determine the tolerance of fiberoptic bronchoscopy without premedication, other than topical anaesthesia.

Methods. 550 patients, 454 men and 96 women, underwent fiberoptic bronchoscopy without sedatives during premedication. They received 1 mg lorazepame per os the night before the procedure. Premedication included topical anaesthesia with lidocaine (2%, 20 cc) and atropine (0.3 mg) intramuscularly.

Results. Most of the 550 patients (98%) tolerated the procedure well, without other premedication. In three patients the procedure had to be stopped due to dyspnea, in three others due to edema of the larynx and in four due to refusal to undergo the examination.

Conclusions. We concluded that bronchoscopy without sedatives during premedication, with the operator remaining in close contact with the patient throughout the procedure, is perfectly acceptable and is without side effects.

Keywords: bronchoscopy, premedication, sedatives.

Introduction

Bronchoscopy without sedatives during premedication is the method proposed by many authors [1] because it can be performed safely and without the side effects of sedation. We applied this method to 550 patients.

Materials and Methods

550 patients, 454 men and 96 women, underwent fiberoptic bronchoscopy for diagnostic reasons. All patients were fully informed about the endoscopy by way of a detailed discussion with the doctor a few days prior to the examination. Every single patient was informed that there was no danger and that the local anaesthetic has an unpleasant taste but that it prevents the pain. All patients were also warned about dysphonia and that they might get the urge to cough with the passing of the fiberscope through the glottis, and the possibility of bleeding after the biopsy.

The endoscopy was carried out in a bronchoscopy room by the same operator

Address for correspondence: Ageliki Sotiri, Department of Pulmonary Medicine, General Hospital of Ioannina "G. Hadjicosta", Kitheronos 36-38 Pl. Koliatsou, Athens 11255, Greece. Tel.: +30-1-2011631. Fax: +30-1-8039525.

who had informed the patient. All patients followed the instructions to avoid food and drink for at least 3 h. In all cases the nasal route was chosen [2]. Electrocardiographic monitoring was performed and supplemental oxygen was administered by nasal cannula. The patients were prepared using 1 mg lorazepame per os the night before the procedure. Pethidine or other sedatives were not used. Premedication included a nasal topical anaesthesia with lidocaine gel (2%), a topical anaesthesia with lidocaine (2%, 20 cc) in the form of a spray from a hand atomiser, and an atropine (0.3 mg) intramuscular injection 30 min before the procedure. The patients were in the lying supine position facing the operator during the procedure. The bronchoscopist remained in close contact with the patient and carefully explained the procedure a step at a time as it happened.

Results

None of the patients experienced any particular anxiety or tachycardia. Almost all of them gave their full and relaxed cooperation, and the procedures were performed without problems. In three patients the procedure had to be stopped due to dyspnea, in three others due to edema of the larynx, and in four due to refusal to undergo the examination.

Discussion

We concluded that bronchoscopy without sedatives during premedication, with the operator remaining in close contact with the patient throughout the procedure, is perfectly acceptable and is without side effects. A successful procedure using this method requires the relaxed cooperation of the patient in order to eliminate fear, pain and anxiety. This is possible through a simple but detailed discussion with every patient. Using this method we are able to dispense with sedatives. Topical anaesthesia alone is almost always adequate [3].

References

1. Colt HG, Morris JF. Fiberoptic bronchoscopy without premedication. A retrospective study. Chest 1990;98(6):1327–1330.
2. Bates M. Fiberoptic bronchoscopy. Thorax 1980;35:640.
3. Pearce SJ. Fiberoptic bronchoscopy: is sedation necessary? Br Med J 1980;281:779–780.

Bronchology and Bronchoesophagology: State of the Art.
H. Yoshimura et al., editors.

Interventional bronchoscopy in the Czech Republic in 1999

Irena Spasova[1], Pavel Barton[2], Vitezslav Kolek[3], Miloslav Marel[4] and Frantisek Bruha[5]

[1]Department of Pulmonary Medicine, University Hospital, Hradec Kralove; [2]Medical Institute Jevicko; [3]Department of Pulmonary Medicine, University Hospital, Olomouc; [4]Department of Pulmonary Medicine, University Hospital Motol, Prague; and [5]Department of Pulmonary Medicine, University Hospital, Plzen, Czech Republic

Abstract. *Background.* In the Czech Republic, bronchoscopy is widely carried out by pulmonologists, otolaryngologists, anesthesiologists and some thoracic surgeons and pediatricians. However, interventional bronchoscopy is performed in several specialized medical centers and is carried out by pulmonologists only. The purpose of our study was to investigate the present status of the interventional bronchoscopy in the adult pulmonological departments in the Czech Republic.

Methods. A mail survey, distributed among pulmonologists in the Czech Republic, has been conducted each year since 1994. The last one was completed in January, 2000. Sixty-six (98%) out of 69 bronchological departments responded. Data from the remaining three departments were obtained by phone.

Results. In the Czech Republic (10 million inhabitants), 69 bronchological departments performed 27,000 bronchoscopic procedures in 1999 (270 bronchoscopies/100,000 Czechs). Thirteen departments performed 847 interventional bronchoscopies. Eight departments performed lasertherapy (201 patients/442 sessions), seven departments carried out intrabronchial brachytherapy (153 patients/328 applications), three departments applied cryotherapy (eight patients/19 procedures), one department used electrocautery (12 patients/13 sessions) and four departments introduced tracheobronchial stents (41 patients/45 stents).

Conclusions. As compared with the Dutch population, the bronchoscopic activity in the Czech Republic was almost three-fold higher. On the other hand, the number of bronchoscopies performed in the Czech Republic has persisted at a constant level between 1994 and 1999. Interventional bronchoscopy created only a small part of routine bronchoscopy (3%). Data indicate a trend in the development of routine vs. specialized interventional bronchoscopists. The need for optimal training in all aspects of bronchoscopy, including rigid instruments and the cost of the technology, are the main reasons for the centralization of interventional bronchoscopy over several large medical institutions.

Keywords: intrabronchial, survey.

Introduction

In the Czech Republic, bronchoscopy is widely carried out by pulmonologists, otolaryngologists, anesthesiologists and some thoracic surgeons and pediatricians. However, interventional bronchoscopy is performed in several specialized

Address for correspondence: MU Dr Irena Spasova CSc, Department of Pulmonary Medicine, University Hospital, Pospisilova 365, 500 05 Hradec Kralove, Czech Republic. Tel.: +420-49-583-6341. Fax: +420-49-583-6226. E-mail: spasova@fnhk.cz centers in the University Hospitals or Medical Institutes and is carried out by pulmonologists only. The purpose of our study was to investigate the present status of the interventional bronchoscopy in the adult pulmonological departments in the Czech Republic.

Methods and Patients

A mail survey, distributed among the pulmonologists in the Czech Republic, has been conducted each year since 1994 [1]. The last one was completed in January, 2000. Sixty-six (98%) out of 69 bronchological departments responded. Data from the remaining three departments were obtained by phone. The questionnaire contained 21 questions regarding bronchoscopic equipment and figures of bronchoscopic procedures in 1999.

Results

In the Czech Republic (10 million inhabitants), 69 bronchological departments performed 27,000 bronchoscopic procedures in 1999 (270 bronchoscopies/ 100,000 Czech). Thirteen departments performed 847 interventional bronchoscopy procedures. Eight departments performed lasertherapy, seven departments carried out intrabronchial brachytherapy, three departments applied cryotherapy, one department used electrocautery and four departments introduced tracheobronchial stents. Two departments were equipped with a autofluorescence device and started examining the pre- and early-malignant changes of the bronchial mucosa.

201 patients (167 patients with malign and 34 patients with benign lesions) were treated with a Nd-YAG laser over 442 sessions. Seventy-nine percent of them were performed under local anesthesia, and 21% of them under general anesthesia. In 153 patients, endobronchial brachytherapy was carried out over 328 applications, in all cases, because of malignancy. Most of the brachytherapies (98%) were applied under local anesthesia. Eight patients underwent endobronchial cryosurgery because of malign endobronchial lesions. Nineteen cryosurgical sessions were carried out, in 89% of cases under general anesthesia. Thirteen electrocautery procedures were performed on 12 patients, five of them because of benign lesions and seven because of malign lesions. All of these procedures were carried out under general anesthesia. Forty-five stents were inserted into 41 patients, in 21 patients because of benign lesions and in 20 patients because of malign lesions. All of the stents were introduced under general anesthesia.

Discussion

Sutedja referred to 15,000 bronchoscopic procedures performed in the Netherlands in 1994 (94 bronchoscopies/100,000 Dutch) [2]. Compared to these figures, the bronchoscopic activity in the Czech Republic was almost three-fold higher. On the other hand, the number of bronchoscopies performed in the Czech Republic persisted at a constant level between 1994 and 1999 [1].

Interventional bronchoscopy created only a small part of the routine bronchoscopy (3%). Data indicate a trend in the development of routine vs. specialized interventional bronchoscopists in the Czech republic. The need for optimal training in all aspects of bronchoscopy, including rigid instruments and the cost of the technology, are the main reasons for the concentration of interventional bronchoscopy over several large medical institutions.

References

1. Marel M, Kolek V, Salajka F, Spasova I, Bruha F. Bronchology in Czech Republic. Abstract of the 9th World Congress for Bronchology, Taipei (Taiwan), 1996, 107.
2. Sutedja G, Festen J, Vandenschueren R, Janssen J, Postmus PE and the Endoscopic Committee of the Dutch Association of Pulmonologists. The pulmonologist practices in the Netherlands. Results of a questionnaire. Eur Respir J 1995;8(Suppl 19):306.

Bronchology and Bronchoesophagology: State of the Art.
H. Yoshimura et al., editors.

Diagnostic bronchoscopy for early detection of lung cancer with positive sputum cytology

Hiroko Tsukada, Toshimitsu Shimbo, Masato Makino, Akira Yokoyama and Yuzo Kurita
Department of Internal Medicine, Niigata Cancer Center Hospital, Niigata, Japan

Abstract. In the Niigata, Prefecture Japan, high risk participants with a smoking index of 600 or higher have been screened by sputum cytology as well as chest X-ray. From 1988 to 1999, 201,131 examinations were performed. Sputum samples were diagnosed as sputum D (markedly or borderline atypical squamous cells or suspicious cells) in 402 cases (0.20%), and sputum E (malignant cells) in 239 cases (0.12%). Of these, 314 primary lung cancers were detected. Of the 197 lung cancer cases diagnosed at our hospital, 137 tumors were centrally located, 157 were squamous cell carcinoma, and 114 were roentgenographically occult. Of these 114 roentgenographically occult cases, 18 exhibited no abnormal findings at the initial bronchoscopy, and 11 out of these 18 were found to have tumors localized beyond the range of view. Those cases which were located distal to segmental bronchi, with only minute findings and less than 10 mm in diameter, were difficult to localize. The bronchoscopic findings of early-stage lesions included thickening and paleness of the surface of bifurcation, and fine granular change of mucosal surface. When lesions are difficult to localize, serial selective brushing and autofluorescence bronchoscopy are useful. Finally, careful follow-up is necessary for cases in which localization has not yet been confirmed.

Keywords: autofluorescence bronchoscopy, localization, mass screening, roentgenographically occult lung cancer, selective brushing.

Background

In the Niigata Prefecture, Japan, in population-based lung cancer screening, high risk participants with a smoking index of 600 or higher have been screened by sputum cytology in addition to chest X-ray. From 1988 to 1999, 201,131 examinations were performed. Sputum samples were diagnosed as having sputum D (sputum specimen that has markedly or borderline atypical cells or suspicious cells) in 402 cases, and as having sputum E (sputum specimen containing malignant cells) in 239 cases. Participants diagnosed with sputum D or E were advised to undergo detailed examination at a hospital. Of these, 314 cases of primary lung cancer and 51 of upper respiratory tract cancer were detected on further examination.

In this article, we examine the process of diagnosis in 197 lung cancer cases with positive sputum cytology diagnosed at our hospital, and also discuss the use-

Address for correspondence: Hiroko Tsukada MD, Department of Internal Medicine, Niigata Cancer Center Hospital, 2-15-3 Kawagishi-cho, Niigata 951-8566, Japan. Tel.: +81-25-266-5111. Fax: +81-25-233-3849. E-mail: htsukada@niigata-cc.niigata.niigata.jp fulness of systematic diagnostic bronchoscopy combining careful observation, autofluorescence bronchoscopy, and serial selective washing and/or brushing.

Patients and Methods

From 1988 to 1999, 197 lung cancer patients with positive sputum cytology were diagnosed at our hospital. All patients were male, with a median age of 69. Ninety-seven patients were diagnosed as having sputum D, and 100 patients as having sputum E. In 137 cases tumors were centrally located, 155 were at clinical stage I, and 157 (80% of all cases) were squamous cell carcinoma. Furthermore, multiple primary lung cancer was found in 20 patients.

At our hospital, patients with sputum D or E are examined by chest roentgenography and bronchoscopy on the first visit. If there are no abnormal findings on chest X-ray and initial bronchoscopy, computed tomography (CT) is then performed. If the lesions are difficult to localize, inspection with autofluorescence bronchoscopy or serial selective washing and brushing is carried out. In cases where localization is not yet confirmed, these patients are carefully followed for at least 2 more years.

Results

Of 197 lung cancer cases diagnosed at our hospital, 114 were found to be of roentgenographically occult type. Of these, 18 exhibited no abnormal findings at initial bronchoscopy, and of these 18 cases with negative bronchoscopic findings, 11 were found to have tumors located beyond the range of view.

Most of the bronchoscopic findings of early-stage lesions that remained within the bronchial wall were minute, these included thickening and paleness of the surface of bifurcation, fine granular change of the mucosal surface, or disappearance of luster.

In the 114 cases of roentgenographically occult cancer, 81 were localized by initial bronchoscopy. In patients with no bronchoscopic abnormalities, more than two bronchoscopic examinations were performed. There was a maximum of nine bronchoscopic examinations carried out in any one patient.

Within the range of bronchoscopic view, all cases but one (which was difficult to localize), were seen to be squamous cell carcinoma. The majority of the lesions in these cases were located in the region distal to the segmental bronchi, and were less than 10 mm in diameter. In addition, nine out of the 11 cases had minute findings, which were difficult to identify as tumors, and were less than 2 mm in height, i.e., of superficial type.

We present examples of cases in which tumors were localized using selective washing and brushing.

First, in 1988 a 72-year-old man was suspected to have squamous cell carcinoma based on sputum cytology results. Roentgenographically, there were no abnormal shadows present, and there were also no positive findings obtained at the first bronchoscopic examination. However, cancer cells were detected in a washing specimen from the right lower lobe. Bronchoscopy was then repeated in order to localize the tumor. At the seventh bronchoscopic examination, the presence of cancer cell clusters indicated that a tumor was present but beyond the range of view of a right B9b. Despite the lack of abnormal findings on bronchoscopy, the right lower lobe was resected in 1990, and histologic examination revealed a 7 mm carcinoma in situ in right B9b.

The second patient was diagnosed in 1997 as having adenocarcinoma based on sputum cytology results. No positive findings were obtained either roentgenographically or at the first bronchoscopic examination. However, cancer cells were then detected in a washing specimen from the left upper lobe, and bronchoscopy was subsequently repeated to localize the tumor. At the fourth bronchoscopic examination, the presence of cancer cell clusters led us to the conclusion that a tumor was present but beyond the range of view of left B3c. Despite the lack of abnormal findings on bronchoscopy, the left upper lobe was resected in 1997, and histologic examination revealed a 12 mm adenocarcinoma of bronchial gland origin.

We now present a case of peripheral type adenocarcinoma localized after a 12 months follow-up evaluation. Based on sputum cytology, a 72-year-old man was suspected to have adenocarcinoma. With initial examination we were unable to detect a tumor. On a chest CT 12 months later an abnormal shadow was noted adjacent to a thoracic vertebra. The right lower lobe was resected in June 1996, and histologic examination revealed a stage I adenocarcinoma.

In cases with only subtle mucosal changes, autofluorescence bronchoscopy is useful. In these cases, even if only a minor mucosal abnormality was found on white light bronchoscopy, the tumor site was identified with the LIFE-system as a well demarcated dark area.

Of 114 patients with roentgenographically occult lung cancer, surgical cure was attempted in 58 of them (51%). The 5-year survival rate, taking into account deaths from all causes, was 73.8%.

Additionally, 55 patients underwent endobronchial brachytherapy with curative intent. Their overall 5-year survival rate was 77%, a result competitive with that obtained with surgery. Our diagnostic approach to early detection is thus seen to have been successful.

Conclusions

In summary, sputum cytology positive, X-ray negative carcinoma may yield only minute abnormal findings or may lie beyond the visibility of a flexible bronchoscope. Therefore, in cases where it is difficult to localize lung cancer, serial selective brushing, autofluorescence bronchoscopy, and careful follow-up should be carried out.

Bronchology and Bronchoesophagology: State of the Art.
H. Yoshimura et al., editors.

Insertion of a gastric tube using a fibrobronchoscope on critical patients

Gui-Qian Wang, Ming Juan Xie, Feng Chi and Ying He
Guangzhou Institute of Respiratory Diseases, Guangzhou, China

Abstract. *Background.* For many critically ill patients, the routine method of gastric tube insertion, through the nose, is unsuccessful. Therefore, the authors created a new method of gastric tube insertion, involving the use of a fibrobronchoscope (BF). From October 1986 to October 1999, 106 patients underwent this new method with a complete success rate. There were 62 males and 44 females. The ages ranged from 13 to 78 years. All patients were critically ill, and the conditions we encountered included severe burns, drug intoxication, the late stages of pulmonary and nasopharyngeal cancers, COPD, ARDS, etc.

Methods. 1) A BF (Olympus BF 4B2, P10, P20,P40 or Pentax FB 15p) was inserted through the nostril under topical anesthesia. The bronchoscope was inserted into the lower esophagus via one side of the piriform recess behind the trachea. 2) The metallic guide was inserted through the biopsy opening of the BF and pushed to the stomach through it. The BF was then removed, while the guide remained inside the esophagus. The siliconized gastric tube was slipped over the metallic guide and pushed into the stomach. Then the guide was removed and the gastric tube was fixed beside the nose.

Results. With the help of the BF, under direct vision, the insertion of nasal gastric tubes became easy manoeuvre and the 106 cases it was tried on had a successful outcome. No complications or side effects occurred.

Conclusions. Using the routine method for the insertion of gastric tubes and tracheal intubation in critical patients, especially comatose, is quite difficult. With the help of a BF, 106 patients successfully underwent this procedure. It is a safe and easy manoeuvre, and extending the use of this method would be worthwhile.

Keywords: fibrobronchoscope, gastric tube, insertion.

Introduction

In clinical practice, physicians have often been unable to insert gastric tubes in critical, especially comatose, patients. In general, this situation has led surgeons to perform gastrostomy for nutritional purposes. For this very reason, the authors created a new method of gastric tube insertion, involving the use of a fibrobronchoscope (BF), thus avoiding gastrostomy. From October 1986 to October 1999, 106 patients successfully underwent gastric tube insertion using this method.

Address for correspondence: Gui-Qian Wang, Guangzhou Institute of Respiratory Diseases, 151 Yan Jiang Road, Guangzhou 510120, China. Tel.: +86-20-83341017. Fax: +86-20-83350363.

Materials

Of the 106 patients, 62 were male and 44 female. Age ranged from 13 to 78 years. Most of the patients were critically ill in medical wards or ICU. The conditions we encountered included big area burns, drug intoxication, COPD, lung cancer, nasopharyngeal cancer, etc. (Table 1).

Instruments

The following instruments were selected: 1) a small-sized adult FB (i.e., Olympus BF 4B2, types P10, P20, P40 or Pentax FB 15p); 2) a metallic guide with a semi-oval or string tip (length: 150 cm, diameter: <2 mm); and 3) a siliconized gastric tube. A small amount of liquid paraffin was also used.

Procedures

1. Atropine (0.5 mg, H) was injected 15 min before the procedure (with the exception of glaucoma cases). Next, 2% lidocaine was sprayed on the pharynx and trachea, 3 times, at 5 min intervals. Then, 0.5 to 2% ephedrine was dropped into the nostril and finally 2% lidocaine was sprayed into the nostril.
2. A BF (size already stated) was then pushed through the nostril to either side of the piriform recess. This was selected as the landmark for the BF to enter the esophageal opening. Under direct vision, the BF was pushed to the lower end of esophagus.
3. The metallic guide was then inserted through the biopsy opening of the BF and pushed to the distal end of it. The BF was withdrawn and the metallic guide remained inside the esophagus.
4. The wall of the distal end of the gastric tube was then swabbed with liquid paraffin. The gastric tube was slipped over the metallic guide and pushed into the stomach. The metallic guide was withdrawn, and finally, the gastric tube was fixed beside the nose.

Table 1. The conditions of the 106 patients who underwent the new method.

Condition	No. of patients
Severe burns	2
ARDS	1
Nasopharyngeal cancer	3
Drug intoxication	1
Lung cancer	11
COPD	88

Results

With the help of the BF, the insertion of a gastric tube was successful in 106 critical patients. No complications nor side effects occurred.

Case Reports

Case 1

A 40-year-old male with, chiefly, 2nd and 3rd degree burns covering 95% of his body surface. The gastric tube was inserted on admission, but unfortunately it came off 1 month after insertion. Another gastric tube insertion using the traditional method was attempted, but failed. Using the new method, the tube was inserted with ease.

Case 2

A 69-year-old male, with a lung infection and ARDS after severe trauma. Complications with profuse hemorrhages of the upper digestive tract occurred. After using artificial respiration and a wide spectrum of antibiotics, the symptoms improved. He was poorly nourished and required gastric tube feeding, but the gastric tube could not be inserted using the traditional method. However, using the new method the insertion of gastric tube was performed without difficulty.

Discussion

1. Many critically ill patients need a nasal gastric tube for nutrition and decompression. For such kinds of patients, this was not an easy job. Formerly, when doctors were unable to insert the gastric tube using the routine manoeuvre, gastrostomy was often adopted as an alternative. In some patients, due to the nature of their condition, gastrostomy could actually become technically difficult. Thus, a new way to insert the gastric tube was in urgent need.
2. It should be emphasized that the new method of gastric tube insertion cannot be used in cases of severe obstruction in the upper esophagus, e.g., esophageal malignancy or benign stricture.
3. If there was any inflammation of the pharynx or piriform sinus, causing esophageal obstruction, this method could only be used after the control of the infection.
4. If there was any cirrhosis of the liver with venous varicosity of the esophagus or other causes of hemorrhages of upper digestive tract, this procedure would have to be done with special caution and would better be continued when active bleeding had stopped.
5. The success of our method means that gastrostomy, carried out for nutritional purposes, is now seldom performed on our patients. We need not worry if

the traditional method of nasal gastric tube insertion fails, because we now have an efficient alternative at our disposal.

Reference

1. Wang G-Q. Gastric tube placement with the insistence of a fibrobronchoscope in critical ICU patient. The 1st International Chinese Congress of Chest Diseases, 1990;353.

©2001 Published by Elsevier Science B.V.
Bronchology and Bronchoesophagology: State of the Art.
H. Yoshimura et al., editors.

Laryngeal nerve blockade for bronchoscopy

Mauro Zamboni, Emanuel Torquato, Walter Roriz, Paulo de Biasi and Edson Toscano
Thoracic Surgery Department, Cancer National Institute/Health Ministry, Rio de Janeiro, Brazil

Introduction

Anesthesia or sedation before bronchoscopy is necessary for facilitating the examination and cooperation of patients, minimizing physiologic responses to irritation of the respiratory tract, and offering safety and comfort during performance of these procedures. Several forms of anesthesia may be used when examining the respiratory airways with rigid or flexible bronchoscopes. We report on our experiences using bilateral superior laryngeal nerve blockade (BSLNB), associated with topical tracheal anesthesia by transcricothyroid membrane puncture.

Materials and Methods

Over a period of 2 consecutive years a prospective study was conducted in 163 adult patients (120 men and 42 women; age range 16 to 83 years; median age of 63.5 years) who underwent bronchoscopy with BSLNB and topical anesthesia by transcricothyroid membrane puncture. These patients were not premedicated and were examined for diagnostic or follow-up purposes.

BSLNB was performed in all patients regardless of the pulmonary disease shown at consultation, purpose of procedure, or type of apparatus. 128 bronchoscopic examinations were performed with a flexible Pentax FB 18X bronchoscope (Pentax Corp., NY), and 28 were performed with a rigid Wolf 400 × 7 bronchoscope (Richard Wolf GMBH, Knittlingen, Germany). The remaining seven patients underwent both rigid and flexible bronchoscopy simultaneously. None of these patients were sedated or subjected to general anesthesia.

Examinations were performed using a modification of the original technique for laryngeal nerve blockade. Patients placed in dorsal decubitus were monitored by pulse oximetry, with oxygen supply offered to those complaining of dyspnea or whenever hypoxemia was evident by oximetry. Following these procedures, the neck was hyperextended to allow a better exposure of anatomical structures.

Address for correspondence: M. Zamboni, Thoracic Surgery Department, Instituto Nacional de Cancer, Rua Sorocaba 464/302, CEP: 22271-110 Rio de Janeiro, Brazil. Tel.: +55-21-537-7638. Fax: +55-21-537-5562.

Ten milliliters of 1% lidocaine (100 mg) was injected with a 13 × 4 mm needle at three application points. The superior horn of the thyroid cartilage was palpated, the carotid vascular-nervous bundle was displaced posteriorly, and the neck was punctured to reach the bundle. After aspiration to ensure that the external carotid artery had not been punctured, 2 mL (20 mg) of anesthetic was introduced in a fanlike distribution; this procedure was also performed contralaterally for completing a bilateral blockade of the superior laryngeal nerve. Topical tracheal anesthesia was achieved by transcricothyroid membrane puncture with 6 mL (60 mg) of anesthetic without using intravenous sedative or oral sedatives before anesthesia. In patients undergoing flexible bronchoscopy, the apparatus was introduced through a nostril, previously anesthetized with 3 to 5 mL of 2% lidocaine gel (60 to 100 mg). Patients having rigid bronchoscopy received four or five applications of a 10% lidocaine spray (40 to 50 mg) at the base of the tongue to suppress the gag reflex, with a maximum dosage of 300 mg of lidocaine.

Results were obtained after separate assessments by the patient and the examiner on the same scale of 0 to 10. Patients' and examiners' assessments were obtained immediately after bronchoscopy by the same endoscopist using the following grades: poor (0 to 3), tolerable (4 to 6), good (6 to 8), and very good (9 to 10), according to the patient's tolerance, cooperation, and degree of comfort and easiness observed by the endoscopist. Results of evaluations of patients and endoscopists were analyzed using a χ test.

Results

Patients were evaluated according to the Karnofsky performance status (PS) scale, on a range from 40 to 100%. In all patients completion of the examination was possible. Laryngeal nerve blockade was not contraindicated, even in patients with cervical alterations, e.g., enlarged thyroid gland or superior vena cava syndrome. In two flexible bronchoscopies (1.2% of 163 patients), a supplemental 10% lidocaine spray in the oropharynx was required. The time elapsed from the administration of anesthesia to the initiation of bronchoscopy varied from 0 to 8 min, with a median of 3 min.

Samples of bronchial washings were collected from almost all patients (150), whereas bronchoalveolar washings were obtained from 13 patients with or without transbronchial biopsy. Regarding patients' evaluations, procedures were considered poor in 3/163 (2%), tolerable in 18/163 (11%), good in 123/163 (76%), and very good in 18/163 (11%). In the examiners' evaluations, procedures were considered poor in 4/163 (2.5%), tolerable in 12/163 (7%), good in 31/163 (19%), and very good in 115/163 (70.5%). The patients' and endoscopists' evaluations were found to be significantly different for the "good" and "very good" categories ($p < 0.001$).

Transitory complications like tracheal bleeding (less than 1 mL in 5/163, 3% of patients) and local hematoma (2/163, 1.2% of patients) did not affect the course of the examination. Some patients suffered from dysphagia (54/163, 33%), whereas others had hoarseness (8/163, 5%) that disappeared after the effect of anesthesia wore off.

Discussion

For several years, topical or general anesthesia has been used in bronchoscopic examinations. An optimum local anesthetic procedure would be one requiring a low dose with safe and tolerable effects both for patients and bronchoscopists. Topical anesthesia through the mouth and oropharynx has been found to be uncomfortable for the patient who must maintain an open mouth and a protruding tongue, causing frequent gagging and coughing and therefore resulting in a more time-consuming anesthetic procedure (15 to 20 min).

A comparison between cricothyroid puncture and topical anesthesia through the bronchocoscope showed that cricothyroid puncture was not associated with complications or with discomfort to patients. Following this study, BSLNB and transcricothyroid puncture was adopted in our institution as the main anesthetic procedure for bronchoscopy in more than 3,000 examinations performed during the past 5-year period.

The patients who were studied were anesthetized with a lidocaine solution, gel and/or spray, without associated premedication, for the purpose of evaluating anesthetic procedures. The issue of sedation for bronchoscopy, particularly flexible bronchoscopy, is a controversial one. Patient anxiety and lack of cooperation, however, make premedication necessary, using drugs like benzodiazepines or with narcotics and atropine to reduce bronchial and oropharyngeal secretions.

Adequate anesthesia is crucial for a successful examination of the respiratory airway. Lidocaine, in several presentations and concentrations, is most frequently used for the upper respiratory tract because of its fast, efficient action and rapid absorption: its half-life in plasma ranges from 30 to 180 min according to its clinical usage. Dosage should not surpass necessary requirements and must not exceed 300 mg, thereby avoiding toxicity and other potential effects like modifying alveolar cell counts and inhibiting bacterial growth. Recent studies have demonstrated that even small amounts of lidocaine, when administered into the respiratory tract, may inhibit bacterial growth and, consequently, affect microbiologic analysis of collected samples.

In the original technique, the superior laryngeal nerve was blocked at the thyrohyoid membrane, but this procedure is complex and prone to failure and complications in inexperienced hands. However, the modification used in our institution makes the procedure safer and easier, even for beginners training in respiratory endoscopy. In a prospective study by Lukomsky et al. of 4,595 bronchoscopic procedures (1,146 using a flexible bronchoscope and topical anesthesia; 3,449 using a rigid bronchoscope and general intravenous anesthesia), complications occurred in 5.1% of the procedures, of which 1.1% were classed as major complications and 4% as minor. A comparison of rigid bronchoscopy and flexible bronchoscopy complications showed significantly higher rates in flexible bronchoscopy complications attributable to the toxic effects of tetracaine, and rigid bronchoscopy complications associated with inadequate general anesthesia. In our experience, complications, when present, resulted from puncturing and infiltration of anesthetic. These were minimized by using thin (13 × 4 mm) needles for laryngeal nerve blockade and puncturing of the transcricothyroid membrane, and by the small amount of anesthetic required for effective anesthesia. Dysphagia, being frequent, transitory, and generally indicative of complete blockade, was found to recede when the anesthetic effects had ceased.

Conclusion

A modified BSLNB procedure has been found to be safely and easily executed. BSLNB associated with tracheal and bronchial anesthesia by transcricothyroid membrane puncture, resulted in excellent conditions for successful and rapid examinations under comfortable conditions for patients and with minimal complications. This procedure has been successfully used in most of our routine examinations.

Bronchology and Bronchoesophagology: State of the Art.
H. Yoshimura et al., editors.

Bronchoscopy yields in the diagnosis of pancoast tumors

Mauro Zamboni, Débora C. Lannes, Walter Roriz, Emanuel Torquato and Edson Toscano
Department of Thoracic Surgery, National Cancer Institute, Health Ministry, Rio de Janeiro, Brazil

Background

We performed this study over a period from 1986 to 1994. The number of patients involved was 50. Ages ranged from 28- to 90-years-old (median = 55.5).

Sex (Fig. 1)

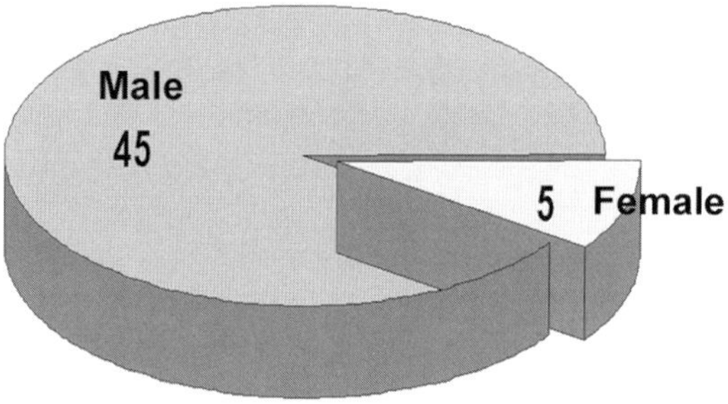

Fig. 1.

Smoking (Fig. 2)

Staging (Fig. 3)

Number of bronchoscopies (n = 23); positive bronchoscopies (n = 5) (Fig. 4)

Address for correspondence: M. Zamboni, Thoracic Surgery Department, Instituto Nacional de Cancer, Rua Sorocaba 464/302, CEP: 22271-110 Rio de Janeiro, Brazil. Tel.: +55-21-537-7638. Fax: +55-21-537-5562.

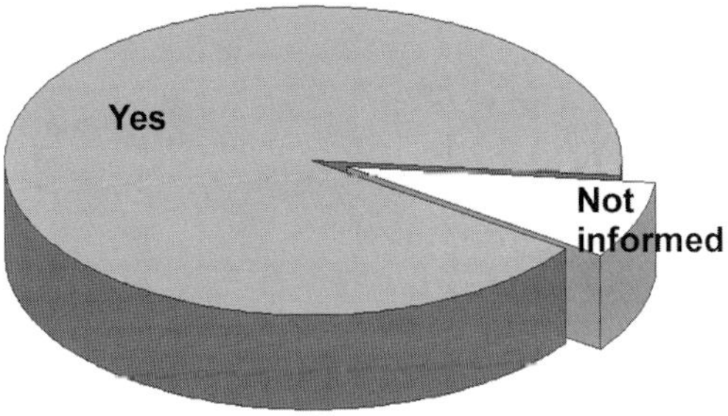

Fig. 2.

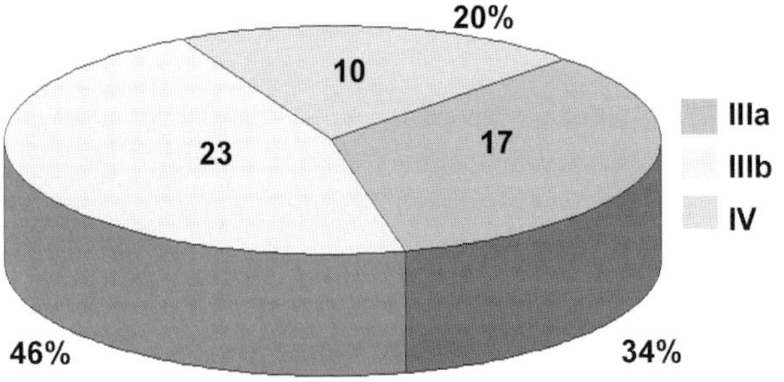

Fig. 3.

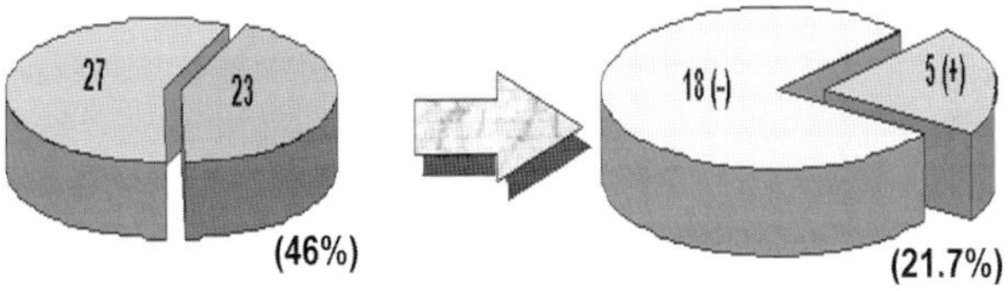

Fig. 4.

Diagnosis (n = 50) (Fig. 5)

Other diagnosis methods (negative bronchoscopies, n = 18) (Fig. 6)

All the patients who underwent bronchoscopy had a pulmonary mass, shown on the chest X-ray they were earlier submitted to.

Bronchoscopy type (Fig. 7)

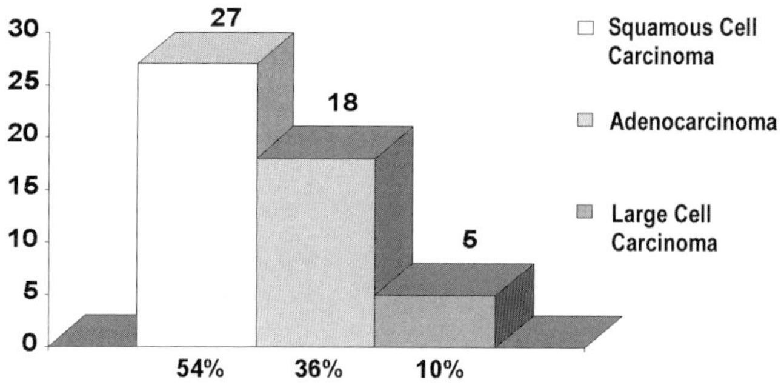

Fig. 5.

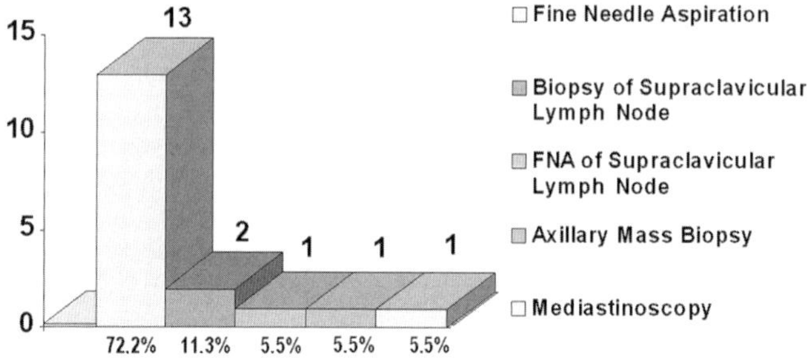

Fig. 6.

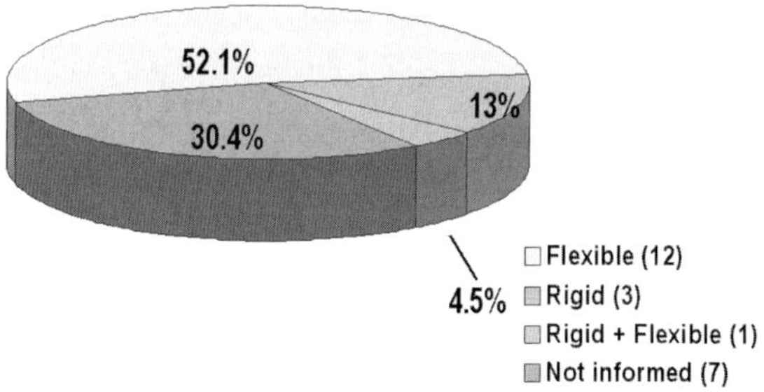

Fig. 7.

Bronchoscopy results (Fig. 8)

Endoscopic findings (abnormal bronchoscopy, n = 5)

Three extrinsic compressions;
One infiltrating lesion;
One vegetating lesion.

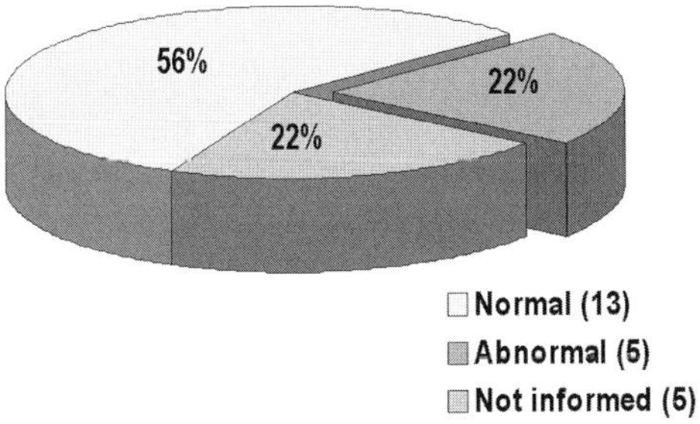

Fig. 8.

Positive endoscopic proceedings

Three bronchial brushing:
- three adenocarcinomas.

Two bronchial lavage:
- one squamous cell carcinoma;
- one adenocarcinoma.

One bronchial biopsy:
- one squamous cell carcinoma.

Conclusion

Bronchoscopy is not a good diagnostic method to use with regard to patients with pancoast tumors because its yield is very low and restricted in patients with endoscopic abnormalities. Of the 23 examinations carried out, only 5 (21%) furnished a positive diagnosis.

Reference

1. Pralash UBS. Advances in bronchoscopic procedures. Chest 1999;116(5):1403–1408.

Bronchology and Bronchoesophagology: State of the Art.
H. Yoshimura et al., editors.

Bronchoscopy yields in the diagnosis of superior vena cava syndrome

Mauro Zamboni, Débora C. Lannes, Walter Roriz, Paulo de Biasi and Edson Toscano

Department of Thoracic Surgery, National Cancer Institute, Health Ministry, Rio de Janeiro, Brazil

Background

This study was conducted over a period from 1986 to 1996. The number of patients involved was 50. Age ranged from 41- to 77-years-old (median = 54.5).

Sex (Fig. 1)

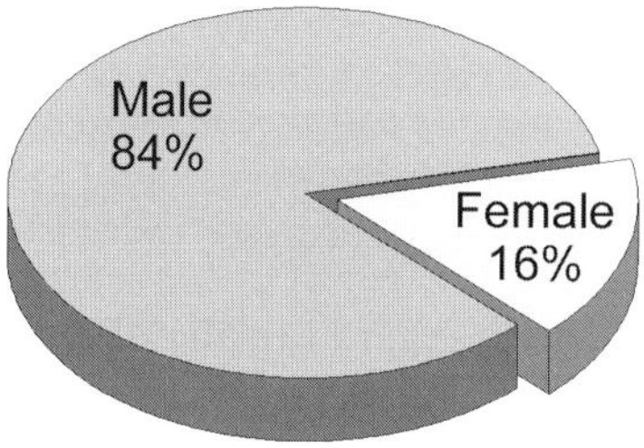

Fig. 1.

Smoking (Fig. 2)

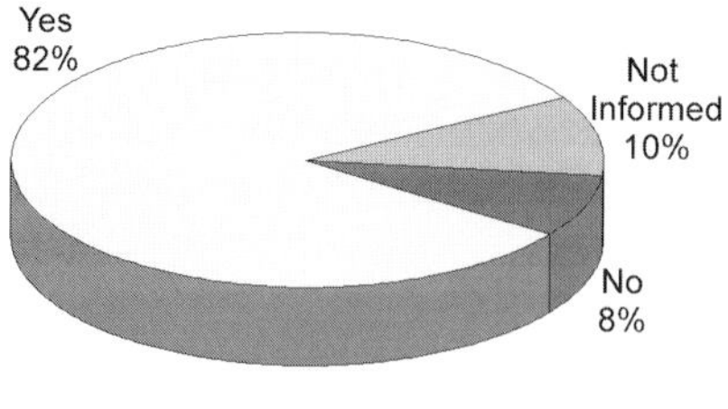

Fig. 2.

Address for correspondence: M. Zamboni, Thoracic Surgery Department, Instituto Nacional de Cancer, Rua Sorocaba 464/302, CEP: 22271-110 Rio de Janeiro, Brazil. Tel.: +55-21-537-7638. Fax: +55-21-537-5562.

Staging (Fig. 3)

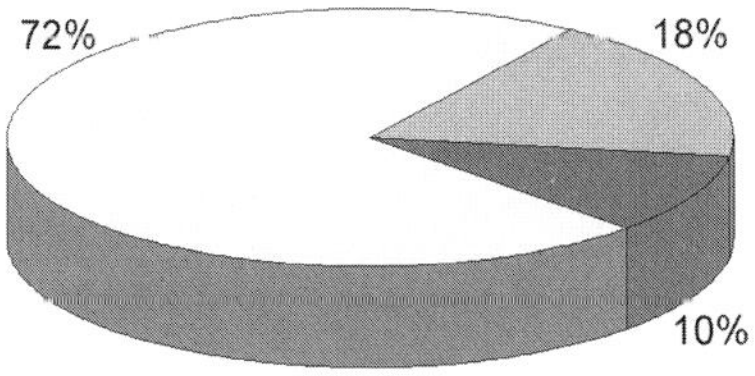

Fig. 3. IIIb: n = 36 (72%), IV: n = 9 (18%), not informed: n = 5 (10%).

Bronchoscopies done (n = 33); positive bronchoscopies (n = 20) (Fig. 4)

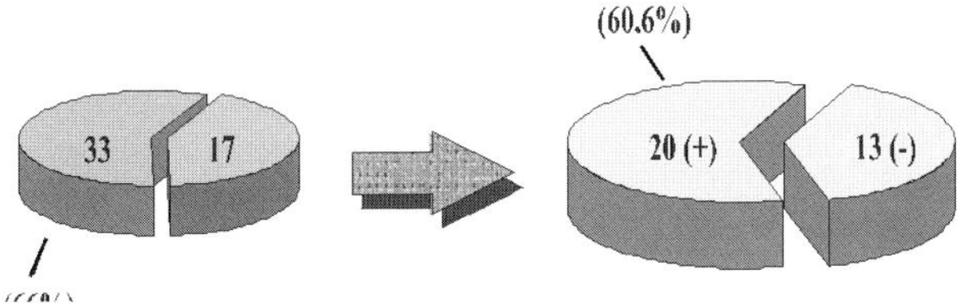

Fig. 4.

Diagnosis (n = 50) (Fig. 5)

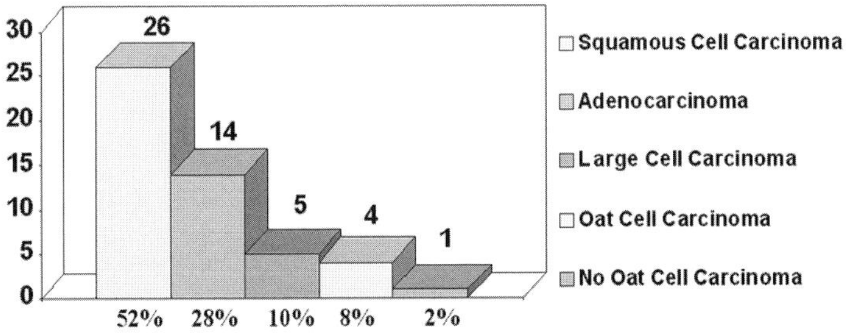

Fig. 5.

Other diagnosis methods (negative bronchoscopies, n = 13) (Fig. 6)

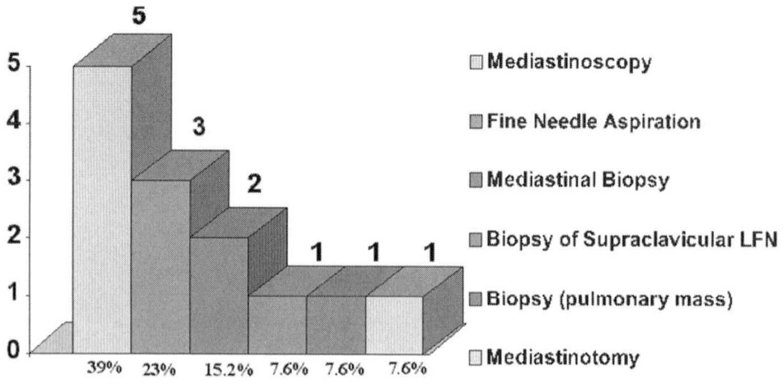

Fig. 6.

Rx images (n = 33)

Pulmonary mass: 22 (66.7%);
Atelectasis: 5 (15.1%);
Mediastinal enlargement: 4 (12.2%);
Pulmonary nodule: 1 (3%);
Not informed: 1 (3%).

Broncoscopy (Fig. 7)

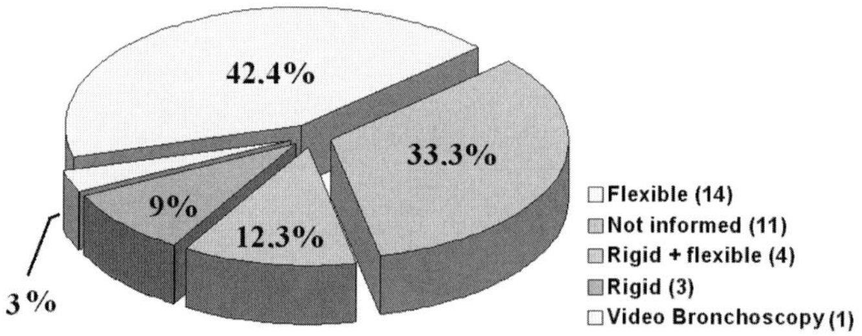

Fig. 7.

Results (Fig. 8)

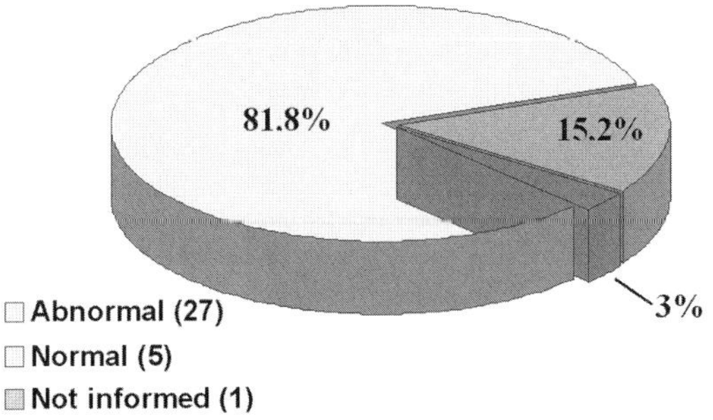

Fig. 8.

Endoscopic alterations (abnormal bronchoscopy, n = 27)

Vegetating lesions: 8
Extrinsic compressions: 7
Infiltrating lesions: 3
Infiltrating lesions + extrinsic compression: 3
Vegetating lesion + extrinsic compression: 2
Vegetating lesion + infiltrating lesion + extrinsic compression: 2
Vegetating lesion + infiltrating lesion: 1
Not informed: 1.

Negative endoscopic alterations (n = 7)

Extrinsic compression: 3 (42.8%)
Infiltrative lesion + extrinsic compression: 2 (28.8%)
Infiltrative lesion + vegetating lesion: 1 (14.2%)
Vegetating lesion: 1 (14.2%).

Positive endoscopic procedures

Fifteen bronchial biopsy:
- eleven squamous cell carcinoma
- two adenocarcinomas
- one large cell carcinoma
- one oat cell carcinoma.

Ten bronchial lavage:
- five squamous cell carcinoma
- four adenocarcinomas
- one oat cell carcinoma.

Six bronchial brushing:
- four squamous cell carcinoma
- one adenocarcinoma
- one oat cell carcinoma.

Conclusion

We conclude that, as our experiment using bronchoscopy produced a yield of 60.6% (20/33) in patients with superior vena cava syndrome, this procedure should be a part of the diagnostic investigation for patients with this syndrome.

References

1. Markman M. Diagnosis and management of superior vena cava syndrome. Cleve Clin J Med 1999;66(1):59–61.
2. Dempke W, Behermannn C, Schuber C et al. Diagnostic and therapeutic management of the superior vena cava syndrome. Med Klin 1999;94(12):681–684.
3. Laguna Del Estal P, Gazapo Navarro T, Murillas Angoitti J et al. Superior vena cava syndrome: a study based on 81 cases. An Med Interna 1998;15(9):470–475.

Central type early stage lung cancer

Bronchology and Bronchoesophagology: State of the Art.
H. Yoshimura et al., editors.

Fluorescence bronchoscopy in the early detection of premalignant and malignant lesions

Kinya Furukawa, Masatoshi Kakihana, Norihiko Ikeda, Tetsuya Okunaka, Hideaki Shimatani, Norihiko Kawate, Chimori Konaka and Harubumi Kato
Department of Surgery, Tokyo Medical University, Tokyo, Japan

Abstract. An autofluorescence endoscopy (SAFE-1000) system has recently been developed. This system is equipped with a conventional xenon lamp with a special bandpass filter as an excitation light source, instead of laser light. The objective of this study was to evaluate whether this simple fluorescence endoscopy system could be as useful as the lung imaging fluorescence endoscopy (LIFE) system in detecting premalignant and malignant lesions of the bronchial tree. A total of 108 cases were studied and biopsies were carried out on 234 sites. Bronchial biopsies were performed at the area of abnormal finding discovered by conventional bronchoscopy (CB) or SAFE-1000, and specimens were then histopathologically investigated. The results of sensitivity for cancer plus dysplasia and dysplasia alone were 74 and 64% by CB, and 89 and 85% by SAFE-1000, respectively. The positive predictive value (PPV) was 64% (CB) and 70% (SAFE-1000). These data showed almost the same results obtained when using the LIFE system with our group. The SAFE-1000 was developed for detection of mucosal autofluorescence without the application of any photosensitizers or use of any lasers. Our results imply the possibility of using this simple device for the autofluorescence diagnosis of subtle bronchial lesions.

Keywords: autofluorescence, early detection, fluorescence bronchoscopy, LIFE, SAFE-1000.

Background

Once roentgenographically occult lung cancer or severe dysplasia is detected by sputum cytology, the lesion must be localized by bronchoscopy since central type early stage lung cancer will not show up as an abnormality on chest X-ray or even on helical computed tomography (CT). However, it is sometimes difficult to locate these lesions by conventional bronchoscopy (CB) alone, even with careful inspection, because early stage lung cancer, especially carcinoma in situ, shows only subtle mucosal changes [1]. Therefore, repeated examinations are sometimes necessary to localize the lesion [2]. Autofluorescence bronchoscopy, i.e., the lung imaging fluorescence endoscopy (LIFE) system, has been developed for patients in this situation and applied clinically. Many reseachers worldwide have proven the utility of this system for the early detection of endobronchial malignancies [3,4]. Recently, the autofluorescence endoscope (SAFE-1000) system has been developed. This system is equipped with a conventional xenon

Address for correspondence: Kinya Furukawa, Department of Surgery, Tokyo Medical University, 6-7-1 Nishishinjuku, Shinjuku-ku, Tokyo 160-0023, Japan. Tel.: +81-3-3342-6111. Fax: +81-3-3349-0326. E-mail: k-furu@tokyo-med.ac.jp lamp with a special bandpass filter as an excitation light source instead of laser light. In this paper, we discuss the usefulness of this simple device as well as that of the LIFE lung system in the detection of premalignant and malignant lesions, and also of autofluorescence bronchoscopy for the screening of abnormal sputum cytology findings.

Materials and Methods

Autofluorescence bronchoscopy

A SAFE system (SAFE-1000, Asahi Pentax Co., Tokyo Japan) was used for this study [5,6]. This system is made up of a camera unit, fiberoptic bronchoscope, excitation light source, PVE filing system, and peripherals. The white light from the 75W xenon lamp is passed through an IR cut filter and then through an excitation filter which specifically passes 420—480 nm excitation light. The excitation light is then transmitted via a light guide to the target area. Images obtained with an objective lens are transmitted via a fiberoptic image guide back to the eyepiece of the endoscope and guided through the prism to the fluorescence filter, which specifically passes a 490—590 nm fluorescence signal. The selected signal is then amplified by the image intensifier, and, by means of a video camera, appears as a fluorescent image on the monitor. Abnormal mucosa showed up as a cold image due to its lack of autofluorescence. It is easy to change between white light and excitation blue light with the changeover switch on the camera unit. This system is also compact and easy to handle.

Subjects

Between January 1997 and December 1999 the subjects were classified into three categories: cases with lung cancer, abnormal sputum findings, and smokers with current symptoms. Bronchial biopsies were performed at the area of abnormal finding discovered by CB or SAFE-1000, and specimens were then investigated histopathologically. A total of 108 cases were enrolled in the study. The 56 cases of lung cancer included 24 squamous cell carcinoma, 26 adenocarcinoma, and four small cell carcinoma. The 32 cases of abnormal sputum cytology findings included one invasive cancer, five early cancers, 17 dysplasias, and nine with unknown origin. The 20 cases of smokers with symptoms comprised six dysplasias and 14 normal or inflammation cases.

Results

We carried out biopsies on 234 sites with abnormal findings discovered by CB, SAFE-1000 or both. A comparison of endoscopic findings with the pathological diagnosis of the biopsy specimens was performed. Invasive cancer was detected at 32 sites, all of which were correctly diagnosed by both CB and SAFE-1000 examinations. Early cancer was detected at 12 sites, of which 10 were recognized by both CB and SAFE-1000 examinations. One site was not recognized by CB, but only by SAFE-1000. Dysplasia was detected at 87 sites: 43 of them were recognized by both CB and SAFE-1000, however, 31 cases (36%) were recognized only by SAFE-1000. Of the normal or inflammation cases, 48% were false positive on SAFE-1000 examinations due to chronic inflammation which caused increased cell layers. The results of sensitivity for cancer plus dysplasia were 74% by CB and 89% by SAFE-1000, and for dysplasia alone they were 64% by CB, and 85% by SAFE-1000. The positive predictive value (PPV) was 64% by CB and 70% by SAFE-1000. The SAFE-1000 data were similar to those obtained by the LIFE system in a previous study by the authors (sensitivity: 95% for cancer plus dysplasia, 90% for dysplasia, PPV: 73%) [3]. In 78 cases we also investigated abnormal sputum cytology cases by additional autofluorescence bronchoscopy using LIFE or SAFE-1000. Using the Japanese classification, Class C (moderate dysplasia), class D (severe dysplasia) and class E (carcinoma) were identified in 28, 22 and 28 cases, respectively.

Discussion

Fluorescence diagnosis can be classified into two groups: photodynamic diagnosis (PDD) using light and a tumor-specific photosensitizer, and autofluorescence diagnosis (AFD). After the pioneering work on PDD by Profio, Doiron et al. [7], Hayata and Kato also examined the possibility of photodiagnosis for central type early stage lung cancer since 1979. We have developed several kinds of laser diagnostic systems using a krypton laser [8], excimer dye laser [9] and diode laser [10]. However, these systems were hampered with problems including skin photosensitization, false positive fluorescence and autofluorescent interference. Therefore, autofluorescence from endogenous chromophores came to our attention. The concept of autofluorescence bronchoscopy is based on the fact that the autofluorescence of abnormal areas is different from that of normal areas. The normal area of the bronchus shows green autofluorescence when excited by blue light, but abnormal areas such as cancer or a precancerous lesion show cold spots due to decreased green autofluorescence [11,12].

Aubin demonstrated that autofluorescence arises from intracellular nicotinamide adenine dinucleotide (NADH), riboflavin and flavin coenzymes [13], and Barenboim showed that collagen and elastin in connective tissue have strong autofluorescence, in the blue-green and yellow spectral regions, respectively [14]. Using an excimer dye laser diagnostic system, autofluorescence showed two emission peaks of autofluorescence appearing at around 450 and 500 nm, which are compatible with the fluorescence spectra of collagen, elastin, NADH and flavin. Autofluorescence decreases following tissue transformation from normal to carcinoma. The basis of this phenomenon can be explained by the following three factors: (1) tissue structure, (2) intracellular metabolism, and (3) increase of microvasculature and blood flow. The thickening of the bronchial membrane decreases autofluorescence from the submucosal layer. In our study, the autofluorescence could be detected from the submucosal layer by fluorescence microscopy, which is composed of collagen and elastin [3]. On the other hand, tumor tissue does not show autofluorescence, and the matrix between cancer cells shows very low autofluorescence. Accelerated intracellular metabolism in cancer cells decreases riboflavin and flavin coenzymes and NADH caused by overproduction of lactic acid through glycolysis. Adachi showed a decrease of autofluorescence intensity following an increase in the ratio of lactic acid to FMN [6]. FAD in tumor tissue was significantly lower than in normal tissue in our study. Recently, Keith et al. [15] demonstrated an increase of microvasculature in dysplastic lesions which might cause decreased autofluorescence because hemoglobin absorbs the excitation light.

In 1991, the LIFE lung system using a He-Cd laser, without any photosensitizer, was developed by Palcic and applied clinically by Lam [11]. Following this, Asahi Pentax developed the SAFE-1000 system, and we started to apply it clinically from 1994 onwards [5]. In recent years, autofluorescence diagnosis has been reported to improve the detection rate of intraepithelial lesions. Lam et al. reported favorable results in their multicenter clinical trial with the LIFE system [4]. Since fluorescence diagnosis is advantageous, we needed to make a cheap, simple and effective device. One advantage of the SAFE-1000 system is that it uses a standard xenon lamp with a filter rather than a laser [5,6]. In the current study, the diagnostic rate of invasive cancer is the same with both CB and SAFE-1000. While fluorescence evaluation does not aim to diagnose advanced cancer, the extent of the lesion could be objectively observed by the SAFE-1000 system. This is useful in the preoperative determination of the resection line or to determine the indications of endoscopic local treatment, such as photodynamic therapy. The sensitivity of detection of cancer plus dysplasia, and dysplasia alone was 74 and 64% with CB, and 89 and 85% with the SAFE-1000 system, respectively. Therefore, using the SAFE-1000 fluorescence bronchoscopy in addition to CB could increase the diagnostic rate by 15 to 20%. This is a promising sign for the early detection of premalignant and malignant lesions.

Conclusion

Autofluorescence endoscopy is useful in the early detection of premalignant and malignant lesions. The results of sensitivity for dysplastic lesions were 51% for CB, 90% for LIFE and 88% for SAFE-1000, respectively. The results of PPD were 64% for CB, 73% for LIFE and 70% for SAFE-1000, respectively. SAFE-1000 is equally as capable at diagnosing premalignant lesions as LIFE. SAFE-1000 is also a convenient and safe system, and does not require a laser light. Our study suggests that autofluorescence diagnosis of subtle bronchial lesions is possible with the simple SAFE-1000 system.

Acknowledgements

The authors wish to thank Prof J. P. Barron at the International Medical Communications Center, Tokyo Medical University, for his support in reviewing this paper.

References

1. Woolner LB, Fontana RS, Cortese DA et al. Roentgenographically occult lung cancer: pathologic findings and frequency of multicentricity during a 10 year period. Mayo Clin Proc 1983; 59:435–466.
2. Cortese DA, Pairolero PC, Bergsralh EJ et al. Roentgenographically occult lung cancer: a 10 year experience. J Thorac Cardiovasc Surg 1983;86:373–380.
3. Ikeda N, Kim K, Okunaka T et al. Early localization of bronchogenic cancerous/precancerous lesions with lung imaging fluorescence endoscope. Diagn Ther Endo 1997;3:197–201.
4. Lam S, Kennedy T, Unger M et al. Localization of bronchial intraepithelial neoplastic lesions by fluorescence bronchoscopy. Chest 1998;113:696–702.
5. Kato H, Okunaka T, Ikeda N et al. Application of simple imaging technique for fluorescence bronchoscope: preliminary report. Diagn Ther Endo 1994;1:79–81.
6. Adachi R, Utsui T, Furusawa K. Development of the autofluorescence endoscope imaging system. Diagn Ther Endo 1999;5:65–70.
7. Profio AE, Doiron DR. A feasibility study of the use of bronchoscopy for localization of small lung tumors. Phys Med Biol 1977;22:949–957.
8. Hayata Y, Kato H, Konaka C et al. Fiberoptic bronchoscopic laser photoradiation for tumor localization in lung cancer. Chest 1982;82:10–14.
9. Kato H, Imaizumi T, Aizawa K et al. Photodynamic diagnosis in respiratory tract malignancy using an excimer dye laser system. J. Photochem Photobiol B Biol 1990;6:189–196.
10. Sheyhedin I, Okunaka T, Kato H et al. Localization of experimental submucosal esophageal tumor in rabbits by using mono-L-aspartyl chlorin e6 and long-wavelength photodynamic excitation. Lasers Surg Med 2000;26:83–89.
11. Palcic B, Lam S, Hung J et al. Detection and localization of early lung cancer by imaging techniques. Chest 1991;99:742–743.
12. Hung J, Lam S, LeRiche JC, Palcic B. Autofluorescence of normal and malignant bronchial tissue. Lasers Surg Med 1991;11:99–105.
13. Aubin JE. Autofluorescence of viable cultured mammalian cells. J Histochem Cytochem 1978;27:36–43.
14. Barenboim GM. Luminescence of biopolymers and cells. NY: Plenum Press, 1969;64–75.
15. Keith RL, Miller YE, Gemmill RH et al. Angiogenic squamous dysplasia in bronchi of individuals at high risk for lung cancer. Clin Cancer Res 2000;6:1616–1625.

Bronchology and Bronchoesophagology: State of the Art.
H. Yoshimura et al., editors.

Our experiences of LIFE (light induced fluorescence endoscope) lung system and PDT (photo-dynamic therapy)

S. Hanzawa, S. Momiki, K. Sasaki, I. Hashizume, N. Kasamatsu, T. Yasui and T. Seto
Hamamatsu Medical Center, Hamamatsu, Japan

Introduction

Following conventional examination by white-light bronchoscope, bronchoscopic examination by LIFE-lung system (Xillix, Canada) was carried out in 15 patients: 14 cases of known lung cancer and one of anamesis of squamous cell carcinoma. In the 14 lung cancer cases, there were significant tumor invasion findings, and in the sqaumous cell carcinoma case, diagnosis of in situ carcinoma was established by biopsy in the abnormal reddish brown area. In eight cases of known lung cancer, dysplastic lesions were detected by biopsy or cytological specimens in suspicious areas. It can be seen, therefore, that the LIFE-lung system can be useful in detecting even metaplastic or precancerous lesions [1,2].

Case 1

This was a case of known lung cancer, a 68-year-old woman with cough symptoms. Her chest X-ray showed a tumor shadow at the left hilus, and sputum cytology subsequently revealed squamous cell carcinoma. Bronchoscopy and LIFE were then performed with the following results: the orifice of the left upper bronchus was normal, but the orifices of Lt. B1 + 2 and 3 were obstructed by tumor. The LIFE diagnosis was abnormal and squamous cell carcinoma was confirmed by biopsy.

Case 2

This was a case of in situ carcinoma. The patient was a 70-year-old woman with cough symptoms, with poor pulmonary function and who was a smoker. She had anamnesis of right tuberculosis and resected lung squamous cell carcinoma. At the left main bronchus a small protrusion was detected by bronchoscopy and the LIFE also showed positive findings in this area. By brushing cytology and

Address for correspondence: S. Hanzawa, Hamamatsu Medical Center, 328 Tomitsuka-cho, Hamamatsu, Shizuoka 432-8580, Japan. Tel.: +81-53-453-7111. Fax: +81-53-452-9217.

biopsy the diagnosis of squamous cell carcinoma in situ was established and PDT was performed. There has been no apparent recurrence since this therapy (1.5 years).

PDT (PDT EDL-1, Hamamatsu Photonics, Japan) was performed in two cases of carcinoma in situ. In one case the carcinoma diagnosis was established in the same way as in Case 2, in the other one the carcinoma was detected by mass screening of sputum cytology. One year after PDT treatment no recurrence had been observed in either case. PDT is one of the most effective therapeutic treatments against hilar early lung cancer, especially in patients with poor pulmonary function.

Case 3

This was another case of carcinoma in situ. A male 74-year-old smoker with pulmonary emphysema and poor pulmonary function showed positive findings in mass screening sputum cytology. The dull angle of bifurcation of the left upper division bronchus was observed by bronchoscopy, and biopsy at this point then showed carcinoma in situ. PDT was performed and no recurrence has been observed in the 1.5 years following this treatment.

Conclusion

This study demonstrated the utility of the LIFE-lung system and the effectiveness of PDT. We believe that a certain level of experience is necessary to correctly analyse the various findings of the LIFE-lung system [3]. In our experience, the differentiation between suspicious areas and abnormal areas was quite challenging. It would be essential to have the experience of at least 20 to 30 malignancy or early cases. As regards the cases where PDT was carried out, the follow-up bronchoscopy study will be requested within a certain period of time to allow detection of any recurrence.

References

1. Lam S et al. Localization of bronchial intraepithelial neoplastic lesions by fluorescence bronchoscopy. Chest 1998;113(3):696–702.
2. Fujisawa T et al. Screening with sputum cytology in the chiba lung cancer program and usefulness of LIFE-system for detection of precancerous and cancerous lesions of the bronchi. (Abstract) 10th World Congress of Bronchology and Bronchoesophagology. Budapest, Hungary.
3. Kato H et al. The role of fluorescence diagnosis in the early detection of high risk bronchial lesion. J Bronchol 1998;5(4):273–274.

Bronchology and Bronchoesophagology: State of the Art.
H. Yoshimura et al., editors.

A 16-year experience of mass screening by sputum cytology

Masami Sato[1], Motoyasu Sagawa[1], Hiroto Takahashi[1], Akira Sakurada[1], Yoshinori Okada[1], Yuji Matsumura[1], Tatsuo Tanita[1], Takashi Kondo[1], Shigefumi Fujimura[1], Kastuo Usuda[2], Satomi Takahashi[2], Yasuki Saito[3] and Kan'ma Kanna[3]

[1]Department of Thoracic Surgery, Institute of Development, Aging and Cancer, Tohoku University, Sendai, Japan; [2]Department of Surgery, Sendai Kosei Hospital, Sendai, Japan; and [3]Department of Thoracic Surgery, Sendai National Hospital, Sendai, Japan

Abstract. We have conducted population-based lung cancer mass screening in Miyagi Prefecture, Japan, since 1982. In this paper we report our results. All screenees were examined by miniature X-ray film. Cytological studies were made for a high-risk group: male screenees whose smoking index was above 600, and who were 50 years of age or more.

From 1982 to 1997, a total of 3,994,285 screenees were examined by miniature X-ray film. Of these, 192,982 (4.8%) were also examined by sputum cytology. 415 patients showed positive cytology, and 437 showed suspected positive cytology.

1,294 lung cancers were detected by X-ray films. 342 primary lung cancers, 55 cancers in otorhinolaryngeal regions, 13 previously diagnosed cancers, four metastatic cancers and one myeloma were detected by sputum cytology. The detection ratio by sputum cytology was 177.2 per 100,000. The ratio by X-ray film was 32.4 per 100,000. The ratios of clinical stages 0–1 were 56.4% by X-ray film and 78.9% by sputum cytology. In patients detected by sputum cytology alone and by X-ray film alone, the 5-year survival was 74.9 and 39.6%, respectively.

In conclusion, sputum cytology is a useful method for early detection of lung cancer.

Keywords: early lung cancer, lung cancer, population-based mass screening, sputum cytology.

Population-based lung cancer mass screening has been conducted in Miyagi Prefecture, Japan, since 1982 [1]. In this paper we have focused on sputum cytology as a screening method.

From 1982 to 1997, a total of 3,994,285 screenees were examined by miniature X-ray film. Of these, 192,982 (4.8%) were also examined by sputum cytology. Cytological studies were made for a high-risk group that consisted of male screenees whose smoking index was above 600, and who were 50 years of age or more. 415 patients showed positive cytology, and 437 showed suspected positive cytology. Of these patients, 786 (92.3%) were examined by bronchoscopy.

Usually, we performed bronchoscopy under topical anesthesia. From September 1986, brushing of all bronchi was carried out when we failed to localize the

Address for correspondence: Masami Sato MD, Department of Thoracic Surgery, Institute of Development, Aging and Cancer, Tohoku University, 4-1 Seiryo-machi, Aoba-ku, Sendai 980-8575, Japan. Tel.: +81-22-717-8526. Fax: +81-22-717-8526. E-mail: m-sato@idac.tohoku.ac.jp

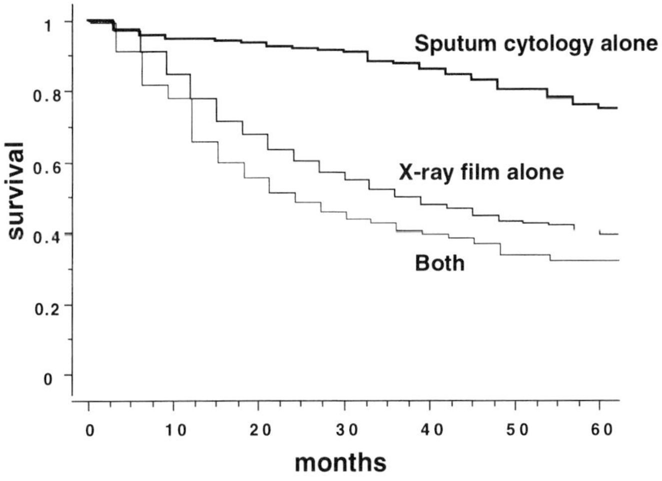

Fig. 1. Survival curves of lung cancer patients according to the detection method in mass screening.

tumor [2]. In November 1997, we introduced the LIFE-lung System at the time of the initial examination.

While 1,294 lung cancers were detected by X-ray films, 342 primary lung cancers, 55 cancers in otorhinolaryngeal regions, 13 previously diagnosed cancers, four metastatic cancers and one myeloma were detected by sputum cytology. After the initial examination, 79 cancers were localized. The detection ratio by sputum cytology was 177.2 per 100,000 cases. On the other hand, the ratio by X-ray film was 32.4 per 100,000. Thus, the ratio by sputum cytology was 5.5 times higher than that by X-ray film.

The ratios of clinical stages 0-1 were 56.4% by X-ray film and 78.9% by sputum cytology. The 5-year survival was 74.9% in patients detected by sputum cytology, 39.6% by X-ray film alone, and 32.7% by both methods (Fig. 1).

In conclusion, sputum cytology is a useful method for early detection of lung cancer, especially squamous cell type.

References

1. Nakada T, Sato H, Saito Y et al. Detection of early lung cancer, results of radiologic and cytologic screening in the Miyagi Program. Tohoku J Exp Med 1987;152:173–185.
2. Sato M, Saito Y, Nagamoto N et al. Diagnostic value of differential brushing of all branches of the bronchi in patients with sputum positive or suspected positive for lung cancer. Acta Cytol 1993;37:879–883.

©2001 Published by Elsevier Science B.V.
Bronchology and Bronchoesophagology: State of the Art.
H. Yoshimura et al., editors.

Growth fraction analysis of early neoplastic and dysplastic lesions in the bronchus

M. Shiba[1], T. Fujisawa[2], K. Shibuya[2] and H. Hoshino[2]
[1]Kimitsu-Chuo Hospital, Kisarazu, Japan; and [2]Chiba University School of Medicine, Chiba, Japan

Introduction

It is suspected that squamous dysplasia is the precursor lesion of squamous cell carcinoma in the bronchial epithelium. Here we report growth fraction analysis, and p-53 oncoprotein and bcl-2 protein accumulation of early squamous cell carcinoma and dysplasia in the bronchial epithelium, using specimens obtained under bronchofiberscopic biopsy.

Materials and Methods

In this study we used biopsy material obtained by bronchoscopic examinations of the patients that showed abnormal sputum cytology in mass screening for lung cancer detection. Immunohistochemical studies were performed using formalin fixed materials that were diagnosed as early cancer or dysplasia. We used antibodies for Ki-67, p-53 oncoprotein and bcl-2 protein for this analysis.

Results

Growth fractions by Ki-67 labeling index were 40.5% in 21 early squamous cell carcinoma, 25.9% in 17 dysplasias and 4.2% in normal mucosa. P-53 oncoprotein was positive in 55.6% in cancers, 56.3% in dysplasias and 0% in normal mucosa. Bcl-2 protein was positive in 46.7% in cancers, 5.9% in dysplasias and 0% in normal mucosa.

Conclusion

An increase in growth fraction, positive rate of p-53 oncoprotein and bcl-2 protein were demonstrated with the progress of normal mucosa, borderline lesions and early cancers.

Address for correspondence: M. Shiba, Kimitsu-Chuo Hospital, 1010 Sakurai, Kisarazu, Chiba 292-8535, Japan. Tel.: +81-766-21-3930. Fax: +81-766-28-2865.

Bronchology and Bronchoesophagology: State of the Art.
H. Yoshimura et al., editors.

Fluorescence bronchoscopy to detect preinvasive bronchial lesions

K. Shibuya[1], T. Fujisawa[1], H. Hoshino[1], M. Baba[1], Y. Saitoh[1], T. Iizasa[1], M. Suzuki[1], M. Otsuji[1], Y. Haga[1], H. Yamaji[1], A. Iyoda[2], T. Toyozaki[2], K. Hiroshima[2] and H. Ohwada[2]

Departments of [1]Surgery and [2]Pathology, Institute of Pulmonary Cancer Research, Chiba University School of Medicine, Chiba, Japan

Abstract. Our aim was to evaluate whether the use of fluorescence bronchoscopy following conventional white-light bronchoscopy examination is useful in the early diagnosis of preinvasive bronchial lesions of the tracheobronchial tree. Patients with abnormal sputum cytology were referred to our institute and examined with both white-light and fluorescence bronchoscopy. All abnormal areas discovered by white-light or fluorescence bronchoscopy examination or both, had biopsy specimens taken for pathological examination. Forty-five lesions were revealed to be preinvasive bronchial lesions. Multicentric lesions were observed in 17 patients in this study. Examination using a fluorescence bronchoscopy, in addition to conventional white-light examination, was found to enhance the detection and localization of preinvasive bronchial lesions.

Keywords: carcinoma in situ, dysplasia.

Background

Centrally arising squamous cell carcinoma of the tracheobronchial tree, especially in heavy smokers, is thought to develop in multiple stages: from squamous metaplasia to dysplasia, followed by carcinoma in situ, and finally invasive cancer. Therefore, a new approach to treating squamous cell carcinoma of the tracheobronchial tree is to detect and eradicate preinvasive bronchial lesions before they become invasive cancer [1,2]. Hence, we conducted a detailed investigation on the use of fluorescence bronchoscopy in the detection of preinvasive bronchial lesions. Preinvasive bronchial lesions were defined as lesions that were dysplasia and carcinoma in situ according to recent WHO criteria [3].

Methods

Patients with abnormal sputum cytology were referred to our institute and examined with both white-light and fluorescence bronchoscopy. Conventional white-light (BF-240, Olympus Optical Corp., Tokyo, Japan) examinations were

Address for correspondence: T. Fujisawa, Institute of Pulmonary Cancer Research, Chiba University School of Medicine, 1-8-1 Inohana, Chuo-ku, Chiba 260-8670, Japan. Tel.: +81-43-222-7171, ext. 5464. Fax: +81-43-226-2172. E-mail: fujisawa@med.m.chiba-u.ac.jp first performed with patients under local anesthesia with sedation by intravenous injection and O^2 inhalation. Areas with abnormal findings were recorded for subsequent biopsy. Fluorescence bronchoscopy (Xillix LIFE – Lung Fluorescence Endoscopy System; Xillix Technologies Corp; Richmond, BC, Canada) examination was then carried out. Biopsy specimens of all suspicious or abnormal areas discovered by white-light bronchoscopy examination, fluorescence bronchoscopy examination, or both, were taken for pathological examination. All of the biopsied specimens were diagnosed by two expert pulmonary pathologists at our institute. Informed consent was obtained from each patient prior to investigation.

Results

Pathological diagnosis of the biopsied specimens

Three biopsies were diagnosed as carcinoma in situ, 42 as dysplasia and 19 as squamous metaplasia. Forty-five lesions were revealed to be preinvasive bronchial lesions.

Multicentric lesions observed in tracheobronchial tree

Multicentric lesions were observed in 17 patients in this study. Fluorescence bronchoscopy showed synchronous lesions of the tracheobronchial tree. Invasive lung cancer and dysplasia were detected in three patients, and in one patient invasive lung cancer, carcinoma in situ and dysplasia were detected. Early hilar lung cancer and dysplasia were detected in two patients. Laryngeal cancer and dysplasia were found in one patient, carcinoma in situ and dysplasia were detected in one patient. Multiple dysplastic lesions were detected in nine patients.

Conclusions

We have found that the use of fluorescence bronchoscopy in addition to conventional white-light examination can enhance the detection and localization of preinvasive bronchial lesions.

References

1. Lam S, MacAulay C. Endoscopic localization of preneoplastic lung lesions. In: Martinet Y, Hirsch FR, Martinet N, Vignaud J-M, Mulshine JL (eds) Clinical and Biological Basis of Lung Cancer Prevention. Basel: Birkhauser Verlag, 1997;231–238.
2. George PJ. Fluorescence bronchoscopy for the early detection of lung cancer. Thorax 1999;54: 180–183.
3. Travis WD, Colby TV, Corin B, Shimosato Y, Brambilla E. Preinvasive lesions. In: Travis WD, Colby TV, Corin B, Shimosato Y, Brambilla E (eds) International Histological Classification of Tumours: Histological Typing of Lung and Pleural Tumours, 3rd edn. Berlin, Heidelberg, and New York: Springer Verlag, 1999;2–5,28–29.

Bronchology and Bronchoesophagology: State of the Art.
H. Yoshimura et al., editors.

Experiences with fluorescence bronchoscopy: D-light AF system

Barna Szima, Imre Mészáros and János Strausz
Pulmonary Institute Törökbálint, Hungary

Abstract. *Background.* Chest X-rays are traditionally performed in Hungary for tuberculosis screening, however, one-third of lung cancers are actually discovered in this way. Further improvements in stage distribution and resectability can be achieved through the introduction of sputum cytology screening and autofluorescence (AF) bronchoscopy.

Methods. In this paper we present our preliminary results using the Storz D-light AF system. It uses a noncoherent excitation light, and detects AF with the help of a built-in filter. After carrying out a white-light bronchoscopy we switch to AF mode and get a real-time image. Normal mucosa show up as green fluorescence component and abnormal mucosa as bluish-reddish.

Results. Between April and December 1999 we performed 80 AF bronchoscopies and took samples for histology in 58 patients. The histological results of mucosal changes showing loss of AF as the only bronchoscopic abnormality were as follows: three normal cases, one scar, four chronic bronchitis, 13 metaplasia, six dysplasia, and two invasive carcinoma.

Conclusions. AF bronchoscopy was useful for the preoperative evaluation of the resection lines, and for bronchial stump and anastomosis control. In cases of a poor AF image, direct observation of the trachea is recommended. Longitudinal follow-up is needed, as well as further investigation of the genetic changes in the high grade preinvasive lesions (moderate, severe dysplasia, carcinoma in situ).

Keywords: autofluorescence, bronchoscopy, D-Light AF, early detection, lung cancer.

Introduction

Lung cancer is the principal cause of deaths by cancer in Hungary. The frequency of lung cancer in men is slightly decreasing with time, whereas the frequency in women is increasing (Fig. 1).

Chest X-rays are performed in Hungary for tuberculosis screening, however, one-third of lung cancers are in fact also discovered in this way. Almost 4 million chest X-rays were performed in 1999 in a network of pulmonary dispensaries. Patients in whom lung cancer is discovered by X-ray screening have been compared to patients where it is discovered by complaints concerning the oncological stages. Fifty-four percent of the patients discovered by chest X-ray were at stage I or II (Fig. 2) [1].

Methods

The D-Light/autofluorescence (AF) system is based on a xenon lamp. In AF

Address for correspondence: B. Szima, Pulmonary Institute Törökbálint, Törökbálint, Munkáccy M.u. 70, 2045 Hungary, Hungary. Tel.: +36-23-335-014. Fax: +36-23-335-012.

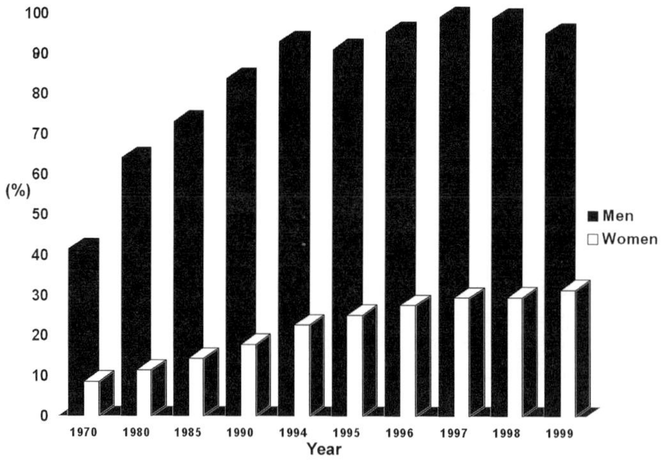

Fig. 1. Incidences of lung cancer in men and women in Hungary (% per 1000).

mode, wavelengths from 380 to 460 nm are used for excitation. For detection, most of the excitation light is blocked by a long pass filter integrated in the eye-piece of the bronchoscope [2].

Results

Between April and December 1999 we performed 80 AF bronchoscopies and took samples for histology in 58 patients. Our indications were as follows: 23 cases of suspected peripheral tumor lesion, five of central lesion, eight of resectability, seven of stump or anastomosis control, three of previous metaplasia, two

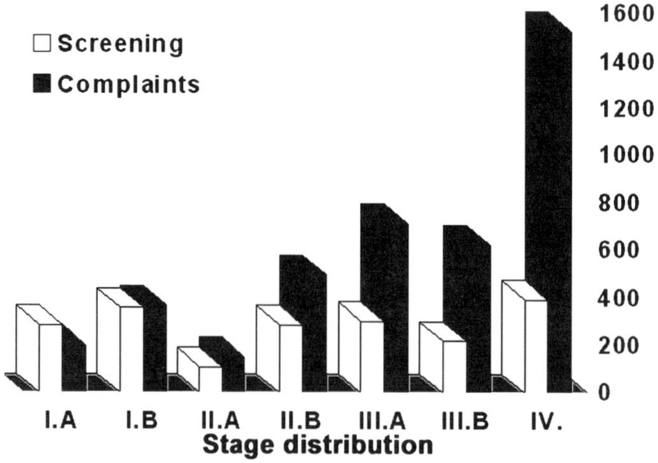

Fig. 2. Distribution of lung cancer stages in 1999 from X-ray screening and patient complaints.

with positive sputum cytology, one with carcinoma in situ, and two with resected benign tumor.

The histology results of mucosal changes showing loss of AF as the only bronchoscopic abnormality were the following: three normal cases, one scar, four chronic bronchitis, 13 metaplasia, six dysplasia, and two invasive carcinoma.

Discussion

The best outcome when treating lung cancer is achieved when the lesion is discovered in the intraepithelial, preinvasive stage. The benefits of AF compared with conventional white-light bronchoscopy have been demonstrated in clinical trials [3,4].

Most of the clinical experiences in this area of research are related to the LIFE-Lung System [5]. The incoherent excitation light of the D-Light/AF system results in a deeper penetration into the tissue and excites fluorescence originating mainly from the submucosa. A higher absorption of light by the thickened epithelium and a reduced fluorescence excitation of chromofores in the submucosa can be the explanation for the contrast between tumor and normal tissue. The color of malignant areas appears bluish-reddish and darkened. In contrast, the color of normal mucosa is dominated by the green fluorescence component. Bronchoscopically malignant tissues are indicated by specific changes in color and disturbance of the relief and fine structure of mucosal surface.

Carcinogenesis is a slow process and is estimated to take 3 to 4 years in dysplasia cases and about 6 months for carcinoma in situ. The proportion of patients in whom invasive cancer will develop from carcinoma in situ is not known, although it has great importance for clinical decision making. We can say that the majority of sites showing carcinoma in situ do progress to invasive carcinoma.

AF bronchoscopy with the D-Light/AF system was useful for the preoperative evaluation of resection lines, and for bronchial stump and anastomosis control in our clinical practice. The increased time taken for bronchoscopy was well-tolerated by the patients, and we did not observe any additional side effects. In cases of a poor AF image (mostly in the trachea), we could not make a correct diagnosis, although we did get a perfect AF image under direct observation without the camera. Longitudinal follow-up in these cases is needed, as well as further investigation of the genetic changes in the high grade preinvasive lesions (moderate, severe dysplasia, carcinoma in situ).

References

1. Pataki G, Megyesi Á, Fehér I. Epidemiological data of the Pulmonary Institutes, 1999. Budapest: Korányi National Institute for Pulmonary Diseases, 2000;73–92.
2. Haeussinger K, Pichler J, Stanzel F et al. Autofluorescence bronchoscopy: the D-light system. In: Bolliger CT, Mathur PN (eds) Interventional Bronchoscopy, vol 30. Basel, Karger: Prog Respir Res, 2000;243–252.

3. Lam S, Kennedy T, Unger M, Miller YE et al. Localisation of bronchial intraepithelial neoplastic lesions by fluorescence bronchoscopy. Chest 1998;113:696–702.
4. Haeussinger K, Stanzel F, Huber RM et al. Autofluorescence detection of bronchial tumors with the D-light/AF. Diagnostic and Therapeutic Endoscopy 1999, vol. 5, 1999;105–112. Respiratory Society Journals Ltd, 1998;22–35.
5. Khanavkar B. Autofluorescence bronchoscopy. J Bronchol 2000;7:60–66.

Bronchology and Bronchoesophagology: State of the Art.
H. Yoshimura et al., editors.

Ultrasonographical approach for diagnosis of depth of invasion in early bronchogenic squamous cell carcinoma

Hiroto Takahashi, Motoyasu Sagawa, Masami Sato, Yasuki Saito, Akira Sakurada, Itaru Ishida, Takeshi Oyaizu, Tatsuo Tanita, Don Boming, Wu Shulin, Chiaki Endo, Yuji Matsumura, Shigefumi Fujimura and Takashi Kondo
Department of Thoracic Surgery, Institute of Development, Aging and Cancer, Tohoku University, Sendai, Japan

Abstract. In order to be able to determine appropriate treatment, it is important to evaluate the depth of invasion of roentgenographically occult bronchogenic squamous cell carcinoma (ROSCC), since ROSCC invading bronchial cartilage cannot be effectively treated by photodynamic therapy (PDT). To evaluate the depth of invasion, we have conducted transtracheo-bronchial endoscopic ultrasonography (TUS).

TUS was performed on 22 ROSCC lesions using a flexible bronchofiberscope, a rotating ultrasound transducer (20 MHz), and an endoscopic ultrasound machine. We ultrasonographically classified the degree of the depth of transmural invasion into two groups; A: "inside of cartilaginous layer" and B: "cartilaginous layer or over". The patients were treated by irradiation, PDT, or surgical resection. Pathological findings were also classified into categories A or B. In order to calculate the sensitivity for evaluating transmural invasion by TUS, the complete recovery (CR) cases and the recurrent cases after PDT were classified into pathological A and B, respectively. Two cases treated by irradiation were excluded from the analysis.

In the evaluation of invasion within cartilage, the sensitivity was 85.7%, the specificity was 66.7%, the accuracy was 80.0%, and the positive predictive value was 85.7%. Using TUS, the decision of treatment modality would be more confident.

Keywords: early lung cancer, photodynamic therapy, roentgenographically occult lung cancer, transtracheo-bronchial ultrasonography (TUS).

Introduction

To determine the appropriate mode of treatment for roentgenographically occult bronchogenic squamous cell carcinoma (ROSCC), it is important to evaluate the depth of cancer invasion. If ROSCC invades over the cartilage, then a considerable number of the patients will have lymph node metastases and photodynamic therapy (PDT) is therefore not effective. In order to evaluate the depth of invasion in ROSCC, we have carried out transtracheo-bronchial endoscopic ultrasonography (TUS) [1,2].

Address for correspondence: Hiroto Takahashi MD, Department of Thoracic Surgery, Institute of Development, Aging and Cancer, Tohoku University, 4-1 Seiryo-machi, Aoba-ku, Sendai 980-8575, Japan. Tel.: +81-22-717-8521. Fax: +81-22-717-8526. E-mail: hiroto@idac.tohoku.ac.jp

Materials and Methods

This study was based on the data obtained from 22 lesions with ROSCC (including multifocal carcinomas detected in one patient) treated from October 1996 to December 1999. The patients were 21 men and one woman ranging from 49 to 79 years in age, and from 550 to 2000 in Smoking Index. The chest X-ray films on admission showed no abnormal shadows in any of the patients.

After the localization of each lesion was established using conventional bronchoscopic observation [3], light-induced fluorescent bronchoscopy (LIFE) [4], or differential brushing of all segmental/subsegmental bronchi [5,6], TUS was performed. Patients received pentazocin, hydroxyzine hydrochloride, and atropine sulfate preoperatively. Arterial oxygen saturation, blood pressure, and electrocardiogram were monitored during examination. Under local anesthesia, TUS was performed using a flexible bronchofiberscope, 1T40 (Olympus, Tokyo), which has a biopsy channel of 2.8 mm. A single rotating ultrasound transducer with a frequency of 20 MHz, UM-BS20-26R (Olympus, Tokyo) was used for TUS, which was 2.6 mm in diameter and with a balloon. The transducer was connected to an endoscopic ultrasound machine, EU-M20 (Olympus, Tokyo), whose motor continuously rotated the transducer, producing a real-time radial image.

To eliminate the air around the transducer for preparing the ultrasonographic observation, 10 to 20 ml of saline was injected preoperatively into a chamber between the transducer and the sheath. Then, the transducer-containing catheter was inserted into the biopsy channel of the bronchoscope and was placed just beyond the tip of the flexible bronchofiberscope. To observe the ultrasonographic image of the bronchial surface, the balloon was enlarged by filling with saline, and was gently attached to the ROSCC. The ultrasound images were immediately available on the monitor in real time and individual freeze-framed images were printed.

We observed the carcinoma and the structure of the bronchial wall ultrasonographically, particularly the bronchial cartilage, and defined the degree of the depth of transmural invasion into the bronchial wall. The degree of transmural invasion was classified ultrasonographically into two groups; A: "inside of cartilaginous layer", and B: "cartilaginous layer or over".

The patients were treated with irradiation, photodynamic therapy (PDT), or surgical resection. Clinicopathological findings and response to treatment were compared with the ultrasonographical classification.

Results

The degree of transmural invasion of 22 ROSCC lesions was determined ultrasonographically. Fourteen lesions were classified into group A and eight into group B (Fig. 1).

In group A, 10 lesions were treated with PDT, resulting in complete response

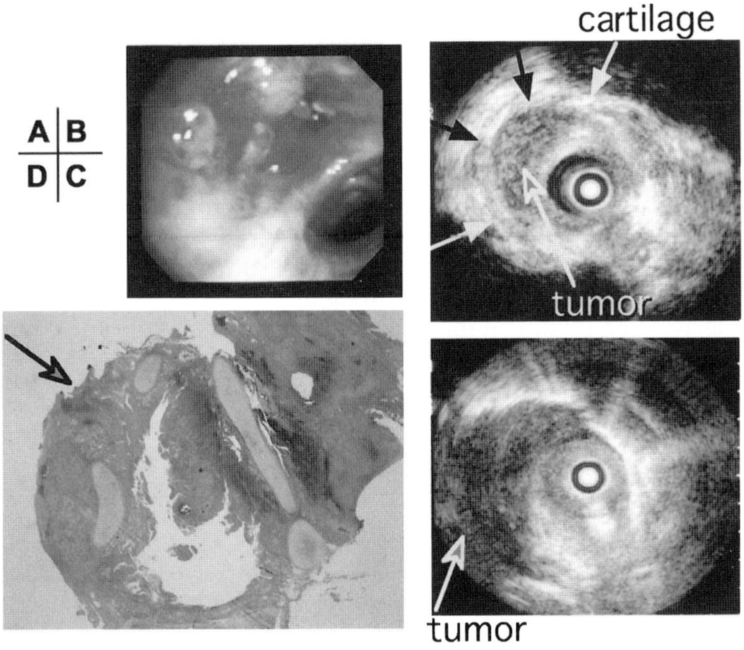

Fig. 1. **A:** Bronchoscopic findings of the tumor revealed an irregular surface and stenosis. **B:** The tumor is hypoechoic on the image obtained by transtracheo-bronchial ultrasonography. In this image, bronchial cartilage was preserved and the depth of invasion was diagnosed as within the cartilage. **C:** However, in another adjacent image, bronchial cartilage was involved with the tumor, and the depth of invasion was diagnosed as being beyond the cartilage. Therefore, this case was ultrasonographically classified into group B. **D:** Histological findings of the tumor revealed that the tumor invaded beyond the bronchial cartilage.

(CR) for nine lesions and recurrence for one lesion. Four lesions were surgically resected and pathological findings revealed that the invasion of three lesions was inside of the cartilaginous layer and the remaining one lesion had invaded beyond the cartilaginous layer.

In group B, four lesions were surgically resected and pathological findings revealed that the invasion of one lesion was inside of the cartilaginous layer and the other three lesions had invaded the cartilaginous layer or further. Two other lesions were treated with PDT, resulting in CR for one lesion and recurrence for one lesion. Another two lesions were treated with irradiation, resulting in CR for both.

In order to assess the efficacy of preoperative evaluation of transmural invasion by TUS, clinicopathological findings and response to PDT were compared with the ultrasonographical classification. In order to calculate sensitivity, the CR and recurrence cases after PDT were regarded as pathological groups A and B, respectively. The two cases treated by irradiation were excluded from the analysis. In the preoperative evaluation of invasion within bronchial cartilage by TUS, the sensitivity was 12 out of 14 (85.7%), the specificity was four out of six (66.7%), the accuracy was 16 out of 20 (80.0%), and the positive predictive value was 12 out of 14 (85.7%).

Conclusion

In the evaluation of cancer invasion within bronchial cartilage, the sensitivity and the positive predictive value of TUS was 85.7%, and the specificity was 66.7%. Using TUS, the preoperative evaluation of invasion depth would be more accurate, and the decision on treatment method would be more appropriate compared with the conventional bronchoscopic observation.

References

1. Takahashi H, Sagawa M, Sato M et al. Transtracheobronchial ultrasonographic endoscopy: a new approach to the diagnosis of bronchial wall invasion and lymphadenopathy caused by lung cancer. J Jpn Soc Bronchol 1997;189–194.
2. Takahashi H, Sagawa M, Sato M et al. Ultrasonographic findings of diseases in peripheral lung fields using transtracheobronchial endoscopic ultrasonography (TUS). J Jpn Respir Soc 1998; 36:857–863.
3. Usuda K, Saito Y, Nagamoto N et al. Relation between bronchoscopic findings and tumor size of roentgenographically occult bronchogenic squamous cell carcinoma. J Thorac Cardiovasc Surg 1993;106:1098–1103.
4. Fujisawa T, Lam S, Sato M et al. Autofluorescence bronchoscopy: principles and clinical applications. Tokyo: Kanehara, 1999.
5. Sato M, Saito Y, Nagamoto N et al. Diagnostic value of differential brushing of all branches of the bronchi in patients with sputum positive or suspected positive for lung cancer. Acta Cytol 1993;37:879–883.
6. Sagawa M, Saito Y, Sato M et al. Localization of double, roentgenographically occult lung cancer. Acta Cytol 1994;38:392–397.

Complications of bronchoscopy – prevention and control

Bronchology and Bronchoesophagology: State of the Art.
H. Yoshimura et al., editors.

Prophylactic use of antibiotics to prevent fever following fiberoptic bronchoscopy

Toshiyuki Kita[1], Kouichi Nishi[1], Miki Abo[1], Takio Ohka[1], Masaki Fujimura[2] and Shinji Nakao[2]
1Department of Internal Medicine, Ishikawa Prefectural Central Hospital, Ishikawa, Japan; and [2]Department of Internal Medicine, Kanazawa University School of Medicine, Ishikawa, Japan

Abstract. *Background.* The prophylactic use of antibiotics to prevent pneumonia and/or fever following fiberoptic bronchoscopy has been applied in many institutions. However, there has been uncertainty as to the clinical indication of the value of prophylactic use of antibiotics as well as how to use antibiotics in fiberoptic bronchoscopy. This study aims to evaluate whether the prophylactic use of antibiotics before fiberoptic bronchoscopy is effective in preventing fever following the procedure.

Methods. Fifty-six patients (45 men and 11 women, mean age 61.5 years) underwent routine fiberoptic bronchoscopy and had their body temperature examined every day. Their blood was taken in order to measure white cell count (WBC) and C-reactive protein (CRP) before the procedure and then 2 days after. Twenty-four patients received 3.0 g sultamicillin tosilate (SBTPC) once 45 min before and once just after the procedure (group A). The other 32 patients received 3.0 g SBTPC once just after the procedure and then once the following morning (group B).

Results. There was no significant difference between the mean value of body temperature, WBC and CRP between group A and group B.

Conclusions. Our results indicate that the prophylactic use of antibiotics before fiberoptic bronchoscopy in the prevention of bronchoscopy-related fever is not more effective than the use of antibiotics only after the procedure.

Keywords: C-reactive protein, fiberoptic bronchoscopy-related fever, white cell count.

Introduction

Many institutions have employed the prophylactic use of antibiotics to prevent pneumonia and/or fever following fiberoptic bronchoscopy [1]. However, the clinical indication of the value of prophylactic use of antibiotics as well as how to use antibiotics in fiberoptic bronchoscopy has been widely uncertain. This study aims to evaluate whether the prophylactic use of antibiotics before a fiberoptic bronchoscopy procedure is effective in preventing fever after the procedure.

Address for correspondence: Toshiyuki Kita MD, Department of Internal Medicine, Ishikawa Prefectural Central Hospital, 153 Nu Minamishinbo-machi, Kanazawa, Ishikawa 920-8530, Japan. Tel.: +81-76-237-8211. Fax: +81-76-238-2337. E-mail: kitatoshi@ipch.kanazawa.ishikawa.jp

Materials and Methods / Patients

The study was carried out on 56 patients hospitalized at the Ishikawa Prefectural Central Hospital who underwent transoral fiberoptic bronchoscopies between October 1999 and May 2000 (Table 1). The procedure was carried out on patients under topical anesthesia: the inhalation of 4% lidocaine and 2% lidocaine sprayed into the oral passage, directly instilled onto the vocal cords, and used as needed on the bronchial mucosa. Endobronchial lesions that were visualized were brushed or biopsied, and peripheral lesions were brushed or biopsied under fluoroscopic control. Bronchoalveolar washing was performed 3 times during the procedure by lavage with nonbacteriostatic 50 ml of normal saline, and aspiration, directly through the instrument.

The patients' axillary temperature was taken just before the procedure and then every day up to 3 days after the procedure. Blood samples were taken, before and then 2 days after the procedure, for the measurement of white blood cell counts (WBC) and C-reactive protein (CRP).

Twenty-four patients received 3.0 g sultamicillin tosilate (SBTPC) 45 min before and then just after the procedure (group A). Thirty-two patients received 3.0 g SBTPC just after the procedure and then once more the next morning (group B). The results were expressed as the mean ± SD. The statistical difference of the results was determined using a paired Student's t test and two factor repeated ANOVA, with a p value of less than 0.05 as the criterion of significance.

Results

The mean value (mean ± SD) of body temperature in group A patients was 36.4 ± 0.43°C 45 min before the procedure, 37.2 ± 0.8°C just after the procedure,

Table 1. Details of patients.

	Group A	Group B
No. of patients	24	32
Mean age (mean ± SD)	61.6 years ± 13.2	61.4 years ± 14.8
Sex (M/F)	17/7	28/4
Incidence of factors:		
Indications for procedure:		
Hemoptysis	6 (25.0%)	7 (21.9%)
Pulmonary mass	7 (29.2%)	16 (50.0%)
Pulmonary consolidation	6 (25.0%)	5 (15.6%)
Other	5 (10.8%)	4 (12.5%)
Bronchoalveolar washing	19 (79.2%)	19 (59.4%)
Bronchial brushing	8 (33.3%)	14 (43.8%)
Bronchial and lung biopsy	6 (25.0%)	6 (18.8%)

Group A patients received 3.0 g sultamicillin tosilate 45 min before the procedure and then just after; group B patients received 3.0 g sultamicillin tosilate just after and then 16 h after the procedure.

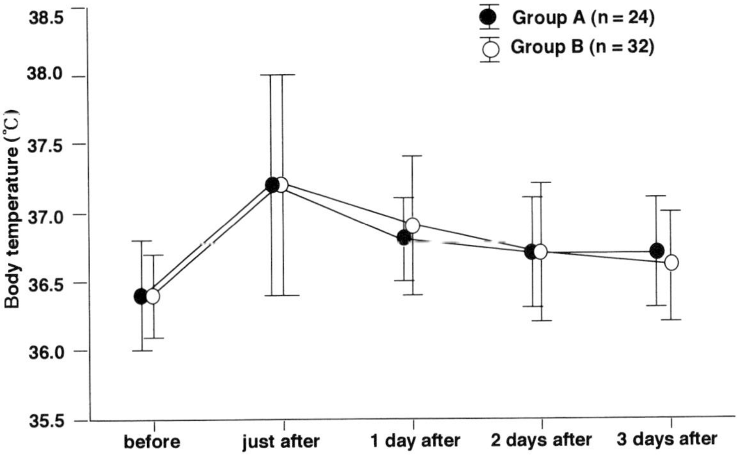

Fig. 1. Time course of highest axillary temperature before, just after and up to 3 days after the procedure (mean ± SD).

36.8 ± 0.3 °C 1 day after, 36.7 ± 0.4°C 2 days after, and 36.7 ± 0.4°C 3 days after. The mean value of body temperature in group B patients was 36.4 ± 0.3°C, 37.2 ± 0.8°C, 36.9 ± 0.5°C, 36.7 ± 0.5°C and 36.6 ± 0.4°C, respectively (Fig. 1). The mean value of WBC and CRP in group A was 7058 ± 2860 (/μL) and 1.4 ± 2.7 (mg/dL), respectively. The mean value of WBC and CRP in group B was 6831 ± 2240 (/μL) and 2.8 ± 3.6 (mg/dL), respectively. There was no significant difference between the two groups.

Discussion

In conclusion, our results suggest that in the prevention of bronchoscopy-related fever, the prophylactic use of antibiotics before a fiberoptic bronchoscopy procedure is not more effective than the prophylactic use of antibiotics only after the procedure.

Reference

1. Robbins H, Goldman AL. Failure of a "prophylactic" antimicrobial drug to prevent sepsis after fiberoptic bronchoscopy. Am Rev Respir Dis 1977;116:325–326.

Congenital abnormalities

Bronchology and Bronchoesophagology: State of the Art.
H. Yoshimura et al., editors.

An adult case of hypoplasia of the middle lobe found during surgery for lung cancer

Minako Fujita, Shozo Fujino, Shuhei Inoue, Keiichi Kontani, Satoru Sawai, Yuji Suzumura and Jun Hanaoka
Second Department of Surgery, Shiga University of Medical Science, Shiga, Japan

Abstract. Pulmonary hypoplasia is detected comparatively often during infancy but tends to be rare in adults. In almost all cases, primary PH in adulthood is indirectly diagnosed on the basis of bronchography, bronchoscopy computed tomography and pulmonary arteriography, however, direct diagnosis based on thoracotomy during life is extremely rare. In this paper we report an adult case of hypoplasia of the middle lobe detected during surgery for lung cancer. In our case, although bronchi and pulmonary vein of the middle lobe were confirmed, there was no trace of the pulmonary arteries.

Keywords: adult, lobar hypoplasia, pulmonary hypoplasia.

Case report

A 55-year-old woman was admitted to our hospital with abnormal shadows seen in the middle lobe and S^6 of the right lung on chest roentgenogram and chest computed tomography (CT). Biopsy on the S^6 shadow with a bronchoscope resulted in the diagnosis of adenocarcinoma and the patient was subsequently hospitalized to undergo surgery. The patient did not smoke and there was no particular history of this condition in her or her family's past.

On admission, there were no abnormal findings from a biochemical examination, examination of lung function or electrocardiogram, apart from slightly low PaO_2 (75.6 torr) on arterial gas chromatography.

Her chest roentgenogram revealed a circular shadow with an irregular margin overlapping the right hilum of lung. On chest CT, a volume loss change with bronchiectasis was seen in the region probably corresponding to the middle lobe. Based on CT findings, the shadow in the middle lobe was considered to be an inflammatory change.

Bronchoscopic findings failed to demonstrate any particular direct abnormality in the right bronchus on first examination, but the bronchus probably corresponding to B^4b showed edematous changes and mild stenosis.

Surgical findings revealed a small, consolidated middle lobe with incomplete lobulation from the upper lobe. Although bronchi and pulmonary veins of the

Address for correspondence: M. Fujita, Second Department of Surgery, Shiga University of Medical Science, Seta-tsukinowa, Otsu, Shiga 520-2192, Japan. Tel.: +81-77-452-0065. Fax: +81-77-455-2765. E-mail: fujitam@skyoto.hosp.go.jp middle lobe were identified, there was no trace of the pulmonary arteries, hence indicating a complete defect. There were no inflammatory findings, e.g., adhesion, observed around the middle lobe, leading to a diagnosis of hypoplasia of the middle lobe (Fig. 1). Consequently, resection of the right middle and lower lobe was performed.

A low magnification histopathologic image of the middle lobe showed an abnormal alignment of the bronchioli, blood vessels and bronchial cartilage, hypoplastic alveoli and ablation, and deciduation of the bronchial mucoepithelia (Fig. 2).

Discussion

Pulmonary development in humans is a dynamic process, occurring from the fourth week of fetal life until about 8 years of age [1]. Arrested development of the lung can be classified into three types [2]: (1) agenesis, in which there is complete absence of one or both lungs, with no trace of bronchial or vascular supply or of parenchymal tissue; (2) aplasia, in which there is suppression of all but a rudimentary bronchus that ends in a blind pouch, with no evidence of pulmonary vasculature or parenchyma; and (3) hypoplasia, in which the gross morphology of the lung is essentially unremarkable but in which there is a decrease in the number or size of airways, vessels, and alveoli. Hypoplasia of the lung may be regarded as primary (idiopathic) or secondary (when it occurs in association with environmental factors or other congenital anomalies that may be implicated in its pathologenesis) [2]. The incidence of primary hypoplasia has been estimated to be one to two cases per 12,000 births [3]. The pathogenesis of primary hypoplasia is even less clear than the secondary form [4]. It may represent an intrinsic defect in lung development as it is not associated with other anomalies by definition.

Clinical findings depend on the degree of pulmonary abnormality. Infants who

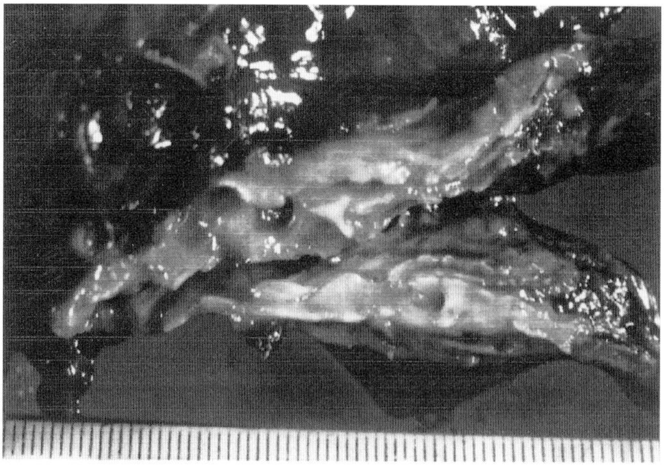

Fig. 1. The raw surface of the middle lobe.

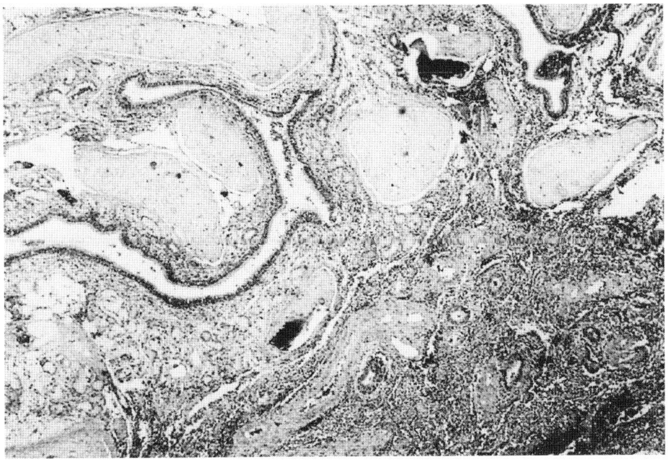

Fig. 2. The histopathologic image of the middle lobe at a low magnification.

have primary pulmonary hypoplasia may experience respiratory distress and are prone to pneumothorax [2]. The condition has been recognized on occasion in adults with chronic respiratory failure [1]. The number of individuals who survive with hypoplasia is greater than agenesis, but the anomalies appear to predispose to respiratory infections, and some patients die before they reach their teens [2,4].

In this case, a surgical finding indicated the onset of hypoplasia in early intrauterine life in the form of something influencing the growth of the lung, e.g., viral infection [5], growth factors [2], hormones [6], intrauterine fluid [7], etc. Lobectomy was carried out because the middle lobe did not demonstrate lung function and may have developed infectious lesions in the future.

References

1. Mas A, Mirapeix R, Domingo C, Sanudo JR, Torremorell MD, Marin A. Pulmonary hypoplasia presented in adulthood as a chronic respiratory failure: report two cases. Respiration 1997;64:240–243.
2. Fraser, Pare. Diagnosis of Diseases of the Chest, 4th edn. W.B. Saunders Company, 1999;597–601,136–144.
3. Fagan DG, Emery JL. A review and restatement of some problems in histological interpretation of the infant lung. Sem Diagn Pathol 1992;9:13.
4. Page DV, Stocker JT. Anomalies associated with pulmonary hypoplasia. Am Rev Respir Dis 1982;125:216–221.
5. Castlman WL. Alternations in pulmonary ultrastructure and morphometric parameters induced by para-influenza (Sendai) virus in rats during postnatal growth. Am J Pathol 1984; 114:322.
6. DiFiore JW, Wilson JM. Lung development. Sem Pediatr Surg 1994;3:221.
7. Adzick NS, Harrison MR, Glick PL et al. Experimental pulmonary hypoplasia and oligohydramnios: relative contributions of lung fluid and fetal breathing movements. J Pediatr Surg 1984;19:658.

Dysphagia

Bronchology and Bronchoesophagology: State of the Art.
H. Yoshimura et al., editors.

Fluoroscopic and manometric findings in a patient with dysphagia after Hunt syndrome

Yuko Matsumura[1], Tetsuya Tanabe[1], Yasuo Ito[1], Yoshihiro Hyodo[1], Naoyuki Kohno[1], Satoshi Kitahara[1], Takehiro Karaho[1] and Yukio Ohmae[2]
[1]*Department of Otolaryngology, National Defense Medical College, Saitama; and* [2]*Tokyo Metropolitan Geriatric Hospital, Tokyo, Japan*

Abstract. In this paper, a case of dysphagia caused by herpes zoster is described. An 82-year-old woman suffered from right otalgia and right facial palsy on 21 May 1999. She was diagnosed with Hunt syndrome and treated accordingly. The right facial palsy improved partially, but hoarseness and progressive dysphagia developed 1 month later. She visited our clinic on 1 July of that year. She was suffering from nystagmus, right facial palsy, right hearing loss and right vocal cord paralysis. Fluoroscopy showed residue of balium in pyriform sinuses, reduced laryngeal closure, cricopharyngeal dysfunction and aspiration during deglutition. Manometry showed weak contractions of hypopharynx and upper esophageal sphincter (UES). The dysphagia and right vocal cord paralysis improved within 4 weeks. Fluoroscopy showed improvement of cricopharyngeal function and aspiration, and recovery of contractions of the level of the vallecula and UES were confirmed from manometry. In our view, herpetic lesions had affected the connecting link between the facial and vagus nerves, and the involvement of vagus nerve had caused weakness of the pharyngeal muscles, therefore aiding the development of dysphagia.

Keywords: cranial nerve involvement, deglutition disorder, herpes zoster, manometry, videofluoroscopy.

Hunt syndrome comprises herpes zoster of the outer ear with lesions of the seventh and eighth cranial nerve [1]. Herpes zoster associated with dysphagia, however, is not commonly seen [2]. In this paper we report one patient suffering from dysphagia who was given a diagnosis of Hunt syndrome.

Case report

The case patient is an 82-year-old woman. She detected a sore throat on 13 May 1999. On 21 May, right otalgia, weakness of the face, hearing loss, and vesicular lesions of the auricle developed. On 25 May, she was diagnosed with Hunt syndrome and began treatment of acyclovir and steroids. Following this initial treatment the right facial palsy partially improved. On 20 June, she was suffering from hoarseness and difficulty in swallowing, and on 1 July 1999 she first visited our clinic.

Address for correspondence: Y. Matsumara, Department of Otolaryngology, National Defense Medical College, 3-2 Namiki-cho, Tokorozawa-shi, Saitama 359-8513, Japan. Tel.: +81-42-995-1686. Fax: +81-42-996-5212.

The following conditions developed in the patient: nystagmus, right facial palsy, right hearing loss, and right vocal cord paralysis. MR imaging revealed no brain mass lesion. Videofluoroscopic examination showed incomplete laryngeal closure, incomplete opening of the upper esophageal sphincter (UES), retention of barium in pyriform sinuses and tracheal aspiration. Manometric examination was carried out to record pressure changes in four standard locations: behind the base of the tongue, at the level of the vallecula, at the level of the hypopharynx, and at the point of UES. These manometric findings in our patient showed a normal coordination of the pharyngeal constrictive wave, low pharyngeal pressure and a short time interval during UES relaxation. Her dysphagia and right vocal cord paralysis were seen to improve within 4 weeks.

Videofluoroscopic examination was performed again on 5 August. Improvement of the laryngeal closure and UES opening were observed, but tracheal aspiration was not. Manometric tracings on 5 August showed elevation in the pharyngeal pressure and the resting pressure of UES. We compared these pressure waves with those of six healthy control cases, ranging in age from 76 to 83 years, for quantitative analysis of swallowing pressure. Manometric tracings were made of 1 ml three swallow of barium liquid in each subject, using barium preparation of 140% w/v. The time period from the onset of UES relaxation to the appearance of peak pressure of the pharynx, peak pressure of the pharynx and UES, duration of UES relaxation, and resting pressure and residual pressure of UES were measured. For statistical analysis, factorial ANOVA was used.

Results

Peaks of pharyngeal pressure showed gradual appearance equally in the manometric tracings of the patient on 12 July and 5 August, and in the controls (Fig. 1A). Although low peak pressure remained at the level of the hypopharynx of the patient compared with controls (Fig. 1B), the peak pressure at the level of the vallecula (Fig. 1C) and UES (Fig. 1D) of the patient on 5 August were higher than those on 12 July. Duration of UES relaxation remained short in the patient compared with the control cases (Fig. 1E). The patient's resting pressure on 5 August was higher than on 12 July (Fig. 1F).

Discussion

We concluded that herpetic lesions had affected the connecting link between the facial and vagus nerves [3], and the involvement of the vagus nerve caused weakness of the pharyngeal muscles, hence instigating dysphagia. Taking into account our case of herpes zoster with dysphagia as well as past reports of similar cases, three of 41 patients showed no improvement of dysphagia [2,4,5], five patients showed aspiration pneumonia [2,5–7], and one of these five died of aspiration pneumonia [5]. We believe that the progress of dysphagia with herpes zoster needs to be carefully monitored in the future.

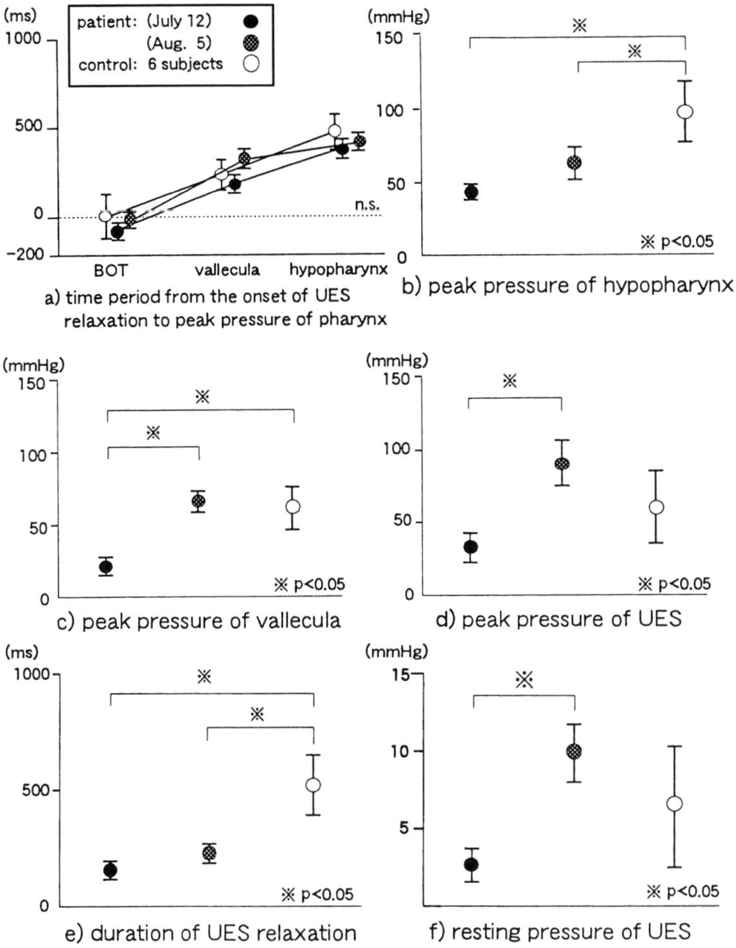

Fig. 1. Comparison of manometric features during swallowing: patient and six controls.

References

1. Hunt JR. The symptom-complex of the acute posterior poliomyelitis of the geniculate, auditory, glossopharyngeal and pneumogastric ganglia. Arch Int Med 1910;5:631–675.
2. Maeda A, Shiojiri T, Tsuchiya K, Watabiki Y. A case of multiple cranial nerve palsy with severe dysphagia due to herpes zoster infection. Clin Neurol 1992;32:524–526.
3. McGovern FH, Fitz-Hugh GS. Herpes zoster of the cephalic extremity. Arch Otolaryngol 1952; 55:307–320.
4. Funakawa I, Terao A, Koga M. A case of zoster sine herpete with involvement of the unilateral IX, X and XI cranial and upper cervical nerves. Clin Neurol 1999;39:958–960.
5. Ogino S, Abe Y, Kitaoku S, Sato S, Irifune M, Matsunaga T. Immunological and virological aspects of Hunt's syndrome associated with multiple cranial nerve paralysises: a case report. Practica Otol 1987;80:585–590.
6. Sato K, Nakamura S, Koseki T, Yamauchi F, Baba M, Mikami M, Kobayashi R, Fujikawa T,

Nagaoka S. A case of Ramsay Hunt syndrome with multiple cranial nerve paralysis and acute respiratory failure. J J Thorac Dis 1991;29:1037–1041.

7. Engstrom H, Wohlfart G. Herpes zoster of the seventh, eighth, ninth and tenth cranial nerves. Arch Neurol Psychiat 1949;62:638–652.

Bronchology and Bronchoesophagology: State of the Art.
H. Yoshimura et al., editors.

Role of anterior tongue as an anchor during swallow

Y. Ohmae[1], M. Sugiura[1] and Y. Matumura[2]
[1]*Tokyo Metropolitan Geriatric Hospital, Tokyo; and* [2]*National Defense Medical College, Saitama, Japan*

Abstract. The contact between the tongue tip and hard palate during swallow plays an important role as an anchor when the central portion of the tongue propels the bolus posteriorly. However, the relationship between the anchoring function of anterior tongue and other elements of the pharyngeal swallow has never been clarified. Simultaneous videofluoroscopic and oropharyngeal manometric examination of oropharyngeal swallowing were performed in eight healthy volunteers with four conditions: 1) control swallow; 2) swallow with stress on anchor function; 3) swallow without anchor function; and 4) effortful swallow. The stress on anchor function and effortful swallow produced a decrease in anterior bulging of the posterior pharyngeal wall (PPW) and an increase in peak pressure at the tongue base, whereas the swallow without anchor function produced an increase in PPW bulging and a decrease in peak pressure at tongue base.

Keywords: anchor, swallowing, tongue, videofluoroscopy.

Background

Deglutitive tongue biomechanics are complex, involving bolus containment, loading, and propulsion. The contact between the tongue tip and hard palate plays an important role as an anchor when the central portion of the tongue propels the bolus during swallow [1]. However, the relationships between the anchor function of the anterior tongue with other oropharyngeal swallowing events have never been investigated and clarified. The aim of this study is to quantify the effects of anchor function on the tongue base movement and other pharyngeal events during swallowing in normal subjects.

Methods

Simultaneous videofluoroscopic and oropharyngeal manometric examination of oropharyngeal swallowing were performed on eight healthy volunteers with the following four conditions: 1) control swallow: each subject completed three swallows with no instruction; 2) swallow with stress on anchor function: pressured contact between tongue tip and palate before and during swallow; 3) swallow without anchor function: no contact between tongue tip and palate before and during swallow; and 4) effortful swallow: squeezing tongue forcefully during

Address for correspondence: Yukio Ohmae MD, Department of Otolaryngology, Tokyo Metropolitan Geriatric Hospital, 35-2 Sakae-cho, Itabasi-ku, Tokyo, Japan. Tel.: +81-3-3964-1141. Fax +81-3-3964-1982.

swallow [2].

Data were analyzed to compare the following: 1) temporal relationships, duration and onset of oropharyngeal events; 2) biomechanical computer analysis of swallowing events: the maximal distance between one point (anterior inferior corner of the second vertebral body) and another opposite point on the surface of the posterior pharyngeal wall (PPW), measured by drawing a line perpendicular to the vertebral column. This distance is the extent of anterior bulge of the PPW [3]; and 3) maximal manometric pressure amplitude at tongue base and hypopharynx.

Results

1. Temporal relationships of oropharyngeal events. The duration of cricopharyngeal opening, laryngeal closure and PPW-base of tongue (BOT) contact were significantly prolonged during the stress swallow on anchor and effortful swallow vs. control swallow, whereas these durations were significantly shorter in the swallow without anchor function vs. control swallow. On the other hand, no significant difference was seen in the timing of oropharyngeal events between the four swallowing conditions.
2. Biomechanical computer analysis of swallowing events. The maximal distance of anterior bulging of PPW during each swallow is shown in Fig. 1. The stress swallow on anchor function and effortful swallow produced a significant decrease in maximal diameter of PPW bulging, and swallow without anchor function produced a significant increase in maximal PPW bulging.
3. Maximal manometric pressure amplitude. Table 1 summarizes the maximal pharyngeal pressure under the four swallowing conditions at tongue base and hypopharynx. The maximal amplitude at the level of tongue base during the stress swallow on anchor function and effortful swallow showed a significant increase vs. control swallow. However, the swallow without anchor caused a

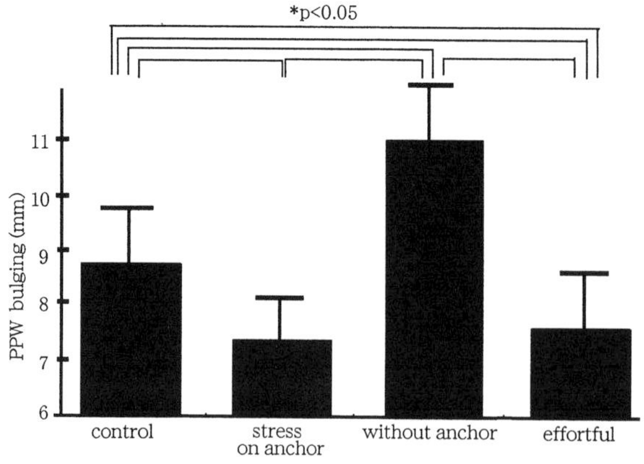

Fig. 1. Maximal anterior bulging of PPW.

Table 1. Maximal pressure amplitude.

	Swallow conditions			
	Control	Stress on anchor function	Swallow without anchor function	Effortful
Tongue base[a]	112 ± 9	138 ± 14	82 ± 8	132 ± 11
Hypopharynx	116 ± 13	119 ± 13	112 ± 12	122 ± 13

[a]$p < 0.05$ ANOVA; data are expressed as mean ± SE mmHg.

significant decrease in maximal amplitude at the tongue base. There was no significant difference in the maximal amplitude for pharyngeal contraction at the hypopharynx.

Conclusions

1. The effects of the anchor function of the anterior tongue during pharyngeal swallow were investigated with videofluoroscopy and manometry.
2. The stress swallow on anchor and effortful swallow produced a decrease in PPW bulging and an increase in maximal pressure amplitude at tongue base, whereas the swallow without anchor produced an increase in PPW bulging and a decrease in maximal pressure amplitude at tongue base.
3. The anchor function of anterior tongue affected the range of the tongue base movement and PPW-BOT contact, i.e., the pressure generator at the level of the tongue base.
4. These findings indicate that instruction of anchor function may create the same effects as effortful swallow, which is designed to increase tongue base movement during swallowing.

References

1. Kahrilas PJ, Lin S et al. Deglutitive tongue action; volume accommodation and bolus propulsion. Gastroenterology 1993;104:152–162.
2. Logemann JA. Noninvasive approaches to deglutitive aspiration. Dysphagia 1993;8:331–333.
3. Fujiu M, Logemann JA. Effect of tongue-holding maneuver on posterior pharyngeal wall movement during deglutition. Am J Speech Lang Pathol 1996;5:23–30.

Bronchology and Bronchoesophagology: State of the Art.
H. Yoshimura et al., editors.

Swallowing disorder due to vagal nerve dysfunction

Miki Saito, Minoru Kinishi, Toshifumi Hasegawa, Masaru Teraoka and Mutsuo Amatsu
Kobe University School of Medicine, Kobe, Japan

Abstract. One of the major functions of the larynx is to prevent aspiration during the pharyngeal phase of swallowing. The vagal nerve plays a major role in achieving a normal swallowing function. In this study we present nine patients with swallowing disorders due to vagal nerve dysfunction. In six patients, parapharyngeal tumors such as neurinoma, paraganglioma and meningioma were removed, and in the remaining three retropharyngeal node dissection was performed. The severity of the postoperative swallowing disorder was evaluated and discussed from the standpoint of: 1) the level of vagal nerve lesion; 2) preoperative compensation; and 3) age factor. As regards the level of vagal nerve lesion, damage to the recurrent laryngeal nerve alone does not cause severe swallowing dysfunction, it is instead damage to the pharyngeal branch and superior laryngeal nerve that cause this disorder. As for the age factor, the subjects of younger age recovered the postoperative swallowing function easily. The presence of preoperative compensation was seen to ease the swallowing disorder.

Keywords: pharyngeal branch, recurrent laryngeal nerve, superior laryngeal nerve, swallowing function.

Introduction

In cases of vagal nerve dysfunction, the level of the vagal nerve lesion affects the swallowing function. The pharyngeal branch provides a motor function to the soft palate and constrictor muscles. The superior laryngeal nerve provides sensory innervation in the supraglottis, and also provides motor function to the cricothyroid muscle. The recurrent laryngeal nerve provides motor function to the intrinsic muscle of the larynx, and sensory innervation in subglottis. This study was designed to evaluate the severity of the swallowing disorder according to the level of vagal nerve lesion and other related factors.

Subjects

Nine patients who complained of swallowing disorder due to vagal nerve dysfunction were recruited in this study. The patients' ages, preoperative diagnosis, level of vagal nerve lesion and other cranial nerve lesion are shown in Table 1.

Address for correspondence: Miki Saito MD, Department of Otorhinolaryngology Head and Neck Surgery, Kobe University School of Medicine 7-5-1, Kusunoki-cho, Chuo-ku, Kobe 650-0017, Japan. Tel.: +81-78-382-6024. Fax: +81-78-382-6039. E-mail: mickey@med.kobe-u.ac.jp

Table 1. Subjects' details.

No.	Age	Preoperative diagnosis	Level of vagal nerve lesion	Cranial nerve lesion
1	21	Neurinoma	A+B+C	
2	46	Neurinoma	A+B+C	
3	62	Neurinoma	A+B+C	Glossopharyngeal nerve, hypoglossal nerve
4	62	Nasopharyngeal cancer	A+B+C	
5	64	Oropharyngeal cancer	A+B+C	Hypoglossal nerve
6	69	Meningioma	A+B+C	
7	71	Submandibular gl. cancer	A+B	Glossopharyngeal nerve, hypoglossal nerve
8	58	Paraganglioma	B+C	
9	72	Neurinoma	C	

A: pharyngeal branch; B: superior laryngeal nerve; C: recurrent laryngeal nerve.

Results

There was a slightly severe swallowing disorder seen in those patients who recovered their swallowing function only by performing vocal cord medialization. In comparison, the swallowing disorders seen in the remaining patients were defined as severe (Table 2).

Discussion

Severity of patients' swallowing disorders was evaluated by considering the factors of age and level of vagal nerve lesion. Lesion of recurrent laryngeal nerve alone dose not cause severe swallowing disorder. However, lesion of the pharyngeal branch and superior laryngeal nerve, which provide the sensory innervation in pharynx and supraglottis, were observed to cause severe swallowing disorders. Regarding the age factor, the subjects of younger age recovered the postoperative swallowing function easily. In this study, those subjects younger than 45 years of

Table 2. Results of patients.

Subject	Functional operation	Diet	Severity
1	Vocal cord medialization	Ordinary	Slight
2	Vocal cord medialization	Ordinary	Slight
3	Vocal cord medialization	Ordinary	Slight
4	Reject	Soft	Slight
5	Myotomy thyrohyoidpexia velopharyngeal closure	Fluid	Severe
6	Myotomy thyrohyoidpexia velopharyngeal closure	Soft	Severe
7	Laryngectomy	Soft	Severe
8	Vocal cord medialization	Ordinary	Slight
9	Vocal cord medialization	Ordinary	Slight

age demonstrated a good recovery of their swallowing function. On the other hand, those subjects older than 65 years of age showed severe disorder when all the branches were damaged.

Bronchology and Bronchoesophagology: State of the Art.
H. Yoshimura et al., editors.

Laryngotracheal separation for intractable aspiration pneumonia

Takayo Yamana, Hiroya Kitano, Masakazu Hanamitsu and Kazutomo Kitajima
Department of Otolaryngology Head and Neck Surgery, Shiga University of Medical Science, Shiga, Japan

Abstract. *Objective.* To confirm that laryngotracheal separation (LTS) is a satisfactory treatment for patients with intractable aspiration pneumonia, even though it does not require tracheoesophageal anastomosis.

Methods. Nine patients with intractable aspiration pneumonia underwent LTS at our institution from 1996 to 1999. Two of them had barium swallow radiography carried out postoperatively.

Results. There was no occurrence of either foul breath or a cough reflex due to pooled secretions in the pouch of the proximal tracheal segment. Barium swallow radiography confirmed that the secretions drained off within 40 min by swallowing or a change in patient position.

Conclusion. We concluded that the pooled secretions in the blind pouch of the proximal tracheal segment would not be a disadvantage of LTS.

Keywords: barium swallow radiography, dysphagia, laryngotracheal separation.

Introduction

Patients with a central nervous system lesion and dysphagia may develop recurrent aspiration pneumonia which is a condition that can be fatal. Surgery is indicated when conservative treatment for intractable aspiration pneumonia fails.

There are several approaches to the surgical management of intractable aspiration. Techniques that completely separate the alimentary and respiratory passages include laryngectomy, laryngotracheal separation (LTS), and tracheoesophageal diversion (TED) [1–4].

TED has been reported to be superior to LTS [1–3]. TED requires a tracheoesophageal anastomosis to prevent foul breath and a cough reflex due to pooled secretions in the blind pouch of the proximal tracheal segment. However, we perform LTS because it is easier than TED. In patients with intractable aspiration pneumonia in whom the general condition is usually poor, it is preferable to perform a simple and definitive procedure. We believe that LTS is therefore superior to TED.

Address for correspondence: Takayo Yamana, Department of Otolaryngology, Shiga University of Medical Science, Seta, Otsu, Shiga 520-2192, Japan. Tel.: +81-77-548-2264. Fax: +81-77-545-7489.
E-mail: yamana@belle.shiga-med.ac.jp

Patients and Methods

Materials

LTS was performed in nine patients with intractable aspiration pneumonia between 1996 and 1999 (Fig. 1). Their ages ranged from 4 to 71 years. In six patients a tracheotomy had previously been performed. In two patients barium swallow radiography was performed postoperatively.

Surgical technique

Under general anesthesia, a horizontal skin incision was made at the superior margin of the existing tracheotomy stoma, or between the third and fourth tracheal rings. The trachea was divided horizontally at the level of the existing tracheotomy, or between the third and fourth tracheal rings. Two tracheal rings were removed from the proximal tracheal stump. The proximal tracheal stump was closed anteroposteriorly as a blind pouch. The tracheal closure was covered with strap muscle flaps based superiorly. The caudal part of the tracheal edge was sutured to the skin, creating a permanent tracheostoma.

Results

In two cases, a small postoperative fistula was noted at the proximal tracheal edge. With local care this closed within 1 month. Neither foul breath nor a cough reflex occurred due to accumulation of secretions in the proximal tracheal pouch. In two cases, barium swallow radiography confirmed that the material that accumulated in the proximal tracheal pouch drained off within 40 min by swallowing or a change in patient position. All the patients were satisfied with the treatment they received.

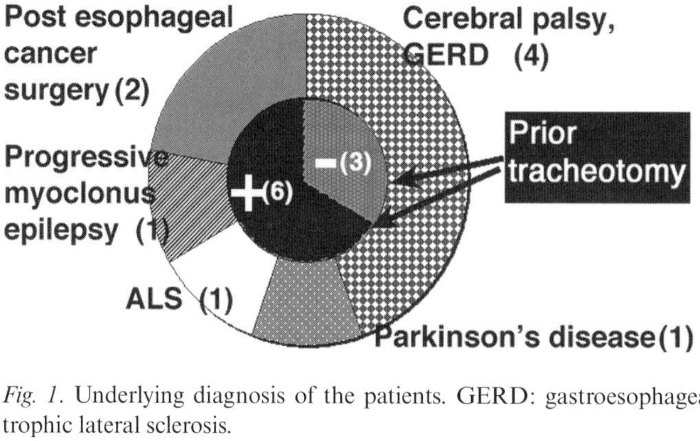

Fig. 1. Underlying diagnosis of the patients. GERD: gastroesophageal reflux disease. ALS: amyotrophic lateral sclerosis.

Discussion

The advantages of LTS include a short operative time period. This is because a tracheoesophageal anastomosis is not required. LTS is not associated with the risk of esophageal fistula, and furthermore, it may be possible to perform LTS under local anesthesia. This can be a significant advantage for patients with impaired respiratory function.

Although there exists the possibility of resulting foul breath and cough reflex due to the accumulation of secretions in the proximal tracheal segment, this was not seen in our patients. Based on postoperative imaging, it appears that the secretions of the oral side of the proximal tracheal pouch drain off within 40 min by swallowing or a change in patient position.

Conclusion

Based on postoperative imaging, it appears that the secretions of the oral side of the tracheal coecum drain off in a brief time. We conclude that LTS is a satisfactory technique for the treatment of patients with intractable aspiration pneumonia.

References

1. Lindeman RC, Yarington CT et al. Clinical experience with the tracheoesophageal anastomosis for intractable aspiration. Ann Otol Rhinol Laryngol 1976;85:609–612.
2. Eisele DW, Yarington CT Jr et al. The tracheoesophageal diversion and laryngotracheal separation procedure for treatment of intractable aspiration. Am J Surg 1989;157:230–236.
3. Kitahara S, Tanabe T et al. Surgical procedure for intractable aspiration. J Jpn Bronchoesophagol Soc 1999;50:603–608.
4. Takano Y, Suga M et al. Satisfaction of patients treated surgically for intractable aspiration. Chest 1999;116:1251–1256.

Electrocautery and microwaves

Bronchology and Bronchoesophagology: State of the Art.
H. Yoshimura et al., editors.

Bronchoscopic electrosurgery for tracheobronchial diseases

Hirohisa Horinouchi, Arifumi Iwamaru, Tomohiro Abiko, Katsuyuki Kuwabara, Mitsutomo Kouno, Masatoshi Gika, Makoto Sawafuji, Masazumi Watanabe, Masafumi Kawamura and Koichi Kobayashi
Department of Surgery, School of Medicine, Keio University, Tokyo, Japan

Background

Intraluminal tumor growth into the airway may cause atelectasis distal to the obstruction or sometimes cause moribund dyspnea. In the case of tracheal involvement, treatment to secure the airway is an urgent and difficult problem because severe symptoms occur only after severe stenosis is revealed.

In the field of bronchoscopy, this intervention has not been routinely performed due to limitations in space for tools. In the fields of gastroscopy and colonoscopy, however, interventional treatment like endoscopic mucosal resection (EMR) and snare polypectomy have become routine treatment modalities. We defined bronchoscopic electrosurgery as the interventional use of high frequency electrical current under bronchoscopic guidance. We have mainly used this intervention with specially developed devices to treat stenotic lesion in major tracheobronchial tree.

Aim

This study was performed to clarify the safety and effectiveness of the bronchoscopic use of high frequency electrical current in a prospective setting. Each procedure was recorded for later analysis.

Patient characteristics

From August 1997 to April 2000, 20 patients underwent bronchoscopic electrosurgery (17 males and three females, age range from 39 to 70 years, average age 60 years). Diseases indicated for bronchoscopic electrosurgery are as follows: two cases of inflammatory granulation at the larynx, one case of inflammatory polyp at the distal bronchus, three cases of primary lung cancer, 10 cases of

Address for correspondence: H. Horinouchi, Department of Surgery, School of Medicine, Keio University, 35 Shinanomachi, Shinjuku-ku, Tokyo 160-8582, Japan. Tel.: +81-3-5363-3806. Fax: +81-3-5363-3493.

lung cancer recurrence which showed involvement of tracheobronchial tree, one case of malignant lymphoma, one metastatic bronchial tumor, one case of bronchial bleeding due to intraluminal invasion of metastatic adenoidcystic carcinoma, one case of tumor invasion from metastatic mediastinal lymph node, and one case of primary osteogenic sarcoma of the lung (Table 1).

Methods

In all cases bronchoscopic electrosurgery was performed either at the Center for Diagnostic and Therapeutic Endoscopy or at the operating room in Keio University Hospital. In the majority of cases the patient was hospitalized in Keio University Hospital and underwent bronchoscopic electrosurgery there.

High frequency electrocoagulators used for this procedure are mainly PSD 10 (Olympus, Japan) or an equivalent apparatus such as USB-30, USB 300 or Valley Lab F240 (Valley Lab, USA). The tools used for this procedure were hot punch biopsy forceps, snare biopsy wire, and a coagulation tip, which were developed especially for bronchoscopic use and distributed by Olympus. The sizes of these tools used varied according to individual cases. Usually tools designed for a 2.3 mm channel were used, and occasionally 2.6 mm diameter tools were also used. All these procedures required secure ground circuit from the patient body. The power of the electrical current was adjusted according to the tools used. For punch biopsy, usually 30 watts was used; for snare resection, 20 to 30 watts were used according to the size and character of the tumor; and for the coagulation tip, 10 to 20 watts were used. In several cases, simultaneous laser ablation was applied. Relief from airway obstruction was attempted in nine patients, in one case hemostasis from intratracheal tumor was attempted, and in another 11 cases biopsy with minimal bleeding was attempted.

Results

In nine patients, tumor protruding into the bronchus prevented a full study of the distal section of the bronchial tree. In these cases, successful hot punch biopsy and/or snare resection of the tumor could be performed and observation of distal side of the tumor became possible.

Table 1.

Disease	No.
Lung cancer (primary)	3
Lung cancer (recurrence)	9
Other tumor	5
Inflammatory granuloma	3
Total	20

In four cases, the main bronchus was almost totally occupied by the tumor, and volume loss or atelectasis of ipsilateral lung was seen. These were treated by snare resection of endobronchial tumor as well as hot punch biopsy. In these cases, there were few complications and a safe procedure was performed in all except one case. One patient with osteosarcoma arisen from right upper lobe developed atelectasis of the right whole lung. Bronchofiberoptic examination showed polypoid tumor occupying the right main bronchus. The patient underwent snare resection, but the treatment failed due to the hardness of the tumor.

There was one case of endobronchial bleeding. Bleeding was observed on the surface of intratracheal metastasis of adenoidcystic carcinoma of the tongue. In this case, blood covered the surface of the tumor preventing effective hemostasis.

Specimens obtained by hot punch biopsy forceps were subjected to both pathological examination, and a cell culture for anticancer drug sensitivity test. In three cases, culture of the cancer cell was successful and the results of the following examination gave feasible treatment choices.

As regards the length of time duration for which electrical current is applied, only less than 1 s is necessary for hot punch biopsy, and a few seconds is enough for snare resection of the endobronchial tumor.

Case report

A 71-year-old female with a history of dilatational cardiomyopathy (DCM) complained of shortness of breath. A chest film at the local medical doctor showed ambiguous left main bronchus and atelectasis of left upper lobe. She underwent bronchoscopy at a local hospital revealing intrabronchial tumor extension. She was then referred to our hospital with suspected intrabronchial malignant tumor. On the day of admission, bronchofiberoptic examination showed a polypoid tumor extending from left main bronchus to lower end of the trachea. On the same day, she underwent the first bronchoscopic electrosurgery without any bleeding. Because of the patient's history of DCM, stepwise resection of the tumor by bronchoscopic electrosurgery was scheduled and three sets of procedures were performed to resect intraluminal polypoid tumor. A final bronchoscopic examination showed the tumor had arisen from left upper lobe without invasion at the orifice (Fig. 1). The patient had undergone left upper lobectomy following systemic mediastinal lymph node dissection. The pathological diagnosis was large cell carcinoma with no lymph node involvement leading pT2N0M0 lung cancer. She is alive, and there has been no apparent recurrence for 18 months following treatment.

Discussion

There are several methods to relieve an obstruction of the tracheobronchial tree. Bronchoscopic electrosurgery is one of these methods though not a well-established one [1,2]. We used this method to treat 20 consecutive patients and

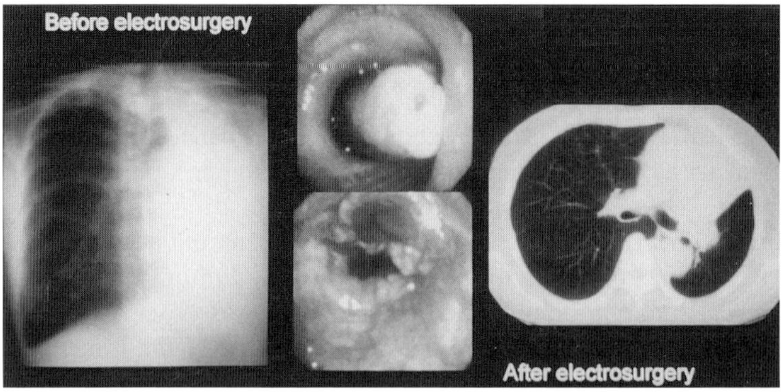

Fig. 1. Right: chest film of 71-year-old female on admission. Middle upper: bronchoscopic view of the tumor: polypoid tumor was protruded into the trachea. Middle lower: after three sets of bronchoscopic electrosurgery, left lower lobe was not involved by the tumor. Left: CAT scan after electrosurgery, airlation of left lower lobe was recovered and tumor was located in left upper lobe.

analyzed the results. Throughout this study, there was no mortality related to this procedure and no major side effects seen. In two cases only we could not achieve a satisfactory outcome. We consider these cases as having been the wrong indication. In our view, indications of bronchoscopic electrosurgery are the following diseases: 1) granulomatous polypoid lesion in tracheobronchial tree, 2) polypoid stenosis and/or obstruction of tracheobronchial tree, and 3) biopsy for easy bleeding tumorous lesion in the airway.

This method could be safely applied from the larynx to subsegmental bronchi. It is an advantageous procedure because laser ablation is sometimes dangerous when the targeted area is located in distal bronchi, as the wall of distal bronchi is thin compared to the effective depth of laser beam. We could reach subsegmental bronchi easily with usual bronchofiberoptic guidance. Although rigid bronchoscopy was advantageous for major tracheobronchial disease, general anesthesia is necessary for this procedure and it is thought to be more invasive than bronchoscopic electrosurgery. The size of the resected specimen was large enough for pathological examination, and debulking of tumor was carried out in a short period of time.

We performed these procedures under local anesthesia with a small premedication dose (mainly opioid derivatives). Preservation of spontaneous breathing is advantageous for those patients with tracheobronchial stenosis/obstruction. There was no smoke generation during the procedure, only a little steam was seen while the electrical current was administered. There is, therefore, no danger of smoke inhalation injury compared to laser therapy. Recovery of resected specimen was one of the problems incurred, and improvement of the device used seems to be necessary. The cost of this procedure is less than using laser therapy, which requires expensive apparatus [3].

Conclusion

Through our preliminary prospective study, bronchoscopic electrosurgery has been seen to be a safe and reliable intervention when applied properly in cases of intrabronchial stenosis or obstruction.

References

1. Sagawa M, Sato M, Takahashi H, Minowa H, Saito Y, Fujimura S. Electrosurgery with a fiberoptic bronchoscope and a snare for endotracheal / endobronchial tumors. J Thorac Cardiovasc Surg 1988;116:177–179.
2. Sheski FD, Mathur PM. Cryotherapy, electrocautery and brachytherapy. Clin Chest Med 1999; 20:123–138.
3. van Boxem TJ, Venmans BJ, Schramel FM, van Mourik JC, Sutedja TG. Radiographically occult lung cancer treated with fiber bronchoscopic electrocautery: a pilot study of a simple and inexpensive technique. Eur Respir J 1998;11:169–172.

Bronchology and Bronchoesophagology: State of the Art.
H. Yoshimura et al., editors.

Bronchoscopic electrosurgery for endotracheal/endobronchial tumors

Motoyasu Sagawa[1], Masami Sato[1], Akira Sakurada[1], Hiroto Takahashi[1], Itaru Ishida[1], Takeshi Oyaizu[1], Tatsuo Tanita[1], Chiaki Endo[1], Yuji Matsumura[1], Shigefumi Fujimura[1], Takashi Kondo[1], Katsuhiko Isogami[2], Toru Hasumi[2], Katsuo Usuda[3], Satomi Takahashi[3] and Yasuki Saito[4]

[1]Department of Thoracic Surgery, Institute of Development, Aging and Cancer, Tohoku University, Sendai; [2]Department of Surgery, Semine Prefectural Hospital, Semine; [3]Department of Surgery, Sendai Kosei Hospital, Sendai; and [4]Department of Thoracic Surgery, National Sendai Hospital, Sendai, Japan

Abstract. Endobronchial tumors sometimes cause stenosis of the major bronchi, which requires prompt palliative treatment. We report here 11 cases of tracheal/bronchial tumors resected by bronchoscopic electrosurgery.

There were seven men and four women, having seven malignant and four benign tumors. The stenosis of the trachea/bronchus was severe in all the patients, except one case with a squamous papilloma. For eight cases the main aims of the electrosurgery were the expansion of the tracheobronchial stenosis, for two cases it was the curative resection of the benign tumor, and for the one remaining case the main aim was the evaluation of carcinoma invasion. Endobronchial electrosurgery was performed under local anesthesia with an electrosurgical unit, a flexible bronchoscope, and a snare or forceps for endobronchial electrosurgery.

An emergent tracheotomy was needed for one case of upper tracheal tumor, and a tracheal resection was required later in another case. Electrosurgery was successfully performed in the remaining nine cases. This technique produced little smoke, and patients' symptoms, such as dyspnea and coughing, were rapidly relieved. Bronchoscopic electrosurgery is a very useful treatment and may be the first choice for cases of polypoid tumor. However, for some tracheal tumors with severe stenosis, preoperative evaluation is very important because a rigid scope may be more useful.

Keywords: bronchial stenosis, bronchofiberscope, electrosurgery, endoscopic surgery, tracheal stenosis.

Introduction

Endobronchial tumors sometimes cause the stenosis of the major bronchi, which requires rapid palliation. For the palliation of stenosis, various different techniques have been specified, e.g., Nd-YAG laser, endoscopic cryosurgery, and subepithelial injection of ethanol [1–3]. We report here 11 cases of endotracheal/endobronchial tumors resected by electrosurgery using a bronchoscope [4–6].

Address for correspondence: Motoyasu Sagawa MD, Department of Thoracic Surgery, Institute of Development, Aging and Cancer, Tohoku University, 4-1 Seiryo-machi, Aoba-ku, Sendai 980-8575, Japan. Tel.: +81-22-717-8521. Fax: +81-22-717-8526. E-mail: sagawam@idac.tohoku.ac.jp

Techniques

Endobronchial electrosurgery was performed under local anesthesia with an electrosurgical unit, a flexible bronchofiberscope/bronchovideoscope, and a snare/scalpel/forceps for endobronchial electrosurgery. Oxygen saturation, blood pressure, and electrocardiogram were monitored during the procedure. An endotracheal tube was placed, except in cases of stenosis of the upper trachea.

We have previously used conventional snares for gastro or colonoscopy. When the length of the tip of the snare is 20 mm, the width of the snare is only 5 mm, although it can be opened wider in a large space. These snares are therefore not suitable for use in narrow spaces, i.e., in the bronchial tree. However, a new snare for endobronchial electrosurgery, which we recently used, can be opened wide even in a narrow space. Here, when the length of the tip of the snare is 20 mm, the width of the snare is 14 mm.

To lasso the polypoid tumor, careful manipulation with a snare was required. Forty watts energy was applied, and the snare was pulled very slowly in order to avoid any mechanical cuts which would cause bleeding. After the polypectomy, the resected specimen was removed with grasping forceps. If possible, any large tumors were cut into a few pieces in order to avoid any difficulties in removing it through vocal folds.

Bronchoscopic findings of the cases

Figure 1 shows the bronchoscopic findings of a 77-year-old male. The left image shows that squamous cell carcinoma is obstructing 90% of the left main bronchus, and the snare is placed at the neck of the tumor. The right image shows the findings after polypectomy. The patient's symptoms of dyspnea and a severe cough were relieved rapidly.

Figure 2 shows a 95% stenosis of the left main bronchus due to endobronchial hamartoma, in a 24-year-old female. With a snare and a scalpel for electrosur-

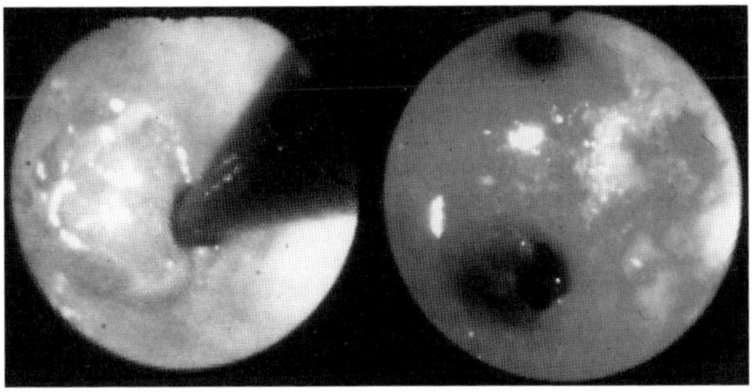

Fig. 1. Bronchoscopic findings revealed squamous cell carcinoma obstructing 90% of left main bronchus and the snare placed at the neck of the tumor (left). After polypectomy, patient's symptoms were relieved promptly (right).

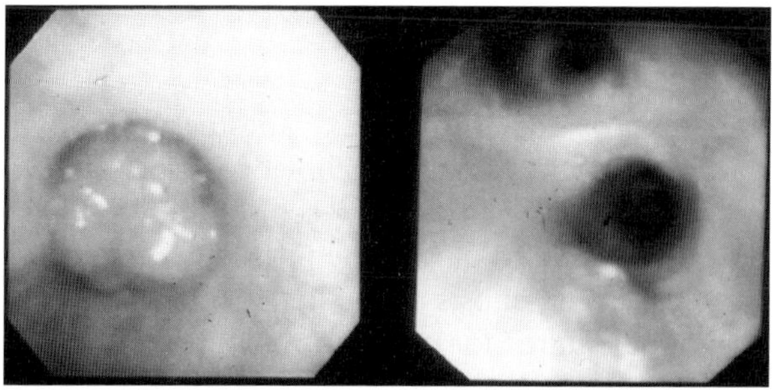

Fig. 2. Bronchoscopic findings revealed 95% stenosis of the left main bronchus. With a snare and a scalpel for electrosurgery, successful resection of the tumor was achieved.

gery, successful resection of the tumor was achieved, and no recurrence has been observed 3 years after the polypectomy.

Figure 3 shows a large endotracheal tumor, obstructing the right main bronchus. Lassoing a snare was very difficult, because the tumor was very large and the base was attached to the front side of the tracheal wall. Therefore, hot-biopsy forceps (endobronchial forceps for electrosurgery) were used. The hot-biopsy forceps were electrified after grasping the base of the tumor. After several episodes of electrification, the tumor was resected safely. The histological diagnosis was leiomyoma, and additional thoracotomy was not required.

Results

Table 1 shows a summary of the 11 cases. Patients had seven malignant and four benign tumors. The stenosis of the trachea/bronchus was severe in all the patients except one case with a squamous papilloma. The main aims of the electrosurgery were the following: the expansion of the tracheobronchial stenosis in eight cases, the curative resection of the benign tumor in two cases, and the evaluation of carcinoma invasion in one case. In two cases with tracheal severe stenosis, this pro-

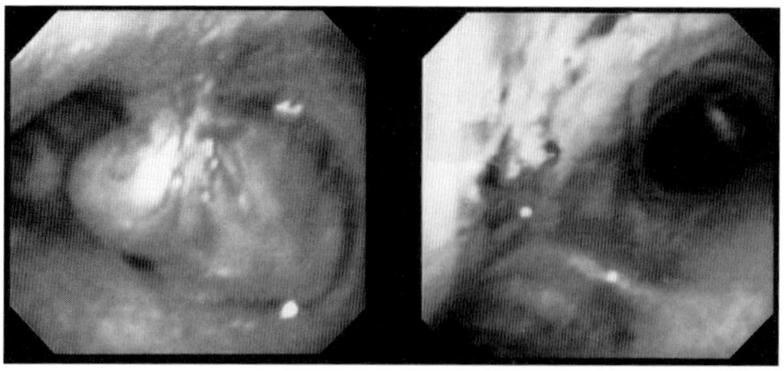

Fig. 3. Bronchoscopic findings revealed a large endotracheal tumor obstructing right main bronchus. After the polypectomy using hot-biopsy forceps, the tumor was almost completely resected, and the base of the tumor was seen at the front wall of the lower trachea.

Table 1. Summary of the cases.

No.	Location of stenosis	Histology	Stenosis	Main treatment aim	Result
1	Trachea	Adenocarcinoma	95%	Expansion of stenosis	Success
2	Trachea	Squamous papilloma	—	Curative resection	Success
3	Trachea	Squamous cell carcinoma	95%	Expansion of stenosis	Failure
4	Trachea	Leiomyoma	95%	Expansion of stenosis	Success
5	Trachea	Mucoepidermoid carcinoma	95%	Expansion of stenosis	Failure
6	Left main bronchus	Squamous cell carcinoma	100%	Evaluation of invasion	Success
7	Left main bronchus	Hamartoma	95%	Curative resection	Success
8	Left main bronchus	Adenocarcinoma	90%	Expansion of stenosis	Success
9	Right intermediate trunk	Neurinoma	100%	Expansion of stenosis	Success
10	Left lower bronchus	Squamous cell carcinoma	95%	Expansion of stenosis	Success
11	Left lower bronchus	Large cell carcinoma	90%	Expansion of stenosis	Success

cedure could not be completed. One patient required tracheal resection on the same day, and the other patient needed emergent tracheotomy. For the rest of the patients our aims were achieved without any complications, and patients' symptoms, such as dyspnea, severe coughing, and stridor, were successfully relieved.

Conclusion

Electrosurgery with a bronchoscope caused little smoke production, took a few min to resect the tumor, and patients' symptoms were relieved promptly. In some benign tumors, additional thoracotomy was not required. This form of treatment could be the first choice for the resection of the polypoid tumor in the bronchial tree. However, for some tracheal tumors with severe stenosis, preoperative evaluation is very important because using a rigid scope might be more appropriate in these cases.

References

1. Jacobson MJ, LoCicero J. Endobronchial treatment of lung carcinoma. Chest 1991;100: 837–841.
2. Marasso A, Gallo E, Massaglia GM, Onoscuri M, Bernardi V. Cryosurgery in bronchoscopic treatment of tracheobronchial stenosis. Chest 1993;103:472–474.
3. Petrou M, Goldstraw P. The management of tracheobronchial obstruction: a review of endoscopic technique. Eur J Cardio Thorac Surg 1994;8:436–441.
4. Themelin D, Duchatelet P, Boudaka W, Lamy V. Endoscopic resection of an endobronchial hypernephroma metastasis using polypectomy snare. Eur Respir J 1990;3:732–733.
5. Gerasin VA, Shafirovsky BB. Endoscopic electrosurgery. Chest 1988;93:270–274.
6. Sagawa M, Sato M, Takahashi H, Minowa M, Saito Y, Fujimura S. Electrosurgery with a fiberoptic bronchoscope and a snare for endotracheal/endobronchial tumors. J Thorac Cardiovasc Surg 1998;116:177–179.

Bronchology and Bronchoesophagology: State of the Art.
H. Yoshimura et al., editors.

Bronchoscopic microwave coagulation therapy for primary and recurrent intrabronchial malignancies

Tatsuya Yoshimasu[1,2], Shoji Oura[1], Teruhisa Sakurai[1], Takako Nakamura[1], Yozo Kokawa[1], Kenji Matsuyama[1], Yasuaki Naito[1], Yugo Nagai[2], Yasuhisa Shioji[2] and Yoshiaki Minakata[2]

Departments of [1]Thoracic and Cardiovascular Surgery and [2]Endoscopy, Wakayama Medical College, Wakayama, Japan

Abstract. Bronchoscopic microwave coagulation therapy (BMCT) was performed for 13 intrabronchial malignancies in our hospital. The malignancies were six small airway lesions (five cases of carcinoma in situ and one case of multiple endobronchial metastasis of carcinoid), and seven cases of airway stenosis due to intrabronchial malignant lesion (four cases of lung cancer and three of esophageal cancer).

Microwave coagulation was performed with 50–100 watts intensity. The BMCT procedure was completed within 1 h in all patients, and we did not experience any complications in any of the patients. Endoscopic CR was obtained in all patients with small airway lesions. Sufficient dilatation was obtained in all airway stenosis patients.

BMCT was a safe and useful procedure for radical treatment of small endobronchial malignant lesion and for relief of malignant airway stenosis.

Keywords: bronchoscopy, carcinoma in situ, lung cancer, microwave coagulation therapy.

Introduction

Bronchoscopic microwave coagulation therapy (BMCT) is a new therapeutic approach to cases of intrabronchial malignant lesion. Microwave coagulation therapy induces tumor coagulonecrosis, and it is now recognized as an efficient treatment for several malignant lesions, e.g., hepatoma, gastric carcinoma, and esophageal carcinoma [1,2].

We applied microwave coagulation therapy under bronchoscopy in the treatment of 13 intrabronchial malignant lesions, and we report this initial experience of BMCT.

Patients and Methods

The patients included five early lung cancer (carcinoma in situ of the central airway), one multiple endobronchial metastasis of carcinoid, and seven cases of

Address for correspondence: Tatsuya Yoshimasu MD, PhD, Department of Thoracic and Cardiovascular Surgery, Wakayama Medical College, 811-1 Kimiidera, Wakayama 641-8509, Japan. Tel.: +81-73-447-2300 ext. 5117. Fax: +81-73-446-4761. E-mail: yositatu@mail.wakayama-med.ac.jp airway stenosis due to intrabronchial malignant lesion (four cases of lung cancer and three cases of esophageal cancer).

Bronchoscopy was performed under modified neuroleptic analgesia (15 mg pentazocine, 5 mg midazolam) and topical administration of 2% lidocaine. Patients breathed spontaneously during the procedure. Microwave coagulation was performed with 50–100 watts intensity.

Results

The whole BMCT procedure was completed within 1 h in all patients, and we did not experience any complications in any patients. Endoscopic CR was obtained in all patients with small airway lesions. There was no local recurrence in these patients during 13 ± 8 months follow-up evaluation period. In all patients with airway stenosis, sufficient dilatation was obtained. However, in five patients, additional therapies such as LASER coagulation therapy, chemotherapy, radiotherapy, airway stent, were needed.

Discussion

Endoscopic microwave coagulation therapy (EMCT) is now recognized as an appropriate treatment for gastric carcinoma, esophageal carcinoma, and colorectal carcinoma [1,2]. It is also effective for the hemostasis of peptic ulcer [1]. The technique is safe and convenient. In our initial experience, there was no inferiority in the usefulness, safety, and convenience of BMCT compared with those treated with EMCT in the gastrointestinal tract.

BMCT was a safe and useful procedure for the radical treatment of small endobronchial malignant lesions and for relief from malignant airway stenosis.

References

1. Tabuse K, Katsumi M, Nagai Y, Kobayashi H, Noguchi H, Egawa H, Aoyama O, Mori K, Yamaue H, Azuma Y, Tsuzi T. Microwave tissue coagulation applied clinically in endoscopic surgery. Endoscopy 1985;17:149–144.
2. Yamaue H, Taimura H, Nagai Y, Johata K, Takifuji K, Iwahashi M, Tsunoda T, Noguchi K. Endoscopic microwave coagulation therapy for villous adenoma of the duodenum; a case report. Gastroenterol Jpn 1991;26:763–768.

Endobronchial tumors

Bronchology and Bronchoesophagology: State of the Art.
H. Yoshimura et al., editors.

Bronchoscopic resection of intraluminal typical carcinoid: long-term outcome

H.E. Codrington, T.J. van Boxem, J.C. van Mourik, P.E. Postmus and G. Sutedja

Department of Pulmonology, Academic Hospital Vrije Universiteit Amsterdam, Amsterdam, The Netherlands

Abstract. We reported previously that intraluminal bronchoscopic therapy (IBT) may provide an alternative for surgical resection in patients with intraluminal typical bronchial carcinoid (ITBC). The long-term outcome of 28 consecutive patients (16 males), in whom ITBC was initially treated with IBT, has been analyzed. In 16 patients (57%, CI: 43–79%; 11 males) IBT was radical. No recurrence has been documented (median follow-up period 46.9 months, range 6.1 to 102.6 months). One patient had an extraluminal residual tumor with slow progression in the last 3 years and refused surgery. In the remaining 12 patients (43%), surgery was performed for residual tumors. Surgery was radical in all cases and tumors were N_0. One patient proved to have atypical carcinoid. The follow-up period of the surgery group was 6.1 to 102.6 months (median 46.9). The average costs, including admission charges, were 6,200 US dollars for surgery vs. 2,500 US dollars for IBT. IBT is a viable, cost-effective alternative for surgery and surgical bronchoplasty and has to be considered at the initial management of patients with ITBC.

Keywords: cost-effectiveness, intraluminal bronchoscopic therapy, intraluminal typical bronchial carcinoid.

Introduction

Various bronchoscopic treatment techniques are currently available for the treatment of patients with intraluminal tumors in the central airways, both for palliation and for treatment with curative intent [2]. We reported previously in a retrospective and in a prospective study, that in a subset of patients with surgically resectable ITBC, IBT may provide an alternative for surgery in terms of complete tumor removal [1]. For ITBC, a parenchyma conserving approach such as surgical bronchoplasty has been accepted as the standard therapy [3–5]. However, this requires considerable expertise. IBT may offer a more practical alternative and is obviously less morbid than surgery. Analyses of the long-term follow-up data and the costs of treatments have been performed.

Address for correspondence: Dr G. Sutedja, Department of Pulmonology, Academic Hospital Vrije Universiteit Amsterdam, P.O. Box 7057, 1007 MB, Amsterdam, The Netherlands. Tel.: +31-20-444-4444. Fax: +31-20-444-4328. E-mail: tg.sutedja@azvu.nl

Patients and Methods

Between June 1991 and January 2000, 28 patients, 16 males, who were referred with the possible diagnosis of ITBC, were entered into this study. All the patients were fully informed about the purpose and limitations of this study [2,6]. Informed consent was obtained. Patients were included when the tumor was accessible using a fiberoptic bronchoscope. IBT, under general anesthesia, was then performed as the initial approach to evaluate the intraluminal tumor mass for accurate staging. Tumor size never exceeded a 2-cm diameter. Extensive biopsies were taken for repeat histological examinations to ensure the typical histology. When feasible, IBT was further applied for the complete eradication of the intraluminal tumor mass, to such an extent that it may enable a less extensive surgical resection. In the cases of residual disease and/or a high resolution CT-scan showing residual extraluminal disease, surgical resection was then carried out.

Results

The median age of the patients was 44 years (range: 18 to 75 years of age). The initial bronchoscopic findings, prior to treatment, are shown in Table 1. Treatment characteristics are also listed. Apart from asymptomatic mild stenosis in one patient during the follow-up period, there were no other complications. There was especially no significant bleeding. In 16 patients (57% CI; 43-79) IBT was radical. The follow-up period was 6.1 to 102.6 months (median 46.9). One patient (No. 21; Fig. 1) had an extraluminal residual tumor behind the dorsal wall of the right main stem bronchus, but refused surgery. Gradual progression was documented after a 3-year follow up. In the other 12 (43%) patients, surgical removal was necessary, and all tumors were N_0 stage. One patient proved to

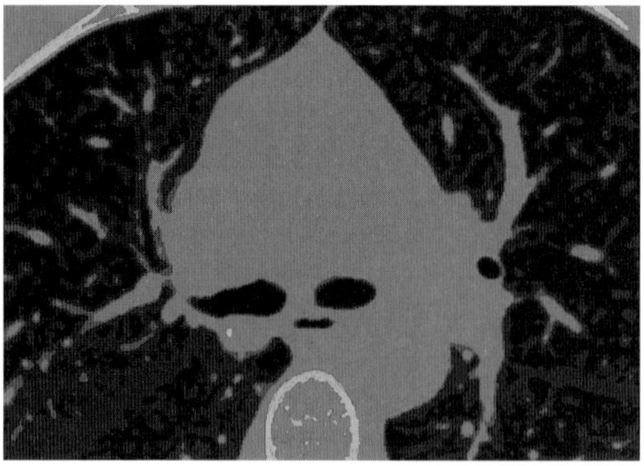

Fig. 1. Patient No. 21, with an extraluminal residual tumor, after bronchoscopic removal of the intraluminal part of the carcinoid tumor was carried out. There is a gradual progression after 3 years. No intraluminal recurrence was apparent on bronchoscopy.

Table 1. Clinical data of patients with an intraluminal typical bronchial carcinoid ⩽ 2 cm in size, initially treated with intraluminal bronchoscopic therapy with curative intent as an alternative to surgery.

No.	Gender	Age	Localisation	BT	Surgery	Hospital stay (days)	Follow-up period (months)
1	M	75	LLL	1x BE		15[a]	47.7
2	M	66	LMB	1x Nd-Yag		3	48.6
3	M	62	LLL	1xNd-Yag 1x BE		3	58.7
4	F	56	LLL	1x BE		1[b]	34.7
5	M	47	BI	2x Nd-Yag		3	70.6
6	M	46	BI	2x Nd-Yag		3	67.9
7	F	47	LMB	2x BE		2	41.2
8	M	49	RUL	1x BE		3	20.8
9	M	42	RUL	1x BE		3	49.7
10	F	41	BI	1x BE		3	57.7
11	M	39	RMB	1x BE		3	60.8
12	M	37	LMB	1xNd-YAG 1x BE		1[b]	36.7
13	M	35	LLL	1x BE		1[b]	43.4
14	M	28	LMB	1x Nd-Yag		3	102.6
15	F	25	LUL	1x Nd-Yag		3	55.7
16	F	18	RUL	1x BE		3	22.0
17	F	67	BI	1x BE		3	23.1
18	M	67	RUL?	1xBE	Lobectomy	7	22.9
19	M	63	RUL?	1xNd-YAG 2x BE	Lobectomy	15	62.1
20	F	60	LUL?	Nd-Yag	Lobectomy	20	67.2
21	F	62	RMB?	1x BE	Refused surgery	3	31.8
22	M	54	BI?	1x Nd-Yag 1x BE	Pneumonectomy	3	10.5
23	F	40	LUL?	1x Nd-Yag	Sleeve-lobectomy #	9	71.3
24	F	37	RUL?	2x BE	Sleeve-lobectomy #	6	8.8
25	M	32	LUL?	2x BE	Lobectomy	9	49.9
26	F	25	RMB?[c]	2x Nd-Yag	Bilobectomy	18	93.6
27	M	28	RML?	1x Nd-Yag	Bilobectomy	6	6.1
28	F	20	LUL?	1x BE	Lobectomy	10	47.7

Abbreviations: M = male; F = female; LLL = left lower lobe; LMB = left main bronchus; BI = bronchus intermedius; RUL = right upper lobe; RMB = right main bronchus; LUL = left upper lobe; ? = distal margin not clearly visible; BT = bronchoscopic therapy; BE = bronchoscopic electrocautery; Nd-Yag = Nd-Yag laser; # = IBT enabled a less extensive surgical resection. [a]longer hospital stay due to poorly controlled diabetes mellitus; [b]outpatient treatment; [c]surgery for stenotic scars.

have an atypical carcinoid. In another patient, no residual carcinoid was found in the resected specimen. In two (18%) of the eleven cases of surgical resections, IBT enabled a less extensive surgical approach. Two sleeve-lobectomies were performed instead of pneumonectomies. The duration of hospital stay was significantly longer in the patients who underwent surgery (9 vs. 3 days IBT). Average treatment costs, including admission charges were 6,200 US dollars vs. 2,500 US dollars for surgery and IBT, respectively.

Discussion

This prospective study was continued after our preliminary data indicated that a subgroup of patients with ITBC may be benefitted by IBT in terms of obtaining a complete response as an alternative to surgical resection [1]. The potential of IBT to completely eradicate occult lung cancer has also been established, as has been recently addressed [2,6]. The success rate of IBT depends strongly on tumor size. Occult, mostly squamous cell cancer $\leqslant$ 3-mm thick and $\leqslant$ 2-cm longitudinal axis length, has been shown to be N_0 tumor. IBT may obtain curative results and therefore serve as an alternative for surgical resection. There is no indication that the technique of IBT is an important determinant of success [6]. As IBT can achieve necrosis of several millimeters deep, we therefore presume that IBT may also play a role in treating ITBC. The relative benign nature of ITBC was an important consideration for justifying surgical bronchoplasty. This has been shown to be feasible, as the size of typical bronchial carcinoid may only allow limited surgical resection [3–5]. In our present series, tumors were intraluminal and never exceeded 2 cm in diameter. High resolution CT scans did not show gross peribronchial tumor involvement [7]. The depth necrosis of several millimeters obtained by IBT is shown to be sufficient for complete tumor eradication in a significant number of patients. We currently use electrocautery, as the probe is more maneuverable, to obtain better results [2,6]. Furthermore, the necrosis caused by electrocautery is very superficial and only several millimeters deep [7]. In case of incomplete bronchoscopic resection, scar formation will not be too extensive and, therefore, not hamper the surgeons when performing a limited resection.

The typical carcinoid behaves differently from the atypical variant [8,9]. This justifies a more conservative approach. Accurate histology is very important. On the other hand, the prognosis of an atypical carcinoid, if completely resected, is not influenced by the radicality of surgery, but by its malignant tendency which may mimic the behavior of a neuro-endocrine tumor to metastasize, such as in small cell lung cancer [9]. IBT, in ITBC, enables us to take extensive biopsies to assure proper histology staging, but at the same time may allow complete tumor eradication. The long follow-up data shows that after complete tumor eradication with IBT, a "wait and see" approach seems justifiable. This may raise the question as to whether the iceberg phenomenon is an important concept in order to justify an immediate surgical intervention. Both extraluminal growth and invisible distal margins are limitations for the success of IBT and in these cases surgical resection is the only alternative.

Conclusion

Intraluminal bronchoscopic treatment is a viable and cost-effective treatment, which is also a good alternative for surgery in a subset of patients with intraluminal typical bronchial carcinoid. The relatively benign nature of this disease justifies a tissue conserving approach such as bronchoscopic surgery and surgical bronchoplasty. Our data showed that in a significant number of the patients (57%, CI: 43-79%) IBT provided an elegant and less morbid approach than the current standard of immediate surgical intervention.

References

1. van Boxem T, Venmans B, van Mourik, Postmus PE, Sutedja G. Bronchoscopic treatment of intraluminal typical carcinoid: a pilot study. J Thorac Cardiovasc Surg 1998;116:402–406.
2. van Boxem TJ, Venmans BJ, Postmus PE, Sutedja TG. Curative endobronchial therapy in early-stage nonsmall cell lung cancer. J Bronchol 1999;6:198–206.
3. Okike N, Bernatz PE, Payne WS, Woolner LB, Leonard PF. Bronchoplastic procedures in the treatment of carcinoid tumors of the tracheobronchial tree. J Thorac Cardiovasc Surg 1978;76: 281–291.
4. Stamatis F, Freitag L, Greschuchna D. Limited and radical resection for tracheal and bronchopulmonary carcinoid tumor. Eur J Cardio Thorac Surg 1990;4:527–533.
5. Schreurs AJM, Westermann CJJ, van den Bosch JMM, van der Schueren RGJRA, Brutel de la Riviere A et al. A 25-year follow-up of 93 resected typical carcinoid tumor of the lung. J Thorac Cardiovasc Surg 1992;104:1470–1475.
6. van Boxem TJ, Postmus PE, Sutedja TG. Photodynamic therapy, Nd-YAG laser and electrocautery for treating early-stage intraluminal cancer. Which to choose? (In press).
7. Sutedja G, Golding RP, Postmus PE. High resolution computed tomography in patients referred for intraluminal bronchoscopic therapy with curative intent. Eur Respir J 1996;9:1020–1023.
8. Arrigoni MG, Woolner LB, Bernartz PE. Atypical carcinoid tumors of the lung. J Thorac Cardiovasc Surg 1972;64:413–421.
9. Travis W, Rush W, Flieder D, Falk R, Fleming M, Gal A, Koss M. Survival analysis of 200 pulmonary neuroendocrine tumors with clarification of criteria for atypical carcinoid and its separation from typical carcinoid. Am J Surg Path 1998;22(8):934–944.

Bronchology and Bronchoesophagology: State of the Art.
H. Yoshimura et al., editors.

A case of endotracheobronchial metastasis of colon cancer successfully treated by laser therapy and endobronchial brachytherapy

Hidehito Kawai, Motoshi Takao, Kouji Onoda, Takatsugu Shimono, Kuniyoshi Tanaka, Hideto Shimpo and Isao Yada
Department of Thoracic Surgery, School of Medicine, Mie University, Tsu, Mie, Japan

Abstract. Seven years ago, a 45-year-old female underwent a left hemicolectomy for the treatment of descending colon cancer. She also underwent partial resection of bilateral metastatic lung cancer both 4 and 2 years ago. She had complained of coughs, hemoptysis and dyspnea for 6 months. Fiberoptic bronchoscopy was performed. Two tumors were detected in the lower trachea and truncus intermedius, which was completely occluded. They were revealed to be tracheobronchial metastases of colon adenocarcinoma. Emergent flexible fiberoptic bronchoscope guided laser therapy was performed under general anesthesia. However, it was also necessary to perform external radiotherapy and endobronchial brachytherapy, because residual viable tumor cells were detected by the bronchoscopic biopsy after laser therapy. Another session of laser therapy was performed to eradicate residual tumor cells which were detected 1 month after radiotherapy. She has been free from tracheobronchial recurrence for 19 months since her first session of laser therapy.

Keywords: brachytherapy, endbronchial metastasis, endtracheal metastasis, KTP laser.

Introduction

Endotracheobronchial metastasis of colon cancer is rare. Here we report a case of endotracheobronchial metastasis of colon cancer, which was successfully treated by laser therapy and endobronchial brachytherapy.

The case

A 45-year-old Japanese female who presented herself at our hospital with complaints of dyspnea, cough and hemoptysis in January 1999. She underwent a left hemicolectomy for the treatment of descending colon cancer. Then she further underwent partial resection of bilateral metastatic lung cancer 4 and 2 years ago. On the chest X-ray, taken on admission, there was a white line which was an atelectasis in the right middle lung field. Ventilatory flow volume analysis showed a pattern of airway obstruction. Fiberoptic bronchoscopy was performed. Two tumors were detected in the lower trachea and truncus intermedius, which

Address for correspondence: Hidehito Kawai MD, Department of Thoracic Surgery, School of Medicine, Mie University, 2-174 Edobashi, Tsu, Mie 514-008507, Japan. Tel.: +81-59231-5116. Fax: +81-59231-2845. E-mail: takao@clin.medic. mie-u.ac.jp

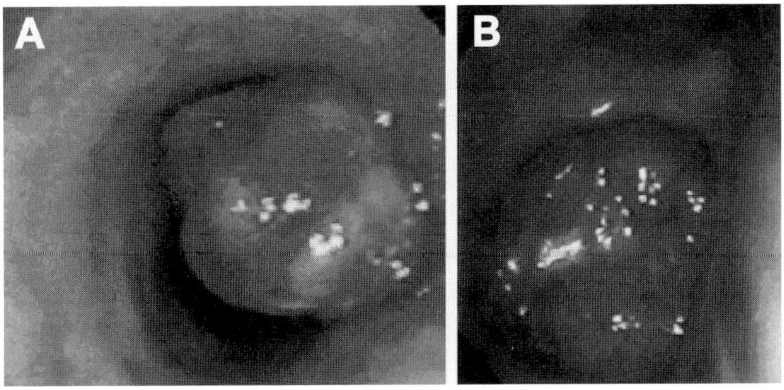

Fig. 1. **A:** An endotracheal tumor was detected in the lower trachea. **B:** An endobronchial tumor was occluding the entrance to the right intermediate bronchus. These tumors were soft and easy to bleed.

was completely occluded (Fig. 1). They were revealed to be tracheobronchial metastases of colon adenocarcinoma. Emergent flexible fiberoptic bronchoscope guided KTP laser therapy was performed under general anesthesia. After this treatment, her symptoms improved remarkably. The endotracheal and endobronchial tumors were almost removed (Fig. 2). However, then she also had to undergo external radiotherapy and endobronchial brachytherapy, because residual viable tumor cells were detected at the truncus intermedius by bronchoscopic biopsy. Another session of KTP laser therapy was performed in order to eradicate the residual tumor cells which were detected 1 month after radiotherapy. She has been free from tracheobronchial recurrence for 19 months since her first session of laser therapy.

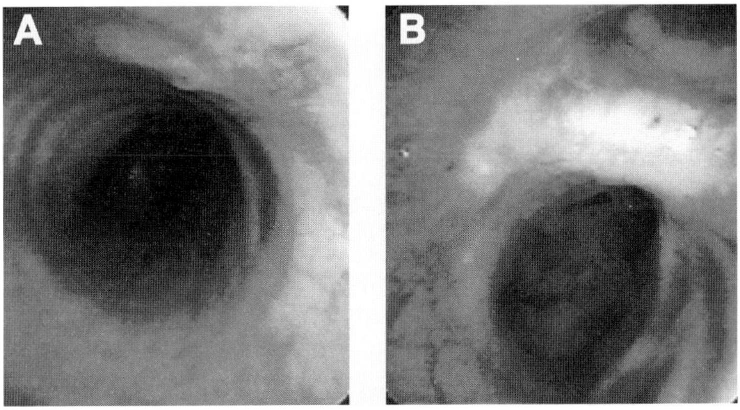

Fig. 2. The postoperative bronchoscopic findings. Both the tumors were almost removed and the airway was no longer obstructed. However, residual tumor cells were detected through fiberoptic biopsy at the truncus intermedius. **A:** Endotracheal. **B:** Endobronchial.

Conclusion

Pelagia Katsimbri states that endobronchial metastasis are less frequent than other types of intrathoracic metastasis [1]. The most common primary sites of endobronchial metastases are the breast, colorectal and uterus. Prognosis is generally poor, averaging 1 to 2 years. Concerning the issue of quality of life, laser therapy and brachytherapy are the treatment of choice for endobronchial metastasis.

Reference

1. Katsimbri PP et al. Endobronchial metastases secondary to solid tumors; report of eight cases and review of the literature. Lung Cancer 2000;28:163–170.

Bronchology and Bronchoesophagology: State of the Art.
H. Yoshimura et al., editors.

Endotracheal/endobronchial metastases: a clinicopathological study with special reference to developmental modes

T. Kiryu, E. Matsui, H. Hoshi and K. Shimokawa
Department of Radiology, Gifu University School of Medicine, Gifu City, Japan

Abstract. *Background.* Endotracheal/endobronchial metastases (EEM) from nonpulmonary neoplasms are rare. However, their definition and developmental modes have not yet been fully elucidated.

Methods. EEM were defined as documented nonpulmonary neoplasms metastatic to the subsegmental or more proximal central bronchus, in a bronchoscopically visible range. The clinical and pathological features of 16 cases were reviewed, with special emphasis on developmental modes. The relationship with the associated bronchus was proposed as follows: Type I: direct metastasis to the bronchus, Type II: bronchial invasion by a parenchymal lesion, Type III: bronchial invasion by mediastinal or hilar LN metastasis, and Type IV: peripheral lesions extended along the proximal bronchus.

Results. Primary tumors included colorectal in six cases, breast in three cases, uterus in two cases, osteosarcoma of the bone in two cases, and maxillary, larynx, and parotid carcinoma in one case. The mean recurrence interval was 65.3 months. The relationship with the associated bronchus was Type I: 5, Type II: 1, Type III: 4, and Type IV: 9 cases. Three patients underwent surgical resection. One patient has remained well for 5 years after their operation. Median and mean survival times were 9 months and 15.5 months, respectively.

Conclusion. The mean recurrence interval was long, at 65.3 months, but the mean survival time was short, at 15.5 months. Type I accounted for only five of 16 cases. Type II was found in only one case. It is thought that this type is a rare form. Type IV affected nine cases. Treatment plans must be individualized, because in some cases, long-term suvival can be expected.

Keywords: developmental mode, endotracheal/endobronchial metastasis, flexible bronchoscopy, prognosis, pulmonary metastasis, recurrence interval.

Introduction

Endotracheal/endobronchial metastases (EEM) from nonpulmonary tumors are uncommon. Some investigators have reported comprehensive studies on this topic [1–3]. However, the frequencies of "endobronchial metastasis" are variable by definition, ranging from 2 to 50% of pulmonary metastases from extrathoracic neoplasms [1–3].

A variety of tumors have been associated with EEM. These include breast, colorectal, renal, ovarian, thyroid, uterine, testicular, nasopharynx, prostate, and adrenal carcinomas, sarcomas, melanomas, and plasmacytomas, although breast [4–6], colorectal [7,8] and renal carcinomas [9–12] predominate [1,13].

Address for correspondence: Takuji Kiryu MD, Department of Radiology, Gifu University School of Medicine, 40 Tsukasa-machi, Gifu City, 500-8705 Japan. Tel.: +81-58-265-1241. Fax: +81-58-265-9028. E-mail: kiryu@cc.gifu-u.ac.jp

The developmental modes have not been fully described previously, and the definition of EEM varies according to the author. One definition includes only direct metastasis to the tracheobronchial wall [13], and the other, secondary involvement, as well as direct invasion [14].

The treatments and management employed in EEM are determined by the histological identification of the primary tumor, its biological behavior, anatomic location, evidence of other metastatic sites, and the patient's performance status [13,14]. It is very important that treatment is individualized [14]. Survival is dependent to a great degree upon the biological behavior of the particular tumor and its responsiveness to the palliative measures available [13].

In this article, we studied developmental modes and proposed the following four developmental conditions in relation to the associated bronchus: Type I: direct metastasis to the bronchus, Type II: bronchial invasion by a parenchymal lesion, Type III: bronchial invasion by mediastinal or hilar LN metastasis, and Type IV: a peripheral lesion extended along the proximal bronchus and assesed as having clinical and pathological features of EEM with special reference to developmental modes.

Patients and Methods

We defined EEM as bronchoscopically visible nonpulmonary tumors metastatic to the the subsegmental or more proximal central bronchus and lesions histologically identical to primary tumors previously documented.

Since January 1990, 38 patients with pulmonary metastasis from extrathoracic malignant lesions were diagnosed by fiberoptic bronchoscopic or surgical procedures, and 16 of them (42.1%) had EEM as defined above, the findings for which form the basis of this article.

The patients' medical records were retrospetively reviewed. Follow-up information was obtained on all patients through medical records. Histological diagnosis was obtained in all cases by direct biopsy with a flexible bronchoscope and reviewed by one of the authors (K.S.) to confirm the diagnosis. Careful histological evaluation was made to establish tissue identity between the primary extrapulmonary tumors and EEM.

We evaluated the recurrence interval from the diagnosis of the primary lesions to the diagnosis of EEM, operability, survival time, and the developmental modes. The developmental modes were assessed according to the following five criteria using chest X-ray, computed tomography, bronchoscopy, and histology: 1) location in the tracheobronchial tree, 2) the number of lesions, solitary or multiple, 3) the laterality of lesions, right or left, 4) the depth of lesions, mucosal invasion or submucosal invasion, and 5) the relationship with the associated bronchus (Type I: direct metastasis to the bronchus, Type II: bronchial invasion by a parenchymal lesion, Type III: bronchial invasion by the mediastinal or hilar LN metastasis, and Type IV: peripheral lesions extended along the proximal bronchus) (Fig 1).

Results

Table 1 shows patient characteristics. In 10 patients free of symptoms, abnormal findings on chest radiographs during the follow-up period were found and they underwent further diagnositic evaluation.

Table 2 shows clinical findings. The time from the diagnosis of the primary nonpulmonary tumors to the diagnosis of EEM was defined as the recurrence interval [13]. The mean recurrence interval for all cases was 65.3 months and the respective primary sites were as follows: colon and rectum (59.4 months; range 1 to 112 months), breast (86.3 months; range 78 to 92 months), bone (63.5 months; range 31 to 96 months), uterus (18.0 months; range 0 to 36 months), maxilla (196 months), larynx (34 months), and parotid (31 months). Although the range was large, a patient with maxilla carcinoma, the histology of which was adenoid cystic carcinoma, had the longest recurrence interval (196 months), whereas a patient with uterus carcinoma, whose histology was adeno-squamous carcinoma, had the shortest (0 months).

The chest radiography images in patients with EEM were quite variable. All patients revealed abnormal findings. These included multiple pulmonary nodules in six cases (37.5%), hilar masses in five cases (31.3%), atelectasis in four cases (25.0%), and mediastinal lymphadenopathy in three cases (18.8%).

Lesions were located in the trachea (five patients; seven lesions), main bronchus (six patients; eight lesions), truncus intermedius (six patients), lobar bronchus (four patients), segmental bronchus (six patients), and subsegmental bronchus (two patients).

Six patients had synchronous, and one metachronous, multiple endobronchial metastases. Two of the six patients with colorectal carcinomas had multiple lesions, one patient had synchronous multiple lesions in the truncus intermedius

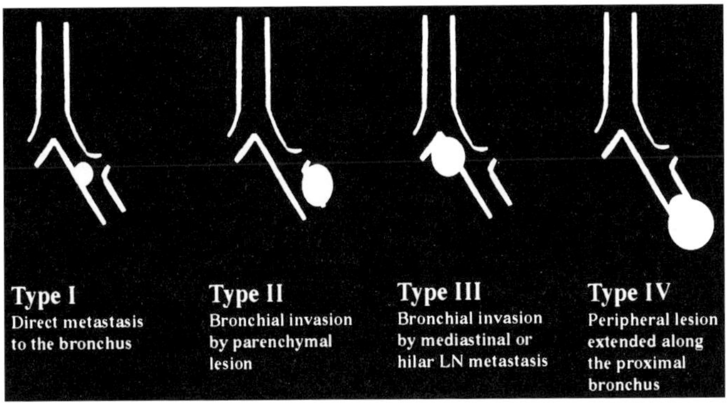

Fig. 1. Four developmental modes of endobronchial metastases and the relationship to the associated bronchus. Type I: direct metastasis to the bronchus; Type II: bronchial invasion by a parenchymal lesion; Type III: bronchial invasion by mediastinal or hilar LN metastasis; and Type IV: peripheral lesions extended along the proximal bronchus.

Table 1. Patient characteristics.

No.	16
M/F	7/9
Mean age (years)	54.0 (15–76)
Symptoms (No.):	
Coughing	5
Dysnea	1
Asymptomatic	10

and segmental bronchus, and the other showed metachronous lesions; one lesion in the left main brochus (40 months after diagnosis of primary site), three lesions in the trachea and two lesions in the right main bronchus (46 months after diagnosis of the primary site). All three patients with breast carcinomas had multiple lesions. One patient with osteosarcoma of the bone and another with uterus carcinoma had multiple lesions.

Twenty of 25 lesions (80.0%), except for seven tracheal lesions, were recognized in the right side and only five lesions in the left side. EEM from colon and rectum cancers, breast cancers, and osteosarcomas of the bone were distributed on both side, but six lesions from uterus, maxilla, larynx, and parotid cancers were seen only in the right side. Nineteen of all the lesions (59.4%) involved the submucosal layer, and only 13 lesions developed in the mucosal layer.

Table 3 shows the relationship between lesions and the associated bronchi as defined above, Type I: five patients (12 lesions), Type II: one patient (one lesion), Type III: four patients (eight lesions), Type IV: nine patients (10 lesions). One patient with rectum cancer had one Type IV lesion in the left main bronchus and five Type I lesions in the trachea and right main bronchus 6 months after surgical resection of the first lesion metachrounously (Figs. 2 and 3). Two of the three patients with breast cancer showed Type I lesions, and one of them demonstrated a marked lymphangitis carcinomatosa in the submucosal layer. Both patients with uterus carcinomas had Type III lesions (Fig. 4). One patient with

Table 2. Clinical findings.

Primary site	No.	Recurrence interval (months)	Operability		Survival (months)	
			Operable	Inoperable	Mean	Range
Colon/rectum	6	1–112 (59.4)	1	6	8.7	2–14
Breast	3	78–92 (86.3)		3	11.0	3–19
Bone	2	31–96 (63.5)	2		36.5	7–66
Uterus	2	0–36 (18.0)		2	1	
Maxilla	1	196		1	31	
Larynx	1	34		1	9	
Parotid	1	31		1	9	
Total	15	0–196 (65.3)	3	14	15.5	1–66

Table 3. Developmental modes of endotracheal/endobronchial metastases and the relationship with the associated bronchi.

Primary site	No.	Type I	Type II	Type III	Type IV
Colon/rectum	5 (13)	1 (5)		1	6 (7)
Breast	3 (8)	2 (5)		1 (3)	
Bone	2 (3)	1			2
Uterus	2 (4)			2 (4)	
Maxilla	1		1		
Larynx	1				1
Parotid	1	1			
Total	15 (31)	5 (12)	1	4 (8)	9 (10)

( ) = No. of lesions.

osteosarcoma of the bone showed both Type I and Type IV lesions in the left lower bronchus synchronously. A patient with maxillary carcinoma had a Type II lesion in the right truncus intermedius, in contact with which a metastatic nodule was recognized in the pulmonary parenchyma (Fig. 5). One patient with parotid cancer had a Type I lesion in the membranous portion of the right main bronchus.

At the time of EEM, nine out of 16 (56.3%) patients had extrabronchial metastatic disease. These extrabronchial metastatic sites included the pulmonary parenchyma (n = 6), pleura (n = 3), brain (n = 3), liver (n = 2), and bone (n = 1).

Three patients, two with endobronchial metastases from osteosarcoma of the bone and one with metastatic colon cancer, had localized endobronchial metastases, but no metastatic lesions in other sites. These three patients underwent surgery; a right lower lobectomy (bone), a left lower lobectomy (bone), and a left lower lobectomy (colon). One patient with metastatic osteosarcoma died of brain

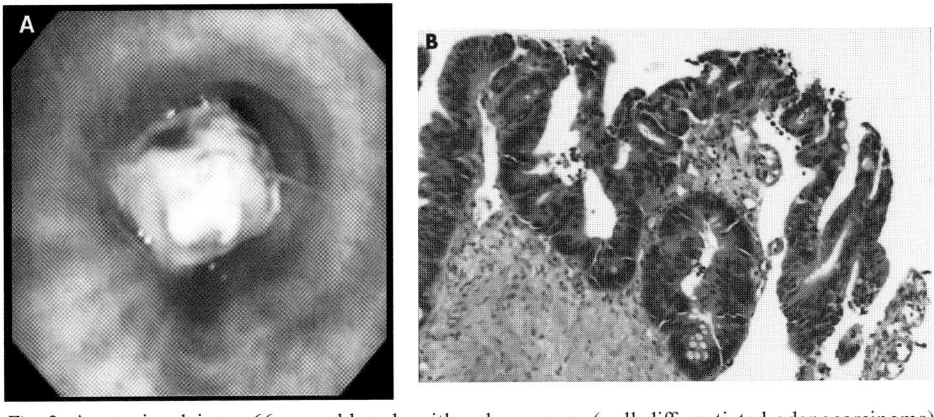

Fig. 2. A case involving a 66-year-old male with colon cancer (well-differentiated adenocarcinoma) Type IV. **A:** Bronchofiberscopy revealed a polypoid lesion covered by necrotic tissue partially obstructing the left main bronchus. **B:** A biopsy specimen of the polypoid lesion revealed papillary growth of neoplastic cells with mucosal invasion. Chest radiography showed left lower lobe atelectasis.

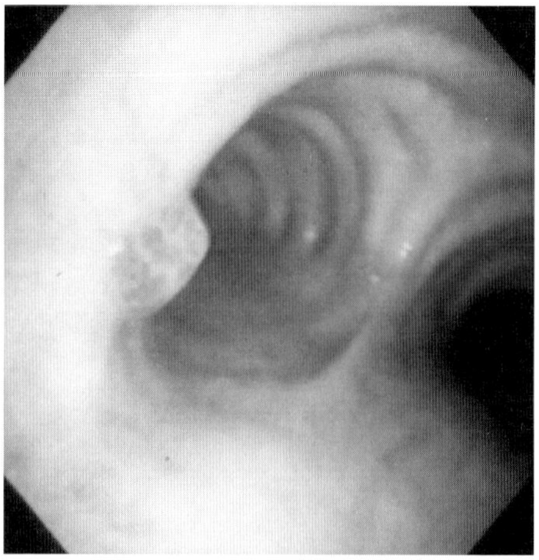

Fig. 3. A case involving a 66-year-old male with colon cancer (same case as in Fig. 2) Type I. Bronchofiberscopy 6 months after surgical resection of the lesion, shown in Fig. 2, revealed multiple small polypoid lesions in the trachea (3 lesions) and right main bronchus (2 lesions). A biopsy specimen of the polypoid lesion revealed papillary growth of neoplastic cells. Chest radiography and computed tomography scans showed no abnormal findings around the tracheal wall.

metastasis 6 months after the operation, and the other patient has remained well for 5 years without any postoperative sign of recurrence. One patient with metastatic colon cancer has survived with recurrence in the tracheobronchial tree 6 months after the operation.

The median and mean survival times from the diagnosis of EEM to death were 9 months (range: 1 to 66 months) and 15.5 months, respectively, and the mean survival times of patients with the respective primary sites were as follows: colon and rectum (8.7 months; range: 2 to 14 months), breast (11.0 months; range: 3 to 19 months), bone (36.5 months; range: 7 to 66 months), uterus (1 month), maxilla (31 months), larynx (9 months), and parotid (9 months). Although the range was wide, a patient with osteosarcoma of the bone had the longest survival time (66 months), whereas a patient with uterus carcinoma had the shortest (1 month) (Table 2).

Discussion

The frequencies of "endobronchial metastasis" are variable, that is, the prevalence depends on how they are defined, ranging from approximately 2 to 50% [1–3,13–18]. If one includes invasion of tracheobronchial structures by parenchymal or lymph node masses, the prevalence rate is higher. However, if they are defined as only direct metastases to the tracheobronchial tree from extrapulmonary lesions, it is much lower. We defined EEM as bronchoscopically visible nonpulmonary tumors, metastatic to the subsegmental or more proximal

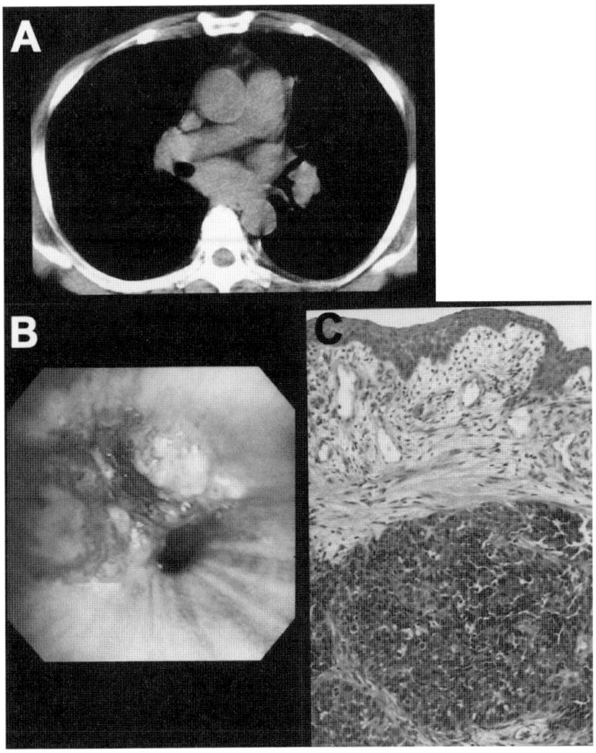

Fig. 4. A case involving a 53-year-old female with uterine cervical cancer (adenosquamous carcinoma) Type III. **A:** A chest computed tomography scan of the truncus intermedius level showed bulky mediastinal lymphoadenopathy located in the carina. **B:** Bronchofiberscopy revealed a sessile, lobulated nodule in the truncus intermedius. **C:** A biopsy specimen of the lesion revealed a neoplastic solid nest in the submucosal layer.

central bronchus and with lesions histologically identical to primary tumors previously documented. In our series, 16 of 38 (42.1%) patients with pulmonary metastasis from extrathoracic malignant lesions had EEM as defined above.

King et al. were the first to emphasize the frequency with which metastatic disease involves the bronchi. They included primary and secondary tracheobronchial tree involvement and did not restrict the order of bronchus. They reported the metastatic involvement of the bronchus, on the basis of pathological studies, in 18.5% of patients (20 of 109 consecutive autopsies) with pulmonary metastatic disease [2]. Braman et al. limited the definition of endobronchial metastases to the involvement of the lobar or main bronchus and reported a 2% prevalence (five of 244 cases) in a autopsy review series [1] Baumgartner defined metastases to the tracheobronchial tree as primary, not secondary, involvement of these structures, and the prevalence rate was approximately 2% [13].

A variety of primary tumors have been associated with EEM, although breast, colon, and renal carcinomas predominate [1,13–16]. In our series, six of 16

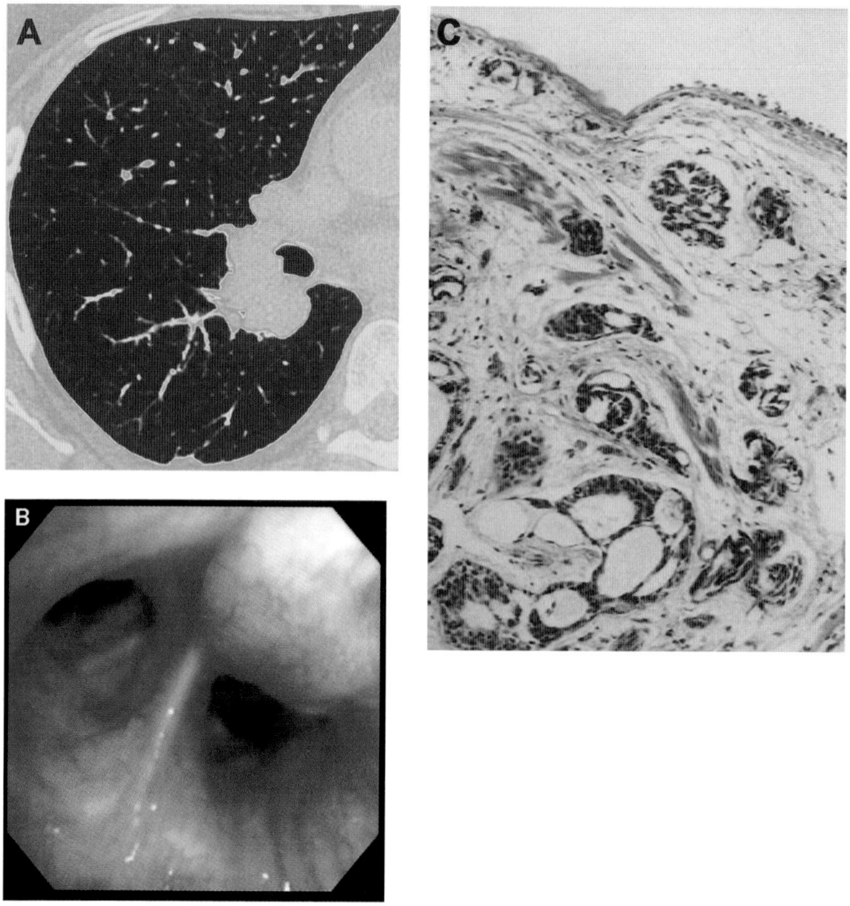

Fig. 5. A case involving a 50-year-old female with maxillary cancer (adenoid cystic carcinoma) Type II. **A:** A chest computed tomography scan of the truncus intermedius level revealed a nodule located in contact with the bronchial posterior wall. **B:** Bronchofiberscopy showed a submucosal nodule in the distal truncus intermedius. **C:** A biopsy specimen revealed cribriform growth by neoplastic cells in the submucosal layer.

patients had colorectal carcinomas, and three of them breast carcinomas. Sarcomas are also capable of causing EEM [19,20], and we reported two patients with endobronchial metastases due to osteogenic sarcomas in this article.

The symptoms and roentgenographic manifestations of patients with EEM were identical to those associated with primary bronchogenic carcinomas [1,13,14]. As a result, it was difficult to differentiate between the two diagnoses on the basis of the symptoms and roentgenological signs alone [14,16]. The most common symptoms are coughing and hemoptysis, with dyspnea and wheezing occuring less often. However, the lesions are asymptomatic in some patients. Heitmiller et al. reported that 52% of their patients were asymptomatic [16]. In our series, 10 of 16 cases (62.5%) were asymptomatic and abnormal shadows were detected with follow-up chest radiography. The roentgenographic findings are quite variable. Patients may present evidence of atelectasis, multiple pulmonary nodules, hilar masses, mediastinal lymphoadenopathy, or a normal chest X-ray film [1,13]. Colletti et al. reported that computed tomography was sensitive in detecting and localizing endobronchial neoplasms, including metastatic lesions and correlated well with bronchoscopic findings [21].

Diagnosis of EEM with fiberoptic bronchoscopy is usually precise [13]. Bronchoscopic results revealed EEM and were diagnostic in all our patients. The histological identification of the tissue can be correlated with previously documented primary tumors or can serve as a guideline for subsequent investigation in those cases in which the underlying tumor has not been identified [13]. Bronchoscopy should be performed early in patients with breast, colon, and renal cancer, who have pulmonary symptoms such as coughing and a normal chest roentgenogram. Extra pulmonary EEM are likely to be found [16].

As has been stated, EEM tend to occur at a significant interval from the diagnosis of the primary tumor, indicating a relatively slow disease progression [13,14]. Baumgartner et al., Katsimbri et al. and Heitmiller et al. reported that the mean intervals from the diagnosis of the primary carcinoma to the diagnosis of tracheobronchial tree involvement were 5.4 years (n = 8), 41 months (n = 8) and 59.9 months (n = 23), respectively. Baumgartner et al. and Salud et al. found that the median interval was 5.0 years and 50.4 months (n = 32), respectively [13–16]. In our series, the mean recurrence interval for all cases was 65.3 months. The longest recurrence interval was 196 months in a patient with maxilla carcinoma, whereas the shortest was 0 months in a patient with uterus carcinoma.

There was no predilection for the airway location in our series, although Heitmiller et al. reported the lobar bronchus was the site in 19 of 23 patients [16]. The primary sites of endotracheal metastases included the breast (two patients), colon (one patient) and uterus (two patients) in our series. Seven of 16 patients had multiple lesions. The primary sites were as follows: the breast (three patients), colon (two patients), bone (one patient), and uterus (one patient). All three patients with breast carcinomas had multiple lesions. Six patients had synchronous multiple lesions, and another patient with colon cancer had metachronous multiple lesions. Of particular interest is the fact that 20 out of 25 lesions, except for seven tracheal lesions (80.0%), were recognized in the right side, but only five in the left side. The cause of this predilection is uncertain.

We also found that 19 of 32 lesions (59.4%) involved the submucosal layer, and 13 lesions developed in the mucosal layer. Schoenbaum et al. stated that tumor cells carried to the lung by the pulmonary arteries or lymphatic channels may enter the peribronchial lymphatics and, after antegrade or retrograde propagation, give rise to a discrete subepithelial deposit of tumor growth in the bronchial wall [22]. Heitmiller et al. reported that deep endobronchial biopsy specimens in 13 patients revealed metastases in the bronchial submucosa, and in nine patients biopsy specimens from exophytic endobronchial tumors revealed only metastatic tumors [16]. They stated that histochemical studies of biopsy specimens from patients with known submucosal involvement failed to show tumors within the submucosal lymphatics or blood vessels, and the most likely explanation was that the metastatic tumor migrated along the lymphatics with subsequent egress into the submucosal space.

We proposed four Types in the relationship between metastatic lesions and the associated bronchi: Type I: direct metastases to the bronchus, Type II: bronchial invasion by a parenchymal lesion, Type III: bronchial invasion by mediastinal or hilar LN metastasis, and Type IV: peripheral lesions extended along the proximal bronchus. As stated by Baumgartner et al., we should estimate EEM by separating primary lesions, direct bronchial wall metastases, and secondary lesions due to invasion of tracheobronchial structures by parenchymal or lymph node masses because of the difference in pathogenesis and clinical significance between each of the lesions [13]. In the four Types proposed by us, primary lesions correspond to Type I, and secondary ones to Type II, III, and IV. In our series, Type I accounted for only five of 16 patients (31.3%): two with breast cancer, one with colon cancer, one with osteogenic sarcoma, and one with parotid cancer. As for secondary lesions, Type II accounted for only one patient with maxillary carcinoma. It is thought that this type is a rare condition. On the other hand, Type IV affected nine of 16 patients (56.3%). It is thought this type is the most common condition.

The treatments and management employed in EEM are determined by the histological identification of the primary tumor and its biological behavior, anatomic location of lesions, evidence of other metastatic sites, and the patient's performance status, and must be individualized [13,15]. Treatments and management include surgical excision, local radiotherapy, especially endobronchial irradiation [23], chemotherapy [13], and transbronchial endoscopic procedures such as, photodynamic therapy, electrocoagulation, forceps, intratumoral ethanol injections, diathermic snares and prosthetic stents, and Nd:Yag laser-debulking therapy [15]. Surgical resection should be confined to patients with localized disease, because most patients have extrabronchial metastatic disease at the time of EEM [15], and mediastinal lymph node metastases are frequently present at the time of postmortem examination [1]. Salud et al. reported that at the time of endobronchial metastases, 20 of 23 (87%) patients had extrabronchial metastatic disease [15], and in our series nine of 16 (56.3%) patients had extrabronchial metastatic disease. Braman also emphasized that mediastinoscopy must be performed to evaluate the possibility of mediastinal involvement before consideration is given to surgical excision of the lesion [1]. However, long survival is expected after surgical resection in some cases with localized disease. In our series, a patient with metastatic osteosarcoma in the left lower bronchus has been alive and well without evidence of recurrence 5 years after a left lower lobectomy.

Survival is dependent to a great degree upon the biological behavior of the particular tumor and its responsiveness to the treatments and management available [13]. Although the recurrence-free interval from diagnosis of primary tumor to the discovery of EEM is almost 5 years, survival after the diagnosis of EEM is poor because it is generally a manifestation of a far-advanced disease stage. Heitmiller et al. reported that the mean survival time from the diagnosis of EEM to death was only 12.5 months (range: 1 to 26 months)[16], and in our series it was 15.5 months (range: 1 to 66 months). However, some studies have reported long-term survival. Ettensohn et al. reported a 21-month mean survival in patients with endobronchial metastases of the breast [6], and Baumgartner et al. reported an overall 32-month mean survival in their patients and concluded that aggressive treatment should be considered in these patients, because survival after treatment in this type of metastatic tumor is not necessarily short [13]. Therefore, it should be emphasized that treatment plans must be individualized, because some patients can achieve long-term suvival [15,16].

If we evaluate survival times according to developmental mode as proposed above, survival times of each Type are as follows: Type I: 14 months, Type II: 31 months, Type III: 2 months, and Type IV: 18 months. Survival time of Type III is the shortest and all three operable cases in our series were Type IV. Although a small number of limited cases were evaluated in our series, the developmental mode of EEM may be one of survival-determinant factors.

We should also pay careful attention to a few clinical problems with EEM. Firstly, the symptoms and roentgenographic manifestations of patients with EEM are indistinguishable from those associated with a centrally located primary bronchogenic carcinoma [1], especially when there has been a long recurrence interval between the occurrence of the primary tumor and EEM, or when the discovery of EEM antedates diagnosis of the primary tumor [13,24]. Gerle and Felson, in a review of endobronchial metastases from renal cell carcinomas, reported that in seven of 17 such patients the metastasis was diagnosed before the primary tumor was identified [12]. Secondly, there are several situations in which bronchial biopsy may not prove diagnostic [1]. Salud et al. stated that no absolute histopathological criteria differentiate primary and secondary tumors, although the clinical setting and immunohistochemical techniques can be useful indicators [15]. Rosenblatt et al. reported that, on occasion, metastatic adenocarcinomas may occur with areas of undifferentiated cellularity interspersed with areas of greater differentiation. This may be a source of confusion and result in an inaccurate diagnosis of undifferentiated bronchogenic adenocarcinoma [18]. Braman et al. also reported that in some instances it may be impossible to differentiate metastatic involvement of the bronchus by an asymptomatic extrathoracic adenocarcinoma from a primary central adenocarcinoma of the lung [1]. Another source of misdiagnosis may arise when a squamous cell carcinomas presents itself as a polypoid endobronchial growth. The histological appearance of the endobronchial biopsy may be so pleomorphic that a mistaken impression of metastatic disease is made. However, the demonstration of carcinoma in situ in the adjacent bronchial epithelium strongly suggests the diagnosis of a primary lung tumor [1,13].

In conclusion, if atypical clinical features are present or an atypical cell type is discovered after biopsy of the lesion, appropriate diagnostic studies should be undertaken to exclude the possibility of EEM from an asyptomatic extrathoracic tumor before definitive therapy is undertaken. Unless careful attention is paid to the clinical, laboratory, and pathological features of each case, a misdiagnosis of primary bronchogenic carcinoma may be made and inappropriate therapy instituted [1].

References

1. Braman SS, Whitecomb ME. Endobronchial metastasis. Arch Int Med 1975;135:543–547.
2. King DS, Castleman B. Bronchial involvement in metastatic pulmonary malignancy. J Thorac Surg 1943;12:305–315.
3. Shepherd MP. Endobronchial metastatic disease. Thorax 1982;37:362–365.
4. Debeer RA, Garcia RL, Alexander SC. Endobronchial metastasis from cancer of the breast. Chest 1978;73:94–96.
5. Albertini RE, Ekberg NL. Endobronchial metastasis in breast cancer. Thorax 1980;35: 435–440.
6. Ettensohn DB et al. Endobronchial metastases from carcinoma of the breast. Med Pediatr Oncol 1985;13:9–13.
7. Carlin BM, Harrell JH, Olson LK et al. Endobronchial metastases due to colorectal carcinoma. Chest 1989;96:1110–1114.
8. Rovirosa Casino A, Bellmunt J, Salud A et al. Endobronchial metastases in colorectal adenocarcinoma. Tumori 1992;78:270–273.
9. MacMahon H, O'Connell DJ, Cimochowski GE. Pedunculated endotracheal metastasis. Am J Roentgenol 1978;131:713–714.
10. Jariwalla AG, Seaton A, McCormack RJM et al. Intrabronchial metastases from renal carcinoma with recurrent tumour expectoration. Thorax 1981;36:179–182.
11. Amer E, Guy J, Vaze B. Endobronchial metastasis from renal adenocarcinoma simulating a foreign body. Thorax 1981;36:183–184.
12. Gerle R, Felson B. Metastatic endobronchial hypernephroma. Chest 1963;44:225–233.
13. Baumgartner WA, Mark JBD. Metastatic malignancies from distant sites to the tracheobronchial tree. J Thorac Cardiovasc Surg 1980;79:499–503.
14. Katsimibri PP, Bamias AT, Froudarakis ME et al. Endobronchial metastases secondary to solid tumors: report of eight cases and review of the literature. Lung Cancer 2000:28;163–170.
15. Salud A, Porcel JM, Rovirosa A et al. Endobronchial metastatic disease: analysis of 32 cases. J Surg Oncol 1996;62:249–252.
16. Heitmiller RF, Marasco WJ, Hruban RH et al. Endobronchial metastasis. J Thorac Cardiovasc Surg 1993;106:537–42.
17. Higginson JF. A study of excised pulmonary metastatic malignancies. Am J Surg 1955;90: 241–252.
18. Rosenblatt MB, Lisa JR, Trinidad S. Pitfalls in the clinical and histologic diagnosis of bronchogenic carcinoma. Chest 1966;49:396–404.
19. Udelsman R, Roth J, Lees D et al. Endobronchial metastases from soft tissue sarcoma. J Surg Oncol 1986;32:145–149.
20. Akiba T, Ujiie H, Takasaki N et al. Endobronchial metastasis from a primary uterine osteosarcoma in a patient with multiple myeloma: Report of a case. Surg Today 1994;24:179–182.
21. Colletti PM, Beck S, Boewell Jr WD et al. Computed tomography in endobronchial neoplasms. Computerized Medical Imaging and Graphics 1990;14:257–262.

22. Schoenbaum S, Viamonte M. Subepithelial endobronchial metastases. Radiology 1971;101: 63–69.
23. Pisch J, Villamena PC, Harvey JC et al. High dose-rate endobronchial irradiation in malignant airway obstruction. Chest 1993;104:721–725.
24. Bourke SJ, Henderson AF, Stevenson RD, Banham SW. Endobronchial metastases simulating primary carcinoma of the lung. Respiratory Medicine 1989;83:151–152.

Bronchology and Bronchoesophagology: State of the Art.
H. Yoshimura et al., editors.

Primary adenoid cystic carcinoma of the trachea: a case report

Jerzy Kozielski and Dariusz Jastrzębski
Department of Pneumonology, Silesian School of Medicine, Zabrze, Poland

Abstract. A case of adenoid cystic cancer of the trachea is described. The chief symptoms of the disease were dyspnea, coughing and a sensation of obstruction in the bronchial tree. During forced expiration under spirometry, the patient lost consciousness. No lesions were found in the rib cage radiograph.

In bronchoscopy, a slit-like constriction of the trachea in the longitudinal axis was found. Diagnosis of the disease was established on the basis of a histological and pathological examination of a section taken from the infiltration in the trachea.

Keywords: primary adenoid cystic carcinoma, trachea tumors.

Introduction

Tumours of the trachea occur only rarely [1]. In 1990 in Great Britain, 44 people died of tracheal tumors. In the same period 803 people died of throat cancer and 34,331 people of lung cancer [2].

Owing to their rare occurrence, tracheal tumours are easily overlooked, especially if their chief manifestation is only, for example, shortness of breath or a cough [3,4]. Considering, however, the indications that call for bronchoscopy which include dyspnea that does not explain the extent of the radiological lesions or a persistent cough, a diagnosis can be made in a short time.

Case description

A 41-year-old patient who was a metal worker by profession and had been a non-smoker for 2 years was admitted to the clinic because of exacerbated shortness of breath. His dyspnea had appeared some 8 months previously. In addition to this, he complained of a cough. The symptoms occurred during inspiration of air. He also reported a sensation of there being an obstruction on his windpipe. The patient had smoked 15 cigarettes a day over a period of 18 years. No lesions were found on physical examination, nor were any abnormalities found in the blood morphology test and the biochemical blood tests. On his admission, spirometry showed FVC 3.29 l (62% pred.), FEV1 2.0 l (46.3% pred.), and PEF 3.32 l (33.9% pred.), with disruptions of the airflow in the small airways (Fig. 1). When performing forced maximal expiration during spirometry the patient sud-

Address for correspondence: Jerzy Kozielski, Department of Pneumonology, Silesian School of Medicine, ul. Koziolka 1, 41-803 Zabrze, Poland. Tel.: +48-32-17-15-608. Fax: +48-32-17-53-015.

SLASKA AKADEMIA MEDYCZNA KLINIKA FTIZJOPNEUMONOLOGII
41-803 Z A B R Z E

ul.Koziolka 1 telefon 171-56-08

Identification	: 867	Age	: 41 Years
Last Name	: [redacted]	Height	: 186 cm
First Name	: [redacted]	Weight	: 86 kg
Date of Birth	: 26:08:1953	Sex	: male
Smoker	:	Ward	: Klinika FT
Physician	: Dr A.K.	Operator	: Dr A.K.

FL-VOL

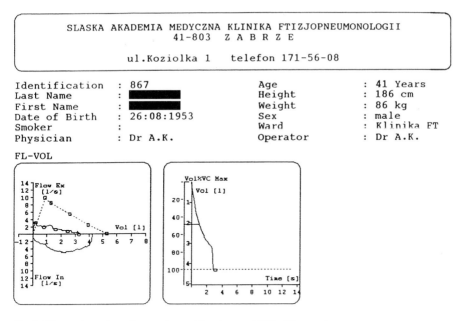

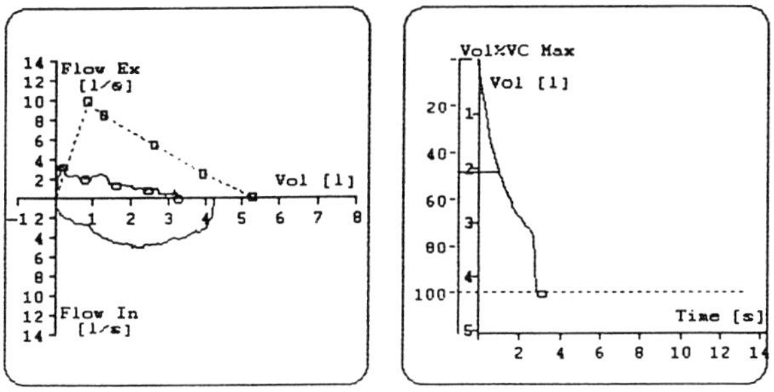

Fig. 1. Flow-volume loop in a patient with primary ACC of the trachea.

denly lost consciousness, which he later described as a sensation that the outflow of air from the airways was blocked. At rest, no abnormalities were found in the gasometric blood test (PaO2 88 mmHg, pCO2 37,6 mmHg), neither were any found in radiology of the rib cage. Fiberoptic bronchoscopy revealed a slit-like narrowing (constriction) 10 cm from the vocal cords, running in the longitudinal axis of the trachea for a length of 1 cm (Fig. 2). On the right side the constricted area had an uneven surface. The mucous membrane in the constricted area was reddened. Apart from the constriction, the bronchial tree exhibited no lesions. Smears and scrapings were taken from the constriction. We did not succeed in taking sections. Histopathological examination of this material showed inflammatory lesions.

A CT examination of this region was conducted; it revealed a slit-like constriction of the trachea at the height of the manubrium sterni over a length of approximately 1.5 cm.

The internal passage of the trachea at the narrowest point measured 4 mm in diameter and 2.4 cm in length. Above and below the lesion the internal passage of the trachea measured 1.8 cm by 2.9 cm. A second fiberoptic bronchoscopy, conducted with puncture of the lesion with a Wang needle, did not permit diagnosis of the disease (Fig. 3). Examination of the supraclavicular lymphatic glands on the right side, made by the Daniels method, showed no pathological blockage. Further fiberoptic bronchoscopy was conducted and this time sections were taken from the lesion. Results of the histopathological examination: infiltratio carcinomatosa – ca adenoides cysticum. In frontal mediastinoscopy no lesions

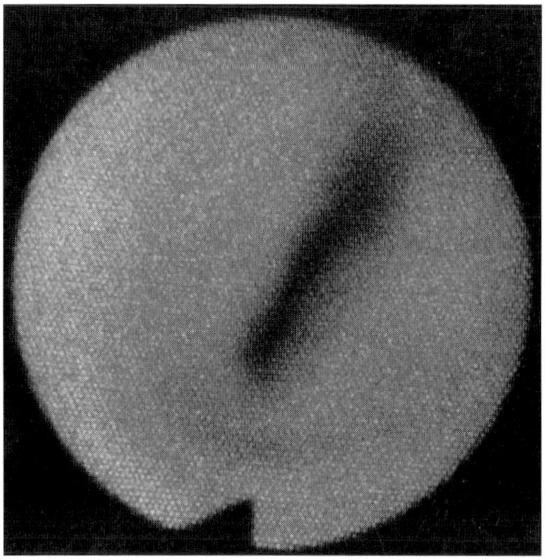

Fig. 2.

were found in the middle thorax. During exploratory surgery it was discovered that tumorous infiltration had spread to, inter alia, the neighbouring tissues of the right brachiocephalic stem. The case was acknowledged to be inoperable. The patient was given a T-type tracheotomy tube, and radiotherapy was begun.

Discussion

Tumours of the trachea that cause constriction of its internal passage lead to disruptions in the cleaning of the bronchial tree, symptoms of build-up of discharge

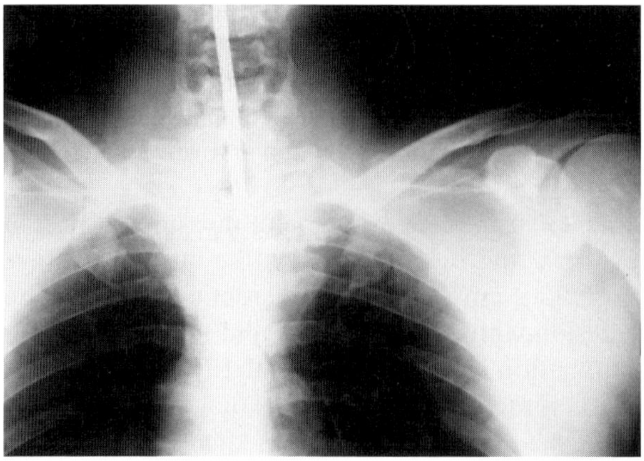

Fig. 3.

below the constriction, and inflammation. The most frequent symptom is, however, shortness of breath (usually severe), coughing and hoarseness [4–6]. Spitting of blood and wheezing often occur. Even a significant narrowing of the trachea – approximately 50% – does not necessarily give all clinical symptoms and audible anomalies [7]. The fact is that clinical symptoms depend, inter alia, on the histological type of the tumour that causes the constriction. For example, spitting of blood usually occurs in epithelial cancer. This is the type of tumour, moreover, that most frequently occurs among tumours of the trachea. Out of 485 of these lesions, the second in frequency of occurrence – accounting for one out of every three of the lesions – is carcinoma adenocysticum (ACC)[8]. This tumour most often occurs in young people [5]. The disproportion between the clinical symptoms and the physical examination, or else between the physical examination and the spirometric and gasometric tests, suggested to us that tracheal lesions were the cause of the patient's discomfort. The expiration flow showed a characteristic result in the test – with a decrease in the peak of expiratory flow. ACC usually develops high up in the trachea and exhibits tuberous swellings and obstructions in the bronchograph [5]. In consideration of the location of these lesions and for fear of taking sections from some of the patients during bronchoscopy, a diagnosis was not arrived at by this method. Despite the thickening of the internal passage of the trachea, we did not succeed in making a diagnosis in our patient using the needle biopsy method. In the diagnosis of lesions located in the trachea the safest method appears to be the use of rigid bronchoscopy as it enables the site of bleeding to be more easily secured and sections to be taken more satisfactorily [9]. CT is an important supplement to this method. In this sort of examination, ACC is visible as masses surrounding the trachea which is becoming constricted due to the thickening of its internal passage [10]. In the treatment of tracheal tumours, radiotherapy is most frequently employed. ACC is a tumour with a better prognosis than epithelial cancer [6,8], since five years after treatment approximately 80% of patients survive. No differences were found in the survival time with this type of tumour as a function of the treatment method. Patients suffering from ACC treated surgically and those treated with radiation lived equally long [8].

References

1. Manninen MP, Antila PJ, Pukonder JS, Karma PH. Occurrence of tracheal carcinoma in Finland. Acta Otolaryngol 1991;111(6):1162–1169.
2. Mortality statistics. England and Words. London: HMSO, 1990.
3. Sekula J, Dobro SW. The trachea tumors diagnosis difficulties. Przegląd Lekarski 1988;45(10): 757–759.
4. Zimmer W, DeLuce SA. Primary tracheal symptoms: recognition, diagnosis and evaluation. Am Fam Physician 1992;45(6):2651–2657.
5. Horvard DJ, Haribhakti VV. Primary tumours of the trachea: analysis of clinical features and treatment results. J Laryngol Otol 1994;108(3):230–232.
6. Manninen MP. Symptoms and signs and their prognostic value in tracheal carcinoma. Eur Arch

Otorhinolaryngol 1993;250(7):3–7.
7. Otto T. Chirurgia zwężeń tchawicy. Pneum Allergol Pol 1991;59(5/6):242–252.
8. Gelder CM, Hetrel MR. Primary tracheal tumours: a national survey. Thorax 1993;48: 688–692.
9. Allen MS. Malignant trachea tumors. Mayo Clin Proc 1993;68(7):680–684.
10. Na DG, Han MH, Chang KH, Yeon KM. Primary adenoid cystic carcinoma of the cervical trachea mimickring thyroid tumour. CT evaluation. J Comput Assist Tomogr 1995;19(4):559–563.

Bronchology and Bronchoesophagology: State of the Art.
H. Yoshimura et al., editors.

Endoscopic resection of an endobronchial renal cell carcinoma metastasis using a polypectomy snare

Seitaro Okamura, Yoshiki Demura, Yoshitaka Totani, Shingo Ameshima, Takeshi Ishizaki and Isamu Miyamori
The Third Department of Internal Medicine, Fukui Medical University, Fukui, Japan

Abstract. We are reporting a case of endobronchial metastasis of renal cell carcinoma. A 76-year-old man was admitted to our section complaining of a high fever and a dyspnea. Four years earlier he underwent a transperitoneal right nephrectomy for renal cell carcinoma. He received postoperative chemotherapy using INF-α. On admission, the X-ray film revealed a total left lung atelectasis. The bronchoscopic examination showed that the main left bronchus was obstructed by a whitish tumor with endoluminal thrombus-like growth. Endoscopic polypectomy using electrosurgery was performed repeatedly. The patient then dramatically improved. No side effects were observed. Histopathological examination identified metastasis from a renal cell carcinoma. This unconventional but simple technique is useful for bronchial deobstruction, when the tumor is accessible with a snare.

Keywords: atelectasis, bronchial polypoid tumor, endobronchial metastasis, endoscopic surgery.

Introduction

Endobronchial metastasis from nonpulmonary carcinoma is uncommon, occurring in only 2 to 5% of patients with cancer at necropsy [1]. Several methods are proposed to treat endobronchial tumors: laser, brachytherapy, intratumoral ethanol injections and photodynamic therapy. There are a few cases in which an electrosurgery snare was reported to have been used [2—4]. Here we report the case of a patient in whom an endobronchial metastatic tumor was endoscopically resected by electrosurgery using a polypectomy snare, and this technique would certainly be proposed as a good alternative to laser or other related methods.

Case report

A 71-year-old man was admitted to the urological section of our hospital, complaining of an abnormal finding in the right kidney on an abdominal echogram. An abdominal echogram and computed tomography showed a low density mass on the right kidney. He was suspected to have renal cell carcinoma and, in May 1993, underwent a transperitoneal right nephrectomy for renal cell carcinoma. He received postoperative chemotherapy using Interferon-α. The follow-up peri-

Address for correspondence: Seitaro Okamura MD, The Third Department of Internal Medicine, Fukui Medical University, Shimoaiduki 23, Matsuoka-cho, Fukui 910-1193, Japan. Tel.: +81-776-61-3111. Fax: +81-776-61-8111. E-mail: seita-o@dj8.so-net.ne.jp od lasting until February 1996 showed para-aortic lymph node metastasis from renal cell carcinoma. He received chemotherapy using Interferon-α and Fluorouracil. In September 1999, the para-aortic lymph node metastasis had increased, thus he was admitted to the urological section of our hospital in order to receive chemotherapy using Interleukin-2.

On 14 November 1999, he was admitted to our section, complaining of a high fever and dyspnea. On percussion and auscultation of the chest, increased dullness and diminished breath sounds were noted in the left lung field. The X-ray film revealed a total left lung atelectasis (Fig. 1). The bronchoscopic examination showed that the left main bronchus was obstructed by a whitish tumor with endoluminal thrombus-like growth (Fig. 2). Biopsy of the lesion was not diagnostic. To improve bronchial obstruction, we decided to perform an endoscopic polypectomy using electrosurgery. A snare designed for the respiratory tract (SD-18C-1, Olympus, Tokyo, Japan) was introduced through a bronchofiberscope (BF P200, Olympus) to lasso the tumor, after which the electrosurgical unit was turned on and the snare was pulled up very slowly (Fig. 3). This procedure was carried out several times. Finally, endobronchial polypectomy was successfully performed without any complications.

The patient's symptoms and the chest X-ray dramatically improved (Fig. 4). Histopathological examination identified metastasis from a renal cell carcinoma.

Discussion

Renal cell carcinoma (RCC) sometime causes an endobronchial metastasis and the growth pattern tends to be in a polypoid pattern [5]. In our case, endobronchial metastasis of RCC grew like thrombus and was the cause of the total

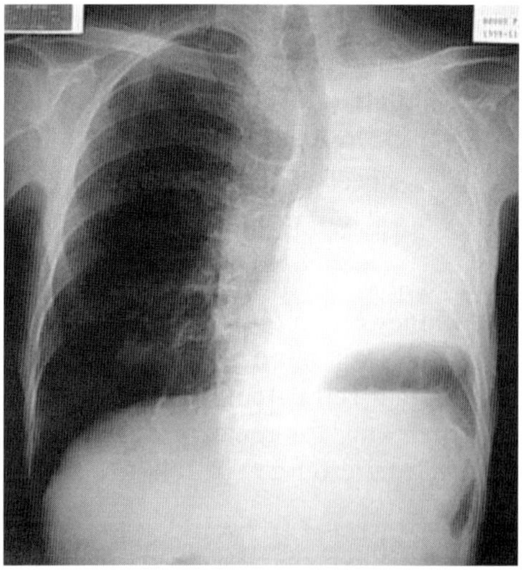

Fig. 1. Chest X-ray film, taken on admission, showing a left total atelectasis.

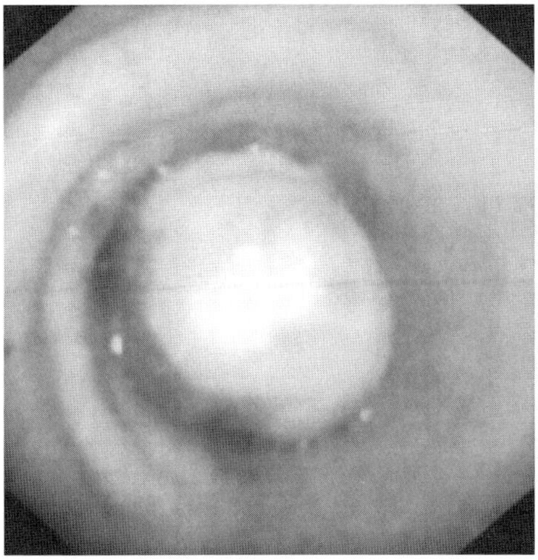

Fig. 2. The bronchoscopic examination showed that the main left bronchus was obstructed by a whitish tumor with endoluminal thrombus-like growth.

atelectasis. There are a few cases in which an electrosurgery snare is reported to have been used [2–4]. Endoscopic polypectomy using an electrosurgery snare is capable of resecting a large quantity of tumor at once and improving the patient's symptoms rapidly. Thus, this technique is particularly useful in emergency situations, for palliative treatment, and generally when the tumor is accessible with a snare.

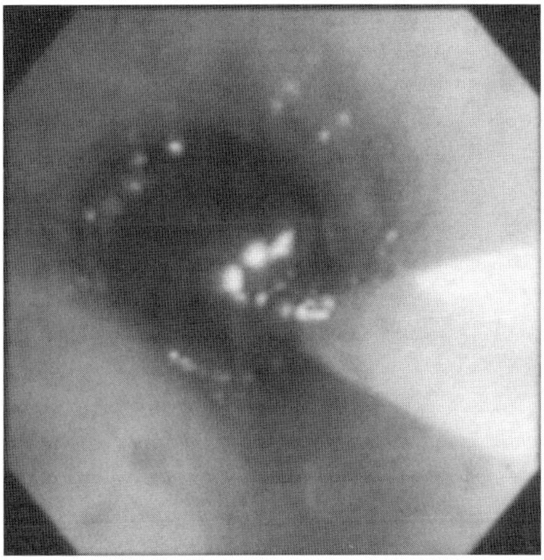

Fig. 3. Endoscopic polypectomy using an electrosurgical snare was performed on 25 Novemder 1999.

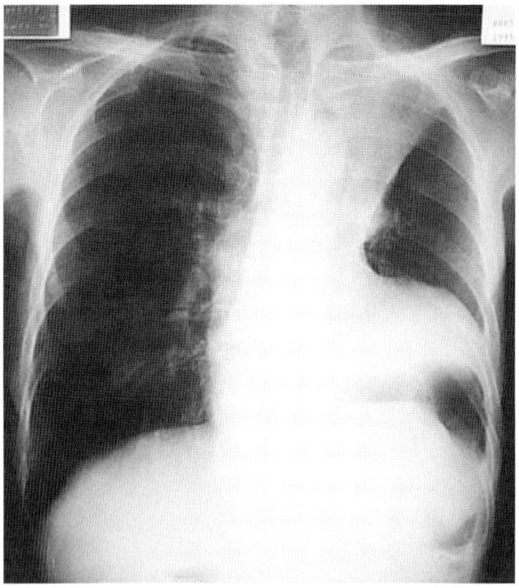

Fig. 4. After polypectomy, the chest X-ray shows a marked improvement of the left total atelectasis.

References

1. Bramman SS, Whitcomb ME. Endobronchial metastasis. Arch Int Med 1975;135:543–547.
2. Ronaldo Adib Kairaka C, Ribeiro Carvalho R, Parada AA, Alves VA, Nascimento Salvida PH. Solitary plasmocytoma of the trachea treated by loop resection and laser therapy. Thorax 1988; 43:1011–1012.
3. Muller LC, Pointer R, Schmid KW, Salzer GM. Endoscopic removal of a pedunculated bronchial lipoma by means of the hot snare. Endoscopy 1989;21:97–98.
4. Themelin D, Duchatelet P, Boudaka W, Lamy V. Endoscopic resection of an endobronchial hypernephroma metastasis using a polypectomy snare. Eur Respir J 1990;3:732–733.
5. Dobbertin I, Dierkesmann R, Kwiatkowski J, Reichardt W. Bronchoscopic aspects of renal cell carcinoma. Anticancer Research 1999;19:1567–1572.

Esophageal cancer

Bronchology and Bronchoesophagology: State of the Art.
H. Yoshimura et al., editors.

Concurrent chemoradiotherapy for advanced hypopharyngeal or cervical esophageal cancer

S. Endo, A. Kida, N. Hamada, Y. Watanabe, H. Nakazato, S. Shigihara, K. Watanabe, K. Ootsuka, S. Suzuki and D. Kobayashi
Department of Otorhinolaryngology – Head and Neck Surgery, Nihon University School of Medicine, Tokyo, Japan

Abstract. *Background.* Chemotherapy is shown to be most effective when delivered concurrently with radiation in patients with untreated advanced-stage tumors. We conducted a concurrent chemoradiation protocol using systemic infusion of Cisplatin (CDDP) and 5-Fluorouracil (5-FU) followed by radical surgery.

Patients and Methods. Thirty-six patients with advanced hypopharyngeal or cervical esophageal cancer received intravenous administration of CDDP (100 mg/m) followed by 120 h of continuous infusion of 5-FU (1000 mg/m/day), and concomitant radiotherapy (200 cGy/day x 20–35 fractions).

Results. The clinical response rate (RR) of the 35 evaluable patients was 33 out of 35 (94.3%). One patient died of aspiration pneumonia. The rate of grade three/four hematological chemotoxicity was 30.6%. Laryngopharyngo- and cervical-esophagectomies were performed in 23 patients, partial resection of the hypopharynx in one patient, and radical neck dissection in another one patient. Among the 33 responsive patients, nine out of 22 (40.9%) were confirmed to have complete responses (CR) from the surgical specimen. The median length of follow-up was 69 weeks. The projected 4-year survival was 53.9%. When those patients who had refused radical surgery for the residual tumor were excluded, 4-year survival rose up to 64.8%.

Conclusions. Concurrent chemoradiotherapy can be safely and effectively applied. Preliminary pathological results indicate the possibility of improving the rate of organ preservation.

Keywords: 5-fluorouracil, cisplatin, organ preservation, survival.

Introduction

Despite recent advances in medical management, including new chemotherapeutic agents, the survival rate of advanced hypopharyngeal and cervical esophageal cancer has not significantly changed. In the hope of obtaining better results, we examined the efficacy of concurrent chemoradiotherapy for patients with these malignancies.

Patients and Methods

All patients with advanced hypopharyngeal or cervical esophageal cancer with-

Address for correspondence: Sohei Endo MD, PhD, Department of ORL-HNS, Nihon University School of Medicine, 30-1 Oyaguchi-kamicho, Itabashi-ku, Tokyo 173-8610, Japan. Tel.: +81-3-3972-8111, ext. 2542. Fax: +81-3-3972-1321. E-mail: sohei@med.nihon-u.ac.jp out distant metastasis who had tolerable renal functioning were included in this study. The regimen consisted of 100 mg/m^2 of Cisplatin (CDDP) followed by 1000 mg/m^2 of 5-Flourouracil (5-FU) for 5 days and concurrent radiation up to 40 to 50 Gy. After this treatment, definitive surgery was planned. Only those patients who refused definitive surgery, were given radiation up to 70 Gy with curative intent.

Results

There were 28 patients with hypopharyngeal cancer, and eight patients with cervical esophageal cancer. In nine out of 36 patients, two cycles of chemotherapy were given concurrently according to the low toxicity and efficacy of the first cycle of chemotherapy. One patient died of aspiration pneumonia during the course of chemoradiotherapy. The delivered radiation doses were 40 to 50 Gy in 27 patients, whereas they were 60 to 70 Gy in eight patients. Among 35 evaluable patients, 16 patients showed clinically complete disappearances of the tumors (CR), 17 had a partial response (PR), and two showed no response (NC). Using the WHO criteria for toxicity, major toxicity was observed in hematologic and GI systems. In the hematologic system, grade three/four toxicity was encountered in 11 (8/3) patients. In the GI system, grade three mucositis was observed in only one patient. Twenty-four out of 35 patients undertook definitive surgery (23 laryngopharyngo- and cervical-esophagectomies, one partial hypopharyngectomy). One patient undertook only radical neck dissection, and another had a neck lymphnode biopsy after complete disappearance of the primary tumor. Six patients refused radical surgery even when their tumor existed after chemoradiotherapy. The remaining four patients, who had less than T4 lesions and achieved CR, were placed under a close follow-up. We were able to preserve the larynx intentionally only in six patients. In histopathological analysis of the surgical specimens, 11 of 24 patients (46.7%) achieved CR. Another 11 had a partial response. As a result, a response rate of 91.7% was seen. All except two patients were followed up until the time of their death. The median length of follow-up was 69 weeks. The projected 4-year survival was 53.9%. When those patients who had refused radical surgery for the residual tumor were excluded, 4-year survival rose up to 64.8%.

Discussion

Chemotherapy is shown to be most effective when delivered concurrently with radiation in patients with untreated advanced head and neck cancer [1]. A prospective study of concurrent chemoradiotherapy using CDDP and 5-FU in esophageal cancer showed complete tumor disappearance in 30% of the resected specimen [2]. Our results confirmed the efficacy of concurrent chemoradiotherapy using CDDP and 5-FU on patients with advanced hypopharyngeal or cervical esophageal cancer.

Conclusions

Concurrent chemoradiotherapy can be safely and effectively applied. Preliminary pathological results also indicate the possibility of improving the rate of organ preservation.

References

1. Al-Meyed S et al. Adjuvant and adjunctive chemotherapy in the management of squamous cell carcinoma of the head and neck region: a meta-analysis of prospective and randomized trials. J Clin Oncol 1996;14:838–847.
2. Leichman L et al. Preoperative chemotherapy and radiation therapy for patients with cancer of the esophagus: a potentially curative approach. J Clin Oncol 1984;2:75–79.

Bronchology and Bronchoesophagology: State of the Art.
H. Yoshimura et al., editors.

Cervical lymph node dissection for thoracic esophageal cancer

Tomoko Hanashi, Misao Yoshida and Yousuke Izumi
Department of Surgery, Tokyo Metropolitan Komagome General Hospital, Tokyo, Japan

Abstract. In order to evaluate the effect of cervical lymph node dissection in surgical treatment of thoracic esophageal cancer, clinico-pathological results were reviewed. 111 patients with thoracic esophageal cancer who underwent esophagectomy with three-field lymph node dissection without preoperative therapy were included in this study.

Results. Patients were classified into three groups: group A: no lymph node metastasis (40% of all patients), group B: metastases in any nodes without the supraclavicular nodes (40%), and group C: metastases including the supraclavicular nodes (20%). The cause-specific 5-year survival rate of group C (34%) was significantly worse than group B (70%) and group A (89%). On the other hand, the cause-specific 5-year survival rate of patients who had lymph node metastases in over eight nodes was worst (22%). They occupied 57% of group C and 7% of group B. In cases who had lymph node metastases in less than seven nodes, there was no significant difference in the 5-year survival rate between groups B and C.

Conclusion. In cases who have total lymph node metastases in less than seven nodes, including metastases in the neck, cervical dissection would probably be effective.

Keywords: esophageal squamous cell carcinoma, number of lymph node metastasis, three-field lymph node dissection.

Introduction

In order to evaluate the effect of cervical dissection in the surgical treatment of thoracic esophageal cancer, the clinico-pathological results of our patients were reviewed.

Subjects

111 patients with thoracic esophageal cancer, who underwent curative esophagectomy with three-field lymph node dissection without preoperative therapy from 1984 to 1999, were included in this study. The depth of cancer invasion was from the submucosa to the adventitia. In this study, supraclaviclar nodes were studied, as they require a cervical approach, while other cervical nodes such as paraesophageal, paratracheal and recurrent laryngeal nerve nodes can be dissected through right thoracotomy. Patients were classified into three groups: group A: no lymph node metastasis (40% of all patients), group B: lymph

Address for correspondence: Tomoko Hanashi, Department of Surgery, Tokyo Metropolitan Komagome General Hospital, 3-18-22 Honkomagome, Bunkyo-ku, Tokyo 113-8677, Japan. Tel.: +81-3-3823-2101. Fax: +81-3-3824-1552.

node metastases in any nodes without the supraclavicular nodes (40%), and group C: metastases including the supraclavicular nodes (20%). There was no significant difference in distribution of the cancer location in each group. However, there were significant differences in the depth of invasion and the number of lymph node metastasis between the three groups. In group A, T1b tumors were more frequent (57%) than in groups B (30%) and C (30%), and T3 tumors were less frequent (32%) than in groups B (57%) and C (61%). As regards the number of lymph node metastasis, patients with one to three nodes occupied 66% in group B and 22% in group C, and patients with over eight nodes constituted 7% of group B and 56% of group C.

Results

The incidence of supraclavicular nodes metastasis was 33% (5/15) when the tumor was in the upper third esophagus, 28% (23/83) in the middle third, and 8% (1/8) in the lower third.

The 5-year survival rate was significantly low in group C (34%) compared with group A (89%) and group B (70%). Therefore, the prognoses of patients with metastasis in the supraclaviclar nodes were significantly poor (Fig. 1).

The 5-year survival rate was 89% in patients without metastasis, 81% in patients with one to three positive nodes, 45% in patients with four to seven positive nodes, and 22% in patients with over eight positive nodes. The postoperative-survival rate declined accordingly as the number of positive nodes increased (Fig. 2). When the total number of positive nodes was equivalent, there was no significant difference noted between the 5-year survival rate of groups B and C (Fig. 3).

The rate of recurrence was high in group C (69%), but if looked at in conjunction with number of positive nodes, it was 12% in patients one to three, 8% in patients with four to seven, and 49% in patients with over eight. The poor prognosis of group C was due to the high incidence of patients who had lymph node metastases in more than eight nodes.

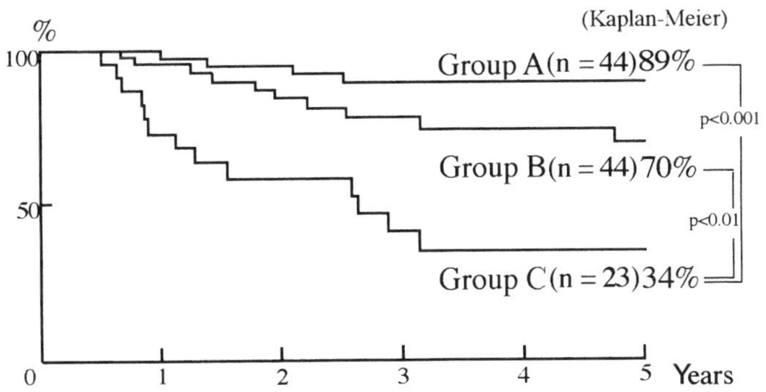

Fig. 1. The cause-specific 5-year survival curves of the three groups.

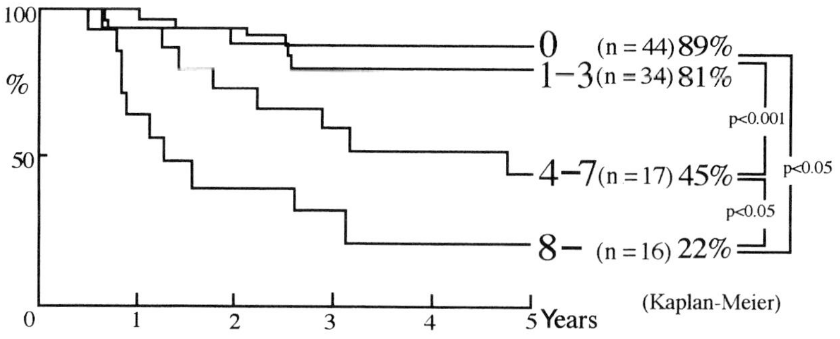

Fig. 2. The cause-specific 5-year survival curves examined in conjunction with the incidence of positive nodes.

Discussion

The incidence of the supraclavicular nodes was 21% of all patients. Therefore, cervical lymph node dissection is important in the treatment of thoracic esophageal cancer, especially in the upper or middle third. The distribution of lymph node metastasis of thoracic esophageal cancer can be revealed by three-field dissection. However, at the same time, the limits of surgical treatment for positive nodes are also evident [1]. It has been said that postoperative survival declines accordingly, as the number of positive nodes increases [2]. In this study, the cause-specific survival rate was good in the patients who had less than three positive nodes, but was poor in the patients with over eight positive nodes. In the cases of patients with four to seven positive nodes, a cause-specific survival rate of about 50% was achieved. In summation, in cases involving patients with cancer of the upper or middle third of the esophagus, with lymph node metastasis in less than seven positive nodes, including supraclavicular nodes, cervical dissection would probably be effective.

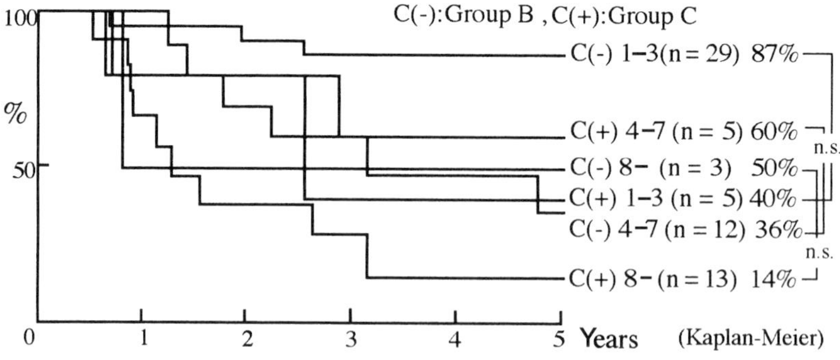

Fig. 3. The cause-specific 5-year survival curve of group C, examined in conjuntion with the incidence of positive nodes.

References

1. Hanashi T, Yoshida M. A study on the optimal lymph node dissection for thoracic esophageal carcinoma according to the stage. Jpn J Gastroenterol Surg 1999;32(10):2474–2478.
2. Yamana H, Kakegawa T et al. Advantage of extended lymphadenectomy for carcinoma of the thoracic esophagus. Jpn J Gastroenterol Surg 1995;28(4):942–946.

©2001 Published by Elsevier Science B.V.
Bronchology and Bronchoesophagology: State of the Art.
H. Yoshimura et al., editors.

The availability of preoperative stenting for severe malignant esophageal stenosis

Yoshiaki Hara, Tomoko Hanashi, Yousuke Izumi, Taro Hirose, Tsuyoshi Kato, Satoshi Ishiyama and Misao Yoshida
Deparment of Surgery, Tokyo Metropolitan Komagome General Hospital, Tokyo, Japan

Abstract. *Background.* In order to evaluate the preoperative application of stent placement in patients with severe esophageal stenosis due to locally advanced squamous cell carcinoma, the clinical results of seven patients were reviewed.

Methods. The subjects were seven patients with severe esophageal stenosis due to advanced esophageal cancer. The mean age was 56 years. Tumors were found in upper third (in two cases), middle third (in three) and lower third (in two) of the esophagus. Esophageal expandable metalic stents (EMS: covered type for five patients, and noncovered for two) were applied. Thereafter, all patients underwent preoperative chemotherapy.

Results. A remarkable improvement in dysphagia was noted in all the patients. There were no severe complications or difficulties during the operations due to the preoperative stent placement of the esophagus.

Conclusion. Preoperative stent placement of the esophagus allowed patients with severe esophageal stenosis to consume food and allowed an improved nutritional condition.

Keywords: esophageal cancer, expandable metalic stent, neoadjuvant therapy.

Introduction

Recent advances in the treatment of esophageal cancer cases, including preoperative adjuvant chemotherapy, improved the operability and prognosis of them. It also elongated preoperative hospitalization and the duration of fasting for patients with severe stenosis of the esophagus. In order to evaluate the preoperative application of stenting in patients with severe esophageal stenosis, due to locally advanced squamous cell carcinoma, the clinical results of eight patients were reviewed.

Subjects and Methods

The subjects were seven patients with severe esophageal stenosis, due to advanced esophageal cancer, consisting of six males and one female. The mean age was 56 years (range: 47 to 66 years). The locations of the tumors in the esophagus were in the upper third in two cases, the middle third three cases, and the lower third

Address for correspondence: Yoshiaka Hara, Deparment of Surgery, Tokyo Metropolitan Komagome General Hospital, 3-18-22 Honkomgome, Bunkyo-ku, Tokyo 113-8677, Japan. Tel.: +81-3-3823-2101. Fax: +81-3-3824-1552.

two cases. All cases received preoperative chemotherapy. Expandable metallic stents (EMS) were introduced before chemotherapy in four cases, during chemotherapy in one case, and after chemotherapy in two cases. Noncovered Ultra-Flex was used in two cases and the covered type in the other five cases (Table 1). The severity of dysphagia before and after stent placement was quantified with a dysphagia grade as follows: grade 0: normal, grade 1: unable to swallow solids, grade 2: unable to swallow semisolids, grade 3: unable to swallow liquids, and grade 4: unable to swallow own saliva [1]. After chemotherapy, all the patients underwent radical esophagectomy.

Results

Severe dysphagia of grade 3 (three cases) or 2 (four cases) was noted before stent placement in all patients, though it improved to grade 1 (five cases) or 0 (two cases), 1 month after stent placement (Fig. 1). Complications encountered, due to stent placement, included chest pain in all cases, high fever in three cases, protracted chest pain in three cases, and heartburn in one case. There were no severe complications, such as migration of the stent, hemorrhage, perforation or fistula formation noted. Case 1 had malignant stenosis in the middle third of the esophagus, and could not swallow semisolids on admission. After stent placement, he was able to swallow solid foods and return home, temporarily for 23 days after chemotherapy, before receiving the radical esophagectomy. Case 2 had esophageal cancer with severe stenosis in the upper third. After he received two cycles of chemotherapy, an esophageal stent was inserted. He could swallow only fluid on admission, however, he was able to consume semisolid foods after the stenting. There were no difficulties encountered during the operations due to preoperative stent placement of the esophagus.

Discussion

Preoperative use of the esophageal stent in esophageal cancer patients, who first receive preoperative chemotherapy, may lead to improved nutritional conditions

Table 1. Patient characteristics.

Cases	Age	Sex	Location	Stent placement[a]	Type of stent
1	47	M	Middle	Before[b]	Noncovered
2	61	M	Upper	After	Noncovered
3	47	F	Upper-middle	During	Covered
4	62	M	Middle	After	Covered
5	48	M	Lower	Before	Covered
6	66	M	Middle	Before	Covered
7	59	M	Lower-middle	Before	Covered

[a]Stent placement refers to before or after chemotherapy; [b]Before chemoradiation therapy.

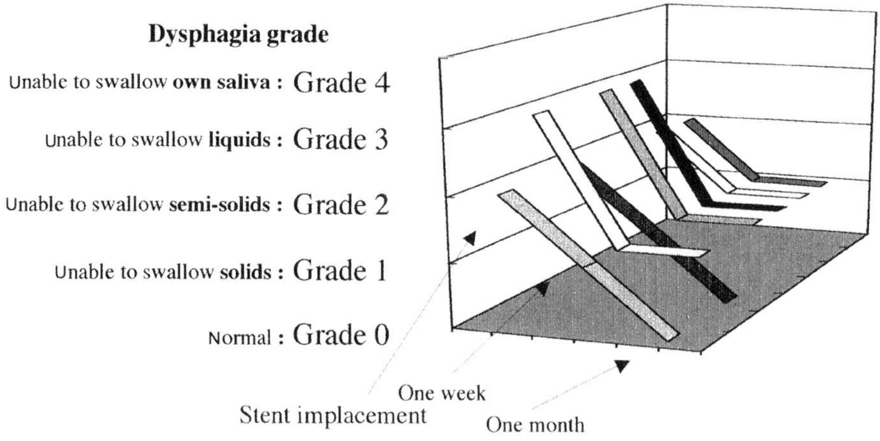

Fig. 1. The improvement of dysphagia.

and quality of life during the preoperative period. On the other hand, esophageal stent placement decreased patients' quality of life in cases with complications. It is controversial as to whether chemotherapy is associated with the increased risk of severe stent-related complications in esophageal cancer patients who were treated with an esophageal stent [2,3]. In our series, chemotherapy before or after stent placement was not associated with the increased risk of severe complications. In conclusion, the preoperative use of an expandable metalic stent in patients with severe stenosis due to esophageal cancer improves dysphagia and allows the consumption of food. Nutritional conditions and the quality of life during the preoperative period may also be improved.

References

1. Raijman I, Walden D et al. Expandable esophageal stents: initial experience with a new nitinol stent. Gastrointest Endosc 1994;40(5):614–621.
2. Kinsman KJ, DeGregorio BT et al. Prior radiation and chemotherapy increase the risk of life-threatening complications after insertion of metalic stents for esophagogastric malignancy. Gastrointest Endosc 1996;43(3):196–203.
3. Raijman I, Siddque I et al. Does chemoradiation therapy increase the incidence of complications with self-expanding coated stents in the management of malignant esophageal stricture? Am J Gastroenterol 1997;92(12):2192–2196.

Bronchology and Bronchoesophagology: State of the Art.
H. Yoshimura et al., editors.

A retrospective study on the sentinel lymph node of esophageal cancer

Yosuke Izumi, Misao Yoshida, Tomoko Hanashi, Taro Hirose, Takeshi Kato, Yoshiaki Hara and Tetsu Ishiyama
Department of Surgery, Tokyo Metropolitan Komagome General Hospital, Tokyo, Japan

Abstract. *Background.* In Japan, it is generally accepted that esohagectomy with three-field dissection improves the prognosis of esophageal cancer. The option of having less tissue removed from the neck, mediastinum and abdomen also reduces the possibility of complications. The idea of the sentinel node is important for appropriate lymph node dissection, especially when less invasive surgery is generally introduced. The aim of this study was to determine whether the idea of the sentinel lymph node can be accepted in esophageal cancer.

Patients and Methods. Nine cases with solitary lymph node metastasis and three cases with cervical lymph node metastasis among fifty cases with submucosal cancer who underwent esophagectomy between 1985 and 1998 were examined retrospectively. All patients underwent esophagectomy with three-field dissection for squamous cell carcinoma of the midesophagus.

Results. Nine cases with solitary lymph node metastasis revealed metastatic areas from the upper mediastinum to the upper abdomen. Two out of three cases with cervical lymph node metastasis also had upper mediastinal lymph node involvement.

Conclusions. The idea of the sentinel lymph node was not supported in this study.

Keywords: esophageal surgery, less invasive surgery, three-field lymph node dissection.

Introduction

The idea of the sentinel node is considered important for optimal lymph node dissection, especially when less invasive surgery is generally introduced. The aim of this study was to determine whether the idea of the sentinel lymph node can be accepted in esophageal cancer.

Patients and Methods

We studied fifty cases with submucosal cancer of the esophagus who underwent esophagectomy with three-field dissection between 1985 and 1998. All patients had squamous cell carcinoma of the midthoracic esophagus. Nine cases had solitary lymph node metastasis and three cases had cervical lymph node metastasis. These twelve cases were examined retrospectively. Figure 1 shows a schematic

Address for correspondence: Yosuke Izumi MD, Department of Surgery, Tokyo Metropolitan Komagome General Hospital, 3-18-22 Honkomagome, Bunkyo-ku, Tokyo 113-8677, Japan. Tel.: +81-3-3823-2101. Fax: +81-3-3824-1552. E-mail: y.izumi-k@komagome-hospital.bunkyo.tokyo.jp

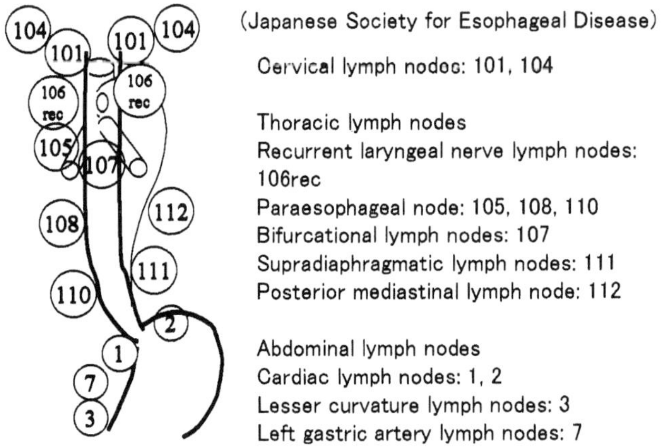

Fig. 1. Number of regional lymph nodes (Japanese classification).

representation of the number of regional lymph nodes according to Japanese classification [1].

Results

Table 1 shows the pathological features of the cases with solitary lymph node metastasis. Nine cases with solitary lymph node metastasis revealed the following metastatic areas between the upper mediastinum and upper abdomen: the recurrent laryngeal nerve nodes (#106recR, #106recL), paraesophageal nodes (#105, #108), bifurcational nodes (#107), posterior mediastinal nodes (#112), cardiac nodes (#1, #2) and left gastric nodes (#7). Nine cases had all of these different regions of lymph node involvement.

Figure 2 shows regions of involved lymph nodes in three cases with cervical lymph node metastasis. One case who had right cervical lymph node metastasis

Table 1. The pathological features of nine cases with solitary lymph node metastasis.

Case	Depth of invasion	ly	v	Involved lymph nodes
1	sm3	+	+	#105
2	sm2	+	+	#7
3	sm3	+	-	#108
4	sm2	+	-	#1
5	sm3	+	+	#112
6	sm2	+	-	#106rec R
7	sm3	+	+	#107
8	sm3	+	+	#106rec L
9	sm1	+	-	#2

sm1,sm2 and sm3: depth of submucosal layer invasion; ly: lymphatic invasion; v: vascular invasion.

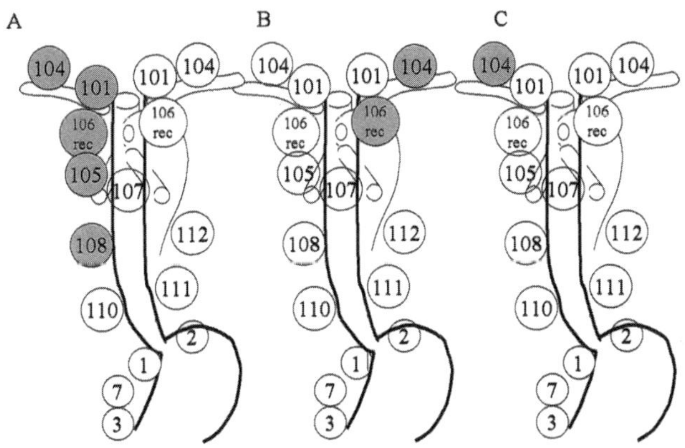

Fig. 2. Three cases with cervical lymph node metastasis.

had involved lymph nodes in the right recurrent nerve lymph node (#106recR). Another case who had left cervical lymph node metastasis had involved lymph nodes in the left recurrent nerve lymph node (#106recL). The other case had involved lymph nodes only in the cervical area.

Discussion

As Fujita reported [2], it is generally accepted, in Japan, that an esophagectomy with three-field dissection improves the prognosis of esophageal cancer. At the same time, it is also often said that the option of having less tissue removed from the neck, mediastinum and abdomen reduces the possibility of complications. Some studies are done to assess whether the thoracoscopic approach could reduce morbidity. However, as Gossot has pointed out [3], the objective benefit of using the thoracoscopic approach has not been reported so far. They concluded that further evaluation of the technique is needed. The sentinel lymph node has been eagerly studied, especially in patients with breast cancer, to avoid the unpleasant side effects of lymphadenectomy [4]. In patients with esophageal cancer, extensive lymph adenectomy can potentially induce fatal side effects. In this study we examined the region of solitary lymph node metastasis of submucosal cancer of the middle third of the thoracic esophagus, to determine where the primary metastatic region is and how we can reduce the area of lymphadenectomy. We found that even submucosal cancer had lymph node involvement from the upper mediastinum to the upper abdomen as a primary metastatic region. This result indicates that three-field lymph node dissection is necessary for a curative operation for submucosal cancer. Shimada [5] reported that RT-nested PCR detected more lymph node metastasis than the pathological or immunohistochemical examination. In our study, two out of three cases with cervical lymph node metastasis also had upper mediastimnal lymph node involvement, although the other case had no upper mediastinal lymph node involvement (Fig. 2A and 2B). This result may change if micrometastasis were examined using recent techniques. At present we cannot indicate that upper mediastinal lymph nodes are sentinel lymph nodes for cervical lymph nodes.

Conclusions

The idea of the sentinel lymph node was not supported in this study. However, it is suggested that submucosal cancer still requires lymph node dissection from neck to around the upper stomach and left gastric artery, even if less invasive surgery is introduced.

References

1. Japanese society for esophageal diseases. Guide lines for the clinical and pathologic studies on carcinoma of the esophagus. Tokyo: Kanehara, 1999.
2. Fujita H, Kakegawa T, Yamana H, Shima I, Tanaka H, Ikeda S, Nogami S, Toh Y. Lymph node metastasis and recurrence in patients with a carcinome of the thoracic esophagus who underwent three-field dissection. World J Surg 1994;18:266–272.
3. Gossot D, Fourquier P, Celerier M. Thoracoscopic esophagectomy: technique and initial results. Ann Thorac Surg 1993;56:667–670.
4. Veronesi U, Paganelli G, Viale G, Galimberti V, Luini A, Zurrida S, Robertson C, Sacchini V, Veronesi P, Orvieto E, Cicco C, Intra M, Tosi G, Scarpa D. Sentinel lymph node biopsy and axillary dissection in breast cancer: results in the large series. J Natl Cancer Inst 1999;91:368–373.
5. Kano M, Shimada Y, Kaganoi J, Sakurai T, Li Z, Sato F, Watanabe G, Imamura M. Detection of lymph node metastasis of esophageal cancer by RT-nested PCR for SCC antigen gene mRNA. Br J Cancer 2000;82:429–435.

©2001 Published by Elsevier Science B.V.
Bronchology and Bronchoesophagology: State of the Art.
H. Yoshimura et al., editors.

Recurrence after esophagectomy with three-field lymph node dissection for submucosal cancer of the esophagus

Tsuyoshi Kato, Yoshiaki Hara, Yousuke Izumi, Tomoko Hanashi and Misao Yoshida
Department of Surgery, Tokyo Metropolitan Komagome General Hospital, Tokyo, Japan

Abstract. *Aim.* The surgical results of submucosal cancer of the esophagus have been improved over the last 10 years. At the same time, there is a small number of patients with postoperative recurrence. The aim of this study was to find the clinico-pathological characteristics of cases with recurrence in order to further improve treatment for submucosal esophageal cancer.

Subjects and Results. Four cases (7.7%) with postoperative recurrence among 52 cases with submucosal cancer treated by esophagectomy and TFD were reviewed. The overall 5-year survival rate of patients who underwent esophagectomy with three-field lymph node dissection (3FD) was 84%, which was significantly better than two-field dissection (2FD, 50%) at our institute. The average number of positive nodes was 4.8 in cases with recurrence and 0.8 in cases without recurrence ($p = 0.0002$). The incidence of marked microvascular permeation was 50% in cases with recurrence and 6% in cases without recurrence ($p = 0.043$).

Conclusion. Postoperative recurrence was noted in 7.7% of all submucosal esophageal cancer cases treated by esophagectomy with three-field lymph node dissection. Clinico-pathological characteristics consisted of a large number of positive nodes or marked microvascular permeations including intramural metastasis. When selecting the appropriate treatment for submucosal cancer of the esophagus, the number of positive nodes and microvascular permeations should be taken into consideration.

Introduction

Esophagectomy with three-field lymph node dissection (3FD) has been the standard operation for submucosal cancer of the esophagus for the last 15 years at our institute. The clinical results of this treatment are excellent. At the same time, there were also a small number of patients who developed postoperative recurrence. The clinico-pathological characteristics of these cases should be examined in order to further improve future treatment.

Subjects

Fifty-two patients with submucosal cancer of the esophagus, who underwent esophagectomy with three-field dissection (3FD), were included in this study.

Address for correspondence: Tuyoshi Kato, Department of Surgery, Tokyo Metropolitan Komagome General Hospital, 3-18-22 Honkomagome, Bunkyo-ku, Tokyo 113-8677, Japan. Tel.: +81-3-3823-2101. Fax: +81-3-3824-1552.

The clinico-pathological characteristics of four patients who developed recurrence after surgery were analyzed.

Results

The overall 5-year survival rate of patients who underwent esophagectomy with three-field lymph node dissection (3FD) was 84%, which was significantly better than two-field dissection (2FD, 50%) at our institute (Fig. 1). The incidence of the postoperative recurrence was noted in 7.7% of all cases. The clinico-pathological characteristics of these cases are as follows: Case 1: a 59-year-old male with two positive nodes and multiple intramural metastases. He developed distant organ metastases in locations such as the lung, liver and bone and died 31 months after the esophagectomy; Case 2: a 58-year-old male with many lymph node metastases. Radical esophgectomy was carried out, including the ligation and resection of the celiac artery in order to remove large lymph node metastases around the celiac axis. He died due to para-aortic lymph node metastases 38 months after the esophagectomy; Case 3: a 57-year-old male with two positive nodes and severe microvascular permeation. He died 8 months after the esophagectomy due to lymph node recurrence in the upper mediastinum; and Case 4: a 62-year-old male with eleven lymph node metastases. He developed lymph node recurrence in the neck 3 months after the esophagectomy.

Discussion

The number of positive nodes is a reliable predictive factor in postoperative prognosis [1,2]. Two patients (50%), with recurrence after esophagectomy, who underwent three-field lymph node dissection had a significantly larger number of positive nodes (cases 2 and 4) in comparison to cases without recurrence. The incidence of severe microvascular permeation, including intramural metastases, was also significantly frequent among patients with recurrence (50%) (Table 1). Patients with recurrence exhibited either of these two factors. The average time

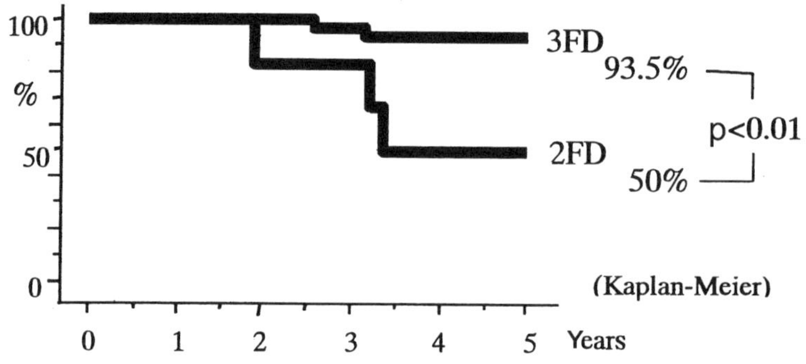

Fig. 1. The effect of three-field lymph node dissection (3FD) on esophageal cancer.

Table 1. Pathological characteristics.

	Number of positive nodes (mean ± SD)		Marked microvascular permeation or intramural metastases (%)	
Recurrence (n = 4)	4.8 ± 4.3	p = 0.0002	50	p = 0.043
Without rccurrence (n = 48)	0.8 ± 1.6		6	

Table 2. Average survival time.

	Average survival (months)	
Recurrence (n = 4)	20	p = 0.06
Without recurrence (n = 48)	64	

of survival in cases with recurrence (20 months) was significantly shorter compared to cases without recurrence (64 months) (Table 2).

Conclusion

In cases with submucosal cancer of the esophagus, esophagectomy with three-field dissection improved the 5-year survival rate. Many lymph node metastases or severe microvascular permeation, including intramural metastases, suggests poor prognosis after radical esophagectomy. These two factors should be seriously taken into consideration when selecting the appropriate treatment for submucosal cancer of the esophagus.

References

1. Junzo S, Koh S et al. Management of the superficial esophageal cancer of the thoracic esophagus as related to clinico-pathological factors and prognosis. Jpn J Gastroenterol Surg 1994; 27(7):1729–1736.
2. Comprehensive Registry of Esophageal Cancer in Japan (1988–1994) 1st edn. The Japanese Society for Esophageal Diseases. Japan, 2000.

Bronchology and Bronchoesophagology: State of the Art.
H. Yoshimura et al., editors.

Chemoradiotherapy with low-dose CDDP and 5FU for locally unresectable hypopharyngeal and upper esophageal cancer

Naoyuki Kohno, Satoshi Kitahara, Etuyo Tamura, Tetuya Tanabe, Manabu Nakanobo, Yasuo Ito, Yasuo Murata, Taichi Furukawa and Yuko Matumura
Department of Otolaryngology, National Defense Medical College, Saitama, Japan

Abstract. We designed the late phase II study of synchronous conventional irradiation with low-dose cisplatin and 5-fluorouracil for the treatment of locally unresectable hypopharyngeal and upper esophageal cancer. The chemoradiotherapy consisted of conventional irradiation with 1.6 to 2.0 Gy/day for 5 days a week, cisplatin (3 mg/m^2) by intravenous infusion for 1 h per day for 5 days a week, and 5-fluorouracil (150 mg/m^2) by intravenous infusion for 24 h per day for 5 days a week. Since 17 patients entered into our study and 16 (94%) patients completed the schedule, treatment compliance was identical. Of the 16 patients evaluable for response, nine had a CR (56%), four had a PR (25%), and an overall response rate of 81% was achieved.

The most frequently observed toxicity was mucositis (75%) and grade III leukopenia occurred in two patients. The responsive patients survived longer (19 months) than the nonresponsive patients (3 months) ($p < 0.001$). This regimen showed a marginal mucous reaction but it was tolerated well. We concluded that this treatment option was effective for locally unresectable hypopharyngeal and upper esophageal cancer.

Keywords: chemoradiotherapy, low dose CDDP and 5FU, unresectable.

Introduction

When dealing with advanced hypopharyngeal and upper esophageal cancer, aggressive surgery and/or radiotherapy has been used as the standard treatment option. Under this treatment the prognosis of patients has been poor, and less than 30% of patients live for more than 5 years. We, therefore, propose the alternative of combining chemotherapy with radiotherapy in order to improve locoregional control [1,2]. Thus, we designed the concomitant conventional irradiation with low-dose cisplatin and 5-fluorouracil for the treatment of unresectable hypopharyngeal and upper esophageal cancer.

Materials and Methods

Patients with histologically proven squamous cell carcinoma of the hypopharynx and upper esophagus, considered to be locally unresectable, were eligible. All patients signed an informed consent before enrollment in the study. All patients

Address for correspondence: Naoyuki Kohno MD, Department of Otolaryngology, National Defense Medical College, 3-2 Namiki, Tokorosawa, Saitama 359-8513, Japan. Tel.: +81-42-995-1686. Fax: +81-42-996-5212.

Table 1. Patient characteristics.

Male/female	13/4
Median age (years)	66 (50–85)
Stage III/IV	8/12
Performance status:	
0	11
1	6
Stage III/IV	2/15
Primary site:	
Hypopharynx	11
Cervical esophagus	6

were required to have an ECOG criterion's performance status of less than two, and an expected survival of greater than 3 months. Staging classification criteria was done according to the Union Against Cancer staging system.

Chemoradiotherapy consisted of conventional irradiation with 1.6 to 2.0 Gy/day for 5 days a week with a total dose of up to between 60 and 70 Gy, cisplatin (3 mg/m^2) by DIV for 1 h per day for 5 days a week, and 5-fluorouracil (150 mg/m^2) by DIV for 24 h per day for 5 days a week. The time of survival was calculated from the first day of treatment on protocol until death or last patient contact. Survival was determined by the Kaplan-Meier Method, and comparison of the time of survival was performed by the Log-rank test.

Results

Patients' characteristics are shown in Table 1. Of the 17 patients who entered the study, one (5%) was not evaluable. The reason for this cases of ineligibility was

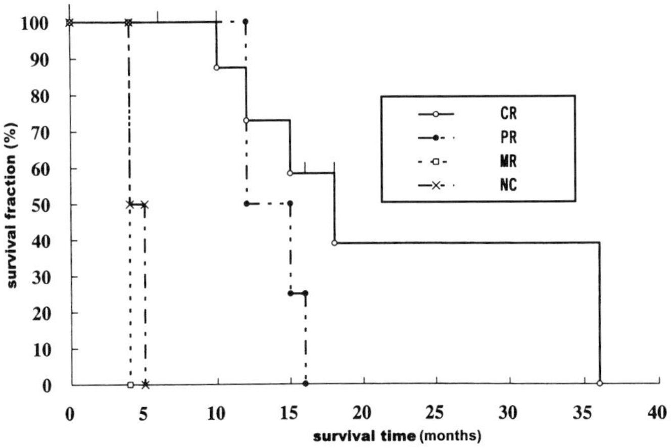

Fig. 1. Survival curves for the responses to the treatment.

Table 2. Toxicities (of the 16 evaluable patients).

Toxicity	Grade I/II	Grade III
Nausea or vomiting	4 (25%)	
Anemia	4	2 (13%)
Leukopenia	4	3 (19%)
Thrombocytopenia	5 (31%)	2
Mucocitis	9 (56%)	3 (19%)
Diarrhea	5	
Alopecia	3	
Renal[a]	2	

[a]Transient increases in serum ceratinine.

protocol violation. Of the 16 patients evaluable for response, nine had a CR (56%), four had a PR (25%), and overall a response rate of 81% was achieved. The median duration of follow-up was 14 months. The responsive patients survived longer (19 months) than the nonresponsive patients (3 months) (Fig. 1). Adverse reactions to this regimen are listed in Table 2. The most frequently observed toxicity was mucositis. Three patients were observed to have Grade III mucositis, but no supportive care, such as enteral nutrition administered through a feeding tube, was required. Myelo suppresion was a major chemotherapy-related side effect. Leukopenia generally occurred 3 weeks after the commencement of chemotherapy. Other toxicities, including alopecia, lassitude, hyponatoremia, and facial edema were all mild and transient. Clinically significant ototoxicity was not observed, nor neurotoxicity or cardiac toxicity.

Conclusions

Since 17 patients entered our study and 16 (95%) patients completed the schedule, treatment compliance was identical.

Our regimen showed a marginal mucous reaction, but it was tolerated well. We conclude that our treatment options were effective on advanced and/or recurrent unresectable head and neck cancer.

References

1. Munro AJ. An overview of randomized controlled trials of adjuvant chemotherapy in head and neck cancer. Br J Cancer 1995;71:83–91.
2. Al-Sarraf M et al. Superiority of chemo-radiotherapy vs. radiotherapy in patients with locally advanced nasopharyngeal cancer. Preliminary results of intergroup randomized study. Proc Am Soc Clin Oncol 1996;15:313.

Gene diagnosis and therapy

Bronchology and Bronchoesophagology: State of the Art.
H. Yoshimura et al., editors.

Adenoviral CTLA4Ig inhibits obliterative airway disease and cell infiltration in rat tracheal allografts

Yusuke Kita[1], Kazuya Suzuki[1], Xiao-Kang Li[2], Hiroshi Nogimura[1], Yoshihiko Kageyama[1], Satoshi Ohi[1], Yasushi Ito[1], Kozo Matsushita[1], Tsuyoshi Takahashi[1], Seiichi Suzuki[2] and Teruhisa Kazui[1]
[1]First Department of Surgery, Hamamatsu University School of Medicine, Hamamatsu; and [2]Department of Experimental Surgery and Bioengineering, National Children's Medical Research Center, Tokyo, Japan

Abstract. *Background.* CTLA4Ig is a soluble recombinant fusion protein that binds to B7 molecules on antigen-presenting cells to block CD28-mediated costimulatory signals and inhibits immune responses. We investigated the effects of systemically administering adenoviral vectors containing CTLA4Ig (adCTLA4Ig) to the obliterative airway disease (OAD) model and examined the infiltrating cells through histopathological studies.

Methods. Tracheal grafts from DA (RT-1^a) or LEW (RT-1^l) rats were transplanted into LEW recipients. The adCTLA4Ig was injected via the recipient's tail vein immediately after grafting. The grafts were removed 7, 14, 21, 28 and 35 days after transplantation for histopathological study. The pathologic scoring criteria and cell infiltration was used for estimation, as described previously [1]. A cryocut section of the frozen piece was double-stained with CD2 and CD25 monoclonal antibodies.

Results. The CD25-positive lymphocyte infiltration in the grafts was remarkably depressed in the adCTLA4Ig-treated group. The allografts on day 28 showed a marked fibrous proliferation and lumenal obstruction, whereas no fibrous change was observed in the syngeneic grafts and CTLA4Ig-treated grafts.

Conclusions. Gene transfer using adenovirus vector achieves efficient transfection into organ cells which contain adenoviral receptors. The adenovirus-mediated CTLA4Ig gene transfer by systemic administration resulted in the remarkable effect of abrogating the OAD in the rat tracheal allografts. The mechanisms can be mediated by inhibiting CD28-associated signal transduction and reducing lymphocyte activity.

Keywords: adenoviral vector, gene therapy, transplantation.

Background

The initiation of a T cell-mediated immune response requires the introduction of antigen-presenting cells (APC) to the T cell receptor (TCR) on helper T cells. Costimulatory signals are also required for T cell activity. The engagement of antigens/MHC with TCR in the absence of costimulatory signals, such as B7/CD28, induces T-cell energy. CTLA4Ig, a soluble recombinant fusion protein that contains the extracellular domain of the CTLA4 and Fc portion of IgG1,

Address for correspondence: Yusuke Kita MD, First Department of Surgery, Hamamatsu University School of Medicine, 3600 Handa-cho, Hamamatsu 431-3192, Japan. Tel.: +81-548-22-9165. Fax: +81-548-22-9165. E-mail: kita21@aqua.ocn.ne.jp strongly adheres to the B7 molecule to block CD28-mediated costimulatory signals and inhibits in vitro and in vivo immune responses.

Obliterative airway disease (OAD) is the most common complication after lung transplantation. The pathologic hallmark of OAD is fibrous small cartilaginous airways along with a variable peribronchiolar inflammatory infiltrate. The chronic inflammation may lead to fibroblast recruitment, extracellular matrix formation, and fibrosis of the bronchioles. This lesion differs from that of acute rejection, which is defined by perivascular mononuclear cell infiltration. A model of OAD, after heterotopical tracheal allografting, in rats undergoes tracheal obliteration, and resembles features of human obliterative bronchiolitis [2]. Mononuclear cell infiltration, denudation of epithelium, fibroproliferation, and obliteration of the airway was subsequently found. These phenomena suggest that a process of graft rejection leads to OAD. In this model, T cells play an important role in the development of disease [1].

Materials and Methods

Adenoviral vector

The adenovirus containing the expression cassette for human CTLA4Ig cDNA or the *Escherichia coli* beta-galactosidase gene (LacZ) was constructed by homologous recombination between the expression cosmid cassette (pAdex/CAhCTLA4Ig) and the parental virus genome.

Experimental groups

Adult male DA (RT-1^a) and LEW (RT-1^l) rats were used as donors and recipients, respectively. The animals were maintained under standard conditions and fed rodent chow and water. Under ether anesthesia, the isolated donor tracheas were transplanted into the subcutaneous pocket in the back of recipients, essentially as described previously [2]. The recipients were divided into the following groups: group 1: DA-to-LEW rats injected with 1×10^9 plaque-forming units (p.f.u.) of control vector, adLacZ (n = 6); group 2: DA-to-LEW rats administered 1×10^9 p.f.u. of adCTLA4Ig (n = 6); group 3: syngeneic grafts (LEW-to-LEW) treated with 1×10^9 p.f.u. of control vector (n = 6); and group 4: syngeneic grafts (LEW-to-LEW) treated with 1×10^9 p.f.u. of adCTLA4Ig (n = 6). The vectors were administered via the recipient's tail vein immediately after grafting. The day of grafting was regarded as day 0 and the grafts were harvested weekly and examined over the course of 49 days.

Histologic studies

The grafts were removed 7, 14, 21, 28, 35, 42 and 49 days after transplantation for histopathological studies. The pathologic scoring criteria was used for estimation, as described previously [1]. For immunohistochemical staining, a cryocut section of the frozen piece was double-stained with CD2 and CD25 monoclonal antibodies.

Results and Discussion

The grafts were removed weekly for histologic study after the transplantation. CD2 was expressed on both resting and activated T cells. CD25 was only expressed on activated T lymphocytes. CD2 and CD25 double-positive lymphocyte infiltration in grafts in group 1 was remarkably depressed in the adCTLA4Ig-treated group (group 2) on day 7 to 14, and the infiltrating levels in group 2 were similar to the syngeneic grafts (groups 3 and 4). The CD25-positive lymphocyte infiltration was prominent until 7 days and then diminished gradually. The control grafts (group 1) showed a marked fibrous proliferation and lumenal obstruction on day 28, whereas no fibrous change was observed in groups 2, 3 and 4 by hematoxylin-eosin staining. DA tracheas treated with adCTLA4Ig (group 2), harvested on day 28, had significantly lower pathologic scores than the control allografts (group 1). No evidence of vector-mediated tissue damage was seen in any graft.

Obliterative airway disease (OAD) is a significant complication which is associated with a T cell response against graft tissue. In rat allografts, the bronchial epithelium starts to express MHC class II antigens during acute rejection and after insufficient cyclosporine treatment [3]. This expression may be induced by locally activated, alloreactive T cells. On epithelial cells, these antigens may stimulate rejection, and become the targets of rejection [4]. The adenoviral vector containing CTLA4Ig-gene markedly inhibited the obliteration of the airway lumen. OAD may be associated with T cell responses against graft tissue.

Monocyte infiltration is a landmark feature of organ rejection. The cellular infiltration is predominantly compromised by macrophages and T lymphocytes, which are responsible for the immunological response to foreign bodies. For this to occur, leukocytes must undergo extravasation, interact with extracellular matrix proteins of the basement membrane, and spread in the graft tissue. AdCTLA4Ig-treatment prevents leukocyte infiltration at the early stage of graft rejection. This result suggests that peripheral leukocytes, especially T lymphocytes, were inhibited by CTLA4Ig-protein and prevented the extravasation. AdCTLA4Ig enabled the persistent gene expression in vivo without repeated administration of the vector. Once the adCTLA4Ig was injected systemically, intrahepatic expression of CTLA4Ig would be prominent. The CTLA4Ig protein might be produced in the gene-transfected hepatocytes and released into blood. Then, eventually, immunosuppressive activity would be induced in the allografts.

Conclusions

The adenovirus-mediated CTLA4Ig gene transfer by systemic administration resulted in the remarkable effect of abrogating the OAD in rat tracheal allografts. The mechanisms can be mediated by inhibiting CD28-associated signal transduction and reducing T lymphocyte activity. The present study demonstrated that adCTLA4Ig-gene transfer into the recipient liver by systemic administration was useful.

References

1. Kelly KE, Hertz MI, Mueller DL. T-cell and major histocompatibility complex requirements for obliterative obliterative airway disease in heterotopically transplanted murine tracheas. Transplantation 1998;66:764–771.
2. Hertz MI, Jessurun J, King MB et al. Reproduction of the obliterative bronchiolitis lesion after heterotopic transplantation of mouse airways. Am J Pathol 1993;142:1945–1951.
3. Romaniuk A, Prop J, Petersen AH et al. Expression of class II major histocompatibility complex antigens by bronchial epithelium in rat lung allografts. Transplantation 1987;44:209–214.
4. Prop J, Jansen HM, Wildevuur CRH et al. Am Rev Respir Dis 1985;132:168–172.

Bronchology and Bronchoesophagology: State of the Art.
H. Yoshimura et al., editors.

The relatively decreased copy number of the p53 gene in lung cancer detected using dual color FISH

Haruhiko Nakamura, Akihiko Ogata, Masaru Hagiwara, Norihito Kawasaki, Tatsuo Ohira, Shunsuke Hiraguri, Makoto Saito, Norihiko Kawate, Chimori Konaka and Harubumi Kato
Department of Surgery, Tokyo Medical University, Shinjuku-ku, Tokyo, Japan

Abstract. For a cell to cell analysis, gene copy number analysis using fluorescence in situ hybridization (FISH) on interphase nuclei is useful. We performed dual color FISH to detect the copy number of the centromere of chromosome 17 and the relative decreased copy number of the p53 gene simultaneously. In 38 lung cancers studied, deletions of the p53 gene were detected in 42.1% of the cases. No significant differences were found in the frequency of the p53 deletion among histologic types or disease stages. The instability of the chromosome 17 copy number was detected in 25%. Deletions of the p53 gene were significantly associated with the instability of chromosome 17 ($p = 0.001$). We concluded that deletions of the p53 gene, detected by FISH, were closely associated with the instability of the chromosome 17 copy number.

Keywords: chromosomal instability, fluorescence in situ hybridization, nonsmall cell lung cancer (NSCLC).

Background

The aberrations of the p53 gene are one of the most frequent abnormalities found in lung cancer cells. In nonsmall cell lung cancers (NSCLCs), 50 to 60% of the tumors have been reported to carry alterations of the p53 gene, while mutations of this gene can be detected in more than 90% of small cell lung cancers. Those p53 gene abnormalities were mainly detected by loss of heterozygosity (LOH) for allelic loss, single strand conformation polymorphism (SSCP) for point mutations or small deletions, and immunohistochemistry (IHC) for altered protein expression.

Since samples for LOH and SSCP are DNAs extracted from cancer tissues, evaluation of the gene abnormalities in an individual cell is impossible. For this purpose, a gene copy number analysis using interphase fluorescence in situ hybridization (FISH) becomes a powerful tool [1, 2]. The relationship between copy number abnormalities and the clinico-pathologic features in lung cancer has not yet been clarified. Thus, we analyzed the copy number of the p53 gene and centromeric signals of chromosome 17 to see the correlaton between the

Address for correspondence: Haruhiko Nakamura MD, Department of Surgery, Tokyo Medical University, 6-7-1 Nishi-shinjuku, Shinjuku-ku, Tokyo 160-0023, Japan. Tel.: +81-3-3342-6111, ext. 5071, 5838, 5845. Fax: +81-3-3342-6154. E-mail: hanakamu@tokyo-med.ac.jp gene copy number abnormalities and clinico-pathologic features of lung cancer patients.

Methods

Touch preparations were made immediately after resection of the tumor; the fresh cut surface of the primary tumor was gently touched to the microscopic slide glasses. A Spectrum-orange-labelled probe for the p53 locus and a Spectrum-green-labelled probe for the centromeric region of chromosome 17 are commercially available and were purchased from the manufacturer (Vysis Inc). In brief, slides were then denatured by incubation with formamide (70% in 2x SSC) at 74°C for 2 min in a water bath. The slides were then dehydrated through ethanol (70% for 2 min, 85% for 2 min, 100% for 2 min). Hybridization solution (10 μl) was applied to each slide, which was coverslipped and sealed with rubber cement. The hybridization solution contained 1 μl of probe in formamide (70%), 2x SSC, and dextran sulfate (10%, Cot1 DNA). After incubation for 16 h at 37°C in a humidified chamber, slides were washed with 2x SSC for 5 min at 74°C. Then DAPI-antifade solution (8 μl) was applied to each spot and coverslipped. 100 cells were counted and when the number of signals of the p53 was less than the number of centromeric signals, those cells were considered to have deletion. When the percentage of deleted cells in the specimen was more than 25%, that tumor was judged to be carrying deletion of the p53 gene. The presence of chromosomal instability (CIN) was judged to be when the sum of percentages of cells that were not carrying the modal copy number of chromosome 17 was more than 25%.

Results

The 38 primary lung cancers consisted of 26 adenocarcinomas, nine squamous cell carcinomas, and three small cell carcinomas, which were all analyzed. In terms of the postsurgical pathological stage, there were 23 in stage I, six in stage II, seven in stage IIIA, and two in stage IIIB. p53 deletion was detected in 16 out of 38 (42.1%) of the patients. The frequency of the p53 deletion is shown in Table 1. No correlation was found between the frequency of the p53 deletion and the stage, histologic type, differentiation grade, or pN factor. However, the p53 deletion was significantly related to the copy number instability of chromosome 17 (χ^2 test, $p = 0.001$). No survival difference was found between the undeleted group and the deleted group (log rank test, $p = 0.4364$).

Conclusions

In our study, deletions of the p53 gene were detected in about 40% of the NSCLC patients. Although abnormalities of the p53 gene have been reported to correlate with a worse outcome in some studies, we did not find any survival differences

Table 1. The p53 gene deletion detected using FISH.

Factors	Frequency of deletion (%)	p value (χ^2 test)
Histologic type:		
Ad	10/26 (38.5%)	
Sq	3/9 (33.3%)	
Sm	3/3 (100%)	0.1025
Pathologic stage:		
I	12/23 (52.2%)	
II	1/6 (16.7%)	
III	3/9 (33.3%)	0.2425
Differentiation:		
W/D	4/10 (40.0%)	
M/D	6/16 (37.5%)	
P/D	3/9 (33.3%)	0.9551
pN factor:		
N0	14/30 (46.7%)	
N1–3	2/8 (25.0%)	0.3701

between the deleted and undeleted groups. However, the presence of chromosomal instability detected in chromosome 17 was closely associated with p53 deletion.

References

1. Virmani A, Tonk V, Gazdar A. Comparison between fluorescence in situ hybridization and classical cytogenetics in human tumors. Anticancer Res 1998;18(3A):1351–1356.
2. Schenk T, Ackermann J, Brunner C, Schenk P, Zojer N, Roka S et al. Detection of chromosomal aneuploidy by interphase fluorescence in situ hybridization in bronchoscopically gained cells from lung cancer patients. Chest 1997;111(6):1691–1696.

Bronchology and Bronchoesophagology: State of the Art.
H. Yoshimura et al., editors.

The effects of calcium on HPV16 gene transcription in cultured laryngeal epithelial cells

Kouichiro K. Tsutsumi, Hiroya Iwatake, Daisuke Kuwabara, Atsushi Hyodo, Takehiko Kobayashi, Izumi Koizuka and Isao Kato
Department of Otolaryngology, St. Marianna University School of Medicine, Kawasaki, Japan

Abstract. The purpose of this study was to examine the effects of calcium on cytokeratin No. 13 (CK13) expression and human papillomavirus type 16 (HPV16) gene transcription in cultured laryngeal epithelial cells (HLEC). We analyzed two types of HPV16-containing HLEC: HPV16-immortalized HLEC (HLEC16) and HPV16-infected cultured laryngeal papilloma cells (HLP16). In the HLEC16, the viral genome was integrated into the host cell chromosomes, while the HLP16 contained the extrachromosomal viral genome. The effects of increasing calcium concentrations on CK13 expression were then evaluated using immunocytochemistry. Both the HLP16 and the HLEC16 responded to an increased calcium concentration by inducing CK13 expression. In HLP16 and HLEC16, the CK13 expression was undetectable at low calcium concentrations (0.1 mM) but became clearly detectable at high calcium concentrations (1.0 mM). The level of viral RNA was elevated in HLP16 with added calcium (1.0 mM) but was similar in HLEC16, grown in either low- (0.1 mM) or high- (1.0 mM) calcium concentrations. These results suggest that a calcium-induced differentiation results in the up-regulation of HPV16 gene transcription in HLP16. The integration of viral genome into the host cell chromosomes may be an important determinant for the differentiation-independent transcription of HPV16 genes.

Keywords: cytokeratin No. 13, differentiation.

Introduction

Human papillomavirus (HPV) gene transcription is closely linked to the differentiation status of infected epithelial cell [1]. A variety of physiological agents, including calcium, regulates the differentiation of cultured epithelial cells [2]. The expression of cytokeratin No. 13 (CK13) can be used as a marker for differentiation in cultured laryngeal epithelial cell (HLEC) [3]. The purpose of this study was to examine the effects of extracellular calcium on CK13 expression and the human papillomavirus type 16 (HPV16) gene transcription in HLEC.

Materials and Methods

We analyzed two types of HPV16-containing HLEC. HPV16 genome was introduced into primary cultured HLEC, and an immortalized cell line (HLEC16)

Address for correspondence: Kouichiro K. Tsutsumi, Department of Otolaryngology, St. Marianna University School of Medicine, 2-16-1, Sugao, Miyamae-ku, Kawasaki, Kanagawa 216-8512, Japan. Tel.: +81-44-977-8111. Fax: +81-44-976-8748. E-mail: tensaikouichiro@msn.com was established [4]. We also obtained cultured papilloma cells (HLP16) from a laryngeal papilloma case. The physical state of HPV16 genome in HLP16 and HLEC16 was evaluated by Southern blot analysis. Bam HI- (one-cut restriction enzyme for 7.9 kb HPV16 genome) digested cellular DNA was hybridized with HPV16 DNA. HLEC16 and HLP16 were cultured in a 0.1 mM low-calcium medium for 48 h. Then the medium was changed for a new low-calcium medium and a 1.0 mM high-calcium medium. Both cells were then cultured for 72 h, the total cellular RNA was isolated, and the level of viral RNA was evaluated by Northern blot analysis. Cells were also fixed, and the CK13 expression was evaluated by immunocytochemistry.

Results

Physical state of HPV16 genome in HLP16 and HLEC16

In HLEC16, the viral genome was integrated into the host cell chromosome. In contrast, HLP16 contained the extrachromosomal viral genome.

Calcium regulation of CK13 expression in HLP16 and HLEC16

Using immunocytochemistry, we evaluated the effect of increasing calcium concentrations on CK13 expression in HLP16 and HLEC16. Both the HLP16 and the HLEC16 responded to an increased calcium concentration by inducing CK13 expression. The CK13 expression was undetectable at low-calcium concentrations (0.1 mM), but became clearly detectable at high-calcium concentrations (1.0 mM).

Calcium regulation of HPV16 gene transcription in HLP16 and HLEC16

Using Northern blot analysis, we evaluated the effect of increasing calcium concentrations (from 0.1 mM to 1.0 mM) on HPV16 gene transcription in HLP16 and HLEC16. HLP16 and HLEC16 were cultured for 72 h in a low-calcium medium (0.1 mM) and high-calcium medium (1.0 mM), and then the total cellular RNA was isolated. The blots were hybridized with the E6/E7 region of HPV16. In order to normalize the quantity of the loaded RNA, blots were rehybridized with the cDNA encoding actin. The level of viral RNA was elevated in HLP16 with added calcium (1.0 mM), but was similar in HLEC16, grown in either low- (0.1 mM) or high- (1.0 mM) calcium concentrations.

Discussion

Our present data suggest two points. Firstly, HLP16 had the extrachromosomal HPV16 genome, and a calcium-induced differentiation might result in the up-regulation of HPV16 gene transcription in HLP16. Secondly, HLEC16 had the integrated HPV16 genome, and the viral genome integration into the host cell chromosomes might be an important determinant resulting in the differentiation-independent transcription of HPV16 genes.

Acknowledgements

This study was supported by Grants-in-Aid for Scientific Research (C) (No. 09671769 and 12671287) from the Japanese Ministry of Education, Science, Sports and Culture.

References

1. Durst M, Glitz D, Schneider A, zur Hausen H. Human papillomavirus type 16 (HPV 16) gene expression and DNA replication in cervical neoplasia: analysis by in situ hybridization. Virology 1992;189:132–140.
2. Yuspa SH, Kilkenny AE, Steinert PM, Roop DR. Expression of murine epidermal differentiation markers is tightly regulated by restricted extracellular calcium concentrations in vitro. Cell Biol 1989;109:1207–1217.
3. Vambutas A, DiLorenzo TP, Steinberg BM. Laryngeal papilloma cells have high levels of epidermal growth factor receptor and respond to epidermal growth factor by a decrease in epithelial differentiation. Cancer Res 1993;53:910–914.
4. Tsutsumi K, Iwatake H, Suzuki T. An experimental model of multistep laryngeal carcinogenesis: Combined effect of human papillomavirus type 16 genome and N-Methyl-N′-nitro-N-nitrosoguanidine. Acta Otolaryngol 1996;522:89–93.

Head and neck cancer

Bronchology and Bronchoesophagology: State of the Art.
H. Yoshimura et al., editors.

Head and neck cancer developing after radical surgery of esophageal cancer

Madoka K. Furukawa[1] and Masaki Furukawa[2]

[1]*Department of Head and Neck Surgery, Kanagawa Cancer Center, Yokohama, Japan; and* [2]*Department of Medical Informatics, Medical Center, Yokohama City University School of Medicine, Yokohama, Japan*

Abstract. We examined nine patients who developed head and neck cancer as asynchronous multiple cancer following radical surgery of esophageal cancer. These head and neck cancer cases included hypopharyngeal cancer in six patients, mesopharyngeal cancer in two patients, and laryngeal cancer in one patient. Treatment consisted of radical irradiation in five of the six patients with hypopharyngeal cancer, however, only one patient with stage II cancer survived without a tumor, and the prognosis was poor in other patients. Among the two patients with mesopharyngeal cancer, one patient underwent radical surgery and survived without a tumor, and the patient with laryngeal cancer recieved radiation therapy, and also survived without a tumor. It is, therefore, necessary to accurately evaluate whether patients can survive radical treatment for metachronously occurring head and neck cancer, and to choose a treatment method in the light of the quality of life (QOL) the patients will have, considering that they are already in poor general condition.

Keywords: asynchronous, multiple cancers, treatment.

Introduction

Recently, with advances in various treatments and diagnostic methods for cancer and the aging of cancer patients, the problem of multiple cancers is being given greater importance [1,2]. The incidence of multiple cancers consisting of esophageal cancer and head and neck cancer is high [3–5], and, in particular, in cases of metachronously occurring multiple cancers, the influence of previous treatment needs to be considered during the determination of the therapeutic strategy [6]. We examined patients who had developed head and neck cancer as asynchronous multiple cancer following radical surgery of esophageal cancer.

Subjects

Between April 1987 and March 1998, 687 patients with head and neck cancer recieved primary treatment at our department, and among them, asynchronous multiple cancers were noted in nine patients who developed head and neck cancer after radical surgery of esophageal cancer. These patients were examined for

Address for correspondence: Madoka K. Furukawa, Department of Head and Neck Surgery, Kanagawa Cancer Center, 1-1-2 Nakao, Asahi-ku, Yokohama 241-0815, Japan. Tel.: +81-45-391-5761. Fax: +81-45-361-4692. E-mail: madoka@yokohama.email.ne.jp the influence of preceding cancer treatment, factors that affect the determination of the therapeutic strategy, and the clinical courses followed during treatment of head and neck cancer as the second cancer.

Results

The subjects consisted of eight males and one female, ranging in age from 56 to 76 years (mean: 65 years). These head and neck cancer cases included hypopharyngeal cancer in six patients, mesopharyngeal cancer in two patients, and laryngeal cancer in one patient. Three patients had stage II cancer, and six patients had stage IV cancer. The interval between the time of surgery on the esophageal cancer and the diagnosis of head and neck cancer was less than 5 years in three patients, 5 to less than 10 years in four patients, and 10 years or more in two patients. In one patient, who developed hypopharyngeal cancer 8 years postoperatively, recurrent cancer of the esophagus was also detected during the diagnosis of hypopharyngeal cancer, however, this was not the case in any of the other patients. Treatment consisted of radical irradiation in five of the six patients with hypopharyngeal cancer, however, only one patient with stage II cancer survived without a tumor, and the prognosis was poor in other patients. Among the two patients with mesopharyngeal cancer, one patient underwent radical surgery and survived without a tumor, and the patient with laryngeal cancer received radiation therapy, and also survived without a tumor.

Conclusion

Patients who have undergone radical surgery for esophageal cancer are frequently in poor general condition due to the influence of previous treatment. It is, therefore, necessary to accurately evaluate whether patients can survive radical treatment for metachronously occurring head and neck cancer, and to choose a treatment method in the light of the QOL the patients will have, considering that they are in already in poor general condition.

References

1. Thompson W, Oddson T, Kelvin F et al. Synchronous and metachronous squamous cell carcinomas of head, neck and esophagus. Gastrointest Radiol 1978;3:123–127.
2. Licciardello J, Spitz M, Hong W. Multiple primary cancer in patients with cancer of the head and neck: second cancer of the head and neck, esophagus, and lung. Int J Radiat Oncol Biol Phys 1989;17:2273–2279.
3. Fitzpatrick P, Tepperman B, de Boer G. Multiple primary squamous cell carcinomas in the upper digestive tract. Int J Radiat Oncol Biol Phys 1984;10:2273–2279.
4. Miyazato H, Tamai O, Tomita S et al. Esophageal cancer in patients with head and neck cancers. Int Surg 1997;82:319–321.
5. Shibuya H, Wakita T, Nakagawa T et al. The relation between an esophageal cancer and associated cancers in adjacent organs. Cancer 1995;76:101–105.

6. Tachimori Y, Watanabe H, Kato H et al. Treatment for synchronous and metachronous carcinomas of head and neck and esophagus. J Oncol 1990;45:43–45.

Bronchology and Bronchoesophagology: State of the Art.
H. Yoshimura et al., editors.

Four cases with laryngeal necrosis after combined chemoradiotherapy for head and neck cancer

Fumihiro Katsura, Yasuhiro Samejima and Eiji Yumoto
Department of Otorhinolaryngology, Kumamoto University School of Medicine, Kumamoto, Japan

Abstract. One severe complication of combined chemoradiotherapy can be the development laryngeal necrosis, when the irradiation field includes the larynx. Of 88 head and neck cancer patients seen over 9 years, four developed laryngeal necrosis (4.6%). The possibility of the development of laryngeal necrosis should be considered in patients who have received irradiation doses of over 67 Gy and develop persistent edema of the larynx.

Keywords: chemoradiotherapy, head and neck cancer, laryngeal necrosis.

Introduction

We have treated head and neck cancer patients with combined chemoradiotherapy for 9 years and attained a relatively high complete-regression rate. However, the risk of certain complications occurring due to this therapy is generally higher compared to that of radiotherapy alone. One severe complication of chemoradiotherapy can be the development of laryngeal necrosis, when the irradiation field includes the larynx. Here, we report four cases of laryngeal necrosis that developed after combined chemoradiotherapy.

Subjects and Methods

During the study period, from 1990 to 1998, 88 patients with head and neck squamous cell carcinomas were treated at our department using combined chemoradiotherapy. Of these, 68 had laryngeal cancer, and 20 had hypopharyngeal cancer. As for the irradiation, the dose was over 60 Gy and the larynx was included in the field. In addition, low-dose cisplatin (CDDP, 5mg/day) was administered intravenously. The diagnosis of laryngeal necrosis was defined as CT findings of cartilage destruction and/or histological proof of cartilaginous necrosis in biopsy specimen.

Address for correspondence: Fumihiro Katsura, Otorhinolaryngology, Kumamoto University School of Medicine, 1-1-1 Honjo, Kumamoto 860-8556, Japan. Tel.: +81-96-373-5255. Fax: +81-96-373-5256.

Results

Based on these criteria, four cases, out of 88 patients (4.6%), were diagnosed to have developed laryngeal necrosis. Table 1 shows the patient characteristics of these four cases. Two cases had hypopharyngeal cancer, two had laryngeal cancer, and none of them had any severe systemic diseases. All of the patients received irradiation of over 67 Gy. Patients 1, 2, and 4 received concomitant chemoradiotherapy along with weekly injections of 5 mg CDDP. Patient 3 received daily injections of 5 mg CDDP and 450 mg 5-FU orally on each irradiated day. During chemoradiotherapy, no severe side effects were observed, and so treatments were completed as planned. All of the patients achieved complete regression of the cancer, however, they continually complaining of dryness, appetite loss, or a sore throat, even after cessation of the therapy.

They were initially managed conservatively, using humidification and oral antibiotics. However, patients 1 and 2 then underwent tracheostomies and eventually laryngectomies because of the progression. Patient 3 suffered from severe pain and dysphagia immediately after irradiation. Intensive conservative treatment, including intravenous injections of antibiotics and steroids, narcotic analgesic, and a gastrostomy, for nutritional purposes, were all carried out several times during the 6 months after the completion of the chemoradiotherapy. Although he was relieved of the severe complaints, without tracheostomy or laryngectomy, his symptoms have remained constant up to the present. Patient 4, who was diagnosed with laryngeal necrosis after 5 months of irradiation, died of a recurrent tumor 5 years later. He occasionally complained of hoarseness and dyspnea but medical treatment relieved his symptoms. However, 4 years later, he was suffering from severe dyspnea, caused by severe laryngeal edema with the fixation of a vocal fold. A biopsy performed using a direct laryngoscope demonstrated recurrence of the tumor. Unfortunately, the diagnosis came too late for a salvage operation due to the extent of invasion. We should have performed an immediate laryngectomy when his symptoms and signs got worse.

Table 1. The patient characteristics of the four cases with laryngeal necrosis.

Case	Age (years)	Gender	Site	Stage	Total dosage used on the larynx (Gy)
1	64	M	Hypopharynx (postwall)	T2N0M0	67
2	74	M	Hypopharynx (pyriform sinus)	T2N0M0	70
3	60	M	Larynx (subglottis)	T2N0M0	70
4	75	M	Larynx (glottis)	T2N0M0	69.4

Conclusions

1. The possibility of the development of laryngeal necrosis should be considered in patients who received irradiation doses of over 67 Gy and developed persistent edema in the larynx.
2. Intensive conservative treatment, including steroids, antibiotics, and hyperbaric oxygen, is essential for patients with laryngeal necrosis. However, if the complaints and signs exacerbate, despite this treatment, a surgical procedure is necessary.

Bronchology and Bronchoesophagology: State of the Art.
H. Yoshimura et al., editors.

A study on the treatment of head and neck cancer accompanied by esophageal cancer

Kiyoaki Tsukahara, Yasuhisa Koyanagi, Tomoyuki Yoshida, A. Masaji Lee, Hitoshi Inoue, Hiroyuki Ito and Mamoru Suzuki
Tokyo Medical University, Tokyo, Japan

Abstract. The incidence of double and triple cancers is on the increase, as have the development of diagnostic technique and therapeutic modality. We studied the clinical course and the effect of treatments for the esophageal cancer cases that accompanied head and neck cancers. Forty-nine esophageal cancer cases, that accompanied head and neck cancers, were treated at our department between 1989 and 1998. Among these, 15 cases were triple cancers. The predominant treatment for synchronous double cancers was end-mural resection or other surgery. One-half the cases involving esophageal cancers preceded by head and neck cancers were operated on and the other half were irradiated and treated with chemotherapy. These results suggest that a periodical follow-up of the upper digestive tract is mandatory, since the majority of the synchronous double esophageal cancers were early stage. High incidence of the esophageal double cancer also suggests that a systemized screening strategy for early detection of a head and neck lesion is urgently needed.

Keywords: asynchronous cancer, conservative treatment, radical treatment, synchronous cancer.

Background

Double and triple cancers have been increasing in recent years as have the development of diagnostic techniques and treatment. However, the most appropriate treatment in such cases has not yet been established. In this study, we examined the treatment methods for double cancer of the head and neck associated with esophageal cancer.

Methods

Of the 513 patients with esophageal cancer, treated at Tokyo Medical University between 1989 and 1998, patients with double cancer of the head and neck were selected as subjects. Double cancer was defined according to the definition of Warren et al. [1] and the additional criteria proposed by Saikawa et al. [2].

Double cancer of other organs was found in 92 (17.9%) of the 513 patients with previously untreated esophageal cancer, and of these, double cancer of the head and neck was found in 49 of the patients (9.6%). Forty-seven of the 49 patients were male and two were female.

Address for correspondence: Kiyoaki Tsukahara, Tokyo Medical University, 6-7-1 Nishishinjunku, Shinjunku-ku, Tokyo 160-0023, Japan. Tel.: +81-3-3342-6111. Fax: +81-3-3226-7030.

Results and Comments

The synchronous esophageal double or triple cancer cases are as follows. Of 19 cases with synchronous double or triple cancer, esophageal cancer was associated with hypopharyngeal cancer in most of the patients (12), and laryngeal cancer in five. Of 21 cases with triple cancer, one case of coexisting gastric and laryngeal cancer, and one case of coexisting gastric and hypopharyngeal cancer were noted. In these patients, the esophageal cancer was detected through a thorough examination of the whole body in the department of otolaryngology. All the esophageal cancers were in the early stage and the treatment method used for all the synchronous double or triple cancer in the esophagus and the head-neck region was radical.

The asynchronous double cancer cases are as follows. Asynchronous double cancer was divided into two types, i.e., cases in which the head and neck case was diagnosed first, and cases in which the esophageal cancer was diagnosed first. Among the patients with double or triple cancer in whom the head and neck cancer was diagnosed first, five had cancers of the hypopharynx and esophagus, and three had cancers of the oropharynx and esophagus. Thus, eight of the 11 (73%) had pharyngeal cancer. In the patients in whom esophageal cancer was diagnosed first, two had cancers of the hypopharynx and esophagus, and one had cancers of the epipharynx and esophagus. Thus, three of the four (75%) had pharyngeal cancer.

The treatment methods used for esophageal cancer in which the head and neck cancer was diagnosed first were as follows: closed evulsion of the esophagus in five cases, radiotherapy and chemotherapy in five cases, and extraction of the esophagus by thoracotomy in one case. Among the patients in whom esophageal cancer was diagnosed first, three were surgically treated by thoracotomy, and one was treated by a closed technique. None of the patients were treated by radio- or chemotherapy.

Among those in whom esophageal cancer was diagnosed first, closed evulsion was only possible in one case (25%), as many of them had advanced diseases. Three (75%) required thoracotomy.

Among the 11 patients in whom esophageal cancer was the secondary cancer, seven were treated radically and four were treated conservatively. Out of the four in whom cancer of the head and neck was secondary, two were treated radically and two conservatively.

In the cases with asynchronous triple cancer, the treatment methods for the patients with two cancers which developed simultaneously are as follows. Synchronous double cancer was diagnosed first in five patients, while single primary cancer of one region was found in three patients.

All five patients in whom synchronous double cancer was diagnosed first could be radically treated. Among the patients with the single primary cancer, only one could be treated radically, while two were treated conservatively.

The treatment methods used for asynchronous double or triple cancer, including those in which two of the three cancers developed simultaneously, are as follows. Among 11 in whom the head and neck cancer was diagnosed first, seven were treated radically. The second cancer was treated conservatively in four cases because of death associated with the treatment, advanced age, advanced esophageal cancer, or bone metastasis. Two of four in whom esophageal cancer was diagnosed first were treated conservatively due to the metastasis to the lung and bone. All patients with triple cancer in whom synchronous double cancer was diagnosed first were treated radically.

Among three in whom the primary cancer was present in the head-neck and the cancer was associated with esophageal cancer, two were treated conservatively because of the advanced head and neck lesion and pulmonary multiple metastases.

The methods of treating asynchronous triple cancer and the reasons for conservative treatment are as follows. Except for the patient with the primary bladder cancer, all had a primary lesion in the head and neck. Among five cases, the third cancer could not be treated radically in three.

The reasons for palliative treatment of the third cancer in these three patients are as follows: the advanced head-neck lesion and bone metastasis, or refusal of surgery.

The survival period after the onset of the last cancer is as follows. Both patients with synchronous triple cancer are still alive.

Except for the two patients with triple cancer, 19 in whom the double cancer developed secondarily were treated radically, but overall, six died within 1 year and nine died within 3 years. However, judging from the gross survival rate (57%), the treatment outcome of esophageal cancer in this study appears to be of an acceptable level. This may be because many of the esophageal cancers were in the early stage.

Among 25 cases with triple cancer in which the single cancer developed secondarily, nine were treated conservatively. It is probably because of this that the gross survival rate dropped to 44%, and 11 died within 3 years. The possible explanations for this include detection of the second or third cancers in more advanced stages, an older age range, and other systemic problems which developed after treatment of the first cancer. For such reasons, in addition to these patients, three more died within just over 3 years after the onset.

Conclusion

The treatment methods for double or triple cancer of the head and neck accompanied by untreated esophageal cancer were examined.

In all cases of synchronous double cancer, cancer of the head and neck was diagnosed first, the esophageal cancer was in the early stage, and all patients were treated radically.

Among the cases with asynchronous double cancer, 11 were only treated conservatively due to local recurrence or distant metastasis after the initial treatment.

These results suggest that long-term and periodical thorough examinations of the whole body are necessary after the development of the first cancer.

We wish to emphasize our recognition of the fact that treatment of asynchronous double or triple cancer is difficult due to the advanced stage of the second or third cancer, advanced age, and other systemic problems encountered after treatment of the first cancer.

References

1. Warren S, Gates O et al. Multiple primary malignant tumors. A survey of the literature and a statistical study. Am J Cancer 1932;16:1356–1414.
2. Saikawa M et al. Multiple primary tumors in head and neck cancer patients. Jpn J Cancer Clin 1998;44(11):1351–1358.

Imaging

Bronchology and Bronchoesophagology: State of the Art.
H. Yoshimura et al., editors.

Virtual CT endoscopy in a case of tracheobronchopathia osteochondroplastica

Kosuke Ishii[1], Yasuyuki Kobayashi[2], Hidetaka Tanaka[1] and Katsumi Takizawa[1]
[1]Department of Otorhinolaryngology and [2]Department of Radiology, Jichi Medical School, Omiya Medical Center, Omiya-shi, Saitama, Japan

Abstract. Remarkable advances in computer-generated graphics have enabled us to observe body structure on the images generated from helical CT data sets. Virtual CT endoscopy is one of these virtual reality methods. Here we report the usefulness of virtual endoscopy in a case of tracheobronchopathia osteochondroplastica accidentally found during endotracheal intubation. The patient was a 68-year-old female for whom a laparotomy, under general anesthesia, was scheduled for cecal cancer. Endotracheal intubation was interrupted due to an osseous protrusion located in the subglottic space. Multiple small nodules were also found on the distal wall of the trachea. Based on three-dimensional CT data, virtual CT endoscopy was performed to demonstrate multiple small nodules on the tracheal wall. Compared with conventional bronchoscopy, virtual CT endoscopy provided more precise images of peripheral bronchi, which could not be produced by real endoscopy, without any burden to the patient.

Keywords: bronchoscopy, computer, CT.

Introduction

Remarkable advances in computer-generated graphics have enabled us to observe body structure on images generated from helical CT data sets. Virtual CT endoscopy is one of these virtual reality methods [1–3]. Here we report a case of tracheobronchopathia osteochondroplastica that was accidentally found during an endotracheal intubation.

Case

The patient was a 68-year-old female who was scheduled to undergo a laparotomy, under general anesthesia, for cecal cancer. However, endotracheal intubation was interupted due to a hard tumor located in the subglottic space. Surgery was postponed after a discussion with otolaryngologists. Symptoms such as stridor and dyspnea had not been noted before surgery. Using bronchoscopy, a bony-hard mass with a white surface was seen protruding from the anterior wall of the subglottis. A small lumen of the airway persisted posterior to

Address for correspondence: Kosuke Ishii MD, Jichi Medical School, Jichi Medical Center, 1-847 Amanuma-cho, Omiya-shi, Saitama 330-8503, Japan. Tel.: +81-48-647-2111. Fax: +81-48-648-5188.

the mass, and it was difficult to observe peripheral bronchi over the stenosis. A horizontal CT of the neck showed that the osseous protrusion in the subglottic space was in close contact with the cricoid cartilage. A chest CT also demonstrated multiple calcifications on the tracheal wall. These findings led us to establish the diagnosis of tracheobronchopatia chondroplastica [4].

Virtual endoscopy

As in this case, diagnostic imaging is very useful in cases of tracheal stenoses where the evaluation of entire airways lesions is necessary, a difficultly bronchoscopy cannot overcome. We performed three-dimensional reconstruction of helical CT images of calcified lesions in the trachea in this case (Fig. 1). Using the technique of virtual endoscopy, we also attempted to observe the inner wall of the 3D-reconstructed trachea and bronchi. The tip of the endoscope was first placed in the supraglottic area, was passed through the glottic space and then guided easily down beyond the protrusion located in the subglottic area. Multiple nodules of various sizes were seen in the distal part of the trachea (Fig. 2). It was clear that protruding lesions were not present in the membranous portion. Compared with conventional bronchoscopy, virtual CT endoscopy provided more precise images of peripheral bronchi, which could not be attained through performing a real endoscope, without any burden to the patient.

Treatment and Course

Ileocecal resection was performed under epidural anesthesia due to the patient

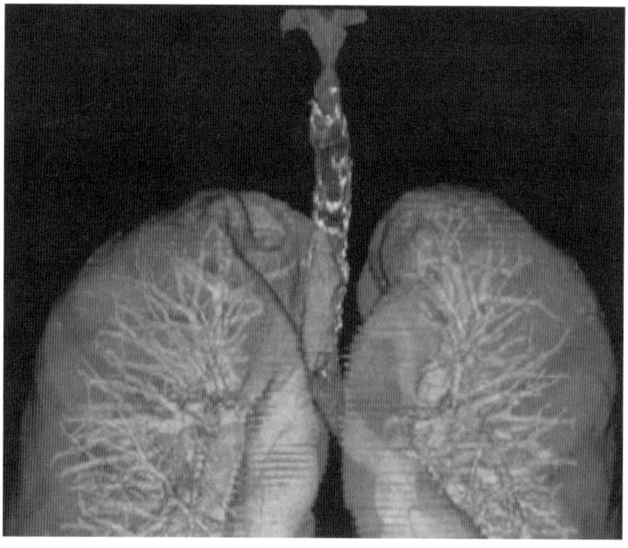

Fig. 1. A three-dimensional image of calcified lesions in the trachea.

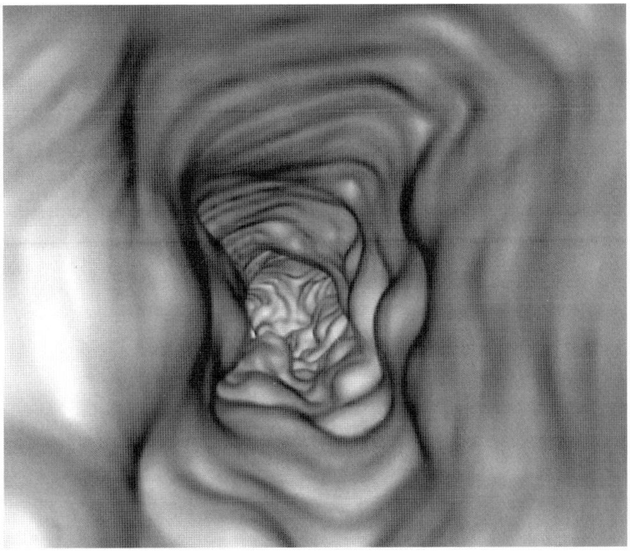

Fig. 2. A virtual endoscopic image of the trachea. Multiple nodules can be seen.

having rejected tracheotomy. As for the tracheobronchopathia osteochondroplastica, she remained under observation owing to the absence of relevant symptoms.

Discussion

As shown in this case, virtual endoscopy is very useful for the observation of trachea with stenosis. After helical CT is performed, the lumen can be observed as many times as required without patient discomfort. However, there are some problems with virtual endoscopy. For example, it is difficult to visualize small or flat lesions, changes in color on the mucosal surface are undetectable, and, of course, biopsy and treatment are impossible. Virtual endoscopy will never replace actual endoscopy. However, advances in computer technology and the clinical significance of virtual endoscopy will increase even further in the future.

References

1. Rubin GD, Beaulieu CF, Argro V et al. Prespective volume rendering of CT and MR images: applications for endoscopic imaging. Radiology 1996;199:321–330.
2. Rubin GD. Techniques of reconstruction. In: Remy-Jardan M, Remy J (eds) Spiral CT of the Chest. Berlin: Springer, 1996;101–127.
3. Vining DJ, Liu K, Choplin RH et al. Virtual Bronchoscopy. Chest 1996;109:549–553.
4. Nienhuis DM, Srakash UBS, Edell ES. Tracheobronchopathia osteochondroplastica. Ann Otol Rhinol Laryngol 1990;99:689–694.

Bronchology and Bronchoesophagology: State of the Art.
H. Yoshimura et al., editors.

The visibility of peripheral bronchi in virtual bronchoscopy from multidetector CT data

Hiroshi Moriya, Masamichi Koyama, Makoto Miyazaki, Hiroshi Honjo and Naoto Hashimoto
Department of Radiology, Fukushima Medical University, School of Medicine, Fukushima city, Fukushima, Japan

Abstract. The visibility of bronchi in virtual bronchoscopy (VB) depends on the collimation thickness of CT. Therefore, the collimation and bronchial imaging using VB were studied. In 10 patients, CT data were acquired with a collimation of 5 mm, and the VB images of lobar to segmental bronchi were obtained. In the another 10 patients, with a collimation of 2 mm, the VB images were obtained up to the entrance (orifice) of the subsegmental bronchus, which is comparable to the level that can be visualized using a conventional bronchoscope. In the remaining five patients, CT data were acquired using a multidetector CT (MDCT) with a collimation of 0.5 mm, and the VB images of the 5th to 10th bronchi were obtained. It was impossible to obtain the images of these peripheral bronchi using a conventional bronchoscope. In conclusion, MDCT with 0.5 mm collimation thickness significantly improved the display of small peripheral bronchi in VB.

Keywords: collimation thickness of CT, fly-through, isotropic voxel, region-growing method.

Background

Virtual bronchoscopy (VB) is a display technique that allows volume data to be observed from within the bronchial tree, which is very valuable in helping the bronchoscopist to visualize the anatomy 3D. However, the visibility of bronchi depends on the collimation thickness of CT. Peripheral bronchi are not visible in VB when using a single-detector CT, compared with actual bronchoscopy. Therefore, we used a multidetector CT (MDCT), which allows isotropic-imaging, and examined the visibility of bronchi in VB from MDCT data.

Materials and Methods

Collimation and bronchial imaging using VB were studied. VB was performed in 25 adult patients with peripheral lung tumors, who were scheduled to undergo transbronchial biopsy using a bronchoscope. CT data were acquired during a single breath-hold. The area extending from the bifurcation of the lobar bronchi to

---

Address for correspondence: Hiroshi Moriya, Department of Radiology, Fukushima Medical University, School of Medicine, Hikarigaoka-1, Fukushima city, Fukushima 960-1295, Japan. Tel.: +81-24-548-2111. Fax: +81-24-549-3789. E-mail: hmoriya@cc.fmu.ac.jp

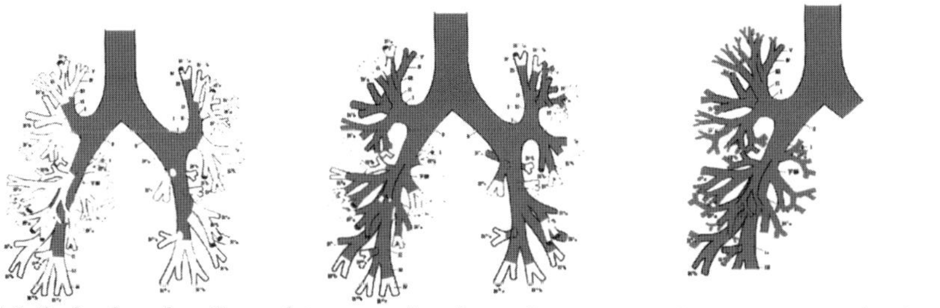

Bronchial display based on 5 mm-data
Based on 2 mm-data
Based on 0.5 mm-MDCT data

Fig. 1. Depicted bronchi on virtual bronchoscopy.

the target lesion was scanned. We used Toshiba Xpress/SX (with a collimation thickness of 5 or 2 mm, 1 s/rotation, single detector, pitch 1; until 1998), and Aquilion MDCT (with a collimation thickness of 0.5 mm, 0.5 s/rotation, 4 detectors, pitch 3; after 1999).

In 10 patients, CT data were acquired with a collimation of 5 mm, in the another 10 patients, with a collimation of 2 mm, and in the remaining five patients, CT data were acquired using MDCT with a collimation of 0.5 mm.

VB was reconstructed at an ALATOVIEW workstation (fly-through software; which employs the polygon method developed by Toshiba and Nagoya University). The volume of the continuous region was semiautomatically extracted using the region-growing method from the tracheobronchial lumen, and VB was used to follow each bronchus to the peripheral limit.

Results

1. VB, with 5 mm collimation, allowed us to obtain the images of the lobar to segmental bronchi, however, the images of the bronchus in the direction of the scan were inferior.
2. VB, with 2 mm collimation, allowed us to obtain images up to the entrance (orifice) of the subsegmental bronchus, which is comparable to the level that can be visualized using a conventional bronchoscope.
3. VB, with 2 mm collimation, allowed us to view more peripheral bronchi (up to about the 5th level), when the bronchi ran perpendicular to the scanning direction, however, when the bronchi ran parallel to the scanning direction, only the branches up to about the 3rd level could be visualized.
4. VB, with 0.5 mm collimation, allowed us to obtain images of the 5th to the 10th bronchi, and images of the bronchi up to the 10th level were frequently obtained in the scan direction. It was impossible to obtain images of these peripheral bronchi using a conventional bronchoscope (Fig. 1, Table 1).

Table 1. The visibility of bronchi in virtual bronchoscopy.

B1a i: 5 6th ii: 7 8th order bronchi	B6a i: 4 7th ii: 5 7th order bronchi
b i: 5–6th ii: 5th	b i: 4–7th ii: 5–8th
B2a i: 4th ii: 5th	c i: 5–7th ii: 4–9th
b i: 5th ii: 5th	B7a i: 4–5th ii: 5–9th
B3a i: 6–8th ii: 6–7th	b i: 3rd–9th ii: 3rd–5th
b i: 6–11th ii: 6–8th	B8a i: 5–8th ii: 4–9th
B4a i: 4th ii: 4–5th	b i: 4–7th ii: 5–7th
b i: 3rd–6th ii: 3rd–6th	B9a i: 4–8th ii: 4–5th
B5a i: 4–5th ii: 6–8th	b i: 5–8th ii: 4–6th
b i: 5–6th ii: 4th	B10a i: 4th ii: 6th

MDCT, with 0.5 mm collimation and 0.5 s/rotation, in the right lungs of five cases.

Conclusion

MDCT, with a 0.5-mm collimation thickness, significantly improved the display of small peripheral bronchi in VB.

Bronchology and Bronchoesophagology: State of the Art.
H. Yoshimura et al., editors.

Virtual bronchoscopy as a roadmap for transbronchial biopsy

Hiroshi Moriya, Masamichi Koyama, Makoto Miyazaki, Hiroshi Honjo and Naoto Hashimoto
Department of Radiology, Fukushima Medical University, School of Medicine, Fukushima city, Fukushima, Japan

Abstract. The definitive diagnosis of lung cancer is frequently based on the results of a transbronchial biopsy. Therefore, we studied the usefulness of virtual bronchoscopy (VB) to simulate actual bronchoscopic procedures. VB was performed in 30 adult patients with lung tumors, who were scheduled to undergo transbronchial biopsy using a bronchoscope. As a result, we could choose the accessible bronchi to the target tumor in all cases. There were no discrepancies between VB images and actual endoscopic images with regard to shape. In conclusion, this technique was effective for identifying the specific bronchus associated with the peripheral lung tumor.

Keywords: lung cancer, mediastinal mass, surface-rendering, transbronchial needle aspiration, volume-rendering.

Background

The definitive diagnosis of lung cancer is frequently based on the results of a transbronchial biopsy. However, in some cases it is difficult to reach small peripheral lesions, and a high degree of technical expertise is also required. Therefore, we have employed virtual bronchoscopy (VB) to simulate actual bronchoscopic procedures in advance. This technique has been found to be effective for identifying the specific bronchus associated with the lesion and for determining the optimal puncture site in bronchoscopic needle biopsy procedures. Therefore, we studied the usefulness of virtual bronchoscopy(VB) in simulating actual bronchoscopic procedures.

Materials and Methods

VB was performed in 30 adult patients with lung tumors, who were scheduled to undergo a transbronchial biopsy using a bronchoscope. CT data were acquired with Toshiba Xpress/SX or Aquilion. The VB was reconstructed on a surface-rendering system (ALATOVIEW workstation; developed by Toshiba and Nagoya University) or a real-time volume-rendering system (work in progress, Toshiba Nasu Works).

Address for correspondence: Hiroshi Moriya, Department of Radiology, Fukushima Medical University, School of Medicine, Hikarigaoka-1, Fukushima city, Fukushima 960-1295, Japan. Tel.: +81-24-548-2111. Fax: +81-24-549-3789. E-mail: hmoriya@cc.fmu.ac.jp

Results

1. We could choose the most accessible bronchi to the target tumor in all cases, and there were no discrepancies between VB images and actual endoscopic images with regard to shape.
2. VB, with 2 mm collimation, allowed us to obtain images of the subsegmental bronchi, and we could choose the most accessible subsegmental bronchi to the lung tumor. VB, with 0.5 mm collimation, allowed us to obtain images of the 5th to the 10th bronchi, and we could choose the most accessible bronchi to the lung tumor on this level as well.

Case 1 (adenocarcinoma showing ground-glass opacity, Fig. 1)

1. Acquisition of helical volume data. CT data were acquired using Aquilion (a multidetector, with a slice width of 0.5 mm, 0.5 s/rotation, pitch 3).
2. Methods for virtual bronchoscopy. VB was performed at an ALATOVIEW workstation, which allows a surface display of the bronchial lumen, and permits the point of view to be adjusted interactively. Segmentation was performed using the threshold technique and the region-growing technique (semiautomatic extraction). The virtual tracheobronchial space and target tumor were generated for simulation.

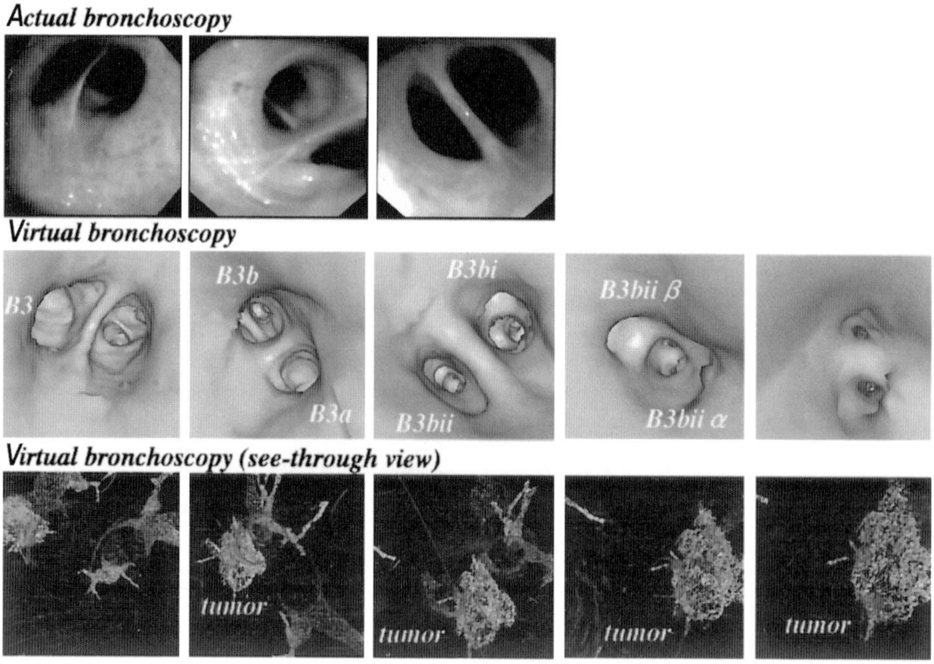

Fig. 1. A peripheral lung tumor.

3. Techniques of virtual bronchoscopy for transbronchial biopsy planning [1–3]. VB was performed before bronchoscopic examination for a peripheral lung nodule. The virtual tracheobronchial space and target tumor were generated for simulation. The peripheral nodule and the peripheral bronchi were visible through the bronchial wall in see-through view (wire-frame images).

Figure 1 shows a case of adenocarcinoma showing ground-glass opacity that could not be clearly visualized by X-ray fluoroscopy. However, preoperative VB allowed us to confirm that the tumor could be reached via the branch running superiorly toward B3biiα or the branch running laterally toward B3biβ. In the actual procedure, biopsy was performed based on the information obtained by VB simulation, and a suitable specimen for pathological diagnosis was successfully obtained.

Case 2 (mediastinal lymphnode metastases of small cell lung cancer, Fig. 2)

1. Acquisition of helical volume data. CT data were acquired using Xpress/SX (a single-detector, with a slice width of 5 mm, pitch 1). CT studies were performed with 100 mL of nonionic contrast medium (Iopamiron 370) injected at a rate of 2 mL/s. The scan delay was 50 s.
2. Methods for virtual bronchoscopy. VB was performed using a real-time volume-rendering system, which allows a volume display of the acquired

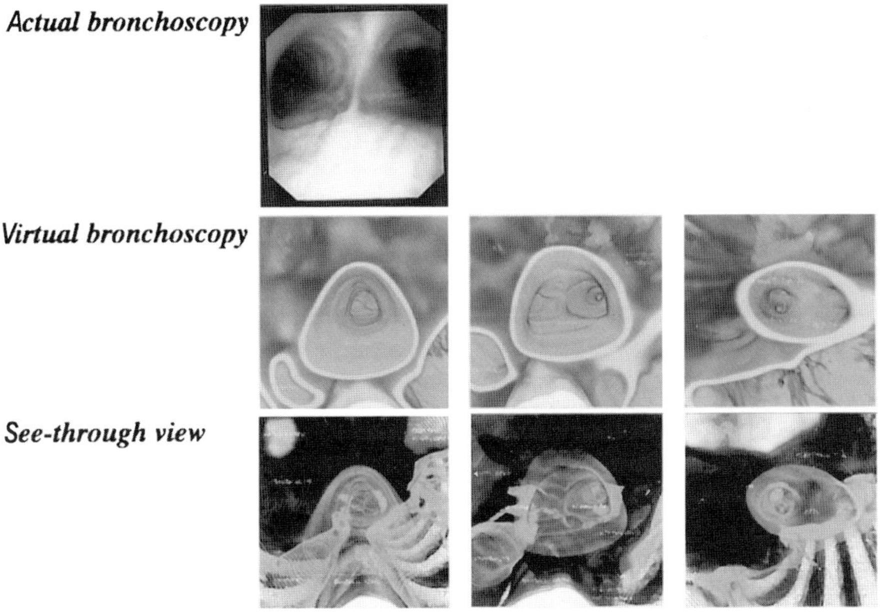

Fig. 2. Enlarged mediastinal lymph nodes.

volume data and permits the point of view to be adjusted interactively. Volume rendering has the advantage of permitting peribronchial tissues to be seen through the bronchial walls. The virtual tracheobronchial space, thoracic vessels, and mediastinal lymph nodes were rendered for simulation (volume rendering parameters can be adjusted to see through the bronchial wall to examine structures external to the lumen).

3. Techniques of virtual bronchoscopy for transbronchial biopsy planning [4,5].

Figure 2 is a case with mediastinal lymph node metastases of small cell lung cancer. VB was performed before transbronchial needle aspiration. The enlarged mediastinal lymph nodes and the large vessels (aorta, right pulmonary artery, superior vena cava, azygos vein) were visible through the carinal wall. We identified a safe and accessible point in the bronchial tree. Transbronchial needle aspiration biopsy was performed through the bronchial wall of the mediastinal side of the right main bronchus, and atypical cells of small cell carcinoma were obtained.

Conclusion

VB is an effective clinical tool for planning transbronchial biopsy procedures in patients with peripheral lung tumors or mediastinal masses.

References

1. Moriya H, Koyama M, Honjo H et al. Interactive virtual bronchoscopy as a guide for transbronchial biopsy in two cases. J Jpn Soc Bronchol 1998;20:610–613.
2. Moriya H, Honjo H, Miyazaki M et al. 3D imaging with an X-ray CT scanner: high-speed multislice CT scanner and 3D image processor. Med Rev 1999;71:2–6.
3. Moriya H, Honjo H, Miyazaki M et al. Clinical experience with the aquilion multidetector CT scanner. Med Rev 2000;72:1–11.
4. Moriya H, Suzuki K. CT bronchoschopic examination using the fly-through methods: virtual bronchoscopy. Med Rev 1999;70:1–8.
5. Moriya H, Miyazaki M, Koyama M et al. Virtual bronchoscopy as a roadmap for transbronchial biopsy procedures. In: Lemke HU, Vannier MW, Inamura K, Farman AG (eds) CARS '99 (International Congress Series No. 1191). Amsterdam: Elsevier, 1999;993.

Bronchology and Bronchoesophagology: State of the Art.
H. Yoshimura et al., editors.

Selective bronchography using iomeprol and carboxymethylcellulose sodium

Yoichi Nakanishi, Koji Inoue, Kanehito Kimotsuki, Taishi Harada, Koichi Takayama, Miiru Izumi, Hiroshi Wataya, Takahiro Minami, Ric Ishibashi and Nobuyuki Hara

Research Institute for Diseases of the Chest, Graduate School of Medical Sciences, Kyushu University, Fukuoka, Japan

Abstract. The aim of this study was to assess the usefulness and safety of bronchography using iomeprol and carboxymethylcellulose sodium (CMC-Na). Firstly, an optimum concentration of CMC-Na was determined by comparing the mixture of iopamidol and different concentrations of CMC-Na. The mixture of iopamidol and 4% CMC-Na had a more substantial amount of viscosity (1,083 cP at 37°C), compared to iopamidol alone (9 cP). Bronchography was performed in 31 patients. The mixture of the contrast medium (4% CMC-Na and iomeprol but not iopamidol) was directly injected through the bronchoscope channel and bronchography was performed. Good quality bronchograms were obtained in 32 out of 35 (91%) cases without the rapid appearance of air alveologram, frequently seen when using iomeprol alone. Dynamic changes in the bronchi, between inspiratory and expiratory phases, were clearly observed in a selected patient group. Side effects were slight and disappeared transiently. In conclusion, bronchography using iomeprol and CMC-Na is a useful and safe approach to detect morphological changes in a tracheobronchial tree.

Backgrounds

Bronchography used be a gold-standard procedure for the evaluation of the morphological changes in a tracheobronchial tree. However, there were several disadvantages, especially when standard bronchographic contrast agents were used. These included technical difficulty, side effects such as, drug allergy or impairment of ventilation, and the obscuration of the bronchoscopic view when the standard media was injected through the channel. Instead, CAT scans were adopted as an alternative method. However, when using a CAT scan, dynamic changes in the bronchi are difficult to observe, the evaluation of relatively peripheral bronchi (4th to 6th bronchi) is impossible, and the diagnosis of congenital anomalies in a tracheobronchial tree is very difficult [1].

Several investigators have reported the usefulness of nonionic contrast media [2,3], but it is difficult to obtain a clear imaging due to its low viscosity. Therefore, we developed the idea of assessing the usefulness and safety of bronchography using a nonionic contrast media and carboxymethylcellulose sodium (CMC-Na).

Address for correspondence: Yoichi Nakanishi, Research Institute for Diseases of the Chest, Graduate School of Medical Sciences, Kyushu University, 3-1-1 Maidashi, Higashi-ku, Fukuoka 812-8582, Japan. Tel.: +81-92-642-5378. Fax: +81-92-642-5389.

Materials and Methods

The nonionic contrast media iopamidol and iomeprol were used. In order to increase the viscosity of the contrast media, sterilized CMC-Na was also used. Preparation of the bronchographic contrast media consisted of mixing the same amounts of iopamidol and CMC-Na together, at the concentrations of 1 to 4%. Then, the viscosity, specific gravity and osmolarity of each mixture was measured. After optimization of the bronchographic media, bronchography was performed. The contrast media were injected through the channel of the bronchoscope.

Results

The physicochemical characteristics of each mixture were determined. Iopamidol alone, had an iodine concentration of 370 mg/ml, a viscosity of 9 cP at 37°C, a specific gravity of 1.41 at 37°C and an osmolarity of 1073 mOsm/kg H_2O. In contrast, the mixture containing nonionic contrast media and 4% CMC-Na, had an iodine concentration of 185 mg/ml, a viscosity of 1083 cP at 37°C, a specific gravity of 1.22 at 37°C and an osmolarity of 548 mOsm/kg H_2O. This mixture was judged to be of optimal usefulness due to its high viscosity and tolerable osmolarity, even though its iodine concentration was a little low.

For bronchography, iomeprol instead of iopamidol was adopted because of its higher iodine concentration. A total of 31 patients underwent a total of 35 bronchographies. There were 16 male and 15 female patients with the median age of 54 years (range: 27 to 75 years). Clinical diagnosis of the patients consisted of bronchiectasis in 13 patients, lung neoplasm in eight and various other methods for the remaining 10. Among 35 bronchographies, all the cases were evaluable and in 32 out of 35 (91%) cases, good quality images were obtained. In one case with Williams-Campbell syndrome and another with Steven-Johnson syndrome, dynamic changes of the bronchi were observed that could not be detected by a CAT scan. Concerning side effects, a transient low grade fever of less than 37.5°C was seen in two cases, a headache in one, flashes in two and nausea in two. However, all of these side effects were only mild and disappeared spontaneously.

Discussion

By adopting a nonionizing contrast medium, we developed a refined method of bronchography. Since this medium was translucent, it did not obscure the bronchoscopic view when it was injected through the channel of bronchoscope, and a clear image was obtained due to its high viscosity and sufficient concentration of iodine. Irritability to the airway was also mild because of the tolerable osmotic pressure. Allergic reactions were few, since the media used were nonionizing media and most of the medium was aspirated off after bronchography. In addition, irreversible alveolar damage, which used to be induced by standard contrast media, did not occur.

In conclusion, bronchography using iomeprol and CMC-Na is a simple, useful and safe approach to detect morphological changes in a tracheobronchial tree.

References

1. Barbato A, Novello Jr A, Zanolin D, Corner P, Talenti E. Diverticulosis of the main bronchi: a rare cause of recurrent bronchopneumonia in a child. Thorax 1993;48:187–188.
2. Morcos SK, Baudouin SV, Anderson PB, Beedie R, Bury RW. Iotrolan in selective bronchography via the fibreoptic bronchoscope. Br J Radiol 1989;62:383–385.
3. Riebel T, Wartner R. Use of non-ionic contrast media for bronchography in neonates and young infants. Eur J Radiol 1990;11:120–124.

Bronchology and Bronchoesophagology: State of the Art.
H. Yoshimura et al., editors.

Real-time observation of the ciliary motion of the bronchial epithelium through a bronchovideoscope

Akira Sakurada, Masami Sato, Motoyasu Sagawa, Hiroto Takahashi, Shulin Wu, Yoshinori Okada, Yuji Matsumura, Tatsuo Tanita and Takashi Kondo
Department of Thoracic Surgery, Institute of Development, Aging and Cancer, Tohoku University, Sendai, Japan

Abstract. Ciliary motion plays a very important role in the human respiratory system. We observed the surface of a surgically resected human bronchus through the stereoscopic zoom microscope, as well as videoscopes specially modified for high-power magnification, which can magnify objects by approximately × 100. By changing the angle of the light-guiding fiber and the objective stage of the stereoscopic zoom microscope, ciliary motion was visualized in the halation of the bronchial surface at a certain angle of incidence. The ciliary motion was recognized as the many fine flickers of light at the magnification of × 100 to × 150, and was recognized as many beating whips at the magnification of × 500. Through the videoscopes, many flickers of light were recognized on the surface of the surgically resected bronchus, using the structure enhancement function of a video image processor. The light flickers were also recognized in the human body through the videoscope. Observation through a novel videoscope, according to our optical method, will enable us to understand the physiological role of ciliary motion in vivo and apply bronchoscopic diagnosis to various disorders.

Keywords: bronchoscope, cilia, magnification, visualization.

The ciliary beats of the bronchial epithelium play an important role in the airway clearance system. However, real-time observation has depended on a phase-contrast or stereoscopic zoom microscope, and most investigations have been performed mainly in vitro [1,2]. In a few reported studies, ciliary activity was measured in vivo by a laser-based light-reflection technique, but visualization of the ciliary motion has not been reported in vivo [3–5]. If the real-time endoscopic observation of ciliary motion in the human body should become possible, it would be very useful for understanding the human airway clearance system and also for detecting a variety of disorders of the respiratory system. Here, we report such real-time visualization of ciliary motion made possible by the use of a specially modified bronchovideoscope.

We used model CF-200Z, model 6C240, and prototypes of the high-power magnification bronchovideoscope (Olympus Optical Co., Ltd.). These videoscopes can magnify objects × 80 to × 100 on a 14-inch TV monitor at a short focal distance, of approximately 3 to 5 mm. We inserted the videoscope into the

Address for correspondence: Akira Sakurada, Department of Thoracic Surgery, Institute of Development, Aging and Cancer, Tohoku University, 4-1 Seiryo-machi, Aoba-ku, Sendai 980-8575, Japan. Tel.: +81-22-717-8526. Fax: +81-22-717-8526. E-mail: sakurada@idac.tohoku.ac.jp bronchial lumen and monitored the image on a 14-inch TV monitor. We were able to recognize the details of known structures, for instance, the winding of the capillary vessels and the irregularities of the surface of carcinoma. The captured image was modified in real time through the structure-enhancement function of a video processor, model CV-240 (Olympus Optical Co., Ltd.). Through careful observation, we were able to recognize fine light flickers in the halation on the bronchial surface.

To clarify whether the fine light flickers, observed with the magnifying endoscope, were ciliary motion or not, we observed the resected human and porcine lungs with a stereoscopic zoom microscope. Approximately 1 cm^2 of bronchial wall was cut from the lung and immediately attached to a small corkboard with pins. We placed the sample on an objective stage, adjustable to various angles, and changed the direction of the light-guided fiber in order to achieve appropriate halation on the bronchial surface. The most efficient angle of incidence for observation was determined. At the magnification of $\times$ 100 to $\times$ 150, fine light flickers were observed in the areas of halation, as observed through the videoscope. We speculate that these images resulted from Fresnel reflection. With increasing magnification up to $\times$ 500, the image was gradually recognisable as many beating whips. In addition, the motion had an almost regular rhythm and a specific direction. According to the appearance and the manner of the motion, we concluded that the image represented metachronal waves of the cilia.

Our results show a possible novel clinical application of the bronchovideoscope to investigate tracheobronchial disorders. It is widely known that atypical squamous cells replace ciliated cells in the early periods of carcinogenesis. With a modified bronchovideoscope, we will be able to distinguish areas where ciliated cells are absent from the surrounding normal areas. This is a new detection method for intraepithelial lesions, that is completely different from all present methods. In addition, we will be able to monitor ciliary activity, which is affected by a variety of disorders, drugs and operative procedures. Our method has enormous advantages over the laser-based light-reflection technique. Although there are some problems to be resolved, such as the stabilization of the image, this method will enable us to understand ciliary motion in the human body.

Acknowledgements

The authors would like to thank K. Kaji, T. Kitano, Y. Morizane, T. Takigawa, T. Suzuki and I. Nakamura (Olympus Optical Co. Ltd.) for their technical assistance.

References

1. Wanner A, Salathé M, O'riordan TG. Mucociliary clearance in the airways. Am J Respir Crit Care Med 1996;154:1869–1902.
2. Sanderson MJ, Dirksen ER. Quantification of ciliary beat frequency and metachrony by high-

speed digital video. Meth Cell Biol 1995;45:289–297.
3. Wong LB, Miller IF, Yeates DB. Stimulation of ciliary beat frequency by autonomic agonists: in vivo. J Appl Physiol 1998;65:971–981.
4. Wong LB, Miller IF, Yeates DB. Nature of the mammalian ciliary metachronal wave. J Appl Physiol 1993;75:458–467.
5. Huberman D. A device for measuring mucociliary activity in the human bronchi during fiber-optic bronchoscopy. Acta Otolaryngol 1993;113:683–686.

Bronchology and Bronchoesophagology: State of the Art.
H. Yoshimura et al., editors.

Usefulness of virtual bronchoscopy using helical CT in clinical practice

Motoshi Takao[1], Akira Shimamoto[1], Takatsugu Shimono[1], Kuniyoshi Tanaka[1], Hideto Shimpo[1], Isao Yada[1], Syuichi Murashima[2] and Kan Takeda[2]
Departments of [1] Thoracic Surgery and [2] Radiology, School of Medicine, Mie University, Mie, Japan

Abstract. *Background.* The recent advances in helical CT and 3-D image processing technology brought in the medical innovation of virtual bronchoscopy, in which the point of view is placed within the airways and the viewing angle is adjusted in the same way as in bronchoscopic examination.
Methods. The reconstructed 3-D virtual bronchoscopic images were compared with conventional CT images or actual bronchoscopic images in seven patients to evaluate the clinical usefulness of virtual bronchoscopy using helical CT.
Results. It was feasible to analyze the inner surface of airway tracts in all examinations. The images had a definite advantage, in that they depicted the bronchial lumen beyond the stenosis, however, the quality of the mucosal surface seen was inferior to that of actual bronchoscopic images.
Conclusions. Virtual bronchoscopic images using helical CT are superior to conventional CT or FOB in providing unique information about longitudinal lesions of the airway tracts and the distal portion beyond the stenosis, although further improvements are needed for obstructive lesions.

Keywords: clinical study, endobronchial lesion, simulation, three-dimensional (3D) CT, tracheobronchial tree.

Background

The recent advances in helical CT and 3-D image processing technology brought in the medical innovation of virtual bronchoscopy, in which the point of view is placed within the airways and the viewing angle is adjusted in the same way as in bronchoscopic examination [1,2].

Methods

The reconstructed 3-D virtual bronchoscopic images were compared with conventional CT images or actual bronchoscopic images in seven patients to evaluate the clinical usefulness of virtual bronchoscopy using helical CT. The helical CT scan cycle consisted of 35 to 40 continuous rotations, each requiring 0.8 s, for a total scanning time of about 30 s. Scans were obtained using a 5-mm X-ray beam width, a 7.5-mm/0.8 s bed sliding speed, and a 1.25 or 2.5-mm reconstruction interval. The patients ages ranged from 7 months to 71 years of age. Tar-

Address for correspondence: Motoshi Takao MD, PhD, Department of Thoracic Surgery, School of Medicine, Mie University, 2-174 Edobashi, Tsu, Mie 514-8507, Japan. Tel.: +81-59231-5116. Fax: +81-59231-2845. E-mail: takao@clin.medic.mie-u.ac.jp get sites were from the trachea to the lobar and segmental bronchi. The nature of target lesions was obstruction in three cases, stenosis in three cases, and anomaly in one.

Results

It was feasible to analyze the inner surface of airway tracts in all examinations (Table 1). The images had a definite advantage, in that they depicted the bronchial lumen beyond the stenosis, however, the quality of the mucosal surface seen was inferior to that of actual bronchoscopic images (Fig. 1). The clinical advantages of virtual bronchoscopy using helical CT are as follows: 1) The evaluation of the airway tracts beyond the severe stenosis is possible, which is not with FOB, and the measurement of the longitudinal distance of airway stenosis or obstruction provide simulation for the airway reconstruction or intervention; 2) The evaluation of airway tracts in critically ill patients or babies who might be at risk using FOB, and patients with multiple traumatic injury (Fig. 2) is feasible; and 3) Reanalysis and reconstruction of images of the target lesion, after examination, is feasible as long as data are saved.

Conclusions

Virtual bronchoscopic images using helical CT are superior to conventional CT or FOB in providing unique information about longitudinal lesions of the airway

Table 1. Patient characteristics of seven cases who underwent virtual bronchoscopy.

Case	Age (years)	Sex	Disease	Site and nature	3D image[a]	Advantage[b]
1	69	M	Lung cancer (preoperative)	Rt. upper br. Obstruction	Good	No
2	60	M	Lung cancer (local recurrence)	Rt.lower br. Stenosis	Excellent	Yes
3	50	F	Lung cancer (postoperative)	Rt. middle br. Obstruction	Good	Yes
4	59	M	Blunt chest injury	Lt. main br. Obstruction	Good	Yes
5	57	M	TAA (postoperative)	Lt. main br. Stenosis	Excellent	Yes
6	0.7	M	Tracheal bronchus	Trachea Anomaly	Excellent	Yes
7	71	M	Lung cancer (postoperative)	Lt. basal br. Stenosis	Excellent	Yes

[a]Excellent: abnormal finding was clearly visualized on 3D image; Good: abnormal finding was visualized on 3D image; and Poor: abnormal finding was not visualized on 3D image. [b]More precise examination was possible compared to FOB. Abbreviations: M: male, F: female, Rt.: right, Lt.: left, br.: bronchus, TAA: thoracic aortic aneurysm, op.: operation.

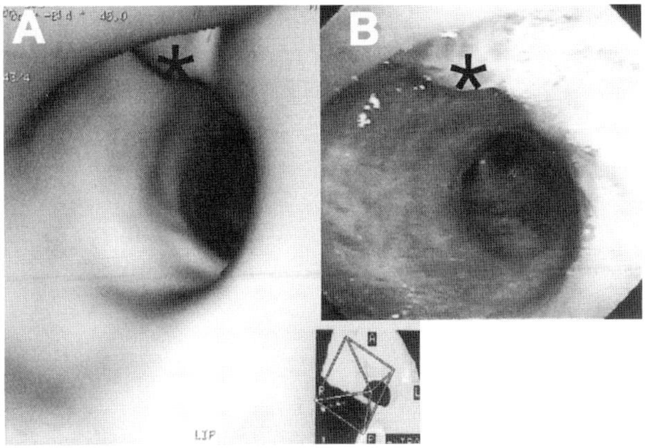

Fig. 1. Squamous cell carcinoma at the orifice of the right upper bronchus (case 1). **A:** Virtual bronchoscopy revealed the patency of airway tracts with fine reproducibility of cartilage crescents and the tumor (*). **B:** The mucosal texture is better visualized using FOB though.

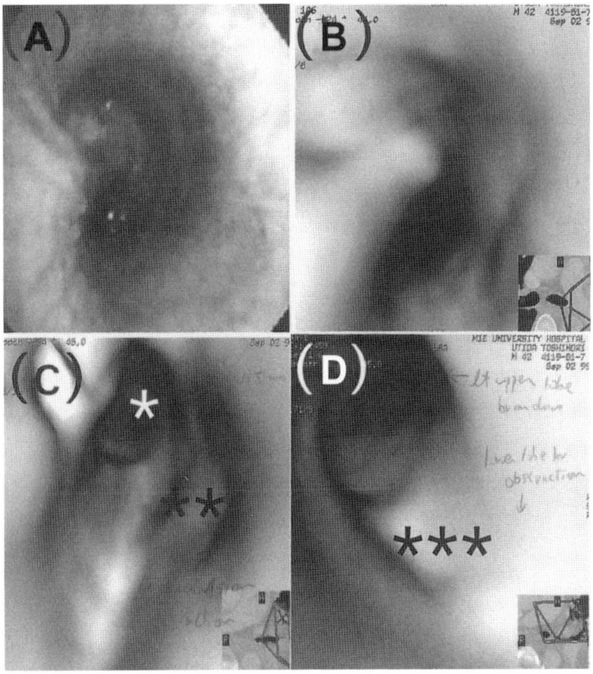

Fig. 2. **A:** FOB was unable to provide information about the distal airway beyond the obstruction of left main bronchus. Virtual bronchoscopy revealed the obstructed left main bronchus (**B**); the patent upper division (*) and the obstructed lingular division (**) (**C**); and the lower bronchus (***) (**D**). This information, suggesting a multiple bronchial injury, made us choose to perform a left pneumonectomy instead of bronchoplasty (case 4).

tracts and the distal portion beyond the stenosis, although further improvements are needed for obstructive lesions.

References

1. Summers RM, Feng DH et al. Virtual bronchoscopy: segmentation method for real-time display. Radiology 1996;200:857–862.
2. Rubin GD, Beaulieu CF et al. Perspective volume rendering of CT and MR images: applications for endoscopic imaging. Radiology 1996;199:321–330.

Bronchology and Bronchoesophagology: State of the Art.
H. Yoshimura et al., editors.

Study of three-dimensional imaging of solitary pulmonary nodules

H. Takekawa[1], M. Noguchi[1], K. Hagiwara[1], M. Maruhashi[1], H. Yokoyama[1], M. Fujii[1], H. Moriyama[2], N. Takizawa[2] and H. Kato[2]
[1]*Tokyo Metropolitan Cancer Detection Center, Tokyo, Japan; and* [2]*Tokyo Medical University, Tokyo, Japan*

Abstract. Helical (spiral) CT is a recently developed method, and CT diagnosis of solitary pulmonary nodules (SPN) using this method has been performed in several institutions [1–6], including ours. We investigated the usefulness of 3D-CT for the diagnosis of SPNs.

Keywords: CT diagnosis, helical CT, peripheral pulmonary nodule, three-dimensional computed tomography.

Introduction

The helical CT scanner, combined with powerful computer hardware, as well as new algorithms for three-dimensional (3D) rendering, has improved the current technical performance of 3D imaging. We investigated the usefulness of differential diagnosis for solitary pulmonary nodules (SPNs) using this new technology.

Materials and Methods

Helical CT scans were obtained using an Xvigor scanner (Toshiba, Tokyo). A helical CT scan with a 2-mm section thickness and 2-mm/s table feed time was performed during a single breath-hold. Each 3D image demonstrated the solitary pulmonary nodules and surrounding structures.

Results

1. In adenocarcinoma, the irregular surface of nodules, pleural indentation and the convergence of peripheral vessels and bronchi could be comprehended spatially (Fig. 1).
2. In hamartoma, the smooth surface of nodules and slight oppression to peripheral vessels and bronchi could be observed (Fig. 2).

Address for correspondence: H. Takekawa, Tokyo Metropolitan Cancer Detection Center, 2-5 Kanda Surugadai, Chiyoda-ku, Tokyo 101-0062, Japan. Tel.: +81-3-3292-2341. Fax: +81-3-3292-0367.

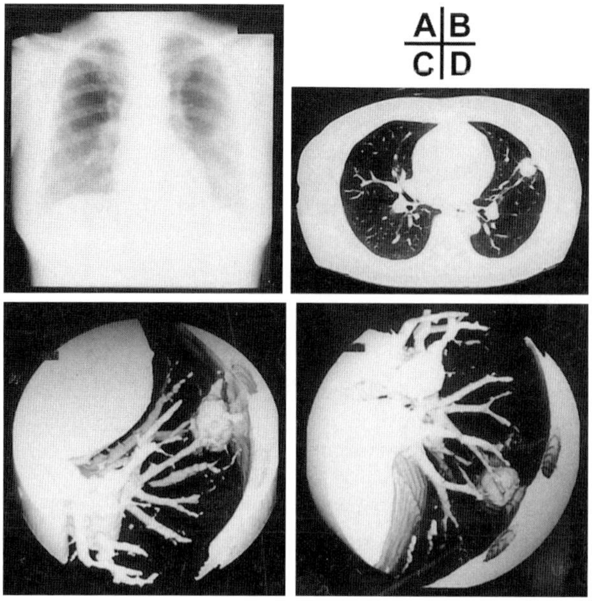

Fig. 1.

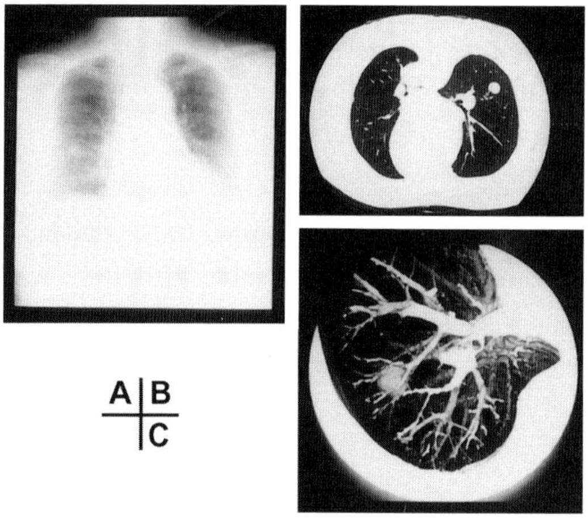

Fig. 2.

3. In AVM, flowing and inflowing vessels of nodules could be observed clearly (Fig. 3).
4. In aspergilloma and nodular lesions in the cavity were comprehended spatially, so fungus ball was strongly suspected (Fig. 4).

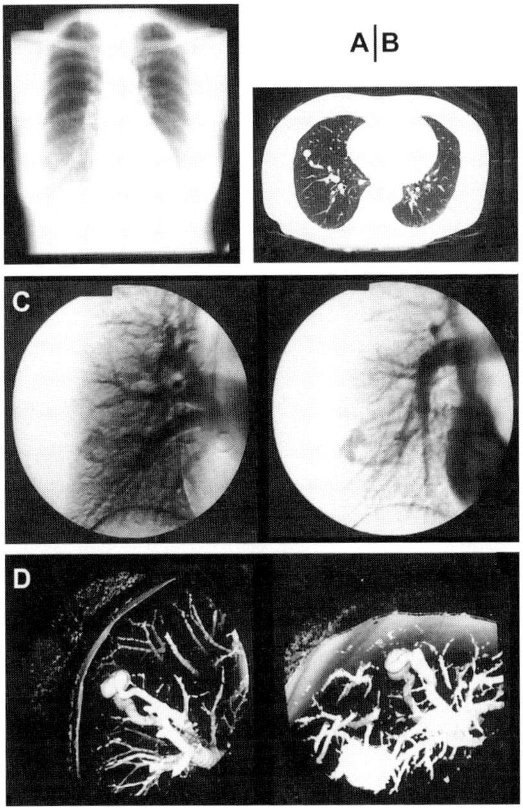

Fig. 3.

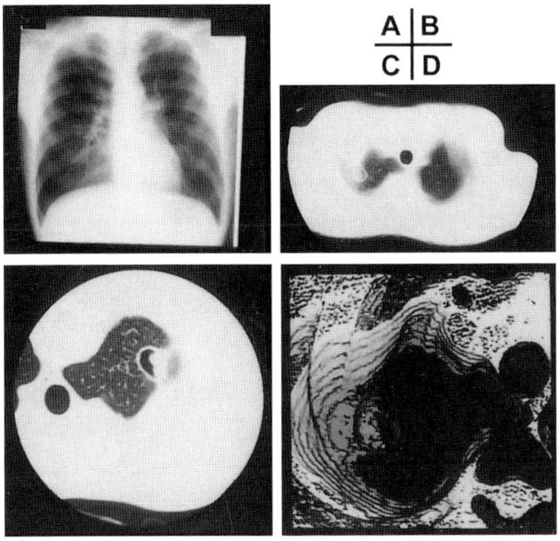

Fig. 4.

Conclusion

3D images offer a quick and comprehensive overview of the spatial extent of solitary pulmonary nodules, and are considered to be useful for differential diagnosis of solitary pulmonary nodules.

References

1. Zwirewich CV, Vedal S, Miller RR et al. Solitary pulmonary nodule: high-resolution CT and radiologic-pathologic correlation. Radiology 1991;179:469–467.
2. Stern RL et al. Three-dimensional imaging of the thoracic cavity. Invest Radiol 1989;24: 282–288.
3. Fishman EK et al. Volumetric rendering techniques; applications for three-dimensional imaging of the hip. Radiology 1987;163:737–738.
4. Siegelmen SS et al. Solitary pulmonary nodules; CT assessment. Radiology 1986;160:307–312.
5. Mori K et al. Three-dimensional computed tomography images of small pulmonary lesions. Jpn J Clin Oncol 1992;22:159–163.
6. Keiko Kuriyama et al. Three-dimensional imaging of focal lung diseases. Jpn J Clin Radiol 1995;40:795–802.

Bronchology and Bronchoesophagology: State of the Art.
H. Yoshimura et al., editors.

Problems with the diagnosis of traumatic pneumothorax using a roentgenogram: an initial classification with CT

Toshiki Tatsumura
Department of Emergency, Toyama Medical and Pharmaceutical University, Toyama, Japan

Abstract. Traumatic pneumothorax is not always easy to diagnose using a radiograph alone. In the present investigation, radiographs failed to diagnose pneumothorax in 22.1% of the cases studied. In contrast, computed tomography (CT) had a 100% diagnostic capability. A preliminary classification of traumatic pneumothorax with CT is proposed.

Keywords: chest injuries, computed tomography, radiograph, traumatic pneumothorax.

Introduction

Traumatic pneumothorax is a disease frequently encountered in daily practise when attending patients with chest injuries. However, not all cases of it can be diagnosed by means of radiographic studies alone. This particular type of pneumothorax has been described as occult pneumothorax and has been discussed by several investigators. Comparative studies of radiography and computed tomography (CT) concerning this type of pneumothorax are scarce, and there are no reports in relation to its classification by CT. The present communication is a preliminary report on the classification of traumatic pneumothorax according to the findings observed from CT examination.

Materials and Methods

The present series consisted of 77 cases of traumatic pneumothorax, and only those cases with simultaneous radiographic study and CT examination were included. There were 48 males and 29 females, with ages ranging from 16 to 78 years (mean: 45.7 years). Traffic accidents were the major causes of trauma (67.5%) followed by falls.

Results

There were three main characteristic patterns of traumatic pneumothorax that were classified using the CT findings, which we have denoted as A, B and C patterns.

Address for correspondence: Toshiki Tatsumura MD, PhD, Department of Emergency, Toyama Medical and Pharmaceutical University, 2630 Sugitani, Toyama 930-0194, Japan. Tel.: +81-76-434-7785. Fax: +81-76-434-5110.

A: only the anterior-portion of the lung is collapsed in this pattern, with the remaining lung expanded to the lateral chest wall. Thus, there was no unoccupied space between the expanded lung and the lateral chest wall (Fig. 1).

In patterns B and C, the lung collapsed away from the lateral chest wall, forming an unoccupied space between the lung and the lateral chest wall.
B: the collapse of the lung is mainly in the anterior-portion, with the remaining lung expanded away from the lateral chest wall.
C: the lung collapsed in an anterior-posterior fashion against the lateral chest wall, different to the other two patterns.

However, some variations in the extent of the collapses in the lungs are observed in each of the described patterns.

The incidences of the three different patterns of traumatic pneumothorax, observed using CT, were A (22.1%), B (50.6%) and C (27.5%). Only those cases with pattern A could not be detected by radiographic studies. In the other two patterns, the existence of pneumothorax was detectable using a radiograph.

Discussion

The results of the present investigation revealed that quite a high percentage of cases of traumatic pneumothorax cannot be detected by a radiograph alone. It is of paramount importance to realize the existence of this type of traumatic pneumothorax, especially to those physicians who are not familiar with this field. If a pattern A traumatic pneumothorax is present, but not recognized, and the

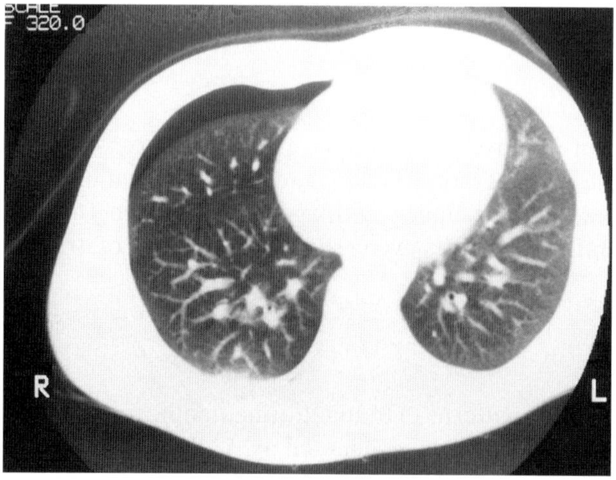

Fig. 1. The axial CT images of pattern A traumatic pneumothorax. The anterior-portion of the lung is collapsed, and the remaining lung is expanded to the lateral chest wall, hence there is no unoccupied space between the lung and the lateral chest wall.

patient is subject to general anesthesia for an emergency operation, or respiratory support is necessary, then tension pneumothorax will occur without notice, giving rise to hazardous complications.

As described above, CT is the most effective means of diagnosis of a pattern A pneumothorax. CT examination should be added to the radiographic study of a patient with chest injury as a routine part of procedure, whenever the condition of the patient allows for such an examination. In particular, regard should be given to patients for whom respiratory support and/or general anesthesia is a necessary measure.

Conclusion

It has been made clear, in the present investigation, that quite a high percentage of traumatic pneumothorax cases cannot be detected solely by radiographic examination. Hence, CT examination together with a routine radiographic examination is necessary in order to avoid any unexpected life-threatening complications.

References

1. Tocino IM, Miller MH, Frederick PR et al. CT detection of occult pneumothorax in head trauma. AJR 1984;143:987–990.
2. Bridges KG, Welch G, Silver M et al. CT detection of occult pneumothorax in multiple trauma patients. J Emerg Med 1993;11:179–186.

Bronchology and Bronchoesophagology: State of the Art.
H. Yoshimura et al., editors.

Observation of the structure of tracheal and bronchial lumens in healthy volunteers by using a newly developed high-magnification bronchovideoscope (side-viewing type)

Hiroki Takahashi, Takayuki Itoh, Masanori Shiratori, Hirofumi Oouchi, Masahiko Nishino, Gen Yamada, Hiroshi Tanaka, Hiroyuki Koba and Shosaku Abe

Third Department of Internal Medicine, Sapporo Medical University School of Medicine, Sapporo, Japan

Abstract. *Background.* The observation of the structure of tracheal and bronchial lumens, in vivo, has contributed to the improvement in clinical diagnosis for many tracheobronchial disorders.

Methods. In order to observe these structures in more detail, we developed a high-magnification bronchovideoscope (side-viewing type), named BF-200HM, in cooperation with Olympus Co. Ltd. (Tokyo). Objects observed by BF-200HM were magnified to approximately × 100 on a 14-inch video-monitor. This magnification rate corresponds to approximately 4 times that of BF-type 200 (Olympus Co. Ltd.), one of the types of bronchovideoscope which are commercially available.

Results. By using BF-200HM in a healthy volunteer, unlike BF-type 200, the distribution of submucosal vessels in intratracheal and intrabronchial lumens clearly showed a palisade-like pattern and branch-like pattern, respectively. Many dips were observed in the surface of the lumens using BF-200HM, but were not found by BF-type 200. These structures may be orifices of bronchial glands.

Conclusions. These results demonstrate that this newly developed high-magnification bronchovideoscope is a useful tool for the evaluation of submucosal vessels and orifices of bronchial glands in vivo.

Keywords: orifices of bronchial glands, submucosal vessels.

Introduction

Development of the bronchovideoscope has enabled us to visualize features of tracheobronchial lumen clearly and conservatively [1,2]. However, even with the use of the bronchovideoscope, it is not so easy to observe fine vessels of under 100 μm in diameter.

In order to observe the finer structure of bronchial mucosa, we developed a high-magnification bronchovideoscope (side-viewing type), named BF–200HM, in cooperation with Olympus Co. Ltd.

Address for correspondence: H. Takahashi, Third Department of Internal Medicine, Sapporo Medical University School of Medicine, South-1 West-16, Chuo-ku, Sapporo 060-8543, Japan. Tel.: +81-11-611-2111, ext. 3241. Fax: +81-11-613-1543. E-mail: htaka@sapmed.ac.jp

Methods

This videoscope is mounted with an objective lens on the lateral side of its distal end. The BF-200HM uses optical magnification, and this prevents the deterioration of the quality of images, which is different from the electric magnification. This provides 40° field of view, 1 to 3 mm depth of field, 6.3 mm distal-end diameter, 5.8 mm insertion-tube diameter, 160°/130° (up/down) of bending capability, 1.2 mm diameter of instrument channel, 550 mm working length, and 820 mm of total length (Fig. 1). We compared BF-200HM with BF-type 200 on their performance.

Results

When compared to the BF-type 200, the BF–200HM scale of magnification was approximately 5 times greater (Fig. 2). The final magnification rate on a 14-inch videomonitor is approximately × 100 actual size. Another merit of this videoscope is that there is less distortion in the margin of the field of view. As shown in Fig. 2, the degree of distortion observed when using the BF-200HM was much less compared to that of BF-type 200. The depth of field (1 to 3 mm) is very shallow when compared to that (10 mm or more) of BF-type 200. Nevertheless, BF–200HM provided clear images, as the surface of its object lens was parallel with the surface of the bronchial lumen.

Healthy volunteers underwent bronchoscopy using BF-type 200 and BF-200HM. Observation using the BF-200HM, unlike the BF-type 200, revealed a difference in the distribution of the submucosal vessels between the trachea and the bronchi. Submucosal vessels in the intratracheal lumen run parallel to one another in a longitudinal direction, which is called a palisade-like pattern. On the other hand, intrabronchial lumens showed a branch-like pattern of submucosal vessels (Fig. 3). Observation using the BF-200HM also revealed many dips in the surface of bronchial and tracheal lumens. The diameters of these

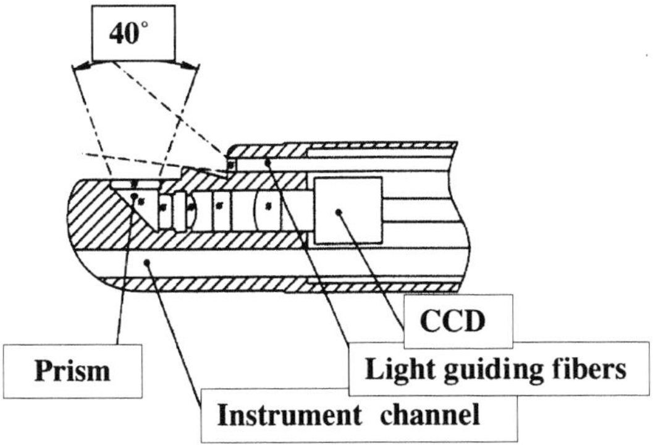

Fig. 1. The distal end of the BF-200HM.

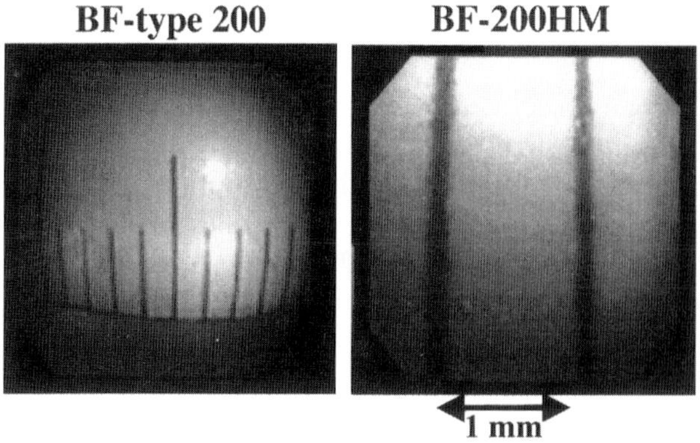

Fig. 2. Magnification rate.

dips were 50 to 100 μm which is almost equal to those of the openings of ducts of bronchial glands. Similar structures were observed in the formalin-fixed bronchial wall, which were removed from a patient with lung cancer, and they were histopathologically confirmed as orifices of bronchial glands (data not shown).

Discussion

The BF-200HM enabled us to observe the surface of tracheal and bronchial lumens at approximately $\times 100$ magnification, compared to actual size. This magnification rate corresponds to 5 times of that obtained using the BF-type 200. By using BF-200HM, we were able to successfully observe small vessels and orifices of bronchial gland ducts. We could identify structures such as vessels and dips at least more than 50 μm in diameter. This new videoscope may be, therefore, a powerful tool for observing the ultrastructure of tracheal and bronchial mucosa due to the benefits of its magnification rate and the fact that it is

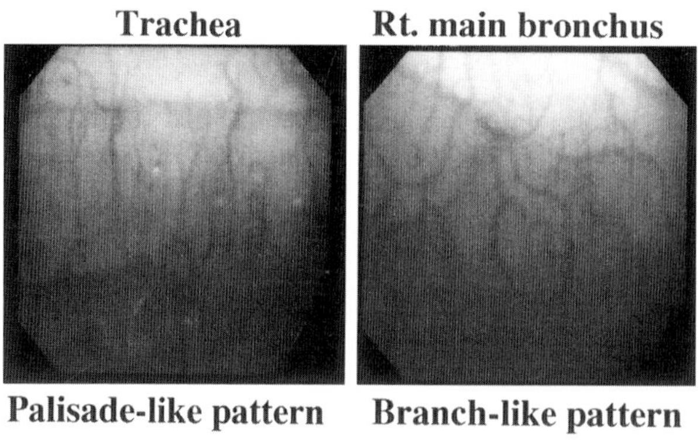

Fig. 3. The distribution of submucosal vessels.

side-viewing. It is expected this development will provide us with new physiological and clinical information.

References

1. Kato H, Kobayashi T, Konaka C. Video (CCD) flexible bronchoscope versus standard flexible bronchoscope: pro videobronchoscope. J Bronchol 1995;2:328–330.
2. Kobayashi T, Koshiishi H, Kawate N, dela Cruz CMA, Kato H. The performance of prototype videobronchoscopes: the Pentax EB-TM1830 and EB-TM1530. J Bronchol 1994;1:160–167.

Bronchology and Bronchoesophagology: State of the Art.
H. Yoshimura et al., editors.

Increased airway vascularity in chronic asthma evaluated by a novel side-viewing highly-magnified bronchoscopy

Hiroshi Tanaka, Gen Yamada, Hiroki Takahashi, Kensuke Oashi, Midori Hashimoto, Shintaro Tanaka and Shosaku Abe
Third Department of Internal Medicine, Sapporo Medical University School of Medicine, Sapporo, Japan

Abstract. This study was aimed to evaluate airway vascularity in asthmatic patients and to examine the usefulness of a side-viewing highly-magnified bronchoscopy, which was newly developed in cooperation with Olympus Co. Ltd. We examined six patients with chronic stable asthma and five control patients. We assessed airway vascularity in three views of the lower trachea in each subject. Morphometric measurements of blood vessels were made from the three tracheal pictures and assessed for 1) vessel area density, which is represented as the fraction (percentage), the number of vessel-overlaid-pixels to the number of pixels per total picture area, and 2) vessel length density which represents the total length of vessels, independent of vessel size. Both vessel area density and vessel length density were significantly ($p < 0.01$) increased in asthmatic patients as compared with control subjects. From these results, we can speculate that airway vascularity in the trachea may increase in chronic asthma patients, and a side-viewing highly-magnified bronchoscopy might be a useful tool to observe the inside of bronchial tree.

Keywords: airway remodeling, angiogenesis, bronchial circulation.

Background

Airway wall remodelling, including submucosal fibrosis, goblet cell metaplasia, glandular hypertrophy, airway smooth muscle hyperplasia and hypertrophy, and angiogenesis is considered to contribute to airway hyper-responsiveness. However, the bronchial circulation has remained an unknown quantity in asthma pathogenesis. This study was aimed to evaluate airway vascularity in asthmatic patients and to examine the usefulness of a side-viewing highly-magnified bronchoscopy, which was newly developed in cooperation with Olympus Co. Ltd.

Methods

We examined six patients with chronic stable asthma and five control subjects with pulmonary diseases without abnormalities in the bronchial tree. We assessed airway vascularity in three views of the lower trachea in each subject. Morphometric measurements of blood vessels were made from the tracheal pictures and

Address for correspondence: Dr Hiroshi Tanaka, Third Dept of Internal Medicine, Sapporo Medical University School of Medicine, South-1 West-16, Chuo-ku, Sapporo 060-8543, Japan. Tel.: +81-11-611-2111, ext. 3239. Fax: +81-11-613-1543. E-mail: tanakah@sapmed.ac.jp

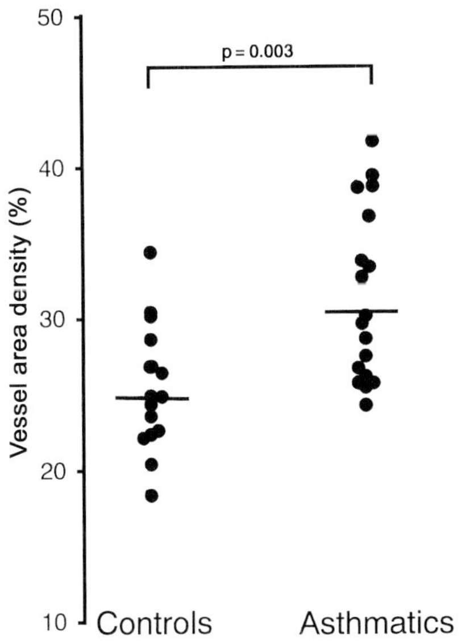

Fig. 1.

assessed following two parameters using Adobe Photoshop ver. 5.0 on a Macintosh computer. One parameter was vessel area density, which is represented as the fraction (percentage), the number of vessel-overlaid-pixels to the number of pixels per total picture area. The second was vessel length density, which represents the length of blood vessels in the given area of tissue and reflects the total length of vessels independent of vessel size.

Results

Both vessel area density (Fig. 1) and vessel length density were increased in asthmatic patients as compared with control subjects ($p < 0.01$).

Conclusions

Airway vascularity in the trachea may increase in chronic asthma patients, and a side-viewing highly-magnified bronchoscopy might be a useful tool to observe the inside of the bronchial tree.

Bronchology and Bronchoesophagology: State of the Art.
H. Yoshimura et al., editors.

The observation of bronchial lesions using a high-magnification bronchovideoscope

Gen Yamada, Takayuki Itoh, Hiroshi Tanaka, Hiroki Takahashi and Shosaku Abe

Third Department of Internal Medicine, Sapporo Medical University, School of Medicine, Sapporo, Japan

Abstract. Recently, we developed a high-magnification bronchovideoscope (side-viewing type) in cooperation with Olympus Co. Ltd. We observed detailed changes in the bronchial mucosa in patients with respiratory disorders using this bronchovideoscope.

We examined eight patients with sarcoidosis, three with primary lung cancer, three with chronic bronchitis, one with allergic bronchopulmonary aspergillosis (ABPA) and five without airway abnormalities (controls). Longitudinally lined, thick mucosa were seen in ABPA, whereas thick whitish mucosa and a few narrow vessels were seen in chronic bronchitis with persistent bacterial infection. Strongly-bound enlarged vessels and ramifying fine vessels were seen in bilateral main bronchi in sarcoidosis. Irregularly winding tumor vessels were seen in lung cancer, and scaly, rough, thick mucosa were seen adjacent to the lung cancer, which suggested submucosal invasion.

A high-magnification bronchovideoscope (side-viewing type) is a useful tool to observe the fine structure of bronchial mucosa.

Keywords: chronic bronchitis, high-magnification bronchovideoscope, lung cancer, sarcoidosis.

Background

Various changes in the bronchial mucosa are seen in respiratory diseases. However, it is difficult to assess the changes in the bronchial mucosa in detail when using a conventional fiberoptic bronchoscope.

Recently we developed a high-magnification bronchovideoscope (side-viewing type) in cooperation with Olympus Co. Ltd. We observed detailed changes in the bronchial mucosa in patients with respiratory disorders through the use of this bronchovideoscope.

Patients and Methods

We examined eight patients with sarcoidosis, three with primary lung cancer, three with chronic bronchitis, one with allergic bronchopulmonary aspergillosis (ABPA) and five without airway abnormalities (controls).

The flexible bronchovideoscope (BF-200HM) is equipped with a charge-

Address for correspondence: Gen Yamada, Third Department of Internal Medicine, Sapporo Medical University, School of Medicine, Chuo-ku South 1 West 16, Sapporo 060-8543, Japan. Tel.: +81-11-611-2111, ext. 3239. Fax: +81-11-613-1543. E-mail: gyamada@sapmed.ac.jp

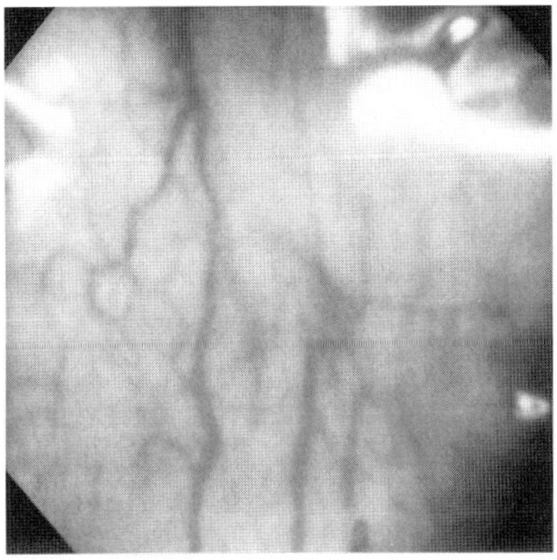

Fig. 1.

coupled device on the frontal side of its distal end. The images of bronchial mucosa were visualized with a magnification of $\times 100$ on a television monitor. We observed the trachea and bilateral main bronchi of these patients under local anesthesia.

Results

We were able to observe detailed changes in the bronchial mucosa, which we were unable to achieve using the conventional fiberoptic bronchoscope.

1. ABPA and Chronic bronchitis. Longitudinally lined, thick mucosa were seen in ABPA, whereas thick whitish mucosa and a few narrow vessels were seen in chronic bronchitis with persistent bacterial infection (Fig. 1).
2. Sarcoidosis. Strongly-bound enlarged vessels and ramifying fine vessels were seen in the bilateral main bronchi in sarcoidosis (Fig. 2).

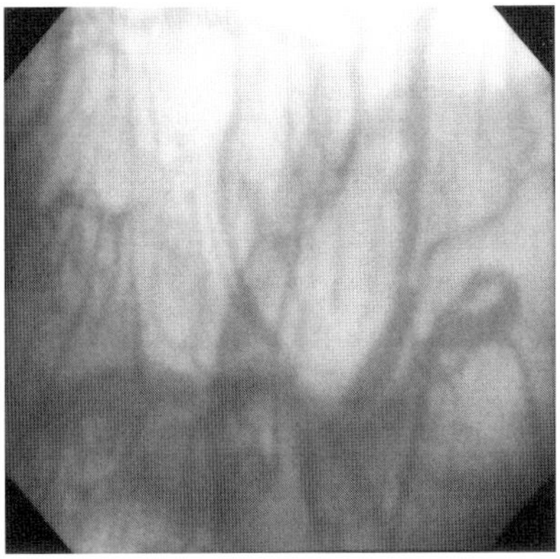

Fig. 2.

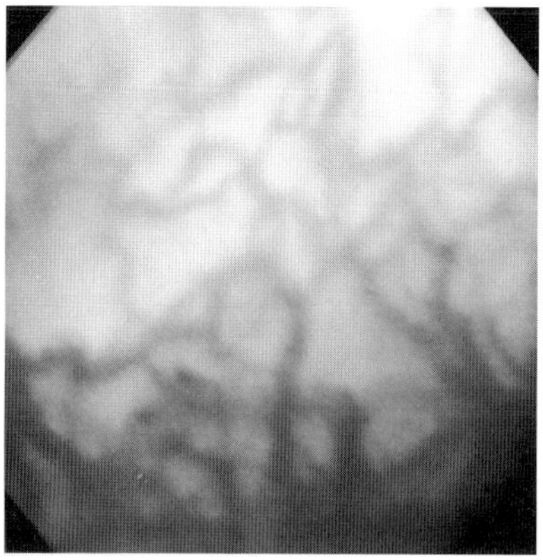

Fig. 3.

3. Lung cancer. Irregularly winding tumor vessels were seen in lung cancer (Fig. 3). Scaly, rough, thick mucosa were seen adjacent to the lung cancer, which suggested submucosal invasion.

Conclusion

A high-magnification bronchovideoscope (side-viewing type) is a useful tool to observe fine structure of bronchial mucosa.

Infectious diseases

Bronchology and Bronchoesophagology: State of the Art.
H. Yoshimura et al., editors.

The value of selologic tests for the diagnosis of active pulmonary tuberculosis

Y. Abe[1], N. Hasegawa[2] and H. Yoshimura[1]

[1]*Department of Thoracic and Cardiovascular Surgery, Kitasato University School of Medicine; and* [2]*Department of Internal Medicine, Cardiopulmonary Division, Keio University School of Medicine, Japan*

Keywords: antigen p-90, IgA, PPD.

Study objective

This investigation was undertaken to assess the effectiveness of the immunoglobulin A antibody (IgA) against the p-90 antigen in the diagnosis of active pulmonary mycobacteriosis, and to compare the results with conventional diagnosis methods [1—3]. We also wanted to evaluate the possibility of these antigens becoming a method of monitoring antituberculosis therapy.

Participants

356 patients and 165 control subjects from our hospital and 52 healthy subjects (not in hospital) were examined (Table 1).

Methods and Results

The detection of the anti-p-90 IgA of sera was performed using an enzyme-immunoassay. The optic density (OD) value observed in subjects in the active mycobacterium tuberculosis (MTB) group was significantly higher than in control groups ($p < 0.001$) (Fig. 1).

There was also a statistically significant difference noted, between the OD value observed on admission and 2 months after the commencement of medication ($p = 0.0003$) (Fig. 2).

The patient group who had extensive lung cavities showed significantly higher OD values (3.810 ± 3.804) than patients without extensive lung cavities (2.040 ± 2.622) and patients with unstable noncavities (1.578 ± 1.912) ($p < 0.05$) (Figs. 3 and 4, Table 2).

However, active MTB could not be statistically discriminated from non-

Address for correspondence: Y. Abe, Department of Thoracic and Cardiovascular Surgery, Kitasato University School of Medicine, 1-15-1 Kitasato, Sagamihara, Kanagawa 228-8555, Japan. Tel.: +81-42-778-8608. Fax: +81-42-778-9840.

Table 1. Group characteristics and the results of the measurement of IgA against Kp-90.

Group	No.	Age mean ± SD	OD mean ± SD	OD 2 (n) mean ± SD
MTB	284	56.2 ± 16.6	2.07 ± 2.54	2.47 ± 3.17[a] (247)
NTM	39	64.7 ± 15.3	1.73 ± 2.42	2.91 ± 3.36 (18)
am	25			
kans	5			
int	6			
fort	2			
chel	1			
OTH	33	65.3 ± 16.8	1.31 ± 1.63	2.24 ± 3.76 (14)
CTL	165	42.3 ± 11.4	0.83 ± 0.86	
CT	52	49.0 ± 6.6	0.48 ± 0.58	

MTB: active pulmonary TB, NTM: nontuberculosis mycobacteriosis, OTH: pulmonary disease without MTB or NTM, CTL: contact with MTB and no findings on chest X-rays, CT: healthy, OD: sera on admission, OD 2: sera 2 months after the commencement of medication; [a]p = 0.0003 between OD and OD 2.

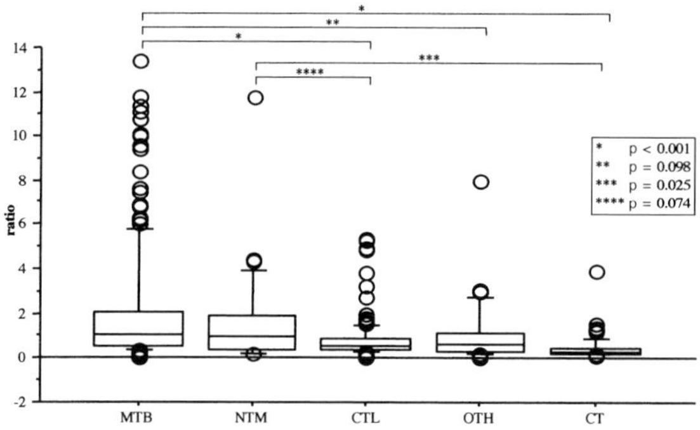

Fig. 1. Distribution of IgA against p-90 antigen levels in the different groups.

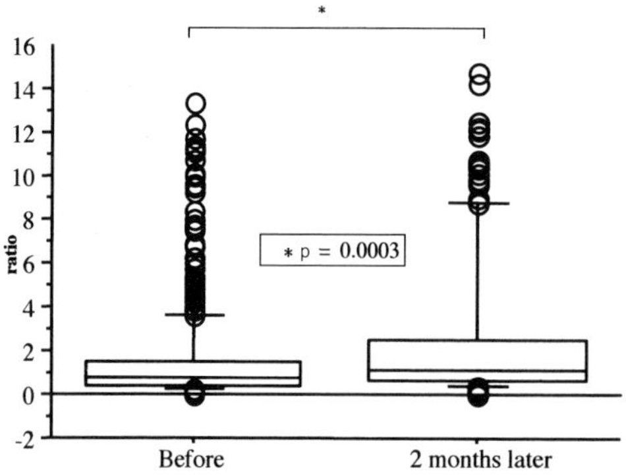

Fig. 2. OD levels in the MTB group before medication and 2 months later, after medication.

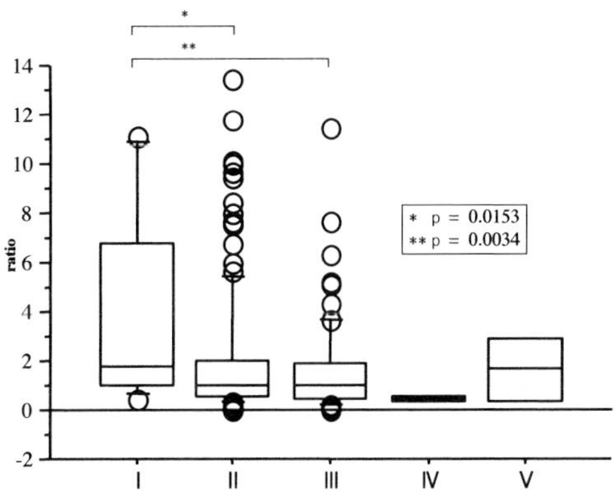

Fig. 3. The OD levels of the different classification types according to the chest X-rays (see Table 2).

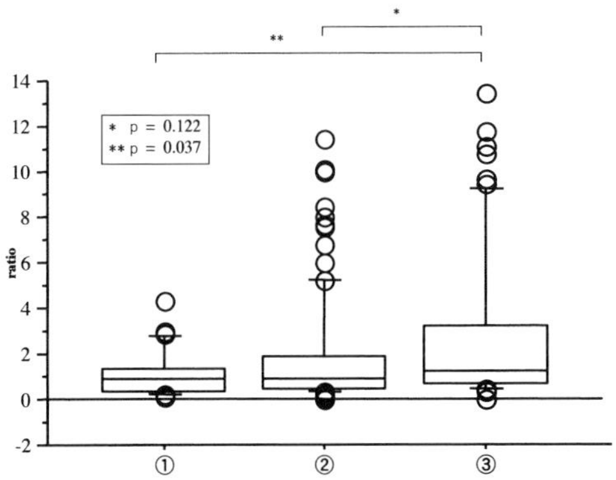

Fig. 4. The OD levels of the different classifications of expansion according to the chest X-rays (see Table 2).

tuberculosis mycobacteriosis (NTM). The sensitivity and specificity values at the cutoff OD value were 84 and 79%, respectively (Fig. 5, Tables 3 and 4). On the other hand, the sensitivity value observed when using the purified protien derivative (PPD) skin test was only 71% in the MTB group.

Conclusion

We were able to discriminate between active pulmonary TB patients and control group subjects based on the IgA-mediated humoral immune response against the antigen p-90, and the results were statistically significant [4]. Two months from the commencement of medication, the OD value had increased, which was again statistically significant. In Japan, all regions have been vaccinated with BCG, so this new method might be a useful alternative to the PPD skin test for discriminating between active and nonactive pulmonary tuberculosis [5].

Table 2. The classification of pulmonary tuberculosis using a chest roentgenogram according to the Japanese society for tuberculosis.

Type:
0: no findings
    There are no findings on a chest X-ray
I: extensive cavities
    The total area of cavities exceeds one-third of the volume of one lung, and the total area of disease expansion is contained within one lung
II: nonextensive cavity
    There is a TB disease shadow, as well as the cavity, but this excludes definition I
III: unstable noncavity
    There is an unstable shadow, but no cavities
IV: stable noncavity
    There is a stable shadow, but no cavities
V: healing
    Findings only indicate healing
Expansion:
1: Area covers less than one-third of one lung
2: Area covers between one-third of, and a whole lung
3: Area exceeds one lung
Laterality:
r: The shadow only exists in the right lung
l: The shadow only exists in the left lung
b: The shadow exists on bilaterally

Table 3. Positive number and sensitivity of conventional methods for the diagnosis of tuberculosis in each of the different groups.

Method	MTB	NTM	OTH	CTL
PPD	201 (71)	23 (58)	15 (45)	101 (3)
Smear	220 (78)	29 (76)		
PCR	234 (82)	25 (64)		
MGIT	270 (95)	39 (100)		

(): sensitivity, MGIT: microgrowth indicator tube, PCR: polymerase chain reactive.

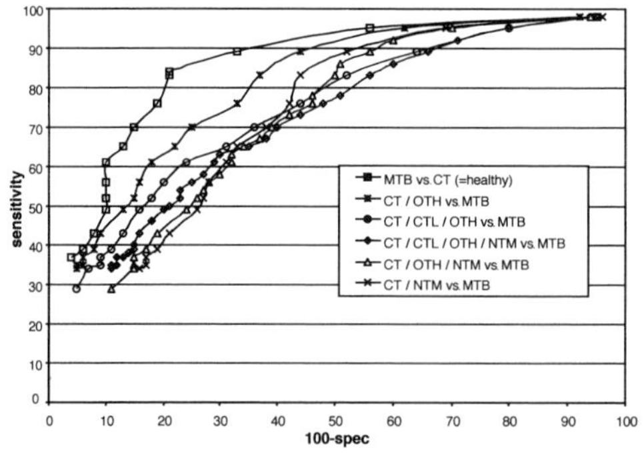

Fig. 5. The reciever characteristic curve of the p-90 serologic test in different matchings of groups.

Table 4. Sensitivity and specificity at cutoff OD values.

MTB vs. CT		
OD value	Sensitivity (%)	Specificity (%)
0.2	98	5
0.3	95	44
0.4	89	67
0.45	86	75
0.5	84	79
0.6	76	79
0.7	70	81
0.8	65	85
0.9	61	90
1	56	90
1.1	52	90
1.2	49	90

References

1. Engvall E, Perlman P. Enzyme-linked immunosorbent assay, ELISA? Quantitation of specific antibodies by enzyme-labeled anti-immunoglobulin in antigen coated tubes. J Immunol 1972; 109:129–135.
2. Daniel TM. Tuberculin antigens: the need for purification. Am Rev Respir Dis 1976;113: 717–719.
3. Nassau E, Parsons ER, Jhonson GD. The detection antibody to mycobacterium tuberculosis by microplate enzyme-linked immunosorbent assay (ELISA). Tubercle 1976;57:67–70.
4. Alifano M, de Pascalis R, Sofia M. Evaluation of IgA-mediated humoral immune response against the mycobacterial antigen p-90 in diagnosis of pulmonary tuberculosis. Chest 1997; 111;601–605.
5. Koshino T, Nishioka S, Fujimura M et al. ELISA for IgG antibody to purified protein derivative (PPD) of patients with pulmonary tuberculosis. Kekkaku 1984;59:621–624.

Bronchology and Bronchoesophagology: State of the Art.
H. Yoshimura et al., editors.

The classification of endoscopical findings of bronchial tuberculosis

Takashi Arai
National Hospital Tokyo Disaster Medical Center, Tokyo, Japan

Abstract. *Background.* We clinically evaluated a new classification system, concerning endoscopical findings of bronchial tuberculosis.

Materials and Methods. 156 lesions were observed in 112 patients.

Results. The new classification consists of six types: Types I to V, and LN. Type I is edema and congestion of the mucosa (nonspecific change). Type II is small intramucosal tubercles covered with normal mucosa. Type III is the findings of ulceration of the mucosa. There are two types of ulcer: Type IIIa (superficial ulcer) and IIIb (granulomatous ulcer). Type IV (granulation) is the granulation protruding from the bronchial wall into the lumen, covered with normal mucosa, which is usually observed during or after chemotherapy. These are the findings of the healing process for Type IIIb. Type V is a scar formation which is the final healing stage of the disease. Sometimes, the scar creates no evident stenosis of the lumen (Type Va), however, it sometimes creates severe stenosis of the lumen (Type Vb). Type LN is the endobroncial change through perforation of the tuberculous peribronchial lymph node.

Conclusion. The new classification of endoscopical findings of bronchial tuberculosis is clinically useful, as it enables us to classify the stages of disease and healing progression, which gives us a better idea of the appropriate treatment needed at each point, and it allows us to better assess how effective different treatments are, and what the process of healing involves.

Keywords: bronchial tuberculosis, bronchoscopy, endobronchial finding.

Object of study

We clinically evaluated a new classification system, concerning endoscopical findings of bronchial tuberculosis.

Materials and Methods

The records and films of bronchoscopic findings, at the time of the initial observation, were reviewed in 112 patients with bronchial tuberculosis examined during the period 1975 to 1986 at Nakano National Hospital in Tokyo.

The patients were divided into three groups according to what stage of treatment they had reached (Table 1). Group A consisted of the patients who had not yet undergone any treatment, group B consisted of the patients who had undergone chemotherapy for more than 3 months, and group C consisted of the

Address for correspondence: Takashi Arai MD, National Hospital Tokyo Disaster Medical Center, Midoricho 3256, Tachikawa, Tokyo 190-0014, Japan. Tel.: +81-42-526-5511. Fax: +81-42-526-5531.

Table 1. Patients with bronchial tuberculosis.

Group	No.	Sex m/f	Age (years) mean/(range)
A: before chemotherapy	63	21/42	44/(20–84)
B: during chemotherapy (> 3 months)	20	7/13	45/(20–69)
C: after chemotherapy	29	9/20	43/(30–70)
Total	112	37/75	44.5/(20–84)

patients who had completed their treatment.

The endoscopical findings of bronchial tuberculosis were classified using the new classification system introduced by the author (Table 2). This new classification system is a modification of the old one that was previously presented by the author in 1988 [1].

Results

156 lesions were observed in 112 patients. The endoscopical findings of bronchial tuberculosis were classified using the new classification sytem (Table 2). The classifications are as follows: Type I is edema and congestion of the mucosa, which is a nonspecific change accompanied by active specific lesions; Type II (intramucosal tubercles) is small intramucosal tubercles covered with normal mucosa. The intramucosal tubercles are seen as small yellow granules through the normal epithelium of the mucosa, which are seen in very early stages of the disease; Type III (ulcer) is the findings of ulceration of the mucosa. There are two types

Table 2. Classification of endoscopical findings of bronchial tuberculosis.

Type I: edema and congestion mucosa (nonspecific)

Type II: intramucosal tubercles

Type III: ulcers
- IIIa: superficial ulcers
- IIIb: granulomatous ulcers

Type IV: granulation
- IVa: nodular granulation
- IVb: polypoid granulation

Type V: scars
- Va: scar without stenosis
- Vb: scar with stenosis

Type LN: perforation of tuberculous lymph node

of ulcer: Type IIIa and IIIb. Type IIIa (superficial ulcer) is the ulceration of Type II, which is covered with a flat white coat. Type IIIb (granulomatous ulcer) is the findings of ulceration with a thick white coat covering the underlying protruding granulations, which sometimes cause a narrowing of the tracheo-bronchial lumen; Type IV (granulation) is the granulation protruding from the bronchial wall into the lumen covered with normal mucosa, which are usually observed during or after chemotherapy. These are findings of the healing process of Type IIIb; Type V (scar) is a scar formation which is the final healing stage of the disease. Sometimes the scar creates no evident stenosis of the lumen (Type Va), however, sometimes it creates a severe stenosis of the lumen (Type Vb); and Type LN is the endobronchial change through perforation of the tuberculous peribronchial lymph node. This type creates granulations in the bronchial wall that have the appearance of lymph node tissue.

The localization of the 156 lesions is shown in Table 3. All of the lesions observed in the trachea were combined with lesions in the bronchus. The distribution of endoscopical findings over the three groups, according to the new classifications, are shown in Table 4.

Type IIIb and IIIa were most commonly observed among group A, while Type V was most frequently seen among groups B and C.

Table 3. The location of the 156 lesions in 112 patients.

Location	Male	Female	Total
Trachea	5	12	17
Left:			
main bronchus	11	36	47
upper lobe bronchus	8	14	22
lower lobe bronchus	2	4	6
segmental bronchus	4	2	6
Subtotal	25	56	81
Right:			
main bronchus	5	12	17
upper bronchus	3	9	12
intermediate bronchus	3	9	12
middle lobe bronchus	2	2	4
lower lobe bronchus	0	1	1
segmental bronchus	7	5	12
Subtotal	20	38	58
Total	50	106	156

Table 4. The distribution of endoscopical findings over the three groups according to the new classifications of bronchial tuberculosis.

Endoscopical findings	Group		
	A	B	C
Type II	6	1	0
Type IIIa	21	1	2
Type IIIb	50	8	5
Type IVa	6	1	1
Type IVb	0	1	0
Type Va	0	0	0
Type Vb	7	14	27
Type LN	4	1	0
Total	94	27	35

Group A: patients before treatment; Group B: patients who have undergone chemotherapy for more than 3 months; and Group C: patients after the completion of treatment.

Discussion

Bronchial tuberculosis was classified endoscopically using the new classifications. Concerning distribution over the sexes, female patients were involved in 2 times the amount of cases than male patients. The most common location of lesions was in the left main bronchus, and was most frequently found in females.

The intramucosal tubercles (Type II) is seen in the early stages of the progression of the disease. This type easily develops into ulcers covered with flat white coats (Type IIIa), and these then develop into granulomatous ulcers covered with thick white coats (Type IIIb). Therefore, Type IIIb is the most commonly observed finding in patients who have not yet undergone treatment. The nodular or polypoid granulations (Type IV) are mostly seen during chemotherapy, and are thought to be the healing stage of Type IIIb.

The scar (Type V) with stenosis is most often seen in cases where chemotherapy has been completed. This is the final stage of healing of granulations.

Conclusion

The new classification of endoscopical findings of bronchial tuberculosis is clinically useful, as it enables us to classify the stages of disease and healing progression, which gives us a better idea of the appropriate treatment needed at each point, and it allows us to better assess how effective different treatments are, and what the process of healing involves.

Reference

1. Arai T. Changes by treatment in bronchoscopical findings of bronchial tuberculosis. J Jpn Soc Bronchol 1988;9:326–331.

Bronchology and Bronchoesophagology: State of the Art.
H. Yoshimura et al., editors.

Bronchoscopy for pulmonary aspergillosis

Akira Fujita[1], Haruyuki Ishii[1] and Hiroshi Yamamoto[2]
[1]Department of Pulmonary Medicine and [2]Department of Thoracic Surgery, Tokyo Metropolitan Fuchu Hospital, Tokyo, Japan

Abstract. Bronchoscopic findings and a diagnostic yield of bronchoscopic procedures in pulmonary aspergillosis were reviewed. Thirty-eight patients were diagnosed on the basis of clinical, radiological, serologic, and microbiologic criteria. Patients with allergic bronchopulmonary aspergillosis were excluded from this study. Bronchoscopic procedures yielded a positive culture in 50% of the patients. The diagnostic results increased to 72% of the patients examined, when performing bronchoscopic procedures and sputum culture together. Nonspecific stenosis of bronchial lumens was the most common abnormality found in bronchoscopic findings. In conclusion, bronchoscopic procedures for microbiologic diagnosis were fair, although the sensitivity was not high in pulmonary aspergillosis.

Keywords: bronchoscopy, pulmonary aspergillosis.

Introduction

Pulmonary aspergillosis is a common fungal disease of the lung in Japan. Obtaining a culture of aspergillus species of respiratory samples is an important tool for the diagnosis of aspergillosis. The purpose of this study was to find out the diagnostic yield of bronchoscopy for pulmonary aspergillosis. In addition, we examined bronchoscopic appearances of pulmonary aspergillosis.

Materials and Methods

We performed a retrospective review of patients with pulmonary aspergillosis undergoing bronchoscopy during a 10-year period (from 1990 to 1999, at Tokyo Metropolitan Fuchu Hospital). The diagnosis of pulmonary aspergillosis was established on the basis of clinical, radiological, and microbiologic criteria, and in some cases with additional serologic tests and/or pathologic findings. Allergic bronchopulmonary aspergillosis (ABPA) was excluded in this study. A total of 38 patients were reviewed, consisting of 27 males and 11 females (ranging from 32 to 80 years of age) with a median age of 65 years. Seventy-four percent of patients complained of hemoptysis or hemosputum. There were four immunocompromised patients. Eighteen patients had aspergilloma, and cavitation with-

Address for correspondence: Akira Fujita, Department of Pulmonary Medicine, Tokyo Metropolitan Fuchu Hospital, 2-9-2 Musashidai, Fuchu-shi, Tokyo 183-8524, Japan. Tel.: +81-42-323-5111. Fax: +81-42-323-9209. E-mail: akifuji@fuchu-hp.fuchu.tokyo.jp out obvious “fungus-ball” was shown on chest X-rays in 10 cases. Three patients developed Aspergillus pneumonia. Cultures for fungi were performed on bronchial lavage and/or brush samples from patients.

Results

Aspergillus spp. was identified in 16 out of 32 bronchial samples (usually bronchial lavages). Of the six patients on whom bronchial or lung biopsy was performed, aspergillus hyphae were revealed in only two cases. There was no difference in overall diagnostic yields between bronchoscopy material and sputum. Eight patients with a negative culture of sputum were diagnosed by bronchoscopy alone. Although bronchoscopic findings for pulmonary aspergillosis were nonspecific, stenosis of bronchial lumens were observed in 14 cases. Severe stenosis such as pinhole bronchus or obstruction was revealed in five cases. Through the bronchoscope, a part of mycetoma or cavity wall could be seen in three patients. Bronchoscopy confirmed the bleeding sites in eight of the 16 cases with hemoptysis. The major sites of bronchoscopic abnormality in patients with aspergillosis were the bilateral upper bronchi and the superior segment bronchus of right lower lobe.

Discussion

The reason why patients with ABPA are not included in this study is that ABPA is an allergic disease which is distinct from other forms of aspergillosis. Bronchoscopic procedures yielded a positive culture in 50% of the patients. This is unexpectedly low. However, eight patients with a negative culture of sputum were diagnosed by bronchoscopy alone. The combination of bronchoscopy and sputum examination achieved a diagnostic advantage. We carried out both culture and antigen tests of bronchial lavage at the same time. The aspergillus antigen test is highly sensitive, but it also detects colonizations or contaminations. According to our experience, the aspergillus antigen test of bronchial lavage has a poor diagnostic value because the specificity is too low. It is suspected that bronchial stenosis has, at least, some relationship to the disease progression, although stenosis of bronchial lumens is not a specific causal factor of pulmonary aspergillosis. Normal clearance mechanisms may be impaired in the involved segments.

Bronchology and Bronchoesophagology: State of the Art.
H. Yoshimura et al., editors.

Serology, PCR and IHC for the detection of *Chlamydia pneumoniae* in patients undergoing bronchoscopy

H. Koyi[1], E. Brandén[1], J. Gnarpe[2], H. Gnarpe[2] and B. Steen[3]
Departments of [1]Respiratory Medicine, and [2]Clinical Microbiology, Gävle Central Hospital, Gävle; and [3]Department of Geriatrics, University of Gothenburg, Gothenburg, Sweden

Abstract. A total of 323 consecutive patients referred for bronchoscopy with suspected lung cancer were investigated for serological markers of chronic *Chlamydia pneumoniae* infection, using throat specimens for the detection of *C. pneumoniae* using PCR and bronchial specimens for detection using IHC. The results were compared to those from healthy blood donors > 50 years of age and with serological data from a cohort of 151 70-year-olds. The rate of positive PCR or IHC detection was unexpectedly low in lung cancer patients. Elevated specific *C. pneumoniae* IgA antibodies were found significantly more often in lung cancer patients. The results suggest that PCR from throat and IHC from bronchial mucosa are of low diagnostic value in lung cancer patients.

Keywords: *Chlamydia pneumoniae*, immunohistochemistry, lung cancer.

Introduction

Chlamydia pneumoniae (Cpn) is an obligate gramnegative intracellular bacterium. It is difficult to culture but may be diagnosed using PCR from throat specimens or by serological analysis with regard to specific IgG-, IgM- and IgA antibodies. Cpn is a common cause of respiratory tract infections [1] and induces the production of matrix metalloproteinases [2]. In 1997, Laurila et al. reported an association between *Chlamydia pneumoniae* infection and primary lung cancer [3]. We recently published a preliminary report of an association between serological markers for chronic *C. pneumoniae* infection and primary lung cancer [4].

The aim of this study was to compare PCR (polymerase chain reaction), IHC (immunohistochemistry) and serology in the diagnosis of Cpn in patients undergoing bronchoscopy.

Materials and Methods

Patients

A total of 323 consecutive patients (181 males, 142 females) were referred for

Address for correspondence: Hirsh Koyi MD, Department of Respiratory Medicine, Gävle Central Hospital, 801 87 Gävle, Sweden. Tel.: +46-26-15-43-28. Fax: +46-26-15-43-22.
E-mail: hirsh.koyi@lg.se

bronchoscopy because of respiratory symptoms or chest X-ray findings suggesting lung cancer (LC) between 1 March 1998 and 28 February 1999. Blood samples and throat specimens were taken before bronchoscopy and biopsies were taken from the bronchial mucosa during bronchoscopy. 107 patients were diagnosed with LC (69 males, 38 females), 216 had other diagnoses (112 males, 104 females). Demographic data are shown in Table 1.

Controls

All consecutive blood donors at the Gävle Central Hospital, over a 1 month period, were asked to answer a questionnaire about their current state of health, medication(s) and smoking habits. Blood was obtained for serological analysis of markers for chronic Cpn infection, and a swab was taken from the retropharyngeal mucosa for detection of Cpn by PCR. A total of 220 blood donors were enrolled in the study. Fifty-two men and 20 women, who were $\geqslant 50$ years of age. Only blood donors > 50 years of age were used for comparison with cases. The median ages were 56 years for the men (range: 50 to 66 years of age) and 55 years for the women (range: 50 to 64 years of age). Another control group was a cohort of 150 randomly chosen 70-year-olds (99 males, 51 females) with only serological analysis available.

Results

Six out of 95 (6.3%) male patients with LC and 16 out of 154 (10.4%) male patients with other diagnoses were PCR+. In female patients, these figures were four out of 36 (11%) and 21 out of 85 (25%), respectively. IHC results were available for 110 males and 93 females. Eight out of 28 (29%) males with LC were IHC+, compared to 17 out of 82 (21%) males with other diagnoses. Females

Table 1. The demographic data of the patients and controls.

	Patients				Controls			
	Males		Females		M bd	F bd	M70	F70
	LC	No LC	LC	No LC				
No.	69	112	38	104	151	61	99	51
Mean age (years)	73	63	72	59	43	41	70	70
Median age (years)	68	66	62	59	44	40	70	70
Current smokers (%)	63.8	42.9	76.3	38.5	16.2	35.5	30[a]	50[a]
Ex-smokers (%)	30.4	25.9	10.5	18.3	22.1	17.7		
Never smoked (%)	5.8	31.3	13.2	43.3	57.1	45.2	70	55

[a]These figures include the amount of both current and ex-smokers. Ex-smoker = 5 years since last smoked.

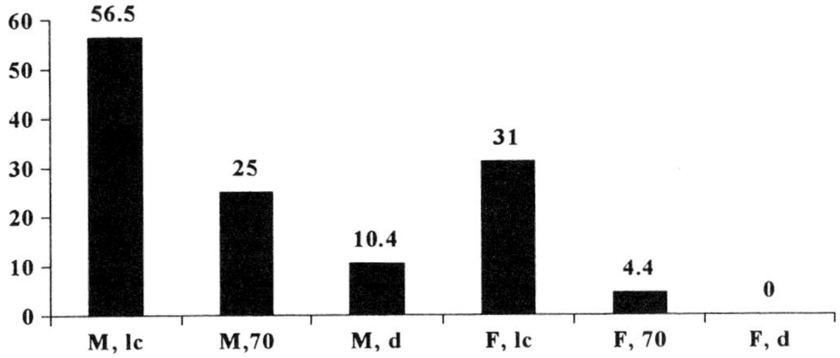

Fig. 1. The prevalence of high titers of specific *C. pneumoniae* IgA antibodies in patients with primary lung cancer and in controls.

with LC were IHC+ in two out of 21 cases (10%) compared to nine out of 72 cases (13%) in females with other diagnoses. Patients with LC had specific Cpn IgA titers significantly more often, > 1 out of 128, than the controls (Fig. 1).

Conclusions

The number of positive PCR and IHC tests were unexpectedly low compared to the number of high antibody titers in serum specimens, demonstrating the low prognostic value of PCR and IHC. The high prevalence of high titers of specific Cpn IgA antibodies in patients with LC suggests that a chronic Cpn infection may be a contributing factor to the development of LC.

References

1. Grayston JT, Campell LA, Kuo CC et al. A new respiratory tract pathogen *Chlamydia pneumoniae* strain TWAR. J Infect Dis 1990;161:618–625.
2. Kol A, Sukhova GK, Lichtman AH, Libby P. Chlamydia heat shock protein 60 localizes in human atheroma and regulates macrophage tumor necrosis factor alpha and matrix metalloproteinase expression. Circulation 1998;98:300–307.
3. Laurila A, Anttila T, Esa Läärä et al. Serological evidence of an association between *Chlamydia pneumoniae* infection and lung cancer. Int J Cancer 1997;74:31–34.
4. Koyi H, Brandén B, Gnarpe J, Gnarpe H, Birgitta A, Hillerdal H. *Chlamydia pneumoniae* may be associated with lung cancer, preliminary report on a seroepidemiological study. APMIS 1999;107:828–832.

©2001 Published by Elsevier Science B.V.
Bronchology and Bronchoesophagology: State of the Art.
H. Yoshimura et al., editors.

The inflammatory process in cases with deep neck infection

H. Nakazato, K. Watanabe, I. Ito, T. Yoshikawa and A. Kida
Department of Otorhinolaryngology – Head and Neck Surgery, Nihon University School of Medicine, Tokyo, Japan

Abstract. The incidence of deep neck infection has generally decreased. However, during the past 3 years, 20 patients were treated in our clinic. Surgical treatments including tracheotomy were applied in 16 cases. Nineteen cases were cured, but one died from a secondary chest abscess leading to sepsis.

It is important to understand the inflammatory process and to be familiar with spread of infection to neck spaces, for the purpose of prompt and adequate management. In order to evaluate the involvement of spaces in detail, CT findings of all cases were reviewed, as CT is most helpful in differentiating which space is involved.

In conclusion, it is suggested that the site of the primary source of infection may affect the extension of inflammation and, moreover, infections originating from each site have a tendency to spread through a few routes from the neck to the mediastinum.

Keywords: clinical potential neck spaces, deep neck infection.

Introduction

It has definitely been shown that antibiotic therapy has greatly changed the clinical course of deep neck infections. While the overall incidence of these infections has greatly decreased, the inadequate use of antibiotics causes local manifestions to be hidden, and these effects may give physicians a false sense of security and delay the timing of appropriate surgical drainage and ultimately lead to the severe complications such as mediastinitis.

During the past 3 years, 22 patients with deep neck infections have been treated in our hospital and one died from a secondary chest abscess. It is not necessarily a rare disease for us. Therefore, it is important to understand the inflammatory process and to be familiar with the spread of infection to neck spaces, for the purpose of prompt and adequate management.

In order to evaluate the involvement of spaces in detail, CT findings of all cases were reviewed, as CT is most helpful in differentiating which space is involved.

Address for correspondence: Hidehisa Nakazato MD, Department of ORL-HNS, Nihon University School of Medicine, 30-1 Oyaguchi-kamicho, Itabasi-ku, Tokyo 173-8610, Japan. Tel.: +81-3-3972-8111, ext. 2542. Fax: +81-3-3972-1321.

Methods

Eight potential neck spaces, which are considered important to evaluate the spread of the infection, were selected from the Levitt's classification [1]. The CT of all patients were reviewed in order to estimate which spaces were involved.

Twenty-two patients with deep neck infection were treated in our hospital from November 1996 to March 2000. Their ages ranged from 33 to 88 years and the average age was 55.2 years. The male/female ratio was 15 to 7.

Results and Discussion

Cases with dental infection as the primary disease generally had a tendency to become worse than cases with a tonsillar infection. The average time spent in hospital in each group was 34 days in the eight cases with dental infection, except for one who died, and 21 days in the seven cases with tonsillar infection. There was a statistically significant difference between the two groups, $p = 0.05$.

One of the reasons for this may be that patients with dental infections were treated with prolonged administrations of inadequate antibiotics in the dental clinic. On the other hand, it is also plausible that cases with tonsillar infections visit the hospital or specialist earlier due to their symptoms, such as trisms or odynophagia.

There are two main routes by which the infection spreads from the focus into spaces, in both dental infection cases and tonsillar infection cases. In cases of dental infection it tends to be through the masticator and parapharyngeal spaces to the mediastinim, and in tonsillar cases it tends to be through the submandibular and anterior visceral spaces to the mediastinum.

Reference

1. Levitt MJ. Cervical fascia and deep neck infections. Laryngoscope 1970;80:409–435.

Bronchology and Bronchoesophagology: State of the Art.
H. Yoshimura et al., editors.

A case of respiratory burn injury showing a marked response to urinastatin

Y. Osakabe and Y. Takahashi
Department of Emergency Center Showa University, Fujigaoka Hospital School of Medicine, Yokohama, Japan

Abstract. A respiratory tract burn is not necessarily related to the severity of the overall burns. Sometimes, during the initial period of a respiratory tract burn, there are no abnormal findings in chest X-rays or blood gases, but the burn is then detected for the first time in the respiratory tract by a sudden deterioration in conditions during the course of treatment for the skin burns. An increasing number of doctors now think it is necessary to observe the respiratory tract by using a bronchoscope immediately after a patient suffers burns, regardless of whether or not there is any symptomatic development in the tract. We report our experience of a case involving a 49-year-old male patient who suffered a respiratory tract burn of the peripheral bronchial type, which seemed to be caused by a smoke inhalation injury. We administered urinastatin (Ur) by way of the respiratory tract with successful results.

Keywords: BAL, respiratory tract burn, Urinastatin (polyvalent enzyme inhibitor).

Respiratory burn injuries [1] are major determinants of the prognosis of patients with burns. Due to the fact that they are not always correlated with the severity of burns, it may be lethal if it is neglected on the first hospital visit. There are differences of opinion as to its treatment. Some researchers report the beneficial effect of steroid therapy [2], while others consider it contraindicative due to the potential increase of infection. We encountered a case of respiratory burn injury, presumably due to smoke inhalation, for which broncho-alveolar lavage (BAL) in conjunction with the administration of urinastatin (Ur) was markedly effective.

Case report: a 49-year-old man was presented with dyspnea. He woke up to find his wooden house burning and his room filled with smoke and a noxious odor. He inhaled a large amount of smoke and was admitted to our emergency center with a sore throat, a cough, difficulty in breathing, and second-degree 5 to 10% burns on both hands. Although there were no burns on his face, bronchoscopy revealed redness and erosions in the respiratory mucosa and a large amount of soot, indicating respiratory burn injury. Each bronchus was injected with 5 mL of 300,000 units of Ur combined with 90 mL of saline solution for 3 consecutive days. At the same time, three sessions of BAL were performed, before and after the completion of the Ur therapy, and after discharge from ICU

Address for correspondence: Y. Osakabe, Department of Emergency Center, Showa University Fujigaoka Hospital School of Medicine, 1-30 Fujigaoka, Aoba-ku, Yokohama 227-8501, Japan. Tel.: +81-45-974-6360. Fax: +81-45-971-1113. E-mail: osa101@mb.infoweb.ne.jp

Table 1. BALF results.

	Admission	After Ur treatment	Twelfth day (outpatient)
TCC $\times 10^4$	0.2	0.4	0.5
Mφ (%)	70	68	99
Seg (%)	30	30	1
Lymph (%)		2	
LTB_4 (PG/Hl.BL)	33.7	17.1	18.7
Neutrophil elastase (MCG/L)	610	15	> 10
Nature of recovered solution	black	colorless	colorless

BALF was conducted at the time of admission, after Ur treatment, and at the time of outpatient checks on the 12th day after the injury. At the time of admission, the patient had quite high values of LTB4 and neutrophil elastase levels compared to the values measured after the administration of Ur and on the 12th day, moreover, the sampled liquid showed a dark color due to soot. After the treatment, both neutrophil elastase and LTB4 values dropped to low levels, and the liquid turned colorless.

(Table 1).

As a result, the lesions in the respiratory mucosa resolved and neutrophils, granulocyte elastase, and LTB4 decreased with time. These results indicate that Ur [3], which along with steroids is commonly used as an antishock agent or polyvalent enzyme inhibitor, should be used actively after respiratory burns due to the minimum amount of side effects it causes in comparison to steroids.

References

1. Teixidor HS, Novick GS, Rubin EF. Pulmonary complication in burn patient. J Can Assoc Radiol 1983;34:264–270.
2. Power SR Jr. Consensus summary on smoke inhalation. J Trauma 1979;19:921–922.
3. Kato M, Arase T, Hayashi S et al. Transbronchial administration of urinastatin in burned patient within halation injury. Anesth Resus 1994;30:291–294.

Bronchology and Bronchoesophagology: State of the Art.
H. Yoshimura et al., editors.

Fiberoptic bronchoscopy in the rapid diagnosis of unknown tuberculosis with the use of NAA tests

Ivan Majer, Mária Švejnochová, Igor Uhliarik, Eva Rajecová, Marta Hájková and Peter Krištúfek

Department of Bronchology, National Institute of Tuberculosis and Respiratory Diseases, Bratislava, Slovak Republic

Abstract. *Background.* NAA tests (nucleic acid amplified tests) directly enable rapid detection RNA or DNA of the Mycobacterium tuberculosis complex in clinical samples. The aim of this study was to estimate the diagnostic utility of fiberoptic bronchoscopy (FOB) in conjunction with the use of NAA tests in the rapid diagnosis of TB in sputum smear negative patients.

Methods. Authors in a retrospective study reviewed the results of NAA tests obtained by examinations of bronchoalveolar lavage fluid (BAL) or bronchoaspirate (BA). During a period of 5 years (1995 to 1999), 2,349 BAL and BA specimens with NAA tests in two, 284 patients were examined.

Results. The Amplicor and PCR (polymerase chain reaction) tests were used in 1,807 samples and the Mycobacterium tuberculosis direct test (MTDT, Gen-Probe) in 542. The NAA test was positive in 91 patients (3.8%), and culture positivity was verified in 77 of them. In the 14 patients with just the NAA test positivity the final diagnosis of TB was accepted in eight cases on the basis of clinical and radiological improvement after 2 months of therapy. In six cases the test was estimated to be a false positive, and there were 12 false negative cases (NAA test negative, culture positive). Sensitivity was 88.5%, specificity 99.3%, positive predictive value 84.8%, and negative predictive value 99.4%.

Conclusions. The findings suggested that the identification of the Mycobacterium tuberculosis complex in bronchoalveolar lavage fluid or bronchoaspirate using NAA tests is a useful method for the rapid diagnosis of TB in patients with negative acid fast bacilli (AFB). Bronchoscopic examination can also exclude other pulmonary diseases.

Keywords: fiberoptic bronchoscopy, NAA tests, tuberculosis.

Introduction

The Slovak Republic can be regarded as a region that is near the top limit of low incidence of TB. The total number of new cases and relapses of all clinical forms and localization of TB was 1,211 in the 1999, i.e., incidence was 22.5 per 100,000 inhabitants. Our commom aim should always be to identify or exclude TB as early as possible. Recent technologic developments make it possible to diagnose tuberculosis more rapidly using NAA tests. The aim of this study was to estimate the diagnostic utility of fiberoptic bronchoscopy (FOB) in conjunction with the use of NAA tests in the rapid diagnosis of TB in sputum smear negative patients. NAA tests directly enable rapid detection DNA or RNA of the

Address for correspondence: Ivan Majer, Department of Bronchology, National Institute of TB and Respiratory Diseases, Krajinská 91, 825-56 Bratislava, Slovak Republic. Tel.: +42-17-40-251-151. Fax: +42-17-45-243-622.

Mycobacterium tuberculosis complex (M. tuberculosis, M. Bovis/bacille Calmette-Guérin, M. africanum and M. microti) in clinical specimens. NAA tests include the Amplicor MT, polymerase chain reaction (PCR) and Mycobacterium tuberculosis direct test (MTDT). These tests enzymatically amplify sequences of a defined DNA/RNA Mycobacterium tuberculosis complex and allow rapid identification in sputum smear negative patients. In our country about 40% of active cases of TB have three negative AFB smears.

Materials and Methods

In this retrospective study we reviewed the results of NAA tests obtained by examination of bronchoalveolar lavage fluid (BAL) or bronchoaspirate (BA). During 5 years (1995 to 1999), 2,349 BAL and BA specimens with NAA tests in two, 284 patients were examined. The sputum smears before FOB were negative or sputum could not be obtained. During the bronchoscopy the suctioned specimen was collected and this was considered to be the BA. When BAL was performed the bronchoscope was advanced and wedged in the area of infiltrate. In patients with diffuse lesions the bronchoscope was wedged in the middle lobe or lingula. The lavage was performed with a total of 100 mL saline solution which was instilled and immediately aspirated. The obtained BAL fluid and BA were sent to the laboratory for an AFB smear, NAA test and culture.

Results

During a period of 5 years (1995 to 1999), 2,349 BAL and BA specimens with NAA tests in two, 284 patients were examined. Amplicor (PCR) was used in 1,807 samples and MTDT (Gene Probe) in 542. The NAA tests were positive in 91 patients (50 males, 41 females, mean age: 54.7 years) (3.8%) and culture positivity was verified in 77 of them (84.6%).

In the 14 patients who only had NAA test positivity, the final diagnosis of TB was accepted in eight cases on the basis of clinical and radiological improvement after 2 months of therapy. In six cases the test was estimated to be a false positive (three cases of lung tumours, two pneumonia and one sarcoidosis verified histologically). In 12 cases the test was estimated to be a false negative (NAA test negative, culture positive). Sensitivity was 88.5%, specificity 99.3%, positive predictive value 84.8% and negative predictive value 99.4%.

Discussion

Flexible bronchoscopy, used in conjunction with NAA tests, for the diagnosis of pulmonary and extrapulmonary tuberculosis has been reported more frequently [1—3]. The sensitivity ranges from 75 to 100%, specificity from 95 to 100%, positive predictive value between 78 and 100% and negative predictive value between 95 and 100% [4]. Our findings suggest that the identification of the Mycobacterium tuberculosis complex in BAL fluid or BA using an NAA test is a useful method for the rapid diagnosis of TB in patients with negative sputum smears. When discrepant results between NAA tests and the culture occur (NAA test positive and culture negative), a clinical follow-up and repeat cultures are necessary to disclose a diagnosis of TB. False negative NAA tests can also occur (NAA test negative and culture positive). Inhibitory substances in respiratory specimens (i.e., blood) can block the enzymatic amplification of DNA/RNA. A negative test result with a positive smear suggests infection with nontuberculous mycobacterium (NTM) or Mycobacterium avium complex. Previously, treatment with antituberculous drugs could affect test results [5]. Bronchoscopic examination is also an important part of being able to exclude other pulmonary diseases.

References

1. Schluger NW, Rom WN. Current approaches to diagnosis of active pulmonary tuberculosis. Am J Crit Care Med 1994;149:264–267.
2. Shah S et al. Rapid diagnosis of tuberculosis in various biopsy and body fluid specimens by the Amplicor Mycobacteriun tuberculosis polymerase chain reaction test. Chest 1998;113: 1190–1194.
3. Kolk AHJ et al. Clinical utility of the polymerase chain reaction in the diagnosis of extra-pulmonary tuberculosis. Eur Respir J 1998;11:1222–1226.
4. Gladwin MT, Plorde JJ, Martin TR. Clinical application of the Mycobacterium tuberculosis direct test. Chest 1998;114:317–232.
5. Moore DF et al. Amplification of rRNA for assessment of treatment response of pulmonary tuberculosis patients during antimicrobial therapy. J Clin Microbiol 1996;34:1745–1749.

Bronchology and Bronchoesophagology: State of the Art.
H. Yoshimura et al., editors.

Bronchoscopic findings of active tracheo-bronchial tuberculosis

Yutsuki Nakajima[1], Yuji Shiraishi[1], Keiichiro Takasuna[1], Naoya Katsuragi[1], Seiji Mizutani[2] and Hideo Ogata[2]
[1]Department of Chest Surgery and [2]Department of Pulmonology, Fukujuji Hospital, Japan Anti-Tuberculosis Association, Kiyose City, Tokyo, Japan

Introduction

Dr Arai, a Japanese thoracic surgeon and bronchoscopist, classified the endoscopic findings of tracheo-bronchial tuberculosis into five types [1]. He observed about 130 cases of them periodically and classified them according to their natural progression and improvement by treatment (Table 1). According to this classification, type 1 is considered to be an early nonspecific change. We re-examined the bronchoscopic findings of our active tracheo-bronchial tuberculosis cases according to Arai's classification, and studied their clinical backgrounds.

Materials and Methods

There were 57 cases of active tracheo-bronchial tuberculosis between 1987 to 1997 in Fukujuji Hospital. These cases accounted for about 3% of the active pulmonary tuberculosis cases admitted to our hospital in the same period. In 53 of these cases the quality of the films of serial bronchoscopic examinations allowed us to study the case in detail. We, therefore, reinvestigated them according to Arai's classification of tracheo-bronchial tuberculosis, analyzed their backgrounds, and in several cases we even followed their improvements during anti-tuberculous chemotherapy on the films.

Results

Out of the 53 cases, 52 had some tuberculous pulmonary abnormalities on initial chest X-ray films. Cavitary lesions were found in five cases, noncavitary infiltrations in 40 (75%) and hilar lymph node enlargements or aterectases in another five. However, regarding the area of pulmonary tuberculous lesions, it was found that in most cases they were not extensively scattered. Usually patients with pulmonary cavitary lesions expectorate abundant tuberculous bacilli in their sputa.

Address for correspondence: Yutsuki Nakajima, Department of Chest Surgery, Fukujuji Hospital, Japan Anti-Tuberculosis Association, 3-1-24 Matsuyama, Kiyose City, Tokyo 204-8522, Japan. Tel.: +81-424-91-4111.

Table 1. Arai's classification system and the number of classified cases according to the initial most advanced lesions.

Type 1: edema and conjestion	–
Type 2: intramucosal tubercle	4
Type 3: ulceration	
a. superficial ulceration	8
b. granulomatous ulceration	36
Type 4: granulation	
a. nodular granulation	1
b. polypoid granulation	2
Type 5: scar	
a. scar without stenosis	–
b. scar with stenosis	2

However, patients with active tracheo-bronchial tuberculosis, even in noncavitary cases, may expectorate quite a few tuberculous bacilli in sputa, as well as the cavitary ones. Actually, 85% (34/40) of noncavitary cases were smear positive in our study (Table 2). At initial bronchoscopic examinations, the most progressed lesions were classified as in Table 1. Ulcerations (type 3) accounted for 83% of total cases, and about four-fifths of type 3 cases, superficial ulcerations, progressed to granulomatous ulcerations with time.

Concerning the locations of advanced granulomatous ulcerations, the most progressive changes of tracheo-bronchial tuberculosis occurred mainly on the mucosa from main through upper bronchial regions on both sides. Furthermore, 89% of these lesions were spreading to more than two major branches. The circumferential extensions of granulomatous ulcerations on the airway wall were over halfway in 24 cases at the initial bronchoscopic examination. In 55% of 36 type 3b cases, the ulceration involved the wall entirely in circumference. Therefore, advanced granulomatous ulcerations complicated various kinds of strictures

Table 2. The relationship between X-ray findings and the detection of TB. Bacilli.

X-ray findings	Material	Smear positive	Smear negative
Cavitary (n = 7)	Sputa	7 (++ ~ +++)	0
Noncavitary (n = 40)	Sputa	31 (++ ~ +++)	3 (all culture +)
	BAL (no sputa)	4 (+)	0
	1st BAL	2 (+++)	0
Enlargement of hilar LN or aterectasis (n = 5)	Sputa	3	2 (all culture +)
Normal (n = 1)	Sputa	0	1 (culture +)
Total		47	6

of the airway. The 33 cases with type 3b included five cases with pinhole strictures and seven cases with almost complete obstructions of the airway at the initial bronchoscopic examination. Due to the existence of several films that were taken periodically, we were able to examine 21 cases with granulomatous ulcerations and observe how they improved with chemotherapy. Following the courses of these cases, only four of 11 cases recovered to type 5a and 5b scars by undergoing antituberculous chemotherapy for a period of 2 months.

Discussion

It is important that the endoscopic classification of tracheo-bronchial tuberculosis reflects the natural progression and improvement of the disease through chemotherapy. In this study we recognize the suitability of Arai's classification for tracheo-bronchial tuberculosis to estimate the natural course of progression and recovery. With regard to backgrounds, many cases without pulmonary cavities expectorated so many tuberculous bacilli, that we had to suspect tracheo-bronchial tuberculosis in noncavitary cases with a smear positive. Arai's type 3b, granulomatous ulceration, is the most advanced lesion, and is sometimes complicated with luminal strictures.

Conclusion

From the results of the study on 53 cases of tracheo-bronchial tuberculosis, we concluded as follows: 1) In about three-quarters of all cases, chest X-ray findings showed noncavitary pulmonary lesions, but 83% of them expectorated abundant Tb. bacilli, as well as the cavitary cases; 2) At the first diagnostic bronchoscopic examinations, ulcerations (Arai's type 3) were recognized in 83% cases, and four-fifths of them progressed to granulomatous ulcerations (Type 3b); 3) The lesions mainly involved the main through upper bronchi on both sides, and various tuberculous abnormalities extended widely on the mucosa of major airways; and 4) From the periodic observations of several cases, antituberculous chemotherapy for 2 months, only improved the granulomatous ulcerations to healing scars in 36% of the cases.

Reference

1. Arai T. Endoscopic classification of bronchial tuberculosis. Kekkaku 1989;64:234.

Bronchology and Bronchoesophagology: State of the Art.
H. Yoshimura et al., editors.

The comparison of culture and PCR examinations performed in sputum and bronchoalveolar lavage for evidence of Mycobacterium tuberculosis

F. Salajka, A. Pokorný, L. Mezenský and A. Hrazdirová
Department of Respiratory Diseases, Masaryk University Hospital, Brno, Czech Republic

Introdution

To establish the bacteriological diagnosis of tuberculosis in smear negative patients, there is favourable experience with performing bronchoscopy and bronchoalveloar lavage (BAL) with subsequent culture examination of the BAL fluid (BALF). The aim of our study was to evaluate the contribution to diagnosis, of BALF examined both in culture and PCR compared with the same set of examinations performed in sputum samples.

Methods

During a period of 45 months, diagnostic bronchoscopy with BAL was performed in all smear negative patients in whom the possibility of pulmonary tuberculosis was too great to be excluded. The results of all patients with a final diagnosis of smear negative active tuberculosis were evaluated in the study. Culture and PCR (Amplicor Roche) examinations in BALF and at least three sputum samples were performed prior to starting the therapy. The results of all three or more sputum samples were assessed together.

Results

Altogether, 163 patients were involved in the final evaluation. Bacteriological (culture) evidence of Mycobacterium tuberculosis was obtained in 87 of them (53%) and the PCR test was positive in 96 patients (59%) (Tables 1—3). The BALF examination exhibited positive results in 24 patients (15%) for culture and 28 patients (17%) for PCR (Table 4). The total sensitivity of the sputum samples was higher than that of the BALF examination — positive results were obtained in 72 patients (44%) for culture and 77 patients for PCR (47%) (Table 5). There were only 25 cases (15%) where BALF produced the only evidence of

Address for correspondence: F. Salajka, Department of Respiratory Diseases, Masaryk University Hospital, Jihlavská 20, 693-00 Brno, Czech Republic.

Table 1. Culture examination in sputum and BALF.

	Sputum +	Sputum -
BALF +	9	15
BALF -	63	76

Table 2. PCR examination in sputum and BALF.

	Sputum +	Sputum -
BALF +	9	19
BALF -	68	67

Table 3. Evidence of Mycobacterium tuberculosis (culture and/or PCR).

	Sputum +	Sputum -
BALF +	9	25
BALF -	82	47

tuberculous etiology in sputum (culture and/or PCR) negative patients; on the other hand, sputum examination was the only confirmation of tuberculosis in 82 (50%) BALF negative patients.

Table 4. Culture and PCR examinations of BALF.

	PCR +	PCR -
Culture +	18	6
Culture -	10	129

Table 5. Culture and PCR examinations of sputum.

	PCR +	PCR -
Culture +	58	14
Culture -	19	72

Conclusion

According to our results, bronchoalveolar lavage showed a surprisingly lower sensitivity in yielding a bacteriological diagnosis compared to sputum in smear negative tuberculous patients. One possible explanation could be that, in our patients, three to five sputum samples were taken and all of these examinations were counted together, regardless of how many positive results were obtained. In addition, performing a PCR examination on the obtained samples (both BALF and sputum) helped to increase the sensitivity of the examination.

Bronchology and Bronchoesophagology: State of the Art.
H. Yoshimura et al., editors.

The role of transbronchial or thoracoscopic biopsy in the diagnosis of pulmonary MAC disease

Kazuhiko Shibata[1], Masahide Yasui[2], Shigeharu Myou[2], Keiichi Mizuhashi[3] and Masaki Fujimura[2]
[1]*Department of Respiratory Medicine, Koseiren Takaoka Hospital, Takaoka;* [2]*Department of Internal Medicine (III), Kanazawa University School of Medicine, Kanazawa; and* [3]*Department of Medicine, Toyama Rosai Hospital, Uozu, Japan*

Abstract. *Mycobacterium avium* complex (MAC) pulmonary disease is increasing in incidence and becoming one of the major problems in respiratory medicine. We have surveyed the 65 cases of pulmonary MAC disease diagnosed from 1995 to 1999 in the northern central (Hokuriku) area of Japan. Among 30 patients who underwent biopsy, epitheroid granulomas were detected in 18. Three were male and 15 were female, with a median age of 67 years, ranging from 53 to 84 years. The method of biopsy was transbronchial in 15 cases and thoracoscopic in three. The species of pathogen were *M. avium* in 12 and *M. intracellulare* in six. Five patients were asymptomatic. The biopsy itself was sufficient to satisfy the bacteriological criteria of ATS statement in seven patients with positive tissue culture. The combination of the biopsy and the bronchoalveolar lavage established the diagnosis in an additional eight patients. Transbronchial or thoracoscopic biopsy has an important role in the diagnosis of pulmonary MAC disease.

Keywords: bronchoscopy, *Mycobacterium intracellulare*, *Mycobacterium avium*, nontuberculous mycobacteriosis, video-assisted thoracoscopic surgery.

Background

Mycobacterium avium complex (MAC) pulmonary disease, especially of so-called nodular-bronchiectasis type in an otherwise healthy individual, is increasing in incidence and becoming one of the major problems in respiratory medicine in Japan, as well as in many other countries. Recently published diagnostic criteria of nontuberculous mycobacteriosis by the American Thoracic Society [1] adopted bronchial lavage and lung biopsy as tools for bacteriological examination. The diagnosis is reinforced if the biopsy specimen demonstrated granuloma or acid-fast bacilli [2]. We investigated the role of transbronchial (TBB) or video-assisted thoracoscopic (VATS) biopsy in the diagnosis of pulmonary MAC disease.

Address for correspondence: Kazuhiko Shibata, Department of Respiratory Medicine, Koseiren Takaoka Hospital, 5-10 Eirakucho, Takaoka 933-8555, Japan. Tel.: +81-766-21-3930. Fax: +81-766-28-2865. E-mail: shibatak@po2.nsknet.or.jp

Subjects

From the survey for definitely diagnosed pulmonary MAC disease in the northern central (Hokuriku) area of Japan from 1995 to 1999, 65 cases were collected.

Results

Among the 65 cases, 30 patients underwent biopsy. Epitheroid granulomas were detected in 18 patients, who then went on to be subjects for further evaluation. There were three male and 15 female patients with a median age of 67 years, ranging from 53 to 84 years. The method of biopsy was transbronchial in 15 cases and thoracoscopic in three. The species of pathogen were *M. avium* in 12 cases and *M. intracellulare* in six. The most common symptoms were cough and sputum, and constitutional symptoms were less common. Five patients were asymptomatic. In all seven patients who underwent mycobacterial examination of the biopsied tissue specimen, the culture yielded a positive result and the biopsy itself was sufficient to satisfy the bacteriological criteria of the ATS statement in these patients. The combination of the biopsy and the bronchoalveolar lavage established the diagnosis in the eight additional patients.

Conclusion

Transbronchial or thoracoscopic biopsy has an important role in the diagnosis of pulmonary MAC disease. Mycobacterial culture of the sample must always accompany the histopathological examination because of the high probability of a positive result.

References

1. American Thoracic Society. Diagnosis and treatment of disease caused by nontuberculous mycobacteria. Am J Resp Crit Care Med 1997;156:S1–25.
2. Tanaka E, Amitani R, Niimi A et al. Yield of computed tomography and bronchoscopy for the diagnosis of Mycobacterium avium complex disease. Am J Resp Crit Care Med 1997;155: 2041–2046.

Bronchology and Bronchoesophagology: State of the Art.
H. Yoshimura et al., editors.

Sputum examination immediately after bronchoscopic procedure for detecting pulmonary tuberculosis

Yuichi Takiguchi[1], Reiko Watanabe[1], Akira Suda[1], Hidetoshi Igari[1], Hiroshi Kimura[1], Kciichi Nagao[2] and Takayuki Kuriyama[1]
[1]*Department of Chest Medicine, Chiba University School of Medicine; and* [2]*Health Sciences Center, Chiba University, Chiba, Japan*

Abstract. *Background.* To improve diagnostic sensitivity of pulmonary tuberculosis, sputum examination immediately after bronchoscopic procedure is sometimes performed.

Methods. The patients consisted of 241 cases that underwent bronchoscopic examination for diagnosis of pulmonary lesions. Bacteriological examinations for mycobacteriosis were carried out on the specimen taken during bronchoscopic procedures and in sputum taken immediately after the bronchoscopic examinations.

Results. Twenty-eight cases were diagnosed as pulmonary mycobacteriosis including 13 pulmonary tuberculosis. Sputum examination immediately after bronchoscopy was useful in only one case among the 28 cases.

Conclusion. The method is not recommended as a routine examination for detecting pulmonary mycobacteriosis, because most of the cases were readily diagnosed by the bronchoscopic procedures alone.

Keywords: nosocomial infection, pulmonary infection, pulmonary mycobacteriosis, pulmonary tuberculosis.

Introduction

Even in a clinical situation in which bronchoscopic examinations are performed mainly for diagnosis of lung cancer and interstitial pneumonia, cases with pulmonary tuberculosis are sometimes interfused. Such cases with unrecognized pulmonary tuberculosis may cause nosocomial spreading of tuberculosis. Therefore, it is essential to detect cases with pulmonary tuberculosis among other pulmonary diseases at the earliest clinical session. In an attempt to improve detection sensitivity for pulmonary mycobacteriosis, sputum examination immediately after bronchoscopic procedures is sometimes performed. This report evaluates its clinical relevance.

Patients and Methods

The patients consisted of 241 successive cases that underwent bronchoscopic

Address for correspondence: Yuichi Takiguchi, Department of Chest Medicine, Chiba University School of Medicine, 1-8-1 Inohana, Chuo-ku, Chiba 260-8670, Japan. Tel.: +81-43-222-7171. Fax: +81-43-226-2176. E-mail: yuichi@med.m.chiba-u.ac.jp examination for diagnosis of pulmonary lesions, including nodular or infiltrative lesions. The 241 cases included 148 outpatients and 93 inpatients. From each patient, specimens were routinely taken by bronchoscopic procedure (e.g., transbronchial fine needle aspiration, transbronchial brushing, bronchial lavage, etc.), and subsequently, sputum taken immediately after the bronchoscopic procedure was also examined. Bacteriological study of the specimens includes direct observation by microscopes with the aid of Ziehl-Neelsen stain, PCR amplification of the DNA of *Mycobacterium tuberculosis*, and 8-week culture.

Results

Twenty-eight patients were finally diagnosed as having pulmonary mycobacteriosis, including 13 cases of pulmonary tuberculosis. As to the incidence according to the roentgenologic appearance, five cases were diagnosed from 115 cases with nodular lesions, 23 cases were diagnosed from 81 cases with infiltrative lesions, and none were diagnosed from 37 cases with diffuse interstitial lesions that needed transbronchial lung biopsy and bronchoalveolar lavage. Methods of the final diagnosis of the 28 cases are shown in Tables 1 and 2.

Discussion

As clearly shown in the Tables, most of the cases with pulmonary mycobacteriosis were already diagnosed by bacteriological examinations taken by pre-bronchoscopic or bronchoscopic procedures. Of the 241 cases who underwent bronchoscopy, sputum examination immediately after the bronchoscopic examination solely yielded a positive result for pulmonary mycobacteriosis in only one case with infiltrative lesion (in this case, atypical mycobacteriosis, see Table 2). Any cases with single nodular or infiltrative lesion would be easily diagnosed by bronchoscopic examination, as presented here. Sputum examination immediately following bronchoscopy might be fruitful for cases with multiple infiltrative lesions in which all of the lesions cannot be examined by the bronchoscopic procedure. In conclusion, sputum examination immediately after bronchoscopic examination gave additional information in only one case among 241 cases, and

Table 1. Methods of final diagnosis for the patients with nodular lesions.

	Lung TB[a] (n = 3)	AM (n = 2)
Pre-BS sputum	0	0
BS procedures	2	1
Post-BS sputum	0	0
(Post-BS sputum alone)	(0)	(0)
CT-guided biopsy	1	1

[a]Pulmonary tuberculosis. AM, atypical mycobacteriosis; BS, bronchoscopy.

Table 2. Methods of final diagnosis for the patients with infiltrative lesions.

	Lung TB[a] (n = 10)	AM (n = 13)
Pre-BS sputum	4	4
BS procedures	9	10
Post-BS sputum	4	4
(Post-BS sputum alone)	(0)	(1)

[a]Pulmonary tuberculosis. AM, atypical mycobacteriosis; BS, bronchoscopy.

therefore, the method is not recommended as a routine examination for distinguishing pulmonary mycobacteriosis from other pulmonary diseases that require bronchoscopic examinations.

Acknowledgements

This work was funded by grants from Chiba Antituberculosis Foundation for medical research.

Laryngeal, pharyngeal and glottic diseases

Bronchology and Bronchoesophagology: State of the Art.
H. Yoshimura et al., editors.

A case of malignant fibrous histiocytoma of the larynx

Masahiko Higashikawa[1,2], Michiro Kawakami[2], Yasuhito Hattori[2], Kazuaki Hashimoto[2], Yuko Suzuki[2], Shigemasa Ikai[3] and Hiroshi Takenaka[1]
[1]Osaka Medical College, Takatsuki; [2]Saiseikai Suita Hospital, Suita; and [3]Higashi-Osaka, Osaka, Japan

Case

A 67-year-old male was suffering from hoarseness. Endoscopic examination demonstrated an irregular mass on the left vocal fold. The tumor was removed and its base was cauterized micro-surgically using a KTP laser under general anesthesia. Pathological examination revealed mild dysplasia. Subsequently, the endoscopic removal was repeated whenever it redeveloped, several times, and pathological diagnosis was mild dysplasia. On 7 July 1999, 22 months after his first consultation, the patient developed dyspnea, that rapidly took a turn for the worse. The tumor had grown to fill the laryngeal space. Pathological examination, using endoscopic, biopsy suggested a nonepithelial malignant tumor. MRI demonstrated that its size had reached over 3 cm in length. We predicted a poor prognosis if the larynx was preserved, and subsequently a total laryngectomy was performed on 1 September. No metastatic lesions were observed. The final definitive diagnosis was malignant fibrous histiocytoma (MFH) of the storiform-pleomorphic type. The patient has remained disease-free after 9 months of follow-up.

Comments

The occurrence of malignant fibrous histiocytoma (MFH) in the head and neck is rare. Only several tens of cases of MFH of the larynx have been reported, and there is still no standard protocol for them because of small number of cases. In the case of a small tumor on the vocal fold, micro-surgical excision with/without laser is successful. On the other hand, cases with a poor prognosis despite undergoing a total laryngectomy have also been called our attention. Fourteen out of 44 patients underwent total laryngectomy, and three out of the 14 died of MFH (Kuwabara et al., 1994). Furthermore, we were unable to preserve the larynx in our case, despite micro-surgical excision with a KTP laser, and it was only a small tumor to begin with.

Address for correspondence: Masahiko Higashikawa, Saiseikai Suita Hospital, 1-2 Kawazono, Suita, Osaka 564-0013, Japan. Tel.: +81-6-6382-1521. Fax: +81-6-6382-2498.

Clinically, our case was suspected to be a malignant neoplasm, due to the redevelopment of the tumor several times, but it was difficult to conclude a definitive pathological diagnosis. One reason for this is that nonepithelial malignant tumors often exhibit various different pathological features. Another reason is the small specimen obtained from the laryngeal tumor. Consequently, rapid growth of the tumor obliged us to undertake total laryngectomy.

In dealing with MFH of the larynx, having a definitive pathological diagnosis at an early stage and having a good idea of the extent of the tumor are indispensable measures needed to improve the curative and preservation of the larynx rates.

©2001 Published by Elsevier Science B.V.
Bronchology and Bronchoesophagology: State of the Art.
H. Yoshimura et al., editors.

CO_2 laser surgery for T1a glottic carcinoma

M. Hirayama, H. Takahashi, K. Yao, K. Inagi, M. Nakayama, K. Nishiyama, T. Makoshi, H. Nagai, J. Yamanaka and M. Okamoto
Department of Otolaryngology, Kitasato University, School of Medicine, Kanagawa, Japan

Abstract. A total of 72 patients with laryngeal cancer (T1a glottis) were treated at the Kitasato University Hospital, between 1984 and 1994. We recommend using CO_2 laser via laryngomicrosurgery when the tumor is located in the membranous portion of the glottis. If the tumor invaded the anterior glottis or posterior glottis, we recommend using radiotherapy. If the tumor mass is bulky, we recommend using combined treatment as discussed below.

The larynx preservation rate was 97.2%. Regarding the 72 patients classified as T1a, laser surgery alone was used in 21 patients. Nineteen of the 21 patients were cured. Radiotherapy alone was performed in 26 patients. Twenty-one of the 26 patients were cured. The combined treatment was performed in 25 patients.

Keywords: CO_2 laser surgery, laryngeal cancer.

Introduction (Fig. 1, Table 1)

A total of 72 patients (69 men and 3 women, age range: 41–79 years, mean age: 61.5 years) with laryngeal cancer (T1a glottis) were treated at the Kitasato University Hospital, between 1984 and 1994. All patients were followed up for more than 5 years (observation period: 5–14 years, average: 7.2 years).

We recommend using CO_2 laser via laryngomicrosurgery when the tumor is located in the membranous portion of the glottis. If the tumor invaded the anterior glottis or posterior glottis, we recommend using radiotherapy. If the tumor mass was bulky, we recommend using combined treatment.

Results (Tables 2 and 3)

At follow-up, 64 of the 72 patients were alive without cancer, while eight patients had died of other causes. The larynx preservation rate was 97.2%.

Regarding the 72 patients classified as T1a, laser surgery alone was used in 21 patients. Nineteen of the 21 patients were cured. Radiotherapy alone was performed in 26 patients. Twenty-one of the 26 patients were cured. The combined treatment was performed in 25 patients (radiotherapy + chemotherapy: 12

Address for correspondence: Masatoshi Hirayama, Department of Otolaryngology, Kitasato University, School of Medicine, 1-15-1 Kitasato, Sagamihara-shi, Kanagawa 228-8555, Japan. Tel.: +81-42-778-8432. E-mail: mhira@d6.dion.ne.jp

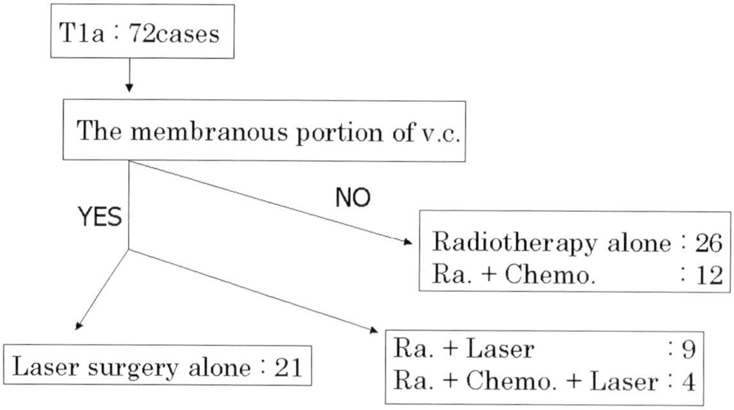

Fig. 1.

Table 1.

· The tumor was located in the membranous potion
  → CO_2 laser via LMS alone
· The tumor invaded the anterior or posterior glottis
  → Radiotherapy
· The tumor mass was bulky
  → Combined treatment (radiotherapy + chemotherapy)

Table 2.

Initial treatment	No. of cases
CO_2 laser via LMS alone	21
Radiotherapy (60 Gy) alone	26
Radiotherapy + chemotherapy (UFT: 300–600 mg)	12
Radiotherapy + laser	9
Radiotherapy + chemotherapy + laser	4

Table 3. Results.

	Complete remission	Local recurrence
Laser	21	2/21
Radiotherapy	26	4/26
Radiotherapy + chemotherapy	12	0/12
Radiotherapy + laser	9	0/9
Radiotherapy + laser + chemotherapy	4	0/4

patients, radiation + laser: nine patients, and radiation + laser + chemotherapy: four patients).

Conclusion

- A total of 72 patients with laryngeal cancer (T1a glottis) were investigated retrospectively.
- Among the cases with laryngeal cancer classified as T1a, laser surgery was indicated only for localized lesion in the membranous portion.
- Laser surgery was also performed for cases with recurrence.

Bronchology and Bronchoesophagology: State of the Art.
H. Yoshimura et al., editors.

Surgical treatment for posterior glottic lesions: our preliminary experience

Masahiro Kawaida[1], Hiroyuki Fukuda[2] and Naoyuki Kohno[3]
[1]Department of Otolaryngology, Tokyo Metropolitan Ohtsuka Hospital, Toshima-ku; [2]Department of Otolaryngology-HNS, Keio University School of Medicine, Shinjuku-ku, Tokyo; and [3]Department of Otolaryngology, National Defense Medical College, Tokorozawa, Saitama, Japan

Abstract. Microlaryngosurgery, using a direct laryngoscope, is the optimal surgical method to remove laryngeal lesions. However, an ordinary laryngoscope does not allow precise observations of the posterior glottic area under inhalation anesthesia, because the tube inserted into the trachea obstructs the surgical field of the posterior glottic area. The tracheal tube must be placed on the tip of the laryngoscope and be moved towards the anterior glottis to allow visualization of the posterior glottis. A prototype model of the direct laryngoscope, capable of manipulating the posterior glottis, was used to accommodate easy positioning of the tracheal tube. This prototype of the laryngoscope is characterized by the concavity on the upper tip portion, which allows easier placement and movement of the tracheal tube toward the anterior commissure.

Keywords: glottic area, laryngoscope, tracheal tube.

Introduction

Posterior glottic lesions are relatively rare in comparison with many other laryngeal lesions, which commonly arise in the anterior glottis. However, a few lesions arise in the posterior glottis. An ordinary laryngoscope does not allow precise observations of the posterior glottis under inhalation anesthesia, because the tube inserted into the trachea obstructs the surgical field of the posterior glottic area. To allow good visualization of this area, a prototype model of the laryngoscope, which has a concavity on the upper tip portion, was manufactured in collaboration with Nagashima Medical Instruments Co., Ltd. The usefulness of this surgical method using this laryngoscope is described herein.

Methods and Technique

Typical posterior glottic lesions are nonspecific granuloma of the vocal process, cysts of the arytenoid, hemangioma, and papilloma. The prototype model of the special laryngoscope was used in microlaryngosurgery for these posterior glottic lesions. This laryngoscope is characterized by the existence of the concavity on

---

Address for correspondence: Masahiro Kawaida, Department of Otolaryngology, Tokyo Metropolitan Ohtsuka Hospital, 2-8-1, Minamiohtsuka, Toshima-ku, Tokyo 170-0005, Japan. Tel.: +81-3-3941-3211. Fax: +81-3-3941-9557. E-mail: kawaida-o@ohtsuka-hospital.toshima.tokyo.jp

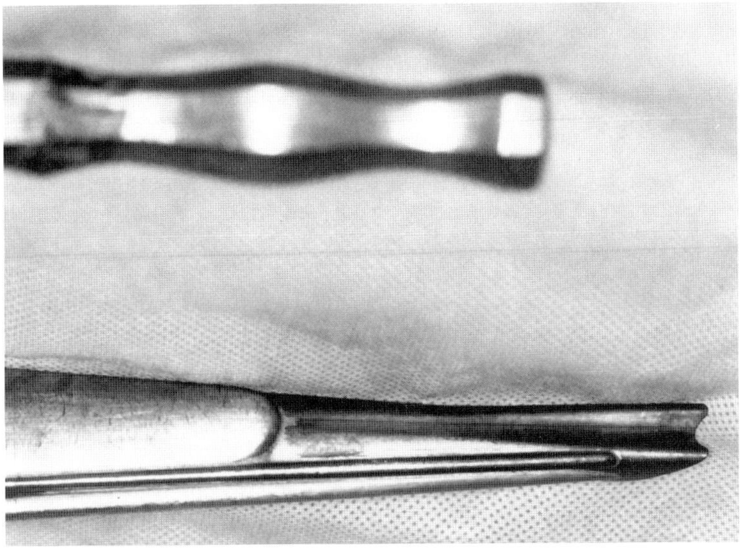

Fig. 1. The upper tip portion of the direct laryngoscope for posterior glottic lesions, manufactured by Nagashima Medical Instruments Co., Ltd.

the upper distal tip, capable of the anterior movement of the tracheal tube (Fig. 1). The tube inserted into the trachea is moved anteriorly, using this laryngoscope, and the surgical field of the posterior glottis is obtained. The lesion is then resected using forceps and scissors.

Results

Good microlaryngosurgical fields of the posterior glottis were obtained using this laryngoscope and it was possible to resect the lesions with forceps and scissors very easily.

There were no recurrences requiring reoperation and the postoperative course was favorable in all patients.

Discussion

Microlaryngosurgery is performed for common laryngeal lesions. Since common lesions arise in the anterior part of the glottis, many laryngoscopes have been developed to obtain surgical fields of the anterior glottis [1,2]. However, because the shape of the tip of an ordinary laryngoscope is tubular, it is impossible to remove the tracheal tube anteriorly. A posterior commissure laryngoscope with a concavity on the upper tip was developed by Ossoff et al. [3]. This laryngoscope was specially manufactured to perform lasersurgery for posterior glottic lesions with a carbon dioxide laser. On the other hand, the laryngoscope used this time has a long, deep concavity that makes it possible to move the tracheal tube toward the anterior glottis. Microlaryngosurgery for posterior glottic lesions was performed with this laryngoscope. Since the proximal end is fine and the concavity is manufactured on its upper tip, it was easy to obtain the surgical field of the posterior glottis.

Conclusion

Although posterior glottic lesions are rare, they should be resected properly. We introduced a prototype of a laryngoscope which makes it possible to move the tracheal tube toward the anterior glottis. Microlaryngosurgery for posterior glottic lesions can be performed easily using this laryngoscope.

References

1. Scalco AN, Shipman WF, Tabb HG. Microscopic suspension laryngoscopy. Ann Otol Rhinol Laryngol 1960;69:1134–1138.
2. Benjamin B. A new adult microlaryngoscope. Ann Otol Rhinol Laryngol 1986;95:207.
3. Ossoff RH, Karlan MS, Sisson GE. Posterior commissure laryngoscope for carbon dioxide laser surgery. Ann Otol Rhinol Laryngol 1983;92:361.

Bronchology and Bronchoesophagology: State of the Art.
H. Yoshimura et al., editors.

Supraglottic laryngeal closure: false vocal cord closure

Satoshi Kitahara, Etsuyo Tamura, Tetsuya Tanabe, Yoko Kitagawa and Yuko Matsumura

Department of Otolaryngology, National Defense Medical College, Tokorozawa, Japan

Abstract. For food intake, long-term dysphagic patients should occasionally be treated with surgery which separates the food passage from the airway. Despite simpler and more definitive procedures already in use, any reversible method to phonation would be welcomed.

We report our method of supraglottic laryngeal closure at the level of false vocal cords. Following the laryngofissure, both false vocal cords were cut down vertically along the edges. In other words, the larynx was separated vertically at the level of the false vocal cords in laryngeal space. Then, the upper and lower parts of false vocal cords were sutured from the back at symmetrical positions. We suture thyroid cartilages to avoid dislocation. No drainage was necessary for the skin suture. We can fiberscopically observe the movement of adduction and abduction of vocal cords through the tracheal stoma.

Eight patients were administered this method of supraglottic laryngeal closure since 1987. In one patient (a 78-year-old male), the glottis was reopened by laser microlaryngosurgery. He successfully reactivated phonation without aspiration for food intake.

Keywords: aspiration, larynx, surgical treatment.

Dysphagic patients who experienced conservative treatment as ineffective, with modification of food textures and/or arrangement of posture during swallowing, are possible candidates for surgical treatment such as laryngeal suspension, or cricopharyngeal myotomy. However, these procedures may be applied to relatively mild cases for whom the insufficient elevation of larynx and/or insufficient opening of esophagus are closely related to their dysphagia. Therefore, those cases with severe dysphagia must be selectively administered laryngo-tracheal diversion [1–3].

From January 1989 to March 2000, 26 cases received laryngo-tracheal diversion to prevent aspiration in our department of Otolaryngology at the National Defense Medical College Hospital. Of these cases, eight were given the procedure of false vocal cord closure. These eight cases consisted of five males and three females (45–78 years of age), and causes were cerebrovascular disease [5], Wallenberg syndrome [1], esophagus cancer resection [1], neck dissection which sacrificed X, XII nerves [1] (Table 1).

Following the laryngofissure, both false vocal cords were cut down vertically along the edges, so that the larynx was separated vertically. Then, the upper and

Address for correspondence: Satoshi Kitahara, Department of Otolaryngology, National Defense Medical College, 3-2 Namiki, Tokorozawa, Saitama 359-8513, Japan. Tel.: +81-42-995-1686. Fax: +81-42-996-5212. E-mail: kita797s@ndmc.ac.jp

Table 1. The cases.

Age (years)	Sex	Cause of aspiration	After operation
78	M	Cerebrovascular disease	Smooth intake
71	M	Cerebrovascular disease	Smooth intake
70	M	Neck dissection sacrificed X, XII nerves	Smooth intake
69	F	Cerebrovascular disease	Smooth intake
65	F	Esophageal cancer resection	Smooth intake
64	M	Cerebrovascular disease	Smooth intake
62	F	Wallenberg syndrome	Smooth intake
45	M	Cerebrovascular disease	Smooth intake

lower parts of false vocal cords were sutured from the posterior commissure to the anterior commissure at symmetrical positions (Figs. 1–3). Surgeons who

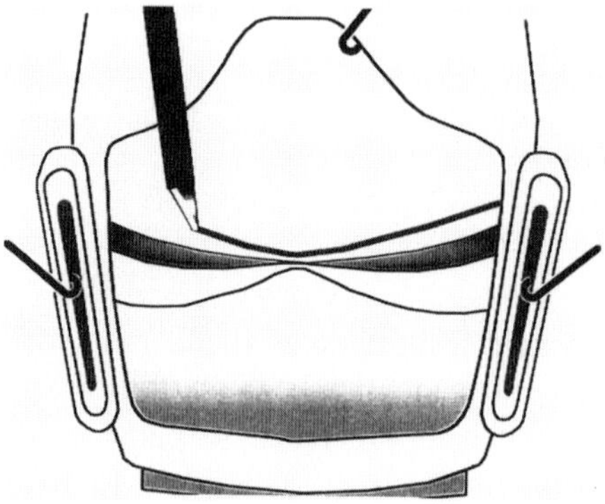

Fig. 1. Following the laryngofissure, both false vocal folds were separated vertically by cutting down along their edges.

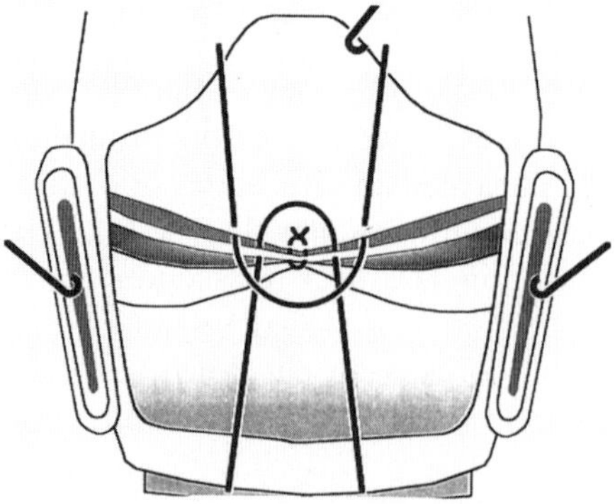

Fig. 2. Upper and lower parts of the false vocal cords were sutured from the posterior commissure to the anterior commissure at the cutting edges.

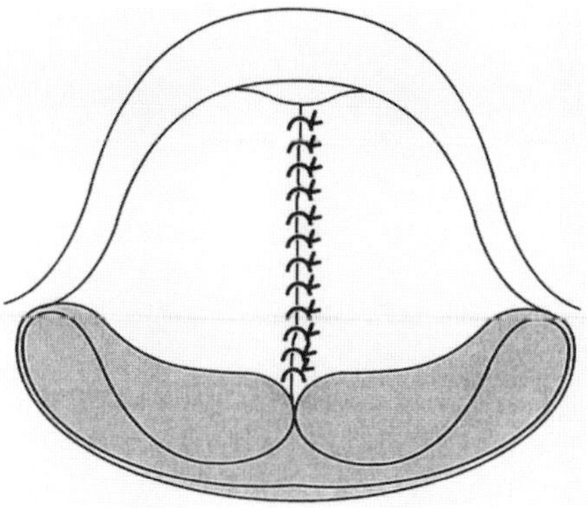

Fig. 3. The larynx was closed at the supraglottic level.

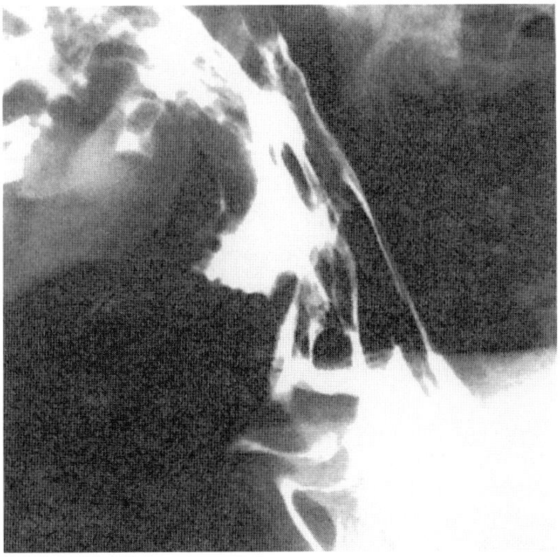

Fig. 4. Preoperative esophageal image of fluoroscopy of a 64-year-old CVA male.

have mastered laryngofissure may also be good at performing false vocal cord closure. If posterior commissure was cut down deeply enough at the level of the false vocal cords, we could prevent leakage.

The outcome showed that all cases succeeded in oral intake, although difficulty from the few posterior sutures is a disadvantage. Figures 4 and 5 show pre- and postoperative esophageal images by fluoroscopy administered to a 64-year-old male who suffered cerebrovascular disease. In one case (78-year-old male), the glottis was reopened by laser microsurgery 5 months after laryngeal closure because he demonstrated successful swallowing without aspiration at esophageal fluoroscopy. His phonation was reactivated [4]. Laryngo-tracheal diversion

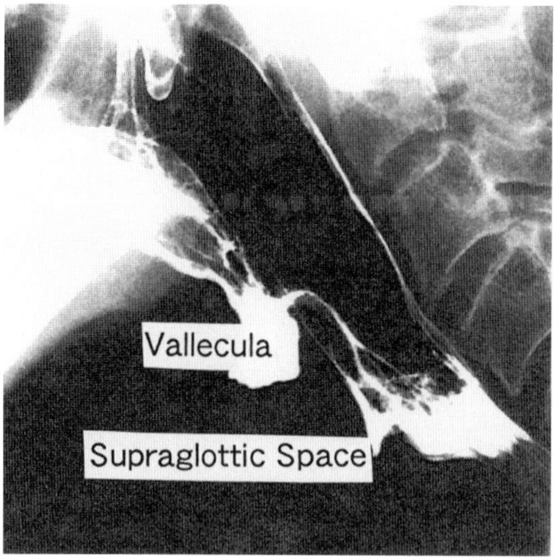

Fig. 5. Postoperative image of the same patient in Fig. 4.

requires operative limitation in each case depending on the location of stoma, causal disease and prognosis of aspiration, etc. However, in cases with an intact larynx, false vocal cord closure is recommendable. It is not only technically easy, but also a reversible procedure with regard to phonation.

References

1. Lindeman RC, Yarrington CT, Sutton D. Clinical experience with tracheoesophageal anastomosis for intractable aspiration. Ann Otol 1976;85;609–612.
2. Montgomery WW. Surgery to prevent aspiration. Arch Otolaryngol 1975;101;679–682.
3. Kitahara S, Tanabe T, Nakanobou M, Karaho T, Matsumura Y, Kitagawa Y, Ohmae Y. Surgical procedure for intractable aspiration. J Jpn Bronchoesophagol 1999;50:603–608.
4. Kitahara S, Ikeda M, Ohmae Y, Nakanobou M, Inoue T, Healy GB. Laryngeal closure at the level of the false vocal cords for the treatment of aspiration. J Laryngol Otol 1993;107:826–828.

Bronchology and Bronchoesophagology: State of the Art.
H. Yoshimura et al., editors.

Bifid epiglottis – a case report

Noriko Morimoto, Nobuko Kawashiro, Fumiko Shishiyama and Nobuaki Tsuchihashi
Division of Otolaryngology, National Children's Hospital, Setagaya, Tokyo, Japan

Abstract. Bifid epiglottis is a rare congenital anomaly often resulting in severe respiratory distress, due to laxity of the cartilage, and chronic aspirations in infants or newborns. Only about 20 cases have been reported in world literature. This anomaly is often associated with other congenital anomalies. The most commonly associated anomalies are hand and/or feet anomalies (~ 90%) while the most severe ones are hypothalamic hamartomas and hypopituitarism.

We present a case of a 5-month-old boy with a bifid epiglottis which was split down to the base in two equal halves. He was referred to our department for aspiration and stridor, and after the operation Hirschsprung's disease was also detected. No other anomalies were detected. Although aspiration has been reported to be rebellious, epigloplasty, which sutures the epiglottic halves together, succeeded in relieving aspiration and stridor and resulted in normal weight gain.

Keywords: associated anomaly, congenital stridor, congenital aspiration.

Introduction

Bifid epiglottis is a rare congenital anomaly often resulting in severe respiratory distress, due to laxity of the cartilage, and chronic aspirations in infants or newborns. Only about 20 cases have been reported in world literature.

Most cases of bifid epiglottis have shown stridor and/or aspiration. When an epiglottis is flaccid, it prolapses into the glottis during inspiration, resulting in inspiratory stridor and dyspnea. We present a case of a 5-month-old boy with bifid epiglottis associated with Hirschsprung's disease.

A case report

A newborn boy was referred to the surgical department for aspiration and abdominal distention, and a diagnosis of Hirschsprung's disease was made. The patient was born of an uneventful pregnancy. At 4 months of age, a radical operation for the Hirschsprung's disease was successfully performed to relieve abdominal symptoms.

However, aggravating aspiration and stridor was noticed after this operation and the patient's symptoms temporarily worsened when he began drinking.

Address for correspondence: Noriko Morimoto MD, Division of Otolaryngology, National Children's Hospital, 3-35-31 Taishido, Setagaya, Tokyo 154-8509, Japan. Tel.: +81-3-3414-8121. Fax: +81-3-3414-9210. E-mail: nmorimoto@nch.go.jp

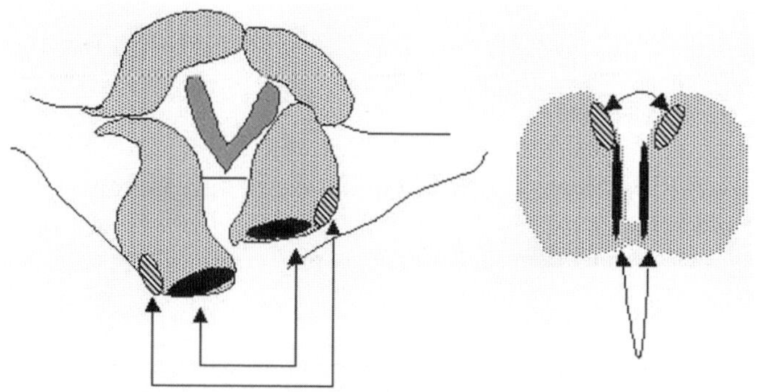

Fig. 1. Each end of of the bifid epiglottis was trimmed and sutured together.

Upper gastrointestinal series reveals significant aspiration. An endoscopic view showed bifid epiglottis which was split down to the base in two equal halves.

After 5 months, since birth, supraglottoplasty was performed under general anesthesia (Fig. 1). A skin incision 5-cm long on the hyoid bone left the hypopharyngeal space open and allowed the base of the epiglottis to be seen. Each end of the epiglottic halves was trimmed and sutured together to give them a normal appearance, by monitoring them through the pharynx using a flexible fiberscope. Over the next 6 months, aspiration and stridor completely disappeared. The child experienced normal growth and development.

Discussion

Bifid epiglottis is often associated with other congenital anomalies [1]. The most common of these are hand and/or feet anomalies (70%), while the most severe are hypothalamic hamartomas and hypopituitarism.

Treatment for bifid epiglottis varies with the symptoms. Some patients were treated conservatively due to the associated anomalies or the expectation of natural recovery and, therefore, their aspiration remained at a constant level. In fact, only three cases [2–4] have been reported to have recovered naturally without any reconstruction. Our management of the epigloplasty succeeded in relieving aspiration and stridor, and resulted in normal weight gain.

References

1. Montreuil F. Bifid epiglottis-report of a case. Laryngoscope 1949;59:194–199.
2. DelMonico ML, Haar JG. Bifid epiglottis. Report of a case. Arch Otolaryngol 1972;96: 178–181.
3. Healy GB, Holt GP, Tucker JA. Bifid epiglottis: a rare laryngeal anomaly. Laryngoscope 1976; 86:1459–1468.
4. Wittig FJ, Hickey SA, Kumar M. Double epiglottis in Weyer's acrofacial dysostosis. J Laryngol Otol 1998;112:976–978.

Bronchology and Bronchoesophagology: State of the Art.
H. Yoshimura et al., editors.

A case of pharyngeal stenosis in recurrent stomatitis

Yasuhiro Murata, Etsuyo Tamura, Jin Adachi, Naoyuki Kohno and Satoshi Kitahara
Department of Otolaryngology National Defense Medical College, Saitama, Japan

Abstract. A 23-year-old woman has suffered from recurrent stomatitis for about 2 years. She visited our clinic on 2 July 1988 due to pain in her throat and mild dysphagia. Ulcering lesion and scar formation in pharyngeal mucosa were seen. Furthermore, a severe web-like stenosis was seen in the lower part of the mesopharynx. The airway was partially obstructed. We could partially observe the epiglottis tip through the remaining space. She was admitted to our hospital for further examinations on 17 March 1999 and had an emergency tracheotomy due to mild dyspnea. The pathological findings of pharyngeal mucosa showed only nonspecific inflammation. Behcet's disease and any other autoimmune disease were clinically ruled out.

Thus, at present, the origin of recurrent stomatitis is unknown. Pharyngoplasty was performed under general anesthesia on 30 April 1999. She was given 300 mg/day Tranilast (a preventing agent for excessive scar formation). As a result, the stenosis of the lower part of mesopharynx was well dilated, and clinical symptoms were remarkably improved. Recurrence of stenosis has not been observed up to the present.

Keywords: nonspecific inflammation, pharyngoplasty, Tranilast.

Case study

This case involves a 23-year-old woman. The chief complaint was pain in her throat and mild dysphagia. Her present illness is recurrent stomatitis, which she has been suffering from for about 2 years. She visited our clinic on 2 July 1998 due to pain in her throat and mild dysphagia. Her medical history includes allergic rhinitis and recurrent aphtha.

At the first examination, we found ulcer formation in her pharynx. Adhesion and deformity of the pharyngeal wall were also observed. Furthermore, a severe web-like stenosis was seen in the lower part of the pharynx. The airway was partially obstructed and through the remaining space, we could partially observe the epiglottis tip. On the other hand, no pathological findings were observed below these lesions.

Histopathological tests revealed nonspecific inflammation with infiltrations of neutrophils and lymphocytes. From immunological examinations no remarkable abnormalities were seen except an increase in IgM.

Address for correspondence: Yasuhiro Murata, Department of Otolaryngology, National Defense Medical College, 3-2 Namiki, Tokorozawa, Saitama 359-8513, Japan. Tel.: +81-42-995-1686. Fax: +81-42-996-5212.

Clinical course

We planned to follow up her condition at the outpatient clinic, however, she had not visited us until 10 March 1999. She came to our hospital because her condition had worsened. At that time, deformity and stenosis in the pharynx were also getting worse. She was admitted on 17 March 1999 for further examination and had an emergency tracheotomy due to mild dyspnea. After tracheotomy, she was given 4 mg of dexamethasone using the tapering method, and Tranilast at 300 mg/day. After administration of these drugs, ulcer formation in the pharynx improved immediately. On 30 April 1999, we performed pharyngoplasty under general anesthesia. Under laryngomicrosurgery, we spread the lower part of the pharynx with Iwamura's laryngoscope, then excised the mucosa of stenotic lesion with microscissors. The margin of the excised mucosa was sutured in order not to adhere. As a result, the narrowing space in the lower part of the pharynx was successfully dilated, and we could observe the larynx easily. Her clinical symptoms were successfully improved, and after closure of tracheostoma, she was discharged on 18 May 1999.

Discussion

Sometimes cases of recurrent stomatitis are encountered. However, pharyngeal stenosis following this stomatitis is comparatively rare [1]. There are some reports concerned with recurrent stomatitis, but the obvious etiology has not been described. Inagi et al. [2] reported 25 cases of recurrent stomatitis. According to this report, the characteristics of this disease were summarized as follows: 1) it is often seen in the 30–40 years age range in men; 2) ulcering lesion appears around the paratine tonsil-paratine arch; 3) mixed lesions of the active ulcer and healing with scar; 4) histopathological findings show only nonspecific inflammation; and 5) the etiology is still unknown, but association with the immune system has been considered.

The case we experienced accorded with these characteristics except for age and sex. Behcet's disease must be considered when recurrent stomatitis is observed. In this case, other symptoms were not confirmed. In addition, HLA B51 was negative. Thus, Behcet's disease was ruled out clinically, and the etiology of recurrent stomatitis presently remains unknown.

As regards therapy, there are some discussions around the use of steroids. In this case, we used Tranilast following the use of a steroid. It is reported that Tranilast was effective for Crohn's disease [3] and Behcet's disease [4]. After administration of this drug, stomatitis improved immediately. Recurrence of stomatitis and stenosis has not been observed up to the present. Thus, it is reasonable to suppose that Tranilast has worked effectively in the prevention of recurrent stomatitis.

In the surgical operation, although collection of stenotic lesion by CO_2 laser was reported [1], we excised the stenotic pharyngeal mucosa by microscissors and sutured the margin of mucosa in order to prevent adhesion. As a result, her clinical course has been successfully stabilized.

References

1. Kaneko M et al. A case of pharyngo-laryngeal stenosis in recurrent aphthous stomatitis. J Jpn Bronchoesophagol Soc 1989;39:348–357.
2. Inagi K et al. Clinical study of intractable recurrent ulcer of the oral cavity and pharynx. J Otolaryngol Jpn 1993;96:1457–1464.
3. Kikuchi T et al. A case of chronic Crohn's disease possibly managed with Tranilast. Jpn J Gastroenterol 1997;94:195–199.
4. Nonomura N et al. A case of pharyngolaryngeal stenosis in Behcet's disease. Auris Nasus Larynx (Tokyo) 1992;19:55–61.

Bronchology and Bronchoesophagology: State of the Art.
H. Yoshimura et al., editors.

The management of a recurrent fibrolipoma of the supraglottic larynx

Tadashi Nakashima, Kikuo Sakamoto, Hirohito Umeno, Yoshihisa Ueda and Tetsuyoshi Umeno
Department of Otolaryngology Head and Neck Surgery, Kurume University School of Medicine, Kurume, Japan

Abstract. We describe a case of a giant fibrolipoma of the larynx that was first treated by a subtotal excision via a lateral pharyngotomy. At the initial surgery, a pedunculated tumor from the left arytenoid occupied the cervical and thoracic esophagus. However, there was a recurrence and the patient suffered from dyspnea. At the second surgery, the masses in the arytenoid and false vocal cord were subtotally removed without damaging the mucosa and the arytenoid swelling almost disappeared.

Keywords: fibrolipoma, larynx, recurrence, surgery.

Introduction

Although lipogenic tumors, such as laryngeal lipoma or fibrolipoma, are histologically benign, they are often thought to be clinically malignant due to a high rate of recurrence over an extended period of time. We report a case of a recurrent giant fibrolipoma of the larynx that was successfully treated by a subtotal excision via a lateral pharyngotomy and submucosal excision.

Patient

A 60-year-old male noticed a voice change and an abnormal sensation in the hypopharynx over a peroid of 4 years. On examination, a white mass was found on the left hypopharynx that reached the left arytenoid process. On a barium-swallowing roentgenogram, there was a tumor of 30-cm in length that reached the thoracic esophagus. The esophagus was markedly dilated by the tumor. CT scan and MRI detected a giant mass that originated from the arytenoid of the larynx suggesting a fat composition of the tumor. A fibreoptic examination revealed a bilobularly pedunculated tumor that ended close to the cardia of the stomach. The tumor was removed under a general anesthesia using a left cervical skin incisional approach. Histologically, the tumor was composed of adipose and fibrous tissues and diagnosed to be a fibrolipoma.

Address for correspondence: Tadashi Nakashima MD, Department of Otolaryngology, Head and Neck Surgery, Kurume University School of Medicine, 67 Asahi-machi, Kurume 830-0011, Japan. Tel.: +81-942-31-7575. Fax: +81-942-37-1200.

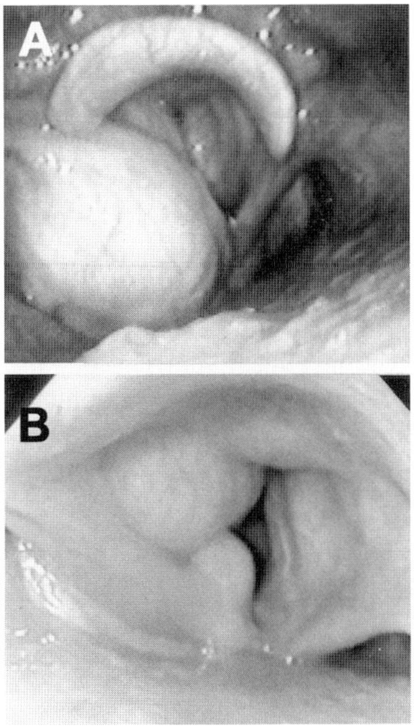

Fig. 1. **A:** Laryngeal fiberscopy of the recurrent fibrolimopa of the left arytenoid. **B:** Postoperative view.

Two years later, the patient noticed the change of voice, again, and dyspnea on exertion. Fibre-optic examination revealed a massive bulging of the left arytenoid (Fig. 1A). A prompt MRI demonstrated a lipogenic tumor not only in the arytenoid but also in the false vocal cord. The same left lateral incision, that had been made at the initial surgery, was used again. After the left thyroid ala was removed, the surface of the lipogenic tumor was exposed along the posterior surface of the thyroid cartilage and the encapsulated tumor was carefully separated from the mucosa of the false vocal cord. In order to avoid damaging the mucosa, direct laryngoscopy was carried out to confirm the orientation of the surgery. Finally, the mucosa of the arytenoid was sutured to the surrounding portions of the thyropharyngeal muscle, and both the lower hypopharynx and the false vocal cord were clearly visualized (Fig. 1B). The postoperative course was uneventful, the patient's dyspnea disappeared and the patient has been followed constantly for more than 12 months. Histologically the tumor was a fibrolipoma.

Discussion

Reports of laryngeal fibrolipoma are very rare. Less than 100 cases existing in the laryngeal region have been reported [1–3]. At the time of diagnosis, most patients are 60 years of age or older [2]. The most common sites of the lipogenic tumor of the larynx are the aryepiglottic fold, vestibular fold and epiglottis. As the tumors are generally solitary, the isolated lipogenic tumor in the larynx, without any systemic manifestations, makes clinical diagnosis extremely difficult. Although the lipogenic tumors are histologically benign, they often show clinically malignant aspects. They sometimes cause a fatal obstruction of the airway due to protrusion into the larynx [4,5]. The present case is the first report of a giant lipogenic tumor that almost reached the cardiac antrum but, fortunately, the tumor was pedunculated in the esophagus. Another problem of benign neoplasms is the frequent recurrence over a long time period [5,6].

Small tumors can be removed endoscopically. Large tumors require external approaches. Lipogenic tumors that exist close to the laryngeal ventricle or false vocal cord require a lateral pharyngotomy or laryngofissure. The pedunculated tumor that extended from the hypopharynx to the cardia of the stomach was removed through a lateral pharyngotomy at the initial surgery. This surgical procedure, however, did not remove the intralaryngeal tumor completely and thus resulted in its potential growth, not only into the arytenoid but also into the false cord. Although the recurrent tumors were successfully extracted, a careful follow-up for any other new lesions is required.

References

1. Di Bartolomeo J, Olsen AR. Pedunculated lipoma of the epiglottis. Arch Otolaryngol 1973;98:55–57.
2. Barnes L, Ferlito A. Soft tissue neoplasms. In: Ferlito A (ed) Neoplasms of the Larynx. London: Churchill-Livingstone, 1993;265–304.
3. Wenig BM. Lipomas of the larynx and hypopharynx: a review of the literature with the addition of three new cases. J Laryngol Otol 1995;109:353–357.
4. Jesberg N. Fibrolipoma of the pyriform sinuses: thirty-seven year follow-up. Laryngoscope 1982;92:1157–1159.
5. Allen MD Jr, Talbot WH. Sudden death due to regurgitation of pedunculated esophageal lipoma. J Thorac Cardiovasc Surg 1967;54:756–758.
6. Trizna Z, Forrai G, Toth B, Banhidy FG. Laryngeal lipoma. Ear Nose Throat J 1991;70: 387–388.

©2001 Published by Elsevier Science B.V.
Bronchology and Bronchoesophagology: State of the Art.
H. Yoshimura et al., editors.

A technical revision of transplantation of fascia into the vocal fold

Koichiro Nishiyama[1], Hajime Hirose[2], Jun Yamanaka[1], Takashi Hiroshimaya[1], Manabu Yokobori[1], Masahiko Takeda[1], Masatosi Hirayama[1] and Makito Okamoto[1]

[1]Department of Otorhinolaryngology, Kitasato University School of Medicine; and [2]Department of Rehabilitation, Kitasato University School of Allied Health Sciences, Kanagawa, Japan

Keywords: autotransplantation, recurrent laryngeal nerve palsy, sulcus vocalis.

Introduction

Tsunoda et al. developed a new surgical method for sulcus vocalis and recurrent laryngeal nerve palsy. It involves the autotransplantation of temporal fascia into the vocal fold. This method is superior to the traditional collagen injection, because the graft is not a foreign body but the patient's own tissue. However, this method has some problems, such as the technical difficulty and a considerably long operating time. We believe that there is still a possibility to improve the technique and save on time required for the surgical procedure.

Methods

We attempted some technical modifications for the transplantation of the fascia into the vocal folds. First, we made a roll-shaped fascia graft. Second, we provided a transplantation site in the vocal fold just medially to the vocal ligament, for which we made an incision as laterally as possible. Third, we prepared a pocket within the lamina propria mucosa of a vocal fold using a special elevator in order to prevent the fall-off of the graft. In addition, we developed a new suturing technique to save operating time.

There are some important tips for the suturing technique. Firstly, this method needs an assistant who pulls one end of the suture with considerable tension while watching the video monitor. Secondly, for the first step of the suturing procedure, both edges of the incised vocal fold mucosa must be penetrated at once. To do this, care must be taken to hold the needle at the most appropriate angle with regard to the curvature of the needle. Thirdly, we use a special probe with a U-shaped tip to slide the knot of the suture toward the vocal folds. Lastly, the procedures were performed under magnification of microscope.

Address for correspondence: Koichiro Nishiyama, 2-6-3-1011 Shonandai, Fujisawa-shi, Kanagawa 252-0804, Japan. Tel./Fax: +81-466-44-7036.

Case

A case of a female patient who had sulcus vocalis and a recurrent laryngeal nerve palsy after a thyroid cancer surgery 2 years ago.

Results

The double voice has improved. The maximum voice retention time has also improved from 7 s before the surgery to 15 s afterwards. The new suturing technique contributes to saving time needed for one suture of the vocal mucosa from 30 min to 3 min. The graft has shown no sign of fall-off ever since.

Bronchology and Bronchoesophagology: State of the Art.
H. Yoshimura et al., editors.

Schwannoma of the larynx: a case report

Y. Noguchi, S. Endo, Y. Abiko, K. Hiroshige, S. Yamaguchi, H. Sekine, K. Ootsuka and A. Kida

Department of Otorhinolaryngology, Head and Neck Surgery, Nihon University School of Medicine, Tokyo, Japan

Abstract. *Introduction.* The head and neck region is frequently involved with Schwannoma, but a Schwannoma of the larynx is rare.

Case report. A 30-year-old female was referred because of a subglottic mass. She had been treated under the diagnosis of bronchial asthma for 6 months. Fiberoptic laryngoscope showed a smooth-surfaced mass just beneath the right vocal cord. Plain CT scan revealed a homogeneous mass in the subglottis. The patient was admitted on the day of first visit and sent to the operating theater on the next day. After establishing the airway through cricothyrotomy, direct laryngoscopic examination and biopsy were carried out. Pathological diagnosis was neurogenic tumor. Two weeks later, the tumor was totally removed through laryngofissure. The postoperative course was uneventful except for persistent cough. On histological examination, the tumor consisted of round or spindle cells. Immunohistochemical staining for S-100 and vimentin was positive in all spindle cells. The diagnosis of Schwannoma with epithelioid pattern was made.

Discussion. Schwannoma of the larynx is a rare tumor and the diagnosis is difficult. Airway management is critical in treating this disease. The most common sites of involvement are aryepiglottic and ventricular folds. Subglottic Schwannoma is extremely rare. Total removal is the treatment of choice.

Keywords: airway stenosis, cough, laryngeal neoplasm.

Introduction

Schwannoma is a benign tumor developing from Schwann cells. The occurrence of Schwannoma is not rare in the head and neck regions, but rare in the larynx. We present a case of this disease that we encountered recently.

Case presentation

A 30-year-old woman was referred to our hospital with a chief complaint of wheezing and dyspnea. Ten months prior to admission, she noticed wheezing and dyspnea on exercise. Three months later, she was seen by a medical doctor at a local hospital, and was diagnosed as having asthma and treated. However, the symptoms were gradually aggravated, such that wheezing and dyspnea occurred even at rest. On the day of admission, plain roentgenogram of the larynx was taken at that hospital, which revealed a mass in the larynx. For fear of

Address for correspondence: Yugo Noguchi MD, Department of ORL-HNS, Nihon University School of Medicine, 30-1 Oyaguchi-kamicho, Itabashi-ku, Tokyo 173-8610, Japan. Fax: +81-3-3972-1321.

airway obstruction, she was immediately referred. With laryngofibroscopy, a reddish-white smooth-surfaced mass was found just below the right vocal cord. On plain CT scan, the well-defined broad-based homogeneous mass was found to have developed from the right side of the subglottis, threatening the airway. The patient was admitted to our hospital on the day of the first visit. On the following day, an operation was performed to secure the airway. After the failure of securing the airway by transoral intubation, emergency cricothyrotomy was performed. Subsequently, the tumor was visualized through rigid laryngoscopy under general anesthesia. An incisional biopsy of the tumor and reduction of the mass by laser vaporization was performed. The pathological diagnosis was benign neurogenic tumor. On the 21st hospital day, total removal of the tumor through laryngofissure was performed. During the operation, the tumor was observed from the lower edge of the right vocal cord down to the level of cricothyroid membrane. Cartilage destruction was not observed. On histopathological examination, proliferation of spindle cells was observed and also partial nuclear palisading, but not typical, was seen. Cellular atypia was lacking. By immunohistochemical staining, vimentin and S-100 protein were positive in tumor cells. Final pathological diagnosis of Antoni type A Schwannoma was made. Postoperative course was uneventful except for an intractable cough, which developed after the initiation of oral intake. No recurrent laryngeal nerve paralysis was observed. The cough was reduced with superior laryngeal nerve block. The cough gradually subsided and disappeared. At 7 months postoperatively, she is free of disease.

Discussion

Schwannoma is a benign tumor developing from Schwann cells. This tumor can occur wherever peripheral nerves are present, but Schwannoma of the larynx is rare [1]. It mostly affects terminal ramifications of the medial branch of the superior laryngeal nerve [2], explaining the supraglottic preferential site of these lesions. Occurrence in the subglottic area as in this case is extremely rare. Regarding the symptoms, no symptoms are observed at the beginning in many cases. This disease can occasionally be found incidentally during health examination. Foreign body sensation in the throat, dysphagia, hoarseness, dyspnea, etc. develop with increasing tumor size. In some case, including our patient, emergency intubation or tracheostomy was performed. In the present case and in some other reports, the cause of dyspnea was mistakenly thought to be asthma. Differential diagnoses are chondroma, lipoma, adenoma, cyst, mucocele, lymphangioma, hemangioma, fibroma, neurofibroma, etc. Each of these tumors is frequently seen as a smooth-surfaced submucosal tumor using a fiberscope. Diagnosis is difficult without excision of the tumor. However, considering the difficulty of biopsy because of location or possible hemorrhage from the tumor, preoperative diagnosis is actually difficult in many cases. Total excision is the choice of treatment. If the size is appropriate, transoral extraction can be performed. If impossible, the external approach should be taken. In the present case, the trans-oral approach was impossible, and laryngofissure was eventually chosen as a curative therapy. Tumor vaporization by YAG laser for the treatment of tracheal Schwannoma was reported. However, application of this method appears to be limited to sufficiently small tumors. The prognosis of this illness is good, and when complete excision is performed, recurrence or malignant change barely occurs. As already mentioned, laryngeal Schwannoma is known to develop from the superior laryngeal nerve in many cases. The superior laryngeal nerve governs the sensation of the larynx. In the present case, intractable cough developed after curative operation. This may be due to irritation of the stump of the superior laryngeal nerve during respiration, after near-total resection of the right medial mucosa of the larynx was performed. The cough gradually ceased, supposedly due to re-epithelization of the laryngeal interior.

Conclusions

A case of laryngeal Schwannoma is presented. Accurate diagnosis and airway management is critical to treat this disease.

References

1. Cummings C et al. Neurogenic tumors of the larynx. Annal Otol Rhinol Laryngol 1969;78: 76–95.
2. Plantet M et al. Laryngeal schwannomas. Euro J Radiol 1995;21:61–66.

Bronchology and Bronchoesophagology: State of the Art.
H. Yoshimura et al., editors.

Laser arytenoidectomy for bilateral median vocal fold fixation

Kiminori Sato, Hirohito Umeno and Tadashi Nakashima
Department of Otolaryngology, Head and Neck Surgery, Kurume University, School of Medicine, Kurume, Japan

Abstract. Submucous CO_2 laser arytenoidectomy was performed in nine cases of bilateral median vocal fold fixation due to bilateral vocal fold paralysis and one case of cricoarytenoid joint ankylosis. All the patients had their airways successfully restored and only minimal voice disturbance associated with this operation.

The surgical procedure used in this study was a modification of Ossoff endoscopic laser arytenoidectomy and consisted of the following four steps for best results: 1) submucous laser arytenoidectomy; 2) widening of the lateral portion of the posterior glottis; 3) membranous portion of the vocal folds left intact; and 4) wound covered with preserved mucosa using fibrin glue.

The advantages associated with submucous CO_2 laser arytenoidectomy using fibrin glue include: 1) restoration of adequate airway with minimal disturbance of voice quality, without aspiration, 2) prevention of granulation or scar tissue formation after surgery which would compromise the airway, and 3) rapid wound healing.

Keywords: airway stenosis, bilateral vocal fold paralysis, cricoarytenoid joint ankylosis, laser surgery.

Background

Many surgical procedures have been established for bilateral vocal fold paralysis to improve airway insufficiency [1–5]. The purpose of these surgical treatments is to restore an adequate airway without disturbing voice quality and swallowing.

Laser arytenoidectomy can be performed via an intralaryngeal approach, which preserves the airway and voice quality without aspiration [2–5]. This method is only slightly invasive and useful for bilateral median vocal fold fixation in bilateral vocal fold paralysis [2–5] and also for bilateral cricoarytenoid joint ankylosis [4,6].

Thornell [1] was the first to conduct arytenoidectomy using an intralaryngeal approach. Ossoff et al. [2] introduced the CO_2 laser for endoscopic arytenoidectomy. At our department, Dr Hirano pioneered endoscopic CO_2 laser arytenoidectomy in 1984. The results of retrospective analysis of our experience [5] indicated some improvements in operative procedures.

Address for correspondence: Kiminori Sato MD, PhD, Department of Otolaryngology – Head and Neck Surgery, Kurume University School of Medicine, 67 Asahi-machi, Kurume 830-0011, Japan. Tel.: +81-942-31-7575. Fax: +81-942-37-1200.

Methods

Submucous CO_2 laser arytenoidectomy was performed in nine cases of bilateral median vocal fold fixation due to bilateral vocal fold paralysis and one case of cricoarytenoid joint ankylosis.

The surgical procedure used in this study was a modification of Ossoff endoscopic laser arytenoidectomy [2] and consisted of the following four steps for best results.

Step 1: submucous laser arytenoidectomy

After exposing the posterior glottis under the microscope, an incision was made along the superior portion of the unilateral arytenoid cartilage from the tip of the vocal process to apex, using a CO_2 laser. Submucous laser arytenoidectomy prevented granulation or scar tissue formation which would narrow the glottis after surgery, thereby accelerating the healing process.

Step 2: widening of lateral portion of the posterior glottis

Following its exposure, the arytenoid cartilage body was vaporized and removed by the laser. Anteriorly, the vocal process of the arytenoid cartilage was vaporized to the posterior macula flava of the vocal fold. Laterally, arytenoid cartilage was vaporized near the muscular process. The body and vocal process of arytenoid cartilage were ablated, exposing the posterior part of the thyroarytenoid muscle. The posterior portion of the thyroarytenoid muscle was then vaporized.

Step 3: membranous portion of the vocal folds left intact

Ideally the membranous portion of the vocal fold should not be vaporized. Only when submucous arytenoidectomy is unsuccessful should the posterior part of the thyroarytenoid muscle beneath the membranous vocal fold be vaporized without removing the vocal fold mucosa.

Step 4: wound covered with preserved mucosa using fibrin glue

The wound was covered with preserved mucosa of the posterior glottis, using fibrin glue. Conserved mucosa must be made as thin as possible by laser vaporization. Pliable thin mucosa covered the wound tightly without any dead spaces. Diffuse postoperative bleeding, as well as crust formation were prevented and there was no granulation or scar tissue formation that would narrow the glottis after surgery, thus promoting wound healing.

Results

All the patients had their airways successfully restored. Eight patients were decanulated. For two patients, there was no closure of the tracheostoma, owing to recurrent thyroid cancer and brain infarction. All the patients could eat normally without aspiration after surgery.

In eight cases, airway resistance was assessed. Seven cases improved and one case showed no change. In five cases, vocal functions were examined. In most of the patients, maximum phonation time, mean airflow rate, fundamental frequency range and sound pressure level range of phonation, pitch perturbation quotient, amplitude perturbation quotient and normalized noise energy showed no significant change postoperatively. These vocal functions indicated that only minimal voice disturbance was associated with this operation.

Conclusion

The advantages associated with submucous CO_2 laser arytenoidectomy using fibrin glue include: 1) restoration of adequate airway with minimal disturbance of voice quality, without aspiration, 2) prevention of granulation or scar tissue formation after surgery which would compromise the airway, and 3) rapid wound healing.

References

1. Thornell WC. Intralaryngeal approach for arytenoidectomy in bilateral abductor paralysis of the vocal cords. Arch Otolaryngol 1948;47:505–508.
2. Ossoff RH, Sisson GA, Duncavage JA, Muselle HI, Andrews PE, McMillan WG. Endoscopic laser arytenoidectomy for the treatment of bilateral vocal cord paralysis. Laryngoscope 1984; 94:1293–1297.
3. Crumley RL. Endoscopic laser medial arytenoidectomy for airway management in bilateral laryngeal paralysis. Ann Otol Rhinol Laryngol 1993;102:81–84.
4. Remacle M, Lawson G, Mayne A, Jamart J. Subtotal carbon dioxide laser arytenoidectomy by endoscopic approach for treatment of bilateral cord immobility in adduction. Ann Otol Rhinol Laryngol 1996;105:438–445.
5. Sato K, Yoshida T, Umeno H, Nakashima T. Laser arytenoidectomy for bilateral vocal fold paralysis. J Otolaryngol Jpn 2000;103:147–153.
6. Sato K, Nakashima T. Laser arytenoidectomy for bilateral cricoarytenoid joint ankylosis. J Jpn Bronchoesophagol Soc 2000;51:40–44.

Bronchology and Bronchoesophagology: State of the Art.
H. Yoshimura et al., editors.

Seven cases of laryngeal tuberculosis and its recent trend in Japan

Hideo Takagi, Satoshi Horiguchi, Takahisa Ami and Mamoru Suzuki
Department of Otolaryngology, Tokyo Medical University Hospital, Tokyo, Japan

Abstract. The incidence of tuberculosis has markedly decreased since the introduction of effective chemotherapy. However, laryngeal tuberculosis has been on the increase in recent years.

Seven cases of laryngeal tuberculosis, treated in our department between 1992 and 1999, are presented in this paper. The tuberculosis involved the vocal cords in four and the epiglottis in three patients. Out of seven patients, six complained of hoarseness, and three complained of pharyngalgia. The chest radiography, sputum test, and purified protein derivative (PPD) were supplemental tools for diagnosis. Chest radiography showed advanced pulmonary disease in six patients. In sputum cytology, four patients were positive for acid-fast bacilli, and three were negative.

Pathological examination is mandatory in order to make a final diagnosis and to rule out malignancies.

Keywords: larynx, pathological examination, PPD, tuberculosis.

Introduction

The incidence of tuberculosis in Japan has decreased owing to the improved living standards, promoted health screening and combined chemotherapy. In recent years, however, tuberculosis has been attracting global attention as a re-emerging infectious disease [1]. In 1997, the number of newly registered patients in Japan increased for the first time in 88 years. Laryngeal tuberculosis is secondary to lung tuberculosis in most cases. The incidence of laryngeal tuberculosis is also anticipated to increase. The purpose of this paper is to call attention of laryngologists to this rare but existing disease.

Methods

Seven patients were diagnosed as having laryngeal tuberculosis at the Department of Otorhinolaryngology, Tokyo Medical University Hospital from 1990 to 1999. The diagnostic criteria include histopathologic changes of caseating granulomas and/or presence of acid-fast bacilli in biopsy specimens. The following were reviewed: 1) age and sex, 2) symptoms, 3) laryngoscopic findings, 4) spu-

Address for correspondence: Hideo Takagi, Department of Otolaryngology, Tokyo Medical University Hospital, 6-7-1 Nishishinjyuku, Shinjyuku-ku, Tokyo, Japan. Tel.: +81-3-3342-6111. Fax: +81-3-3346-9275. E-mail: hideo32@tokyo-med.ac.jp tum analysis for detection of acid-fast bacilli, 5) chest X-ray findings, and 6) histopathologic examinations.

Results (Table 1)

We treated two patients with chemotherapy, and the remaining five patients were referred to the Tuberculosis Center. One patient (case 6) had granulomatous lesions on the epiglottis. Another (case 2) had lesions localized within the left vocal cord. Both received a three-drug combination regimen consisting of INH and REP with EB or SM for 1 year. The granulomatous lesions disappeared following chemotherapy in both patients. However, hoarseness persisted in the patients with vocal cord lesion after treatment.

Discussion

In Japan, the incidence of lung tuberculosis has recently increased. From this fact, the increase of laryngeal tuberculosis is anticipated.

According to recent reports, granulomatous lesions confined to the vocal cords are predominant, with the chief complaint being hoarseness. Six out of seven patients complained mainly of hoarseness, and three complained of pharyngalgia. Consistently with other reports, all patients showed granulomatous lesions. The epiglottis was involved in three of the seven patients. Granulomatous lesions arouse special attention for differential diagnosis from laryngeal cancer. Pharyngalgia and deglutition pain are rare symptoms in laryngeal cancer, while they are frequent in tuberculosis.

The diagnosis of laryngeal tuberculosis is established when a biopsy specimen exhibits caseous necrosis, Langhans' giant cells, and epithelioid cells, and/or tubercle bacilli are detected by acid-fast staining such as Ziel-Neelsenn staining. However, detection of the bacteria sometimes fails, and hence, the purified pro-

Table 1.

Case	Age (years)	Sex	Chief complaint	Site of lesion	Examination of sputum	Chest X-ray
1	24	F	Hoarseness	Unilateral vocal cord	(–)	Infiltration
2	48	M	Lump in throat	Epiglottis-interarytenoid area	(–)	Calcification
3	26	F	Hoarseness, pharyngalgia	Epiglottis	(+)	Infiltration
4	53	F	Hoarseness, pharyngalgia	Bilateral vocal cords	(+)	Infiltration
5	41	M	Hoarseness	Bilateral vocal cords	(+)	Cavitation
6	67	F	Hoarseness	Unilateral vocal cord	(–)	Atelectasis
7	21	F	Hoarseness, pharyngalgia	Epiglottis	(+)	Cavitation

tein derivative (PPD) test, chest X-ray, and sputum smear and culture examinations are necessary. The PPD test is a simple immunological test with a high positivity rate. All of our seven patients were positive for PPD. However, since BCG vaccination has become common in Japan, positive PPD does not necessarily indicate an active tuberculous disease. Laryngeal tuberculosis is usually associated with lung tuberculosis [2]. To diagnose lung tuberculosis, chest X-ray is a simple, but useful tool. In our series, advanced pulmonary disease was diagnosed in six patients using simple chest X-ray.

Although the diagnosis of tuberculosis requires the detection of tubercle bacilli from bacteriological sputum test, culture from the sputum usually takes 4–8 weeks and detectability is said to be 80% at maximum. Even in patients with an abnormal chest X-ray which was highly suspicious of active lung tuberculosis, no tuberculosis bacillus was detected from the sputum smear and culture. Taking this into consideration, we believe that whenever laryngeal tuberculosis is suspected, pathological examination of biopsy specimens is essential in addition to a bacteriological test.

Recently, the polymerase chain reaction (PCR) technique has enabled detection of tubercle bacilli in specimens within 1–2 days without culturing bacteria. This method speeds up the process of making a diagnosis. However, PCR is often negative even when tubercle bacilli are detected in biopsy specimens. The PCR method reportedly has a high sensitivity and specificity of at least 95% in smear-positive specimens. In contrast, in smear-negative cases the sensitivity decreases to 45–75%, while the specificity remains 95% or more. Furthermore, PCR often shows a false positive. Considering this, final diagnosis should be made using a combination of biopsy, PCR method, and conventional bacteriological examination, in addition to the clinical course and findings.

Conclusion

1. Although laryngeal tuberculosis is rare, the incidence is now anticipated to increase.
2. The PPD test, chest X-ray, and examinations of sputum should be performed on all patients when laryngeal tuberculosis is suspected.
3. Pathological examination is mandatory to make a final diagnosis and to rule out malignancies.

References

1. World Health Organization. Global Tuberculosis Control: WHO Report, 1999. Geneva, Switzerland: World Health Organization; 1999.
2. Auerbach O. Laryngeal tuberculosis. Arch Otolaryngol 1946;44:191–201.

Bronchology and Bronchoesophagology: State of the Art.
H. Yoshimura et al., editors.

An excessive atelocollagen injection into unilateral paralysed vocal fold

Satoru Takenouchi[1], Tsuyoshi Takenouchi[2] and Reiko Takenouchi[3]
[1]*Takenouchi ENT Clinic, Kyoto:* [2]*Department of Otolaryngologoy, Tokyo Medical University: and* [3]*Department of Otolaryngologoy, School of Medicine, Nihon University, Tokyo, Japan*

Abstract. *Background.* To counteract hoarseness and dysphagea caused by aspiration due to unilateral vocal fold paralysis, an intrafold injection of atelocollagen was performed on eight patients during the past 9 years. Three cases had aspiration pneumonia preoperatively. As atelocollagen is readily absorbable, 3% density and excessive amounts (2 to 3 ml) were used.

Methods. The intrafold injection of atelocollagen was performed percutaneously through the cricothyroid membrane at the anterior section of the neck after a 1% xylocaine local anesthesia injection was first carried out. Under the video-endoscopic monitor of the larynx, a 1-ml injection of the 3% atelocollagen was started at the lateral part of the vocal process of the arytenoid cartilage to adduct the paralysed vocal fold to the median position, and an additional 1 ml was injected into the median and anterior parts of the paralysed vocal fold. A further 0.5 to 1 ml, in excess, was injected until the entire rand of the affected vocal fold returned to the median position.

Results. After the injection, the patients displayed good airways, were competent at swallowing without aspiration and were able to maintain a better quality of voice for a longer duration.

Conclusion. Atelocollagen is said to be easily absorbable, but the use of it in excessive amounts, at 3% density solution, showed it to be capable of maintaining vocal muscle volume for a longer duration.

Keywords: aspiration, hoarseness, percutaneous injection, video-endoscopic monitoring.

Introduction

To counteract hoarseness and dysphagea caused by aspiration due to unilateral vocal fold paralysis, a percutaneous intrafold injection [1] of atelocollagen [2], under a video-endoscopic monitor, was performed on eight patients (four males and four females, ranging in age from 60 to 75 years) during the past 9 years.

Patients

All cases showed breathy hoarseness, and three cases complained of dysphagea due to aspiration, which developed into aspiration pneumonia. The causes of unilateral vocal fold paralysis were multiple brain infarction (one case), long-term intubation due to an unconscious state caused by a heart attack (one case), left-associated laryngeal paralysis involving the 9th, 10th and 11th cranial nerves (1 case), post a left thyroidectomy (one case), post a total left lung lobectomy

Address for correspondence: Dr S. Takenouchi MD, Takenouchi ENT clinic, 1-1 Higashino-cho, Murasakino, Kita-ku, Kyoto 603-8232, Japan. Tel.: +81-75-431-8476. Fax: +81-75-431-8474.

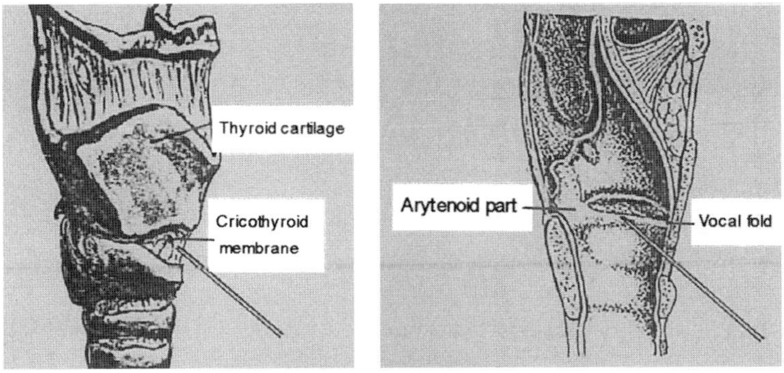

Fig. 1. A percutaneous intrafold injection of atelocollagen through the cricothyroid membrane at the anterior section of the neck under a video-endoscopic monitor of the larynx.

(one case) and idiopathy (three cases). In all cases, the left vocal folds were atrophic and stayed in the intermediate position, and it remained a glottal crevice in spite of the over-adduction of the normal side at a time of phonation. Three dysphagea cases showed phlegm or mucopurulent sputum inflow into the glottice and trachea. The mean maximum phonation time was only 4.2 s (2.5 to 6.8 s) and the mean phonatory airflow rate was 624 ml/s (280 to 950 ml/s).

Methods

A density of 3% and excessive amounts (2 to 3 ml) of atelocollagen were used (Figs. 1 and 2). The intrafold injection was carried out percutaneously through

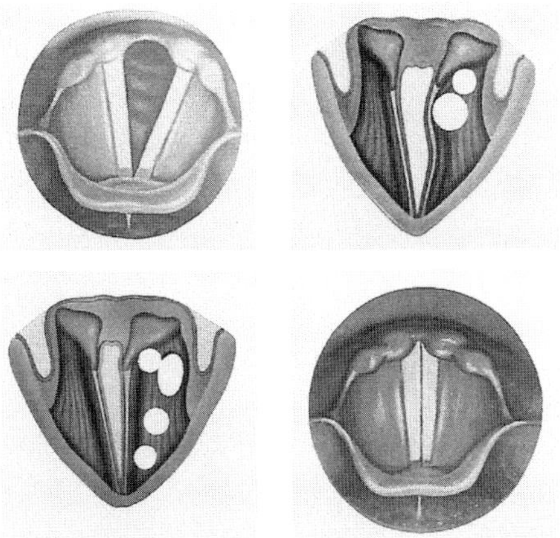

Fig. 2. The needle tip is inserted at the lateral part of the vocal process of arytenoid cartilage, and 1 ml of atelocollagen is injected to adduct its vocal process. Another 1 ml is injected into the middle and anterior parts of the affected vocal fold to bring it to the median position.

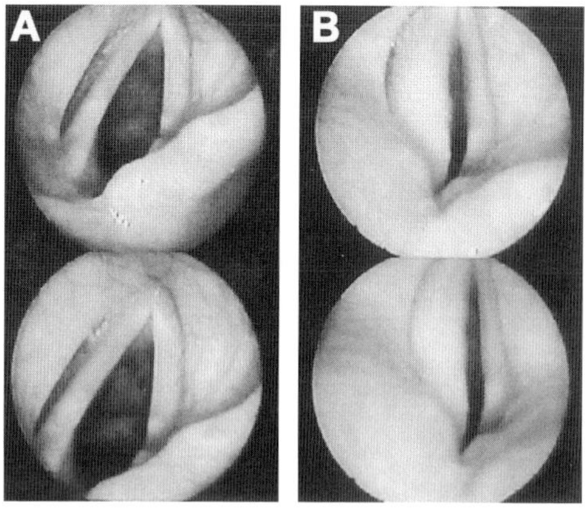

Fig. 3. Preinjection. The left vocal fold was atrophic and stayed in the intermediate position remaining a glottal crevice, in spite of the over-adduction of the other vocal fold at the time of phonation, and showing breathy hoarseness and phlegm inflow into the trachea during inspiration. **A:** Inspiration. **B:** Phonation.

the cricothyroid membrane at the anterior section of the neck. Under a video-endoscopic monitor of the larynx, a 1-ml injection of the 3% atelocollagen was started at the lateral part of the vocal process of the arytenoid cartilage to adduct the paralysed vocal fold to the median position, and an additional 1 ml was injected to the median and anterior parts of paralysed vocal fold. A further 0.5 to 1 ml, in excess, of atelocollagen was injected when the entire rand of the vocal fold returned to the median position.

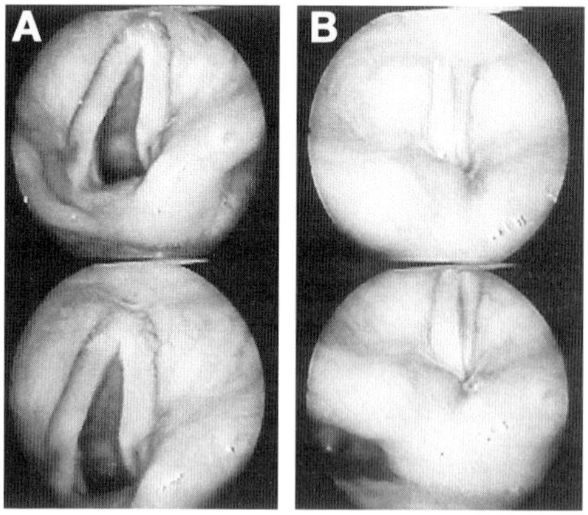

Fig. 4. Postinjection. After the injection, the glottice was completely closed during phonation and produced a good quality of voice, and prevented aspiration at the time of swallowing. **A:** Inspiration. **B:** Phonation.

Results

After the injection (Figs. 3 and 4), the patients displayed good airways, were competent at swallowing without aspiration and were able to maintain a better quality of voice for a longer duration. The mean maximum phonation time was 20 s (12 to 40 s) and the mean phonatory airflow rate recovered to 160 ml/s (80 to 200 ml/s) postoperatively.

Conclusion

Atelocollagen is said to be easily absorbable [3], but the use of it in excessive amounts (2 to 3 ml), at a 3% density solution, showed it to be capable of enabling patients to maintain both their competence in swallowing and a better quality of voice for 3 to 8 years.

References

1. Hiratio M et al. Transcutaneous intrafold injection for unilateral vocal fold paralysis, functional results. Ann Rhinol Laryngol 1990;99:598–604.
2. Tamura E. Basic study of implants for vocal fold augmentation. Larynx Jpn 1994;6:122–129.
3. Yumoto E et al. Long-term results of intracordal collagen injection. Larynx Jpn 1995;7: 111–116.

Bronchology and Bronchoesophagology: State of the Art.
H. Yoshimura et al., editors.

Laser surgery for early glottic carcinoma

Tetsuya Tanabe, Manabu Nakanoboh, Masami Ogura, Taichi Hurukawa, Yuko Matsumura, Etsuyo Tamura, Naoyuki Kohno and Satoshi Kitahara
Department of Otolaryngology, National Defense Medical College, Saitama, Japan

Abstract. Ninety-four cases of early glottic carcinoma (45 cases of T1a, 26 cases of T1b, and 23 T2 cases, with N0 M0 in all cases) that had been treated with CO_2 or KTP laser between April 1982 and December 1998 were reviewed. The histologic diagnosis was squamous cell carcinoma in all cases. The laser excision or ablation of the tumor was carried out by microsurgical technique under general anesthesia. After laser surgery, biopsy specimens were obtained from several sites of the resected area. When residual tumor was suspected, laser surgery was repeated or radiotherapy was performed. The survival rate was 100% for T1 cases and 96% for T2 cases. The voice preservation rate was 98% for T1a, 85% for T1b, and 74% for T2 cases, and vocal function was satisfactorily preserved for daily life. The results led to the following conclusions: 1) about 90% of patients with glottic T1 carcinoma were cured by laser surgery alone; 2) lesions involving the anterior commissure can be treated with laser surgery, and 3) combination therapy of laser surgery and radiation for glottic T2 carcinoma improves the voice preservation rate.

Keywords: laryngeal cancer, laser.

Introduction

The CO_2 and KTP lasers have been widely used as an adjunctive tool in the treatment of benign and malignant tumors in the head and neck area. This paper presents our experience with 94 patients on whom laser was used via laryngomicrosurgery for excision or vaporization or both of early glottic carcinoma.

Subjects and Methods

The subjects consisted of 94 previously untreated patients who had early glottic laryngeal cancer (88 men and six women) and underwent laser surgery between April 1982 and December 1998. The TNM classification was 45 cases of T1a, 26 of T1b, 23 of T2, and N0 M0 in all cases.

Under general anesthesia the lesions were treated with a laser to resect or vaporize the tumor. Noncontact irradiation with a micromanipulator was most commonly performed, but with a KTP laser, contact irradiation with a handpiece was concomitantly carried out. A continuous wave with a focused beam with a power of 10–15 Watts was mostly employed to excise the lesion in the

---

Address for correspondence: Tetsuya Tanabe, Department of Otolaryngology, National Defense Medical College, 3-2 Namiki, Tokorozawa, Saitama 359-8513, Japan. Tel.: +81-42-995-1686. Fax: +81-42-996-5212.

shortest time possible. Vaporization of the remaining tissue was also conducted as required. Laser excision or vaporization was carried out by conventional microsurgical technique when the tumor was in the membranous part of the vocal cord. For posterior lesions, the ventilation tube was pressed forward with the tip of the scope to obtain visualization of a wider surgical field. When sufficient excision in the direction of the laryngeal ventricle was required, the false cord was first excised and then the tumor was excised. Resection or vaporization was performed as far as the thyroid cartilage in cases of tumors in the anterior commissure. After laser surgery, biopsy specimens were obtained from several sites of the resected area for histopathologic examination. When residual tumor was suspected, laser surgery was repeated or radiotherapy was performed.

Results

In the initial treatment, the larynx was preserved in 45 (100%) of the 45 patients with T1a, 24 (92%) of the 26 T1b patients, and 20 (87%) of the 23 T2 patients. Recurrence was observed in one T1a, two T1b, and three T2 patients and they underwent subsequent laryngectomy. The voice preservation rate was 98% for T1a, 85% for T1b, and 74% for T2 cases, and vocal function was satisfactorily preserved for daily life.

The observation period varied from 2 to 18 years. Only one patient, who had a T2 tumor, died as a result of the tumor. The 5-year disease-specific survival rate was 100% for T1 cases and 96% for T2 cases.

Discussion

It has been almost 30 years since the CO_2 laser was first used in the treatment of laryngeal tumors [1]. Many studies have recently reported that laser treatment is indicated only for tumors localized in the membranous portion of the vocal cord.

In our department, laser surgery is employed as a rule for T1 glottic tumors as the first treatment of choice [2]. Some patients received prophylactic combined postoperative radiotherapy between 1982 and 1996. For the period 1987 to 1998, 89% of the patients with T1 tumors were cured by laser surgery alone. Including the four patients who underwent combined radiotherapy, 98% were cured, and their larynges were preserved, indicating an excellent result.

The advantages of laser surgery include a shorter treatment period without the complications of laryngopharyngitis or irradiation-induced cancer, and reduced cost. Vocal function is a minor problem after treatment. Reports that compare the voice of T1 patients who had radiotherapy and that of those who had laser treatment indicate more favorable results for the former [3]. However, long-term observation confirms that satisfactory vocal improvement may be obtained even in highly advanced vocal disorder cases. Nevertheless, vocal function is satisfactory in patients who have undergone laser surgery, and they experience little trouble in everyday life.

Laser surgery alone may not be indicated for the treatment of T2 cases. The fact that only four patients were cured by laser surgery alone in the present study suggests that in cases with T2 glottic laryngeal cancer, more than laser surgery is required to attain cure. In T2 cases, laser surgery can be performed to debulk the tumor before radiotherapy or in those cases in which the tumor is still present after radiotherapy. The cure rate of the T2 cases with laryngeal preservation was 74%. Compared with the cure rate of the T2 cases treated by radiotherapy alone, the result was equivalent or better. Laser therapy is assumed to have achieved a satisfactory result.

Conclusion

About 90% of patients who had glottic laryngeal cancer classified as T1 were cured by laser surgery alone. Even when the tumor could not be completely eliminated, it was possible to cure the patients by combined radiotherapy and preserve the larynx.

With laser surgery alone, it is difficult to cure patients with T2 glottic laryngeal tumors. However, if radiotherapy is performed after reducing the tumor by laser surgery, even patients for whom irradiation was not originally indicated may be cured. Laser surgery may also contribute to the cure of radiation-resistant tumors when the residual tumor has been reduced to the T1 stage.

References

1. Strong MS et al. Laser surgery in the larynx: early clinical experience with CO_2 laser. Ann Otol Rhinol Laryngol 1972;81:791–798.
2. Inouya T et al. Carcinoma of the larynx: role of laser surgery. Trans Am Broncho-Esophagol 1995;75:209–215.
3. Hirano M et al. Vocal function following carbon dioxide laser surgery for glottic carcinoma. Ann Otol Rhinol Laryngol 1985;94:232–235.

Bronchology and Bronchoesophagology: State of the Art.
H. Yoshimura et al., editors.

Hyperfractionated radiotherapy of T2 glottic carcinoma for the preservation of the larynx

Ichiro Tateya[1], Hisayoshi Kojima[1], Shigeru Hirano[1], Ken-ichi Kaneko[1] and Kazuhiko Shoji[2]
[1]*Department of Otolaryngology, Kyoto University Hospital, Sakyo-ku, Kyoto; and* [2]*Department of Otolaryngology, Shimane Prefectural Central Hospital, Izumo, Shimane, Japan*

Abstract. To preserve the laryngeal function in cases of T2 glottic carcinoma, we performed hyperfractionated radiotherapy on 21 cases with T2 glottic carcinoma from 1992 to 1999. The total dose administered ranged from 72 to 74.4 Gy. After radiation, two cases had neck lymph nodal recurrences, but both were salvaged by radical neck dissection. Only one case had local recurrence. She died of lung metastasis. No major complications, such as laryngeal necrosis, were seen in any of the cases. Statistical processing was performed, based on the Kaplan-Meyer method, with the results being that the 5-year-survival rate was 95.2% and the 5-year-laryngeal preservation rate was 95.2%. Hyperfractionated radiotherapy was useful for preserving the larynx in cases of T2 glottic carcinoma.

Keywords: hyperfractionation, laryngeal preservation, T2 glottic cancer.

Introduction

To preserve the larynx, when treating T2 glottic cancer, we have been performing twice-a-day radiation therapy (hyperfractionation) on 21 patients since 1992. In this study, we evaluate the effectiveness of hyperfractionation from the viewpoint of laryngeal preservation.

Materials and Methods

Prior to 1992, our hospital performed once-a-day radiation therapy for the treatment of T2 glottic cancer, with a total dose of 66 Gy. If radiation was ineffective at 40 Gy, surgical treatment was carried out. After 1992, to improve the local control rate, twice-a-day radiation therapy was performed, with two fractions of 1.2 Gy/day up to a total dose of 72 to 74.4 Gy. The duration of treatment was between 40 and 57 days (45.6 days on average). Twenty-one cases of T2 glottic squamous cell carcinoma were treated with hyperfractionation from 1992 to 1998. Kaplan-Meyer estimates were used for the analysis of the survival and laryngeal preservation rates. Follow-up periods lasted for between 1 and 8 years (average: 37 months).

Address for correspondence: Ichiro Tateya, Department of Otolaryngology, Kyoto University Hospital, Sakyo-ku, Kyoto 606-8504, Japan. Tel.: +81-75-751-3346. Fax: +81-75-751-7225.
E-mail: tateya@hs.m.kyoto-u.ac.jp

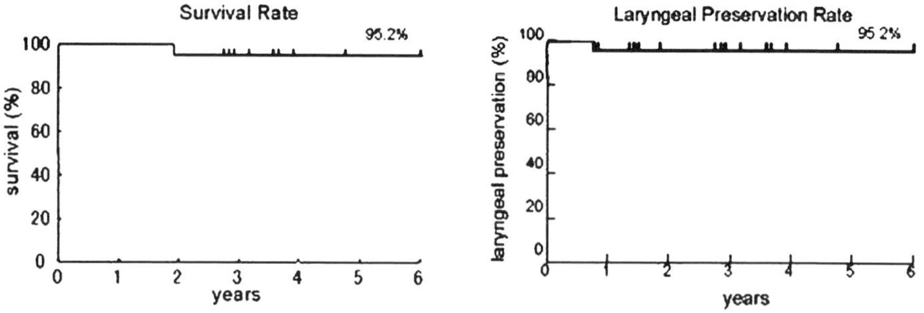

Fig. 1.

Results

The 5-year-survival rate was 95.2% and the 5-year-laryngeal preservation rate was 95.2% (Fig. 1). All cases, except for one, were treated successfully and no local recurrences occurred. One case had severe mucositis and radiation had to be interrupted for 10 days. In this case, local recurrence occurred 6 month after radiation and the patient died of lung metastasis. No major complications, such as laryngeal necrosis, were seen in any of the cases. Two cases had neck lymph nodal recurrences, but both were salvaged by radical neck dissection.

Discussion

Early glottic carcinomas are highly curable using once-a-day radiation therapy with 5-year-survival rates ranging between 80 and 95% for glottic T1 carcinoma, and between 80 and 90% for glottic T2 carcinoma. However, the 5-year-laryngeal preservation rate for T2 glottic cancer is not good enough between 60 and 70% [1,2]. From the end of the 1980s onwards, hyperfractionated radiation therapy was begun as the new standard treatment for cases of head and neck cancer, especially for advanced cases. Concerning early glottic cancer, Burke et al. [3] reported a local control rate of 80% in 10 cases of T2 glottic cancer treated with hyperfractionation in 1990. Fein et al. [4] also reported the effectiveness of hyperfractionation for T2 glottic cancer with a local control rate of 91% in 35 cases. We were also able to achieve a good 5-year-laryngeal preservation rate (95.2%). Thus, hyperfractionation can be considered to be useful for preserving the larynx in the treatment of T2 glottic cancer. In the one case of exception, radiation was interrupted due to severe mucositis and local failure occurred. Nishimura et al. [5] reported the disadvantage of a prolonged radiation period for the survival rate of T1 glottic cancer. This case may suggest that it is important to continue radiation therapy during treatment.

References

1. Harwood AR, Beale FA, Cummings BJ et al. T2 glottic cancer; an analysis of dose-time-volume factors. Int J Radiat Oncol Biol Phys 1981;7:1501–1505.
2. Sakata K, Aoki Y, Karasawa K et al. Radiation therapy in early glottic carcinoma; uni- and multivariate analysis of prognostic factors affecting local control. Int J Radiat Oncol Biol Phys 1994;30:1059–1064.
3. Burke DH, Peters LJ, Goepfert H et al. T2 glottic cancer. Arch Otolaryngol Head Neck Surg 1990;116:830–835.
4. Fein DA, Mendenhall WM, Parsons JT et al. T1-2 squamous cell carcinoma of the glottic larynx treated with radiotherapy: a multivariate analysis of variables potentially influencing local control. Int J Radiat Oncol Biol Phys 1993;25:605–611.
5. Nishimura Y, Nagata Y, Okajima K et al. Radiation therapy for T1,2 glottic carcinoma: impact of overall treatment time on local control. Radiother Oncol 1996;40:225–232.

Bronchology and Bronchoesophagology: State of the Art.
H. Yoshimura et al., editors.

Surgical treatment for severe aspiration with epiglottic closure

Shuji Yokoyama, Makoto Kano, Mutsumi Watanabe, Naofumi Kuwahata and Iwao Ohtani
Department of Otolaryngology, Fukushima Medical University School of Medicine, Fukushima, Japan

Abstract. We performed the present study to determine how diastasis of the epiglottis can be prevented, following epiglottic closure. The form of the epiglottis was classified into two groups for measurement. In both groups, the epiglottis was divided into four equal sections. The amount of tension placed on the thread was measured at three different times: prior to the incision; median incision; and reversed Y incision. In group 1, the tension prior to any incision decreased upon the completion of the median incision. Furthemore, when we compared the decrease in tension from the median incision to the completion of the reversed Y incision, tension decreased at the upper, middle and lower points. In group 2, no significant difference was observed in decreased tension values using a median incision only, nor using the reversed Y incision. We observed an obvious difference during surgery with regard to the relationship between tension and the form of the epiglottis. In the present study, we identified that incision was necessary to prevent diastasis and that only a median incision effectively decreased tension. However, the reversed Y incision was even more effective in decreasing tension at the middle and lower points.

Keywords: diastasis, dysphagia, epiglottic closure, incision.

Background

A variety of surgical procedures can be performed to prevent refractory aspiration pneumonia. One method, first performed by Biller et al., is a procedure that involves suturing the epiglottis into a rolled state to prevent aspiration after total glossectomy [1]. The tip of the epiglottis remains unsutured, leaving a small opening so that phonation is preserved. We performed the epiglottic closure (a modification of Biller et al.'s method) as described in case reports by Tanabe et al., in which dysphagia was associated with cerebrovascular disease, neuromuscular disorders, or was the postoperative condition of cerebral tumor excision [2]. Phonation can be easily achieved using this surgical technique, by closing the tracheal foramen with the finger at the time of expiration, although a permanent tracheal stoma is necessary. Furthermore, this procedure is advantageous because ingestion can be begun without preparatory exercises for deglutition. However, the sewn epiglottis has resulted in postoperative diastasis in some cases, which required repeated surgery. We, therefore, carried out the present study to determine how diastasis of the epiglottis can be prevented, following epiglottic closure.

Address for correspondence: Shuji Yokoyama MD, Department of Otolaryngology, Fukushima Medical University School of Medicine, 1 Hikarigaoka, Fukushima 960-1247, Japan. Tel.: +81-24-548-2111. Fax: +81-24-548-3011. E-mail: shu-zo@fmu.ac.jp

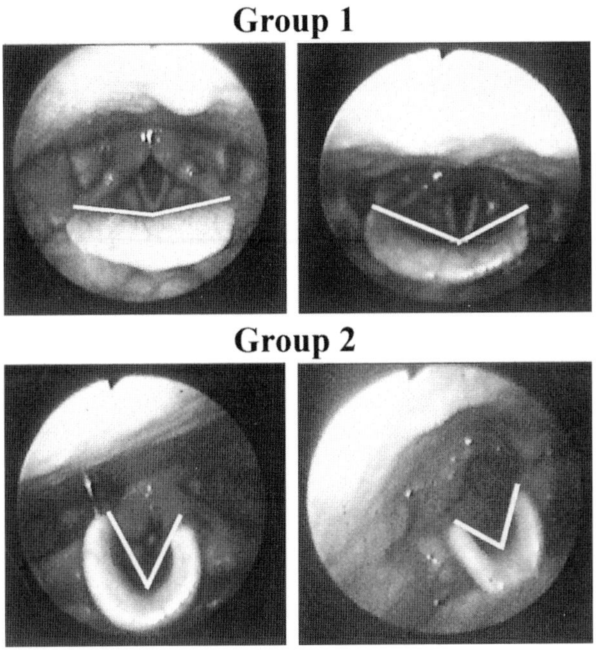

Fig. 1. The classification of the epiglottis.

Materials and Methods

We examined the larynxes of 10 males, ranging in age from 49 to 74 years, who were diagnosed as having carcinoma of the oral, pharyngeal or laryngeal structures. The form of the epiglottis was classified into two types for measurement: group 1 consisted of five patients who had angles of more than 90°, formed by the center of epiglottis and the rise of the left and right aryepiglottic folds; and group 2 consisted of five patients who had this angle at less than 90° (Fig. 1). In both groups, the epiglottis was divided into four equal sections, from the tip to cuneiform tubercle, to establish four measurement points: the upper point, middle point, lower point and cuneiform tubercle (Fig. 2). A silk thread was pulled through the peripheral region of the left and right epiglottic cartilages and tightened so that they came into contact at the median line. The amount of tension placed on the thread was measured at three different times: prior to the incision; after placing a vertical incision along the median line of the epiglottic cartilage (median incision) (Fig. 3); and after transforming the median line into an "upside-down" Y-shaped incision from the bottom of the median incision (reversed Y incision). All measurements were made using a FORCE GAUGE meter (A and D company) and the measured values were shown as absolute values.

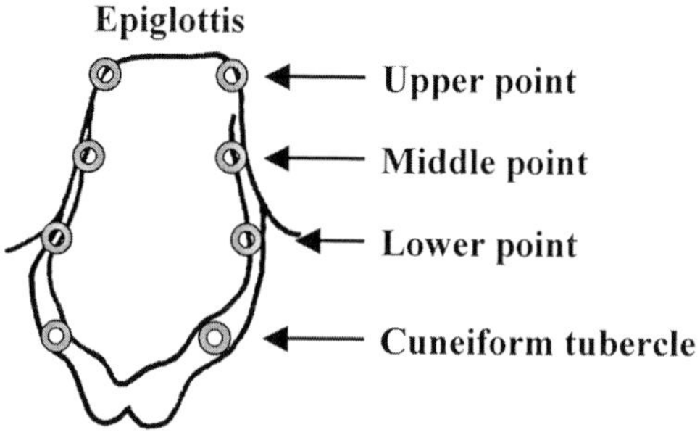

Fig. 2. Measurement points on the epiglottis.

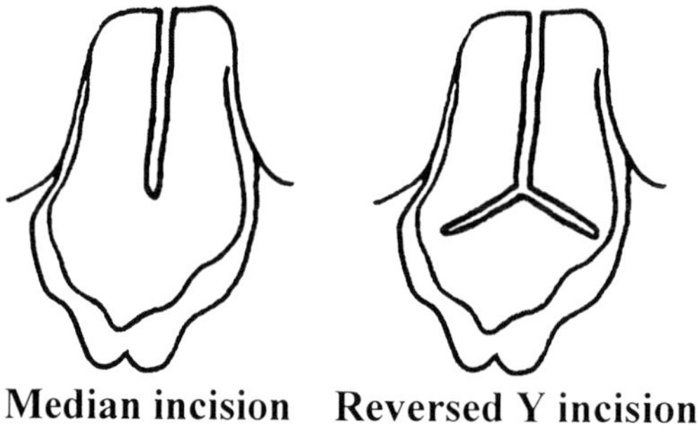

Fig. 3. Epiglottic incision (median and reversed Y incisions).

Results

Comparison between group 1 and group 2 prior to incision

In group 1, the mean tension was 71.8 g at the upper point, 122.2 g at the middle point, 76.2 g at the lower point, and 13 g at the cuneiform tubercle. Similarly, in group 2, the mean tension was 12 g at the upper point, 12.8 g at the middle point, 7.2 g at the lower point, and 6.8 g at the cuneiform tubercle. The tension at the upper, middle and lower points differed significantly between groups 1 and 2, but was not significantly different at the cuneiform tubercle (Fig. 4).

Comparison between the type of incision and the tension produced in group 1

In group 1, the mean tension, prior to incision, decreased upon the completion of the median incision as follows: 71.8 g → 21 g (70.8%) at the upper point; 122.2 g → 36.8 g (69.9%) at the middle point; 76.2 g → 37.2 g (51.2%) at the lower point; and 13 g → 9.7 g (25.3%) at the cuneiform tubercle. The mean tension of the median incision decreased further upon completion of the reversed Y incision: 21 g → 10.8 g (48.5%) at the upper point; 36.8 g → 17.4 g (52.7%) at the middle point; 37.2 g → 19.6 g (47.3%) at the lower point; and 9.7 g → 5.7 g (41.2%) at the cuneiform tubercle (Fig. 5).

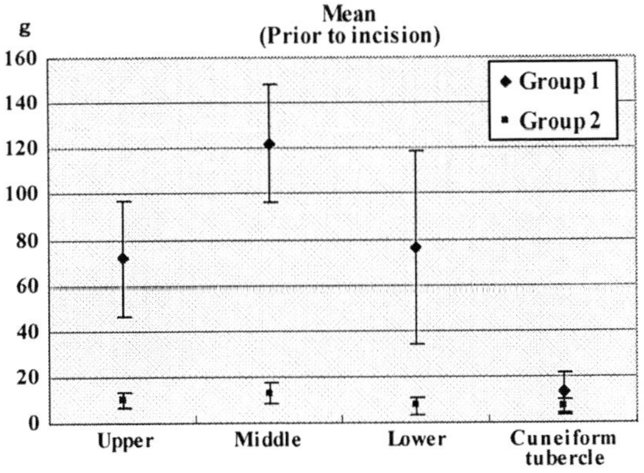

Fig. 4. Comparison between the two groups, prior to incision, at each measurement point.

Comparison of the type of incision and the tension produced in group 2

In group 2, the mean tension, prior to incision, decreased upon the completion of the median incision as follows: 12 g → 6.8 g (43.3%) at the upper point; 12.8 g → 6.8 g (46.9%) at the middle point; 7.2 g → 6 g (16.7%) at the lower point; and 6.8 g → 5 g (26.5%) at the cuneiform tubercle. The mean tension of the median incision decreased further upon completion of the reversed Y incision: 6.8

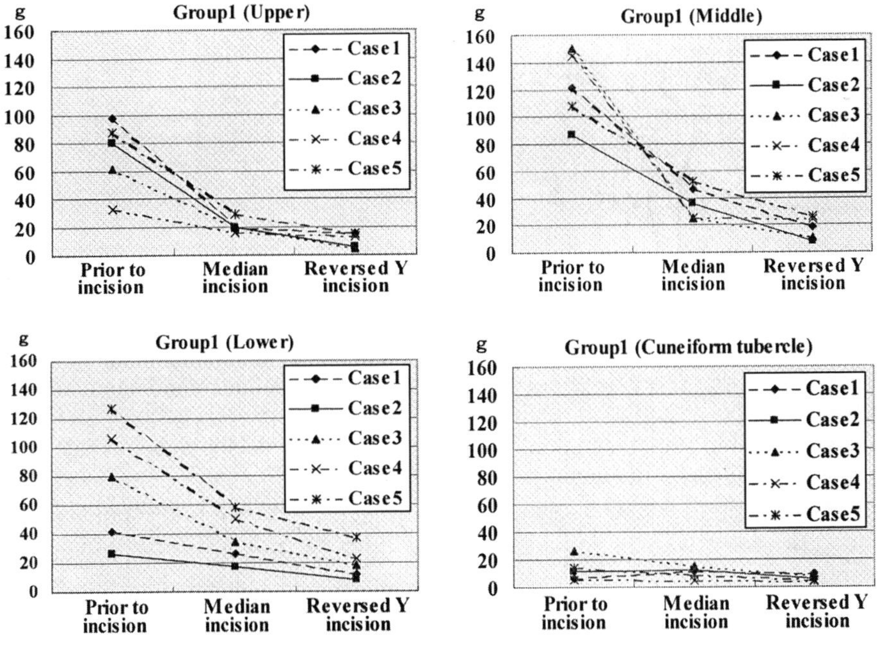

Fig. 5. Comparison of tension, after incision, in Group 1 (upper, middle and lower points, and the cuneiform tubercle).

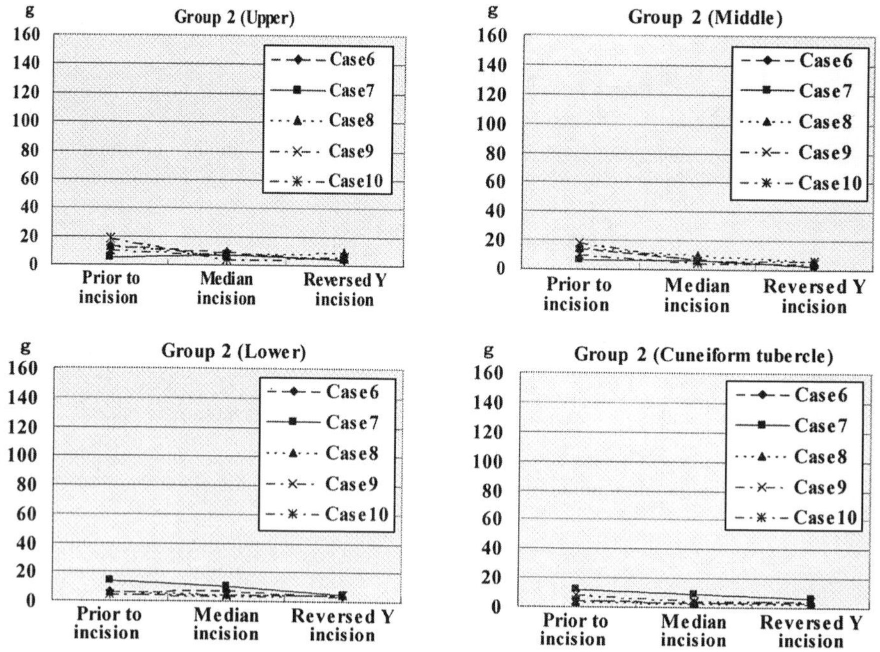

Fig. 6. Comparison of tension, after incision, in Group 2 (upper, middle and lower points, and the cuneiform tubercle).

g → 5 g (26.5%) at the upper point; 6.8 g → 4.6 g (32.4%) at the middle point; 6 g → 5 g (16.7%) at the lower point; and 5 g → 4.5 g (10%) at the cuneiform tubercle (Fig. 6).

Discussion and Conclusion

The most reliable surgical intervention for central dysphagia is laryngeal closure or total laryngectomy, known as Lindeman's operation (separation of the trachea and larynx) [3]. We perfomed the epiglottic closure (a modification of Biller et al.'s method) to prevent aspiration in cases of central dysphagia and preserve phonation in order to maintain patient's quality of life. However, epiglottal diastasis occurred in three out of six cases (upper point, 1; middle and lower points, 2) in which we performed the modification of Biller et al.'s method and repeated surgery was required. Meiteles et al. reported that making an additional vertical incision in the epiglottic cartilage prevents postoperative diastasis [4]. In the present study, we examined the relationship between the form of the epiglottic cartilage and the tension produced by the elasticity of the cartilage, by suturing, and the effect of the incision on the decrease in tension.

Epiglottic form and tension

A variety of epiglottal forms exist, although only two forms, matched evenly between the groups, were examined in the present study. The tension in group 1 was significantly higher at the upper, middle and lower points compared to group 2; a difference of 7 to 10 times. On the other hand, the absolute value of tension was low (15 g) or even less in both groups at the cuneiform tubercle, representing a nonsignificant finding. This, therefore, suggests that the elasticity of the cartilage is weak in both forms at this point. The tension was over 100 g in group 1 at the upper, middle and lower points, but was particularly high at the middle and lower points; the site at which diastasis became a clinical problem.

Incision of epiglottic cartilage and decreased tension induced

Group 1
The tension, prior to any incision, decreased by 60 g or less at the upper point and by 40 g or less at the middle and lower points, upon completion of the median incision. This incision could maintain this decreased tension. Furthermore, when we compared the decrease in tension from the median incision to the completion of the reversed Y incision, the tension decreased by a further 20 g or less at the upper point and 40 g or less at the middle and lower points. Decreased tension was particularly conspicuous at the middle and lower points, indicating that the reversed Y incision was a useful surgical procedure. On the other hand, at the cuneiform tubercle, the decrease in tension was negligible.

Group 2
Prior to any incision, the tension was 15 g or less and was at a baseline value. No significant difference was observed in decreased tension values when using only a median incision, nor using the reversed Y incision. We, therefore, believe that there are few advantages to incising the epiglottic cartilage in patients with this type of epiglottic cartilage.

Adaptation of surgical procedure that decreased tension and indications for use

We observed an obvious difference during surgery with regard to the relationship between tension and the form of the epiglottis. Accordingly, clinicians should consider the form of the patient's epiglottis when deciding whether to use the adapted surgical technique to prevent diastasis, particularly in light of our results in group 2 patients, which indicate that surgery is unnecessary in the epiglottis of the Ω type. The points on the epiglottis were found to produce different tensions, and group 1 patients clearly showed that the tension at the upper, middle and lower points were high. In the present study, we identified that incision was necessary to prevent diastasis and that only a median incision effectively decreased tension. However, the reversed Y incision was even more effective in decreasing tension at the middle and lower points.

References

1. Biller HF, Lawson W, Beak S. Total glossectomy; a technique of reconstruction eliminating laryngectomy. Arch Otolaryngol 1983;109:69–73.
2. Tanabe M. A surgical treatment for aspiration preserving phonatory function. Jpn Bronchoesophagol Soc 1992;43(4):348–352.
3. Lindeman RC. Diverting the paralysed larynx — a reversible procedure for intractable aspiration. Laryngoscope 1975;85:157–180.
4. Meiteles LZ, Kraus W, Shemen L. Modified epiglottoplasty for prevention of aspiration. Laryngoscope 1998;103:1395–1398.

Bronchology and Bronchoesophagology: State of the Art.
H. Yoshimura et al., editors.

Laryngeal carcinoid tumors: a report of three cases

T. Yoshikawa, S. Endo, K. Watanabe, H. Oomori, S. Ogawa and A. Kida
Department of Otorhinolaryngology – Head and Neck Surgery, Nihon University School of Medicine, Tokyo, Japan

Abstract. *Introduction.* Carcinoid tumors of the larynx are rare, however, the number of reports of them has increased over recent years. We present three cases of carcinoid tumors of the larynx encountered at our university hospital.

Patients. Case 1: a 51-year-old male was admitted with the chief complaint of hemoptysis. Resection of the tumor, in conjunction with the adjacent cricoid cartilage and trachea, and the simultaneous reconstruction of the airway was performed. The serum 5-HIAA level increased remarkably.

Case 2: a 57-year-old male was seen to have a small tumor in the arytenoid. Vertical hemilaryngectomy and neck dissection were performed in order to remove the tumor. During the course of the follow-up, multiple lung metastases developed. He remains alive with this disease.

Case 3: an 80-year-old female was seen to have a large mass in the laryngeal aspect of the epiglottis, extending to the anterior commissure. Tumor resection and laser evaporation, followed by external irradiation was carried out. She died of another disease.

Conclusion. Because regional recurrences and distant metastases occur frequently in carcinoid tumors, care should be taken to manage these lesions.

Keywords: distant metastasis, laryngeal neoplasm, surgery.

Introduction

Carcinoid tumors belong to the group of neuroendocrine tumors of epithelial origin, i.e., neuroendocrine carcinomas. These neoplasms usually occur in the gastrointestinal tract or bronchial system, but are very rare neoplasms in the larynx. Recently, the number of reports of these lesions has been on the increase. We present three cases of laryngeal carcinoid tumors encountered at our university hospital.

Case presentation

Case 1

A 51-year-old male smoker with chronic renal failure was admitted with hemoptysis. Broncho-fiberscopic examination revealed a small tumor in the posterior

Address for correspondence: Takuma Yoshikawa MD, PhD, Department of ORL-HNS, Nihon University School of Medicine, 30 Oyaguchi-kamicho, Itabashi-ku, Tokyo 173-8610, Japan. Tel.: +81-3-3972-8111, ext. 2542. Fax: +81-3-3972-1321. E-mail: takuma@med.nihon-u.ac.jp lateral wall of the larynx. There was no cervical adenopathy. Resection of the tumor and the involved cricoid cartilage and adjacent trachea was performed. The pathological diagnosis was a typical carcinoid tumor. He is now free of disease.

Case 2

A 57-year-old male smoker was being followed under chronic otitis media. On his follow-up visit, laryngo-fiberscopic examination revealed a small mass in the left arytenoids. There was no cervical adenopathy. Excisional biopsy of the tumor was performed through rigid laryngoscopy. The pathological diagnosis was an atypical carcinoid tumor. Vertical hemilaryngectomy and radical neck dissection were performed. During the follow-up, multiple lung metastases developed. He remains alive with this disease.

Case 3

An 80-year-old female smoker was admitted to our university hospital due to a continuous sore throat. On laryngo-fiberscopic examination, a large mass arising in the laryngeal aspect of the epiglottis, extending to the anterior commissure was found. The tumor was mostly removed through rigid laryngoscopy. The tumor bed was vaporized by laser. The pathological diagnosis was an atypical carcinoid tumor. Postoperative irradiation was performed up to 60 Gy. She died of an intercurrent disease. Postmortal examination showed a local residual tumor, but neither regional nor distant metastasis.

Discussion

Epithelial neuroendocrine tumors of the larynx are classified into three categories: the typical carcinoid tumor, atypical carcinoid tumor, and small cell carcinoma [1]. The epiglottis and supraglottis are considered as the most frequent locations for these tumors. These tumors are almost always positive for epithelial markers, such as cytokeratin and EMA, and general neuroendocrine markers, such as chromogranin and NSE. They are also positive for calcitonin.

A typical carcinoid tumor of the larynx is an extremely rare neoplasm, and there are only 13 well-documented cases [2]. Patients were usually men (male: female ratio is 12:1) in their sixth to eighth decades who were heavy cigarette smokers. These tumors are usually nonfunctional. The overlying epithelium is usually intact. Microscopically, mitoses, pleomorphism and necrosis are lacking. Argyrophil stains are characteristically positive, and argentaffin stains often negative. The usual management is conservative surgery and the 5-year-survival rate is nearly 100%.

An atypical carcinoid tumor is the most frequent nonsquamous carcinoma of the larynx, with approximately 300 cases thus far reported in literature. Macroscopically, the tumor appears as a nodular, polypoid, pedunculated subepithelial lesion, with or without ulceration of the overlying surface epithelium. Microscopically, the tumor cells are usually polygonal, with amphophilic to eosinophilic cytoplasm and a centrally or eccentrically placed nucleus, often with hyperchromasia and prominent nucleoli. Mitoses are frequent. The presence of lymph node metastases or distant metastases confirm the aggressiveness of the lesion. A marked elevation of the serum 5-HIAA level is considered to be pathognomonic for carcinoid tumor. Surgery is the choice of treatment for an atypical carcinoid, with accompanying neck dissection. The tumor is usually not radiosensitive. In a comprehensive review, the cumulative survival was 48% after 5 years and 30% after 10 years [3].

References

1. Ferlito A et al. A review of neuroendocrine neoplasms of the larynx: update on diagnosis and treatment. J Laryngol Otol 1998;112:827–834.
2. McBride LC et al. Case study of well-differentiated carcinoid tumor of the larynx and review of laryngeal neuroendocrine tumors. Otolaryngol Head Neck Surg 1999;120:536–539.
3. Shanmugaratnan K et al. Histological typing of the upper respiratory tract. International histological classification of tumors, 2nd edn. New York: Springer-Verlag, 1991.

Laryngeal reflex and palsy

Bronchology and Bronchoesophagology: State of the Art.
H. Yoshimura et al., editors.

An experimental study of laryngeal reflexes to superior laryngeal nerve stimulation

Kwang-Moon Kim, Young-Ho Kim and Jung-Pyoe Hong
Department of Otorhinolaryngology, Yonsei University College of Medicine, Seoul, Korea

Abstract. The laryngeal protective reflex is a glottal closure triggered by tactile receptors, in the glottic and supraglottic mucosa, which evoke the reflex contraction of the laryngeal muscles. When this reflex is exaggerated or hypersensitive, it may be responsible for disorders such as spasmodic dysphonia, idiopathic laryngospasm and sudden infant death syndrome, etc. In 1987, a method was described in which the average electrical activity was recorded from the brain stem of a paralysed cat, following the electrical stimulation of the superior laryngeal nerve (SLN). It was termed the laryngeal brain stem response (LBR). Although the LBR has been studied in several species of animals, the generator source of each wave has not yet been precisely demonstrated. There have been numerous reports about the generator source of LBR peaks. In my institute, we also recorded the far-field brain stem activity and waveforms in cats and dogs. In cats, the near-field brain stem activity was recorded, as well as the far-field activity, in the same experimental setup. Mean latencies, configurations and the reproducibility of each wave were demonstrated. Using these results, we were able to speculate about the generator sources of each wave.

Keywords: generator source, laryngeal reflex.

Introduction

Among the physiologic functions of the larynx, the protective reflex is phylogenetically primitive, but imperative. This reflex is triggered by tactile receptors in the glottic and supraglottic mucosa, which evoke reflex contraction of laryngeal muscles. It protects the lung against the entrance of anything but air. However, this reflex, if exaggerated or hypersensitive, may be responsible for several disorders, including spasmodic dysphonia, idiopathic laryngospasm, gastroesophageal reflux and sudden infant death syndrome, etc. [1]. In 1987, Isogai et al. [2] recorded the average electrical activity in paralyzed cats, from the recurrent laryngeal nerve and brain stem simultaneously, following the electrical stimulation of the superior laryngeal nerve (SLN). They termed the far-field brain stem activity the laryngeal brain stem response (LBR). Many investigators have now recorded the LBR in various different animals and we carried out the same experiment with cats and dogs [3]. Although there have been numerous reports about the generator sources of the LBR peaks, no reports were made recording the far- and near-field potentials in the same experimental setup considering possible

Address for correspondence: Kwang-Moon Kim, Department of Otorhinolaryngology, Yonsei University College of Medicine, P.O. Box 8044, Seoul 120-752, Korea. Tel.: +82-2-361-8483. Fax: +82-2-393-0580. E-mail: kmkim97@yumc.yonsei.ac.kr intraspecies variations.

In this context, we designed a study to compare the near-field with the far-field brain stem activity in the cat under the same experimental conditions. We also compared the waveform and latencies of LBR peaks recorded by the above two techniques. Finally, we speculated on the generator sources of LBR peaks through the comparison of our data with those of prior reports.

Materials and Methods

Twenty adult cats weighing 2.0 to 3.5 kg were used. They were divided into two groups of 10 each. One group was used for the far-field technique, and the other for the near-field technique, to record the brain stem evoked response.

For the far-field recording of the LBR in group I, a needle electrode was inserted into the posterior epilaryngeal wall and other electrodes were inserted in the paravertebral muscle at the level of third cervical vertebra as a reference electrode and into the anterior neck muscle as a ground.

For the recording of near-field LBR in group II, an active electrode was inserted into a solitary tract nucleus and nucleus ambiguus, according to the coordinates of stereotaxic atlas of the cat brain.

Results

In the far-field technique, the stimulation of the SLN evoked five positive and five negative waves with reproducible latencies. The positive waves were labelled P1 through P5, and negative waves N1 through N5 in order of their appearance. All the other waves showed reproducibility, but the N5 wave was only observed to have reproducible latencies in two cats.

In four cats, from the far-field technique group, the LBR peaks were recorded after sectioning the vagal trunk above the nodose ganglion.

In the near-field technique, reproducible waves were recorded in the latency range of 1.59 to 4.49 ms at the nucleus solitarius region. These waves corresponded to waves P2, N2, and P3 recorded by the far-field technique. Waves after N3 were not reproducible. The near-field potentials were recorded at the nucleus ambiguus region. However, only P2 was reproducibly recorded (in five cats). All the other waves were not reproducible.

Discussion

Our results suggest that P1, N1 and P2 waves from far-field recording originate from the vagus nerve. P2, N2 and P3 waves are thought to originate from the nucleus solitarius, on comparison of the far- and near-field data.

Transection of the vagal trunk above the nodose ganglion eliminated all waves except P1, N1, and P2. Transection of the SLN, proximal to the stimulating electrode, eliminated all waves except the triggering artifact. These results suggest that the earlier waves are generated by the ipsilateral vagus nerve and that the waveforms obtained in this study can be regarded as neural activity evoked by SLN stimulation. Other reasons are as follows: 1) the initial peak occurred after SLN stimulation in each observation, 2) consistent responses to stimuli of alternating polarity suggest that these waves are nonrandom activities triggered by SLN stimulation, 3) transection of the SLN abolished all the peaks except the stimulus artifact, and 4) the fact that the waveforms persisted under complete muscular paralysis suggests a neurologic origin.

There have been many experiments performed on animals, however, very few studies have been performed on human subjects. In 1990, Yamashita [4] reported that the LBR of humans can be obtained via the transcutaneous insertion of hooked wire electrodes around the SLN area. Although we also tried to record the waveform of LBR in human subjects, we could not pick up any meaningful or reproducible waveforms in our three subjects.

References

1. Sasaki CT, Suzuki M. Laryngeal reflexes in cat, dog and man. Arch Otolaryngol 1976;102: 400–402.
2. Isogai Y, Suzuki M, Saito S. Brainstem response evoked by the laryngeal reflex. In: baer T, Sasaki C, Harris KS (eds) Laryngeal Function in Phonation and Respiration. Boston, Mass: College Hill Press, 1987;71–79.
3. Kim KM, Kim GR, Yoon JH, Cho JI, Kim CK, Park YJ. Experimental study of laryngeal brain stem response evoked by the electrical stimulation of superior laryngeal nerve in cat. Korean J Otolaryngol 1992;35:328–333.
4. Yamashita T. Larynx-evoked brain stem response on human. Larynx Jpn 1990;2:130–135.

Bronchology and Bronchoesophagology: State of the Art.
H. Yoshimura et al., editors.

The effects of neurotrophic factors on the regeneration of recurrent laryngeal nerves in rats

Masahiro Komori[1], Eiji Yumoto[2], Masamitsu Hyodo[3], Seiji Kawakita[3], Takahiko Yamagata[3] and Tetsuji Sanuki[3]

[1]*Department of Otolaryngology, Kosei General Hospital, Mihara-shi, Hiroshima;* [2]*Department of Otolaryngology Head and Neck Surgery, School of Medicine, Kumamoto University, Kumamoto; and* [3]*Department of Otolaryngology, School of Medicine, Ehime University, Onsen-gun, Ehime, Japan*

Abstract. *Background.* Although several neurotrophic factors (NTFs) have been demonstrated to be beneficial to regeneration after nerve injury, there has been little information on the roles of NTFs following the denervation of the recurrent laryngeal nerve (RLN). We investigated the effects of NTFs on the process of regeneration of the RLN.

Methods. After the transection of the left RLN, a silicone tube was placed between the nerve stumps and filled with one of the following solutions: nerve growth factor (NGF), ciliary neurotrophic factor (CNTF), basic fibroblast growth factor (bFGF) or phosphate buffer saline (PBS) as a control. Electromyographical and histological evaluations were conducted 3 weeks after the transection.

Results. Recovery of the evoked electromyographic response was facilitated by local administration of NGF or bFGF. The number of regenerating nerve fibers was increased by CNTF and bFGF. The myelinated nerve fibers were facilitated by bFGF. The decrease in size of the motor neuron in the nucleus ambiguus, due to the transection, was prevented by NGF and bFGF.

Conclusions. This study has possible important clinical implications for a therapeutic management of injured RLN through the use of NTFs, particularly bFGF.

Keywords: atrophy of neuron, nerve sprouting, nerve injury, nerve regeneration, nucleus ambiguus.

Introduction

It has been recognized that vocal cord movement could not recover entirely, even if electromyographic analysis of recurrent laryngeal nerve (RLN) palsy cases demonstrated normal firing patterns of the intrinsic laryngeal muscle [1]. This incomplete recovery of the vocal fold movement, following the RLN injury, may be caused by atrophy of the muscle and the misdirection of the reinnervated nerve fibers [1,2]. Furthermore, atropy and the degeneration of muscles occur irreversibly more severely in proportion to the longer period of denervation. In addition, neurons are also degenerated irreversibly. In short, there is little hope of the recovery of the vocal fold movement if the reinnervation of the RLN occurs following a prolonged period of the denervation of the RLN. Therefore,

Address for correspondence: Masahiro Komori MD, Department of Otolaryngology, Kosei General Hospital, 3-3-28 Minami, Mihara-shi, Hiroshima 723-8686, Japan. Tel.: +81-848-63-5500. Fax: +81-848-62-0600. E-mail: komori@m.ehime-u.ac.jp shortening the period of dennervation might prevent the irreversible degenerative change of the intrinsic laryngeal muscle and motor neurons.

Neurotrophic factors (NTFs) are necessary for the development and survival of the neuron [3,4]. Although several NTFs have been demonstrated to be beneficial to neural regeneration after nerve injury [2], there is little information on the roles of NTFs following the denervation of the RLN. In the present study, we examined the in vivo effect of three NTFs (nerve growth factor, NGF [5], ciliary neurotrophic factor, CNTF [6] and basic fibroblast growth factor, bFGF [7]) on the regeneration of denervated RLN.

Materials and Methods

Surgical procedures

Thirty-nine male rats, weighing between 240 and 280 g, were anesthetized using an intraperitoneal injection of sodium pentobarbital (30 mg/kg body weight). The left RLN was transected at the level of 10 mm from the lower edge of the cricoid cartilage and a 2-mm length of the nerve segment was removed. The gap was bridged with a silicone tube (Fig. 1). The space in the tube was filled with each of the NTFs (final concentrations: 0.5 nmol/l and 5 nmol/l). Ten rats were used for each of the NTF studies, i.e., NGF (Mouse 2.5 S NGF, Collaborative, Inc.), CNTF (Rat CNTF, Pepro Tech, Inc.) and bFGF (Human bFGF, SIGMA, Inc.), five rats for the vehicle study, and four rats for normal study.

Electromyographical study

Three weeks later, two hooked-wire electrodes were inserted into each of the bilateral thyroarytenoid muscles through the front of the thyroid cartilage. Each of the bilateral RLNs were electrostimulated at 15 mm from the lower edge of the cricoid cartilage. Evoked action potentials in the thyroarytenoid muscle were recorded.

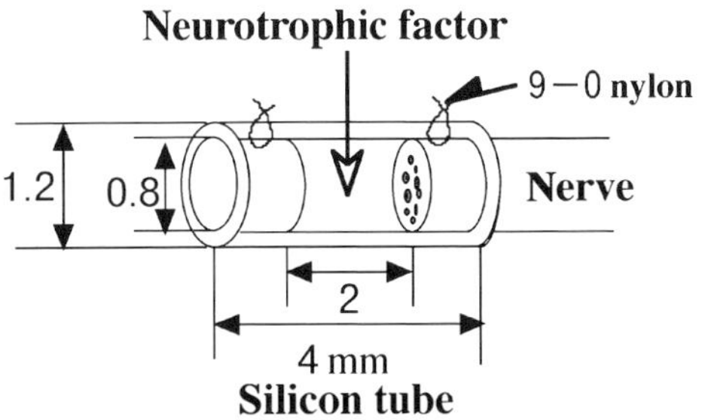

Fig. 1. Treatment of the nerve with a silicon tube.

Table 1. The latency of evoked action potentials.

	Vehicle (ms)	NGF (ms)	CNTF (ms)	bFGF (ms)
	3.23 ± 0.20			
0.5 nmol/l		2.71 ± 0.24	3.20 ± 0.39	2.57 ± 0.12[a]
5 nmol/l		2.48 ± 0.12[a]	3.20 ± 0.37	2.44 ± 0.23[a]

The high concentration groups of NGF and bFGF had shorter latencies than that of the vehicle group ([a]$p < 0.05$, n = 5–6) (Mean ± SE).

Histologic study

The regenerated nerve funiculus at the midportion of the tube were embedded in epoxy resin. Semithin cross-sections of 0.5 μm thicknesses were cut and stained with toluidine blue. For quantification, the numbers of regenerated nerve fibers were measured using analytical software.

To investigate the morphological changes of the neurons from the nucleus ambiguus (NA), the brain stem was embedded in paraffin. Serial cross-sections of 10 μm thicknesses were sliced from the cranial top of the nucleus hypoglossi to the caudal end of the nucleus olibaris inferior, and stained with cresyl violet. The cross-sectional areas and numbers of neurons in every 5th section were measured.

Results

Evoked action potentials could be recorded in all rats of the all groups. The latencies in the groups of high concentration of NGF and bFGF were shorter than those of vehicle, while the latencies in the groups of low concentration of NGF and CNTF were almost the same as those of vehicle (Table 1).

The total number of regenerated nerve fibers was the largest in the group of high concentration of bFGF, then in the group of low concentration of bFGF, followed by the group of low concentration of CNTF (Fig. 2). The differences between the total numbers of regenerated nerve fibers in all the groups and the vehicle group were significant. The bFGF groups had significantly more myelinated nerve fibers than any other group (Fig. 3).

In the NA, the average count of neurons for each group is about 200. There was no significant difference among the number of neurons measured in each group. The ratio of neurons larger than 400 μm^2 in the NGF and bFGF groups was almost the same as that of in the normal group, while those in the vehicle and CNTF groups were lower than those in the other groups (Fig. 4). The ratio of neurons larger than 400 μm^2 in the NGF and bFGF groups was significantly higher than that in the vehicle group.

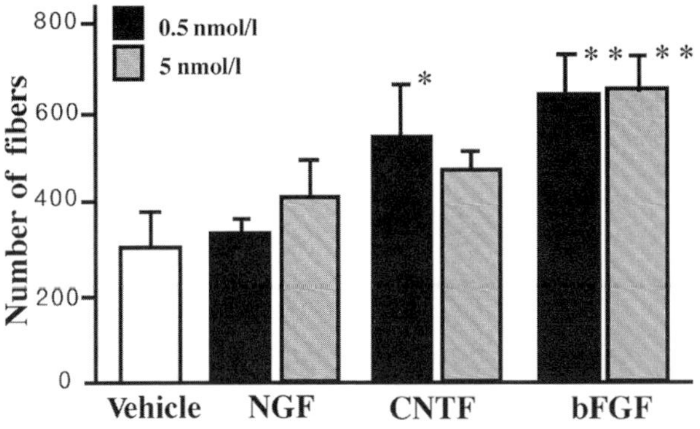

Fig. 2. The total number of regenerated fibers. The total number of regenerated nerve fibers was most abundant in the high concentration of bFGF group, then in the low concentration of bFGF group, followed by the low concentration of CNTF group. The differences between the total numbers of regenerated nerve fibers between all the groups and the vehicle group were significant (*$p<0.05$, **$p<0.01$, $n = 4–5$) (Mean ± SE).

Discussion

Regeneration of the motor nerve is divided into four headings: nerve sprouting, axonal elongation, reinnervation, and myelination. The increase of regenerated nerve fiber means the increase of nerve sprouting, because the number of regenerated nerve fibers is the sum of myelinated and unmyelinated sprouting nerve fibers. The promotion of axonal elongation, reinnervation and myelination resulted in the increase of myelinated nerve fibers, and the latency of evoked action potential is evaluated electromyographically as one side of the function of nerves. Shortening the latency of the thyroarytenoid muscle suggests that NGF

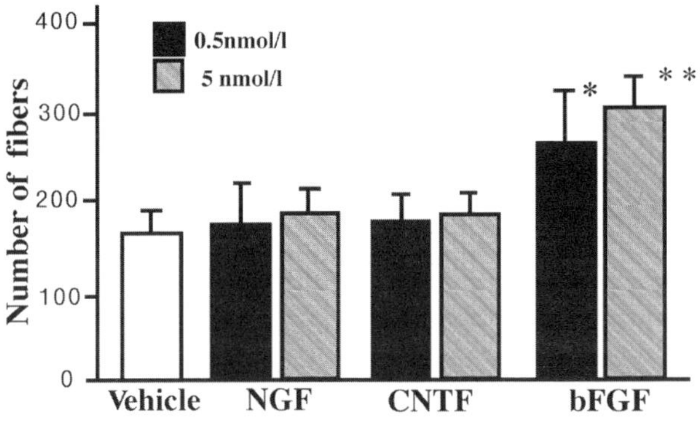

Fig. 3. Number of myelinated regenerated fibers. The myelinated nerve fibers in the bFGF groups were significantly more numerous compared to any other group (*$p<0.05$, **$p<0.01$, $n = 4–5$) (Mean ± SE).

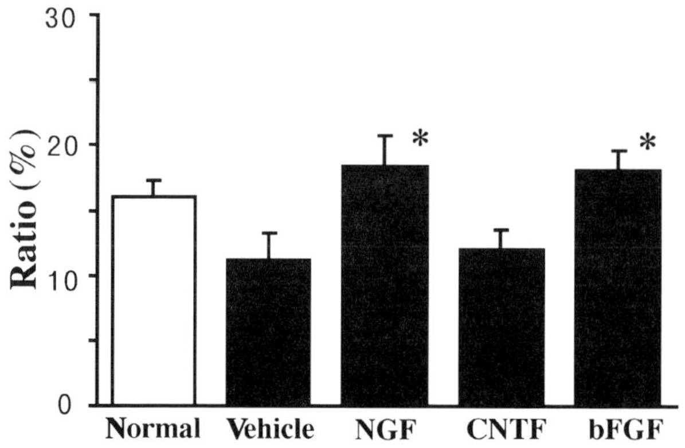

Fig. 4. Ratio of neurons larger than 400 μm^2. The ratios of neurons larger than 400 μm^2 in the NGF and bFGF groups were significantly higher than that of the vehicle group (*$p < 0.05$, n = 4) (Mean ± SE).

and bFGF promoted regeneration of motor nerve fibers of RLN. The increase of regenerated nerve fiber suggests that CNTF and bFGF promoted nerve sprouting and the increase of myelinated nerve fiber suggests that bFGF also promoted axonal elongation and myelination.

The NA contained a mixture of neurons of various sizes [8]. Small neurons are interneurons and large neurons are motor neurons. The area of motor neurons in the NA of a rat is 300 ~ 500 μm^2, considering past studies, including retrograde transport material [9]. Most neurons larger than 400 μm^2 were, therefore, consisdered to be motor neurons. The decrease in neurons larger than 400 μm^2 in the vehicle group meant that the motor neurons became atrophied due to the transection of the RLN. Thus, it was suggested that NGF and bFGF had the effect of preventing atrophy of motor neurons in the NA because the ratios of larger neurons, of over 400 μm^2, in the NGF and bFGF groups did not decrease.

This study has an important clinical implication for the therapeutic management of injured RLN, i.e., the use of NTFs, particularly bFGF.

References

1. Hiroto I, Hirano M, Tomita H. Electromyographic investigation of human vocal cord paralysis. Ann Otol Rhinol Laryngol 1968;77:296–304.
2. Siribodhi C, Sundmaker W, Atkins JP et al. Electromyographic studies of laryngeal paralysis and regeneration of laryngeal motor nerves in dogs. Laryngoscope 1963;73:148–164.
3. Korsching S. The neurotrophic factor concept: a re-examination. J Neurosci 1993;13:2739–2748.
4. Purves D. The trophic theory of neural connections. Trends Neurosci 1986;9:486–489.
5. Levi-Montalcini R, Hamburger V. Selective growth-stimulating effects of mouse sarcoma on the sensory and sympathetic nervous system of the chick embryo. J Exp Zool 1951;116:321–362.
6. Barbin G, Manthorpe M, Varon S. Purification of the chick eye ciliary neuronotrophic factor. J Neurochem 1984;43:1468–1478.

7. Bohlen P, Baird A, Esch F et al. Isolation and partial molecular characterization of pituitary fibroblast growth factor. Proc Natl Acad Sci USA 1984;81:5364–5368.
8. Schade JP. On the volume and surface area of spinal neurons. In: Eccles JC, Schade JP (eds) Progress in Brain Reseach 11, Organization of the Spinal Cord. Amsterdam: Elsevier publishing Co., 1964;261–277.
9. Portillo F, Pasaro R. Location of motoneurons supplying the intrinsic laryngeal muscle of rats. Horseradish peroxidase and fluorescence double-labeling study. Brain Behav Evol 1988;32: 220–225.

Bronchology and Bronchoesophagology: State of the Art.
H. Yoshimura et al., editors.

Basic FGF in the nucleus ambiguus following a recurrent laryngeal nerve injury

Tetsuji Sanuki[1], Eiji Yumoto[2], Seiji Kawakita[1], Masahiro Komori[3], Kazumi Motoyoshi[1] and Masamitsu Hyodo[1]

[1]Department of Otolaryngology, School of Medicine, Ehime University, Onsen-gun, Ehime; [2]Department of Otolaryngology Head-Neck Surgery, School of Medicine, Kumamoto University, Kumamoto; and [3]Department of Otolaryngology, Kosei General Hospital, Mihara-city, Hiroshima, Japan

Abstract. *Background.* The aim of this study was to examine basic fibroblast growth factor (bFGF) immunoreactivity in the nucleus ambiguus (NA) after three different RLN injuries.

Methods. Thirty adult rats underwent a crushing of the left RLN (group A), 30 underwent a transection of the left RLN (group B), and 30 underwent a transection of the left RLN and had both nerve stumps covered with silicone caps (group C). The bFGF in the NA was assessed as the ratio (O/U) of the positive areas on the left and right. O/U was measured 1, 3, 7, 14, and 28 days after injury. Three rats served as controls.

Results. O/U in the control group was approximately one. O/U was elevated on day 7 in group A, on days 3, 7, and 14 in group B, and on day 3 in group C. O/U in group B was greater than that in group A on days 14 and 28. Maximal bFGF immunoreactivity was lower in group C than in groups A and B.

Conclusions. This endogenous bFGF might contribute to preventing lesion-induced neuronal death. Blockage of axonal regeneration might suppress bFGF production in the NA. Further understanding of the roles of bFGF after RLN injury may contribute to the prevention of neuronal death and the facilitation of axonal regeneration.

Keywords: axonal sprouting, immunohistochemistry, nerve transection, nerve crush, reinnervation.

Introduction

In adult rats, administering bFGF to the site of nerve injury or the nucleus prevented neuronal death after nerve transection [1,2]. Chen et al. [3] showed that local treatment with the bFGF-neutralizing antibody or an antagonist for the bFGF receptor caused a decrease in the number of regenerated axons and suppressed the growth of regenerating axons following facial nerve transection, indicating a neurotrophic role of endogenous bFGF. However, bFGF expression in the nucleus following varying degrees of nerve injury has not been elucidated.

The purpose of this study was to determine the bFGF expression in the NA after three different nerve injuries in adult rats.

Address for correspondence: Tetsuji Sanuki MD, Department of Otolaryngology, School of Medicine, Ehime University, Shigenobu-cho, Onsen-gun, Ehime 791-0295, Japan. Tel.: +81-89-960-5366. Fax: +81-89-960-5368. E-mail: sanuki@m.ehime-u.ac.jp

Materials and Methods

Ninety-three adult Wistar rats were used in this study. In group A (n = 30), 1 mm of the left RLN, at the level of the seventh tracheal ring, was crushed with needle forceps, for 5 s (Fig. 1A). In group B (n = 30), 5 mm of the left RLN was resected at the same level (Fig. 1B). In group C (n = 30), the left RLN was resected similarly, but both nerve stumps were covered with sterile silicone caps (Fig. 1C). In group D (n = 3), the left RLN was exposed without further treatment.

On days 1, 3, 7, 14, and 28, after the procedure, the rats in groups A, B, and C were anesthetized, and then perfused transcardially with 4% paraformaldehyde in 0.1 M PB. The brainstem was harvested and postfixed in the same fixative. The medulla oblongata including the NA, which innervates the RLN was serially cut in a cryostat. The sections were processed for an immunohistochemical stain using anti-bFGF mouse antibody. The sections were processed for biotinylated rabbit antimouse IgG-1 antibody and further processed with avidin-biotin-horseradish peroxidase complex. The sections were stained with a solution of 3,3-diaminobenzidine.

Each pair of sections were observed under a microscope equipped with a digital camera. Microscopic images of the medulla oblongata including the NA were imported into a personal computer. The NIH Image was used to quantitatively determine the expression of bFGF immunoreactivity. The numbers of pixels positive for bFGF immunoreactivity on the operated (O) and unoperated (U) sides were counted. The quantity of bFGF expression was represented as O/U.

The data were represented as means ± SD. Student's paired and unpaired t tests

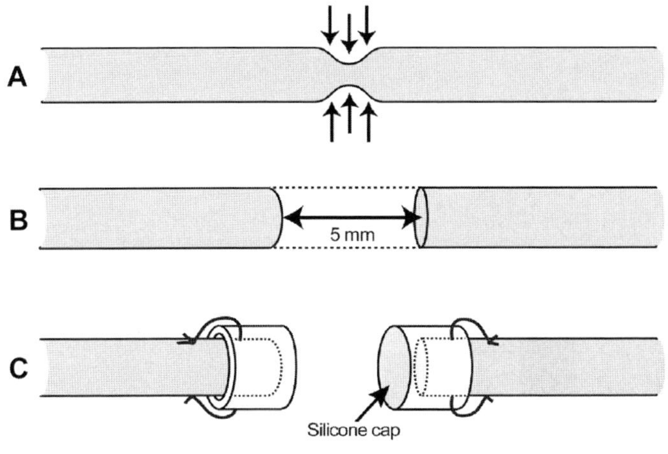

Fig. 1. Procedures used to produce recurrent laryngeal nerve injury. **A:** Group A: 1 mm of the left RLN was crushed with needle forceps for 5 s at the level of the seventh tracheal ring. **B:** Group B: 5 mm of the left RLN was resected at the level of the seventh tracheal ring. **C:** Group C: 5 mm of the left RLN was resected at the level of the seventh tracheal ring and both nerve stumps were covered with sterile silicone caps.

were used to compare the bFGF immunoreactivity between the operated and unoperated sides in the same group and among three groups, respectively. A p value of less than 0.05 was taken as the level of significance.

Results

In group D, O/U was 1.03 ± 0.89, indicating the same level of bFGF expression in the NA bilaterally.

In group A, O/U was greater than 1.0 on days 1, 3, and 7. However, statistical significance was only observed on day 7 when O/U was 2.33 ± 0.77 (Fig. 2). Subsequently, O/U decreased to approximately 1.0.

On day 1, after the procedure, in group B, O/U did not show a significant increase. Then, O/U increased and peaked at 6.92 ± 0.93 on day 14. There was a significantly higher bFGF expression on the operated side on days 3, 7, and 14. O/U decreased to 1.62 ± 0.28 on day 28, with no significant difference between O and U (Fig. 3).

In group C, O/U was 1.75 ± 0.65 on day 3, indicating a significantly increased O. The O/U was less than 1.0 from day 7 onwards (Fig. 4).

O/U was compared among groups A, B, and C (Fig. 5). O/U was greater in group B than in group A on days 14 and 28, and significantly greater than in group C on days 7, 14, and 28. O/U was greater in group A than in group C on days 7 and 14. There were no significant differences in the value of O/U between groups A and B on day 7 or between groups A and C on day 28.

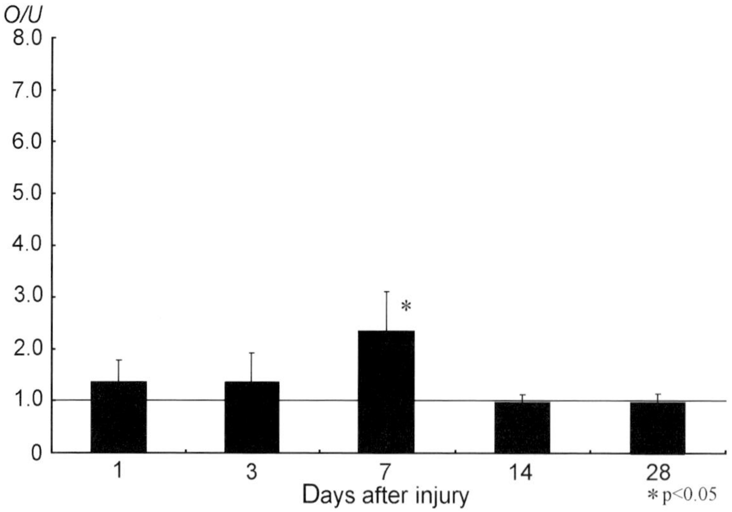

Fig. 2. bFGF expression after nerve crush. The height of each shaded box represents an average value of O/U, and the vertical bars indicate the SD (n = 6 for each observation period). O/U was increased on days 1, 3, and 7. However, only the increase on day 7 was statistically significant ($p < 0.05$, Student's t test).

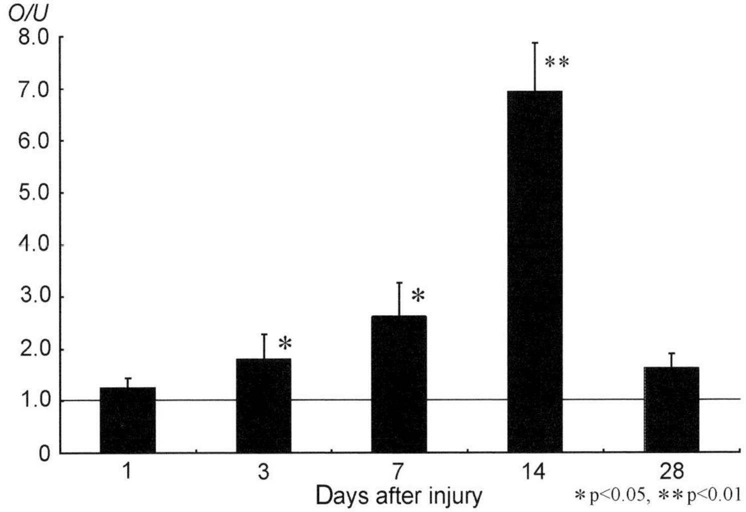

Fig. 3. bFGF expression after nerve transection. There was no significant difference between O and U on days 1 and 28. O/U indicated a significantly higher bFGF expression on the operated side on days 3, 7 ($p < 0.05$, Student's t test), and 14 ($p < 0.01$, Student's t test) after the procedure.

Discussion

We examined bFGF expression in the NA after three different nerve injury treatments in adult rats. High bFGF expression in the NA after RLN injuries in groups A and B demonstrated elevated production of endogenous bFGF.

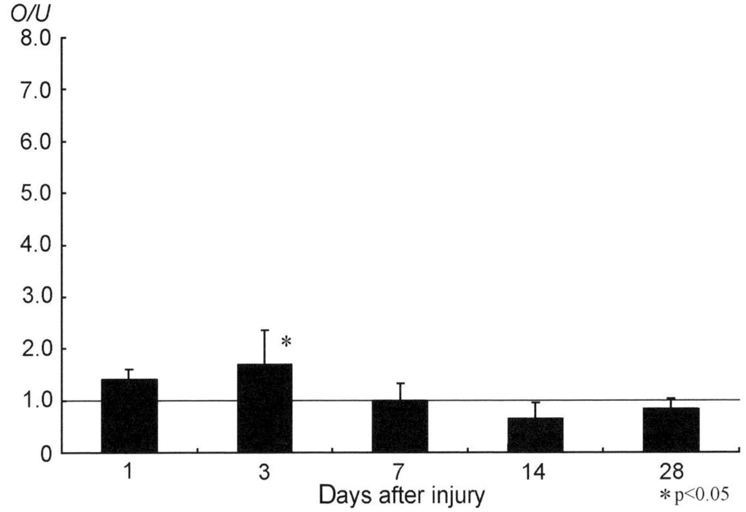

Fig. 4. bFGF expression after nerve transection and capping. O/U was 1.75 ± 0.65 on day 3, indicating a significantly increased O ($p < 0.05$, Student's t test). O/U was less than 1.0 from day 7 onwards.

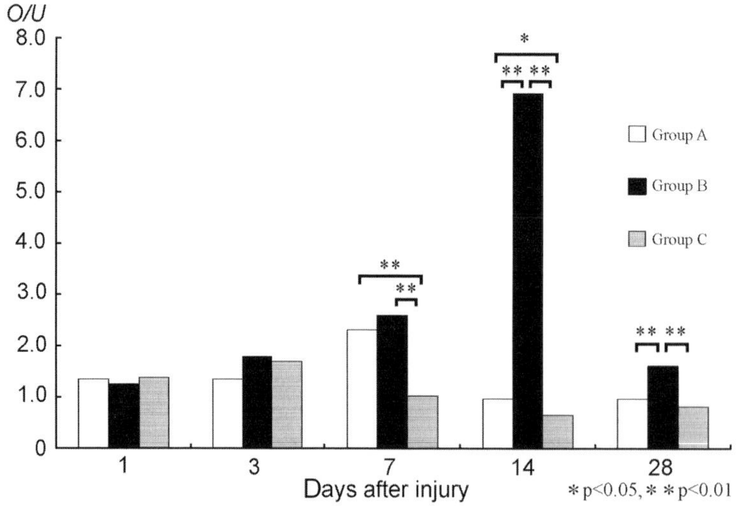

Fig. 5. Comparison of O/U among groups A, B, and C. O/U was significantly greater in group B than in group A on days 14 and 28 ($p < 0.01$, unpaired Student's t test) and than in group C on days 7, 14, and 28 ($p < 0.01$, unpaired Student's t test). O/U was larger in group A than in group C on days 7 and 14 ($p < 0.01$ and $p < 0.05$, respectively, unpaired Student's t test).

The bFGF expression was significantly greater in group B than in group A. Using adult rats, Huber et al. [2] reported a higher level of bFGF mRNA in the hypoglossal nucleus following hypoglossal nerve injury in the nerve transection group compared to the crush group. These findings suggest that increased bFGF in the nucleus should be closely associated with the severity of nerve injury. Severe damage to the nerve requires a longer time for reinnervation, resulting in a higher risk of neuronal death. Therefore, higher bFGF expression in the nucleus is necessary for neuronal survival.

In group C, silicone caps fixed on the nerve stumps prevented reinnervation of the transected nerve. The maximal level of bFGF expression was significantly lower in group C than in groups A and B. These differences may be explained in the following way. Axonal sprouting begins approximately 3 h after nerve injury, and the regenerating axons gradually grow for 5 days, irrespective of the presence or absence of their target [4]. Increased bFGF expression in the motoneuron is considered indispensable for motoneuron regeneration and survival. It increases exclusively in the early stage of regeneration. After reinnervation or neuronal death occurs, bFGF expression decreases in the motoneuron. bFGF of peripheral origin may be transported to the nucleus by axonal flow. Since the silicone caps blocked axonal flow from the stump in group C, bFGF expression may have been suppressed in the NA.

Acknowledgements

The authors would like to thank Dr Seiji Matsuda and Dr Kiyofumi Gyo for their valuable comments on this work.

References

1. Grothe C, Meisinger C, Hertenstein A, Kurz H, Wewetzer K. Expression of fibroblast growth factor-2 and fibroblast growth factor receptor 1 messenger RNAs in spinal ganglia and sciatic nerve: regulation after peripheral nerve lesion. Neuroscience 1997;76:123–135.
2. Huber K, Meisinger C, Grothe C. Expression of fibroblast growth factor-2 in hypoglossal motoneurons is stimulated by peripheral nerve injury. J Comp Neurol 1997;382:189–198.
3. Chen YS, Murakami S, Gyo K, Wakisaka H, Matsuda S, Sakanaka M. Effects of basic fibroblast growth factor (bFGF)-neutralizing antibody and platelet factor 4 on facial nerve regeneration. Exp Neurol 1999;155:274–283.
4. Tomatsuri M, Okajima S, Ide C. Sprout formation at nodes of Ranvier of crush-injured peripheral nerves. Restor Neurol Neurosci 1993;5:275–282.

Bronchology and Bronchoesophagology: State of the Art.
H. Yoshimura et al., editors.

Indication of arytenoid rotation and thyroplasty for unilateral laryngeal paralysis

Hidetaka Yoshihashi, Kiyoshi Makiyama, Chie Suzuki, Akinori Kida and Masayuki Sawashima
Department of Otolaryngology, School of Medicine, Nihon University, Tokyo, Japan

Abstract. Arytenoid rotation, thyroplasty type I and intracordal collagen injections are all forms of treatment for unilateral laryngeal paralysis. In our clinic, arytenoid rotation is indicated in patients who have a wide glottic space during phonation or who have an extreme gap between the levels of bilateral vocal cords, thyroplasty is indicated in patients who have moderate or mild insufficiency of glottic closure, and an intracordal aterocollagen injection is chosen in order to increase the vocal cord volume.

In the present study, phonatory function test results were analyzed in patients treated by thyroplasty type I and arytenoid rotation. Our indication criteria were considered to be basically valid. At the same time, it was suggested that the indication of surgery should respond flexibly to individual needs.

Keywords: expiratory lung pressure, glottic space, mean flow rate, phonatory function.

Introduction

Arytenoid adduction, thyroplasty type I and intracordal collagen injections have all been performed to treat unilateral laryngeal paralysis. We have established indications to determine the best surgical procedure for each patient. To evaluate the validity of our surgical indications, phonatory function test results were compared between preoperative conditions.

Surgical indications

Figure 1 shows a flow chart for the determination of surgical procedures.

Subjects

The subjects consisted of 25 patients with unilateral laryngeal paralysis who underwent phonatory function tests using the phonatory function analyzer PS77E before and after thyroplasty surgery or arytenoid adduction. Postoperative data were obtained 1 or 2 months after surgery.

Address for correspondence: Hidetaka Yoshihashi, Department of Otolaryngology, Nihon University Surugadai Hospital, 1-8-13 Kanda-surugadai, Chiyoda-ku, Tokyo 101-8309, Japan. Tel.: +81-3-3293-1711. Fax: +81-3-3294-3199. E-mail: ent.hide@jc4.so-net.ne.jp

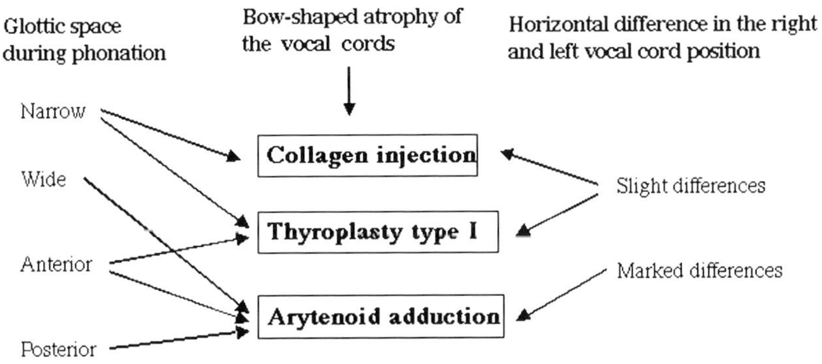

Fig. 1. Flow chart for the determination of surgical procedures.

Results

Figure 2 shows the phonatory function test results of the patients treated by the two different procedures. A comparison of the obtained data, before and after surgery, was made in cases where the difference in fundamental frequency was 20 Hz or smaller. Analyses were performed on the parameters of mean flow rate (MFR), expiratory lung pressure, expiratory aerodynamic power (the product of expiratory lung pressure and MFR), airway resistance (the expiratory lung

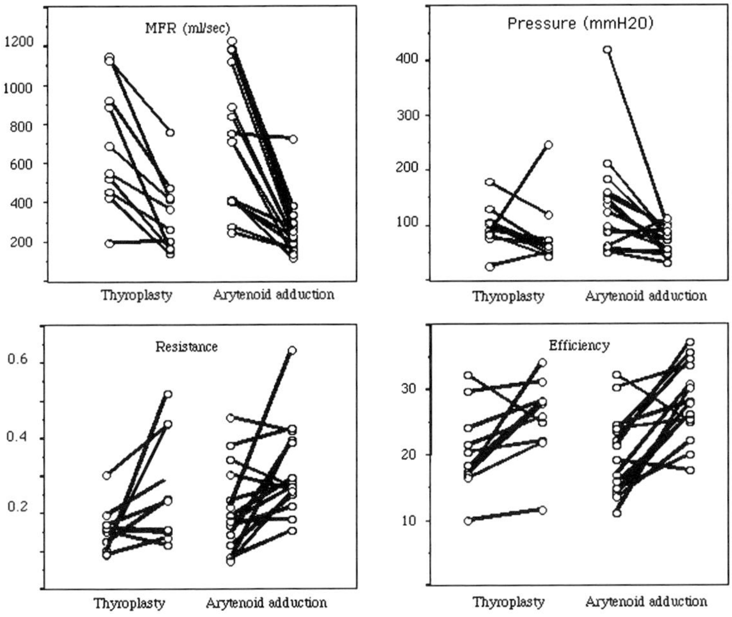

Fig. 2. Phonatory function assessments before and after surgery.

pressure per MFR quotient), and phonatory efficacy (the loudness of voice per expiratory aerodynamic power quotient) [1–3]. Compared with preoperative values, mean flow rate, expiratory lung pressure, and expiratory aerodynamic power decreased after surgery in most cases.

In the present study, phonatory function test results were analyzed in patients treated by thyroplasty type I or arytenoid adduction. Our indication criteria were considered to be basically valid. At the same time, it was suggested that the indication of surgery should be altered based on the patient's condition and disease course. We should respond flexibly to individual needs.

References

1. Shimazaki N, Makiyama K. Aerodynamic assessment of organic voice disorders using the airway interruption method. Practica Otologica 1995;88(Suppl78):39–52.
2. Makiyama K, Makiyama Y, Kida A. Effects of glottal space during phonation on phonatory function in subjects with recurrent laryngeal nerve paralysis. Nihon Univ J Med 1997;39(1): 1–13.
3. Makiyama K, Kida A, Sawashima M. Evaluation of expiratory effort on dysphonic patients on increasing vocal intensity. Otolaryngol Head Neck Surg 1998;118(5):723–727.

Laryngeal speech

Bronchology and Bronchoesophagology: State of the Art.
H. Yoshimura et al., editors.

Light emitting diode laryngo-stroboscope

Tadashi Ishimaru, Kazuhira Endo, Takaki Miwa and Mitsuru Furukawa
Department of Otolaryngology, School of Medicine, Kanazawa University, Kanazawa, Japan

Abstract. The xenon lamp laryngo-stroboscope is a useful piece of equipment for diagnosing diseases of the vocal cord. However, it is heavy and requires a high-voltage power supply. We created a light-emitting diode (LED) laryngo-stroboscope to overcome the drawbacks of the xenon lamp stroboscope. The LED laryngo-stroboscope is constructed of a micro CCD camera with a LED stroboscope. When the probe is inserted into a subject, via the mouth, it is possible to obtain a stroboscopic video view of the vocal cords. The LED laryngo-stroboscope is a new light-weight, battery-operable instrument for laryngology.

Keywords: CCD, endoscope, larynx, vocal cords.

Introduction

It is difficult to observe vocal cord movement due to its speed. Therefore, a stroboscope [1–3], high-speed movie [4,5] and high-speed video [6] were applied for the observation of the vocal cords. The stroboscope is a particularly useful piece of equipment for diagnosing diseases of the vocal cord. The xenon lamp light source of the stroboscope is sizable and requires a high-voltage power supply. The laryngo-stroboscope is also heavy to lift and expensive. As a solution to these problems, we constructed a laryngo-stroboscope with a light-emitting diode (LED) light source (Table 1).

Materials and Methods

The LED stroboscope is composed of a probe and a control unit (Fig. 1). The probe is equipped with LEDs and a small charge couple device (CCD) video camera is inserted into the pharynx via the mouth (Fig. 2). As the red LED is pulsed synchronously to the vibration of the vocal cords, the stroboscopic vocal cord movement is observed via the CCD video camera, as stroboscopic observation is monochrome under a red LED. The frequency of LED pulses is manually controlled by the processor. In nonstroboscopic mode, a white LED is used and color video laryngoscopy is possible.

Address for correspondence: Dr Tadashi Ishimaru, Department of Otolaryngology, School of Medicine, Kanazawa University, 13-1 Takaramachi, Kanazawa 920-8640, Japan. Tel.: +81-76-265-2413. Fax: +81-76-234-9265.

Table 1. LED vs. xenon. The characteristics of the LED and xenon lamp strobocopes.

	Type	Voltage (V)	Weight	Observation	Color	Cost
LED	Solid state	2–3	Light	CCD	Red	Cheap
Xenon	Tube	1000–1500	Heavy	Endoscope + CCD	White	Expensive

Results

A 25-year-old man with normal vocal cords was observed. Vocal cord movement was observed using the stroboscope and was displayed in slow motion via a TV monitor (Fig. 3).

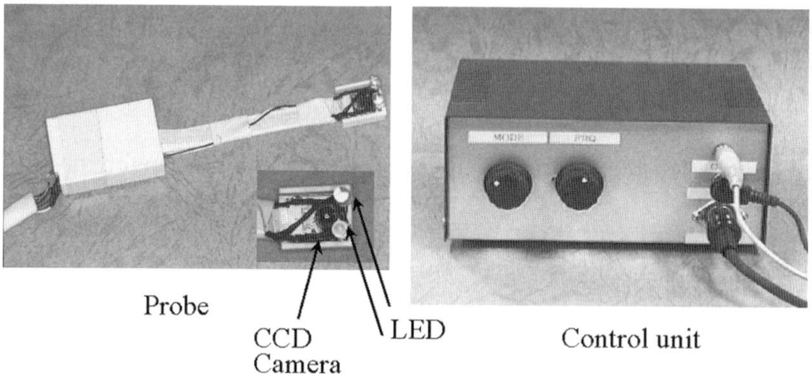

Fig. 1. An external view of the LED laryngo-stroboscope. The system is composed of a probe and a control unit. The CCD camera and LEDs are located in the tip of the probe. The control circuit and batteries are inside the control unit.

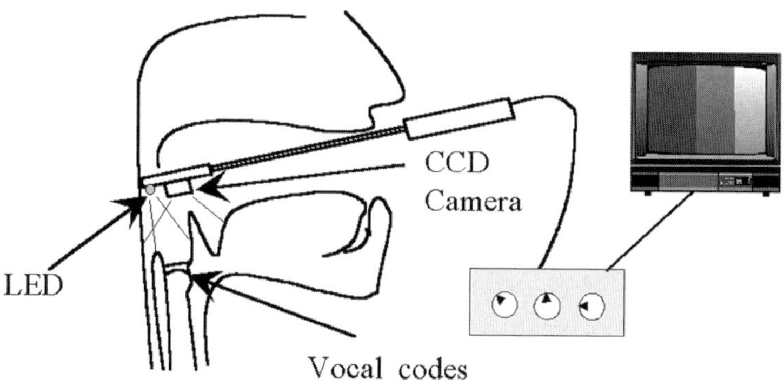

Fig. 2. How to use the LED laryngo-stroboscope. The LED laryngo-stroboscope is inserted into the pharynx via the mouth and the stroboscopist observes the vocal cords on a monitor.

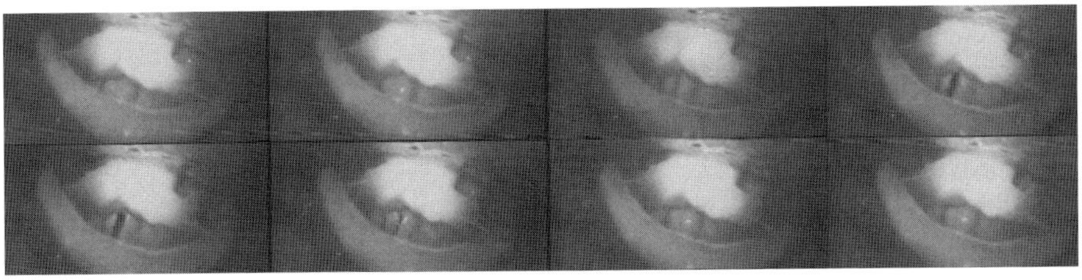

Fig. 3. LED stroboscopic observation. The movement of the vocal cords. One cycle of movement, composed of eight pictures, left to right and upper to lower, is visible.

Discussion

Though the amount of light emitted by the LED is not powerful enough for observation of the vocal cords via an endoscope, a direct CCD camera view, without the endoscope, resolved the problem of insufficient LED light power. Only monochrome observation was performed by our LED stroboscope as the aim of stroboscopy is the observation of vocal cord movement, not of vocal cord color. Monochrome observation is not considered to be a detriment. Replacing the red LED with a white LED may make color LED laryngo-stroboscopy possible.

The high voltage of the xenon lamp is sometimes dangerous. The LED requires only a few volts of power and is, therefore, very safe for the subject and the stroboscopist. As the LED is made of a semiconductor, it has a long life. The xenon lamp, made of a glass tube, is more easily broken and has a shorter life than the LED. The cost performance of the LED laryngo-stroboscope is also superior to the xenon lamp laryngo-stroboscope. The xenon lamp laryngo-stroboscope is thought to be 5 times as expensive as the LED one. Though the LED laryngo-stroboscope has some weak points, it is expected that these will be resolved in the near future, as semiconductor technology becomes further developed.

References

1. Oertel MJ. Das Laryngo-stroboskop und die laryngo-stroboskopishe Untersuchung. Arch Laryngol Rhinol 1895;3:1–16.
2. Schonharl E. Die Stroboskopie in der praktischen Laryngologie. Stuttgart: Georg Theme, 1960.
3. von Leden H. The electric synchron-stroboscope. Its value for practicing laryngologist. Ann Otol Rhinol Laryngol 1961;70:881–893.
4. Fransworth DW. High-speed motion pictures of human vocal cords. Bell Laboratories Records 1940;18:203–208.
5. Hirano M, Yoshida Y, Matsushita H, Nakajima T. An apparatus for ultra-high-speed cinematomography of the vocal cords. Ann Otol Rhinol Laryngol 1974;83:12–18.
6. Hirose H. High-speed digital imaging of vocal fold vibration. Acta Otolaryngol 1988;458: 151–153.

Bronchology and Bronchoesophagology: State of the Art.
H. Yoshimura et al., editors.

The regional blood flow to the human vocal cords when at rest and after phonation

Yoshihiro Iwata[1], Toshihiro Ohyama[1], Noburo Inazuka[1], Seiji Sugiura[1], Kenji Takeuchi[2], Shouji Saito[2], Hiroshi Kadoyama[2], Kensei Naito[2], Hitoshi Toda[3] and Tatuyoshi Okada[3]

[1]Hekinan Municipal Hospital, Hekinan; [2]Department of Otolaryngology, Fujita Health University, Toyoake; and [3]JA Chita Kousei Hospital, Mihama, Chita, Aichi, Japan

Abstract. Much attention has been paid to the blood flow to the vocal cords (VBF) at rest, during phonation, and after smoking. However, it is difficult to perform continuous noninvasive measurements in humans. In this study, we measured VBF continuously in 15 volunteers with normal vocal cords by using a laser blood flow meter (ALF 21 Advance Co.), which is a sensitive technique for determining the changes in VBF. A history of smoking did not significantly influence the increase in VBF associated with phonation. However, the VBF was found to decrease immediately after smoking. Longer phonation was associated with a longer recovery time of the VBF.

Keywords: blood flow, normal human vocal cord, phonation, smoking.

Background

Several studies have suggested, using changes in the oxygen use tension to estimate blood flow, that during phonation, ischemic changes occur in the lamina propria and muscularis layer of the vocal cords [1–3]. There are similar reports from studies using the microsphere surface technique to estimate blood flow [3,4]. However, these techniques cannot continuously record the changes in the blood flow to the vocal cords. The use of a blood flow meter to estimate the blood flow is an invasive and complex method. This method has been used to study blood flow to the nasal mucosa [5–7]. In this study, a laser blood flow meter was used to measure the blood flow to the vocal cord mucous membrane (VBF). Since sampling was performed in cycles 10 Hz higher than the pulse rate, the changes in the blood flow with each pulse could be determined. We measured the changes in VBF associated with ordinary phonation, higher pitched phonation and prolonged phonation, and recorded the recovery times under each of these conditions. Since it is believed that smoking influences the VBF, we also measured an after smoking condition.

Address for correspondence: Yoshihiro Iwata MD, Hekinan Municipal Hospital, 3-6 Heiwa, Hekinan, Aichi 447-8502, Japan. Tel.: +81-566-48-5050. Fax: +81-566-48-5065.
E-mail: yiwata@fujita-hu.ac.jp

Table 1. Subject characteristics.

Sex (male/female)	15/0
Median age (years)	31
Smoking status (never/current)	7/8

Methods

We measured the VBF in 15 volunteers with normal vocal cords according to the following procedure (Table 1):

1. Adequate local superficial anesthesia administered to the nasal cavity, pharynx and larynx.
2. The probe was placed vertically on the surface of the central portion of the vocal cord visualized via a flexible fiberoptic laryngoscope (Fig. 1). The VBF was recorded continuously by a laser blood flow meter (ALF21 Advance Co.).
3. The mean VBF was evaluated before, 5 to 10 s after, and 1 min after 1 min of continuous and ordinary phonation (Fig. 2). Similar measurements were made after 1 min of high-pitched phonation, 5 min of ordinary phonation, and after smoking. The recovery time was calculated for each of the conditions. The Student's t test was used for comparison between groups, and a probability value of less than 0.05 was considered to denote the statistical significance.

Results

The blood flow to the oral mucous membrane was 23.4 to 38.4 ml/min/100 g (mean 31.3). In the quiet state, nonsmokers' VBF were 22.4 to 35.8 ml/min/100 g (mean 27.6), and smokers' VBF were 16.1 to 26.8 ml/min/100 g (mean 21.3). Blood flow to the oral mucous membrane was significantly higher than VBF ($p < 0.02$).

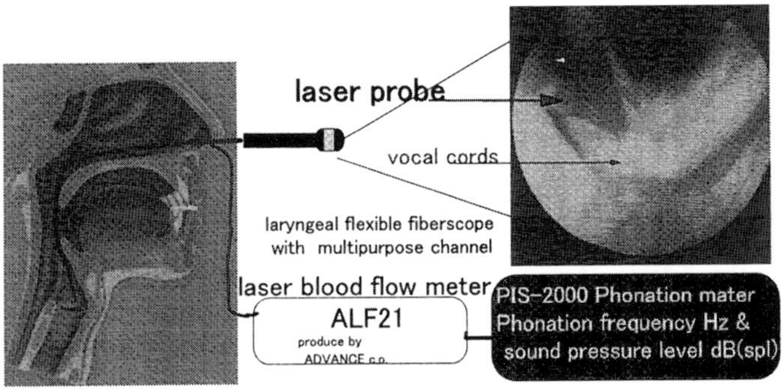

Fig. 1. Methods.

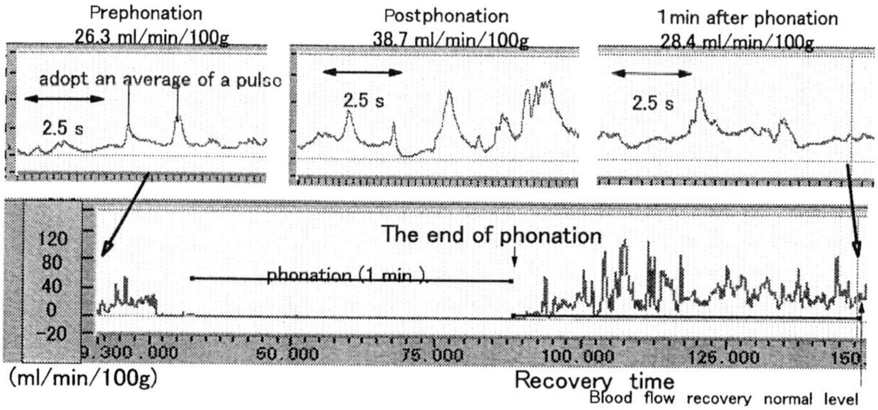

Fig. 2. Sample display of VBF.

Ordinary phonation for 1 min (Fig. 3)

Immediately after ordinary phonation for 1 min, the VBF increased (mean for nonsmokers: 67.4 ml/min/100 g, mean for smokers: 50.5 ml/min/100 g, average: 61.2 ml/min/100 g). The values returned to those of the quiet state within 1 min. There were no significant differences between the values of VBF immediately after 1-min phonation in smokers and those in nonsmokers. However, the VBF immediately after 1-min phonation was significantly higher than that before phonation ($p<0.05$) and that at 1 min after the phonation ($p<0.05$).

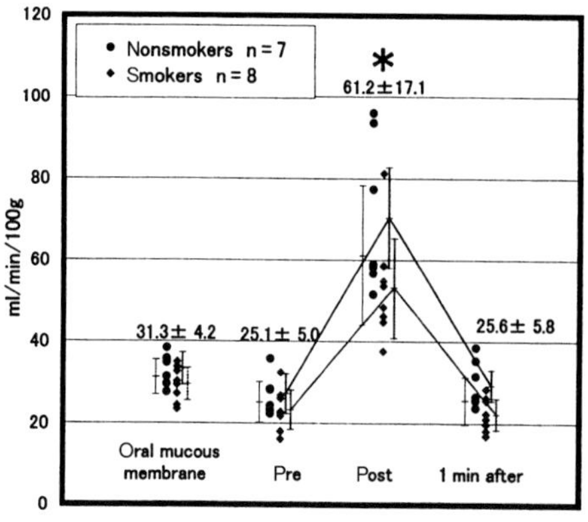

Fig. 3. Change in VBF associated with phonation for 1 min. Pre and post ordinary phonation for 1 min.

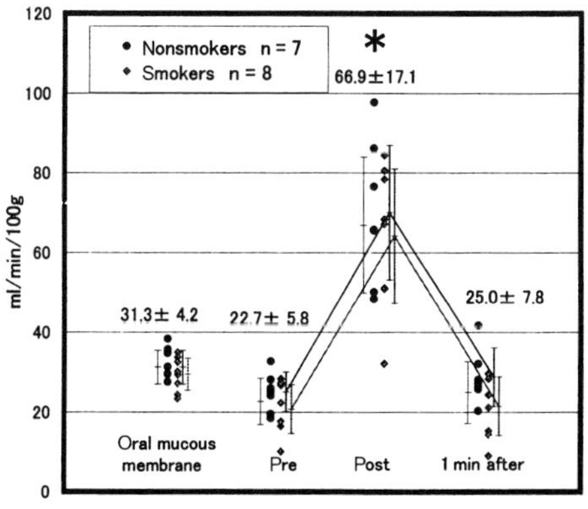

Fig. 4. Change in VBF associated with high-pitched phonation. Pre and post high-pitched phonation for 1 min.

High-pitched phonation for 1 min (Fig. 4)

Immediately after high-pitched phonation for 1 min, the VBF increased (mean for nonsmokers: 67.9 ml/min/100 g, mean for smokers: 63.0 ml/min/100 g, average: 64.5 ml/min/100 g).

Ordinary phonation for 5 min (Fig. 5)

Immediately after ordinary phonation for 5 min, the VBF increased (in nonsmokers it ranged from 44.0 to 96.5 ml/min/100 g, mean 67.7 ml/min/100 g). The VBF value after ordinary phonation for 5 min was significantly higher than the values recorded before phonation and those recorded after 1 min of phonation ($p < 0.01$).

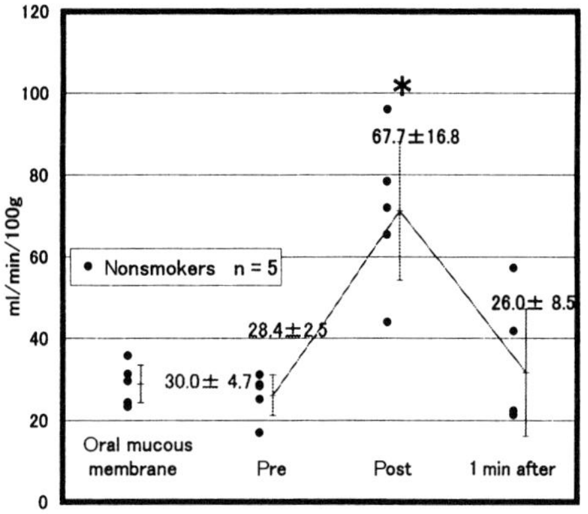

Fig. 5. Change in VBF associated with phonation for 5 min. Pre and post ordinary phonation for 5 min.

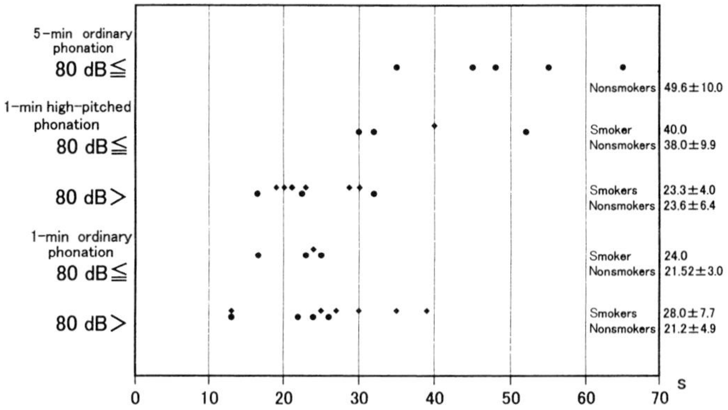

Fig. 6. Recovery time of VBF after phonation.

Recovery time of VBF after phonation (Fig. 6)

The recovery time after ordinary phonation for 1 min and high-pitched phonation for 1 min, ranged from 13 to 31 s (mean: 21). The recovery time after ordinary phonation for 5 min ranged from 45 to 65 s (mean: 50). Thus, the recovery time after 5-min phonation was longer than that after 1-min phonation.

The influence of smoking on VBF (Fig. 7)

VBF was measured after the subject smoked one cigarette. The VBF in eight smokers ranged from 20.4 to 41.8 ml/min/100 g (mean: 28.9) before smoking. The values after smoking ranged from 10.8 to 25.2 ml/min/100 g (mean: 18.3). The difference between the pre- and postsmoking VBF in the smokers was significant.

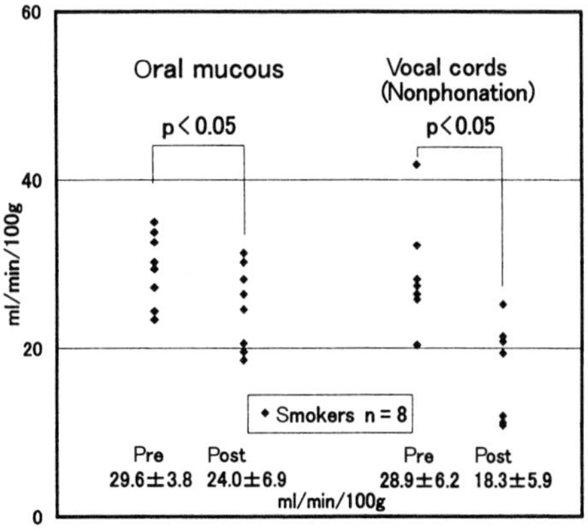

Fig. 7. Influence of smoking on VBF.

Discussion

Hirano et al. [8] and Matsuo et al. [9] carefully described the microvascular anatomy of the vocal cord. The vocal cord mucous vibrates with high frequency, and much attention is paid to the blood flow to the vocal cords. David et al. [4] measured the blood flow to the vocal cords by means of the microsphere surface technique. They determined a blood flow of 11.9 cc/min in canine vocal cords, and also demonstrated that the blood flow increased to 71 cc/min in association with phonation [5], which is consistent with our own results with regard to increased VBF associated with phonation.

In general, the vocal cords of smokers are congested. Thus, it was expected that the blood flow to the vocal cords, when smoking, might be increased. However, there was no significant difference in VBF in the quiet state between smoking and nonsmoking in this study.

Conclusions

1. Phonation requires an increase of VBF.
2. Longer phonation requires more recovery time of VBF.
3. A smoking history did not affect VBF with regard to phonation in this study.
4. However, the VBF reduced immediately after smoking.

Acknowledgements

This presentation is based on the joint research of the Fujita Health University and the Hekinan Municipal Hospital. I would like to express my sincere appreciation and gratitude to my colleagues, my hospital and the late Prof Shigenobu Iwata.

References

1. Hirano M. Structure of the vocal fold in normal and disease states. ASHA Rep 1981;11:11–27.
2. Hirano M. Phonosurgery: basic and clinical investigation. Otologia (In Japanese) 1975;21(Suppl 1): 254–260.
3. Hiroto I, Toyozumi Y, Tomita H et al. An experimental study on the circulation of the vibrating vocal fold. J Otolaryngol Jpn 1969;72:884–888.
4. Arnstein DP, Berke GS, Trapp TK, Bell T. Regional blood flow of the canine vocal cord: the microsphere surface technique. Otolaryngol Head Neck Surg 1990;103:371–376.
5. Arnstein DP, Berke GS, Trapp TK, Natividad M. Regional Blood flow to the canine vocal fold at rest and during phonation. Ann Otol Rhinol Laryngol 1989;98:798–802.
6. Ohyama M, Furuta S, Kurono Y et al. Reflectance spectrophotometric studies on mucosal pathology of the upper airway. Laryngoscope 1982;92:1168–1172.
7. Olsson P, Bende M, Ohlin P. The laser Doppler flowmeter for measuring microcirculation in human nasal mucosa. Acta Otolaryngol 1985;99:133–139.
8. Hiroto I, Toyozumi Y, Tomita H. An experimental study on the circulation of the vibrating vocal fold. J Otolaryngol Jpn 1969; 72:884–888.

9. Matsuo K, Masamichi O, Tomita M, Maehara N, Umezaki T, Shin T. An experimented study of the circulation of the vocal fold on phonation. Arch Otolaryngol Head Neck Surg 1987;113: 414–417.

Bronchology and Bronchoesophagology: State of the Art.
H. Yoshimura et al., editors.

Vocal fold vibration in unilaterally atrophied larynges

Joji Kobayashi[1], Eiji Yumoto[2] and Masamitsu Hyodo[1]
[1]*Department of Otolaryngology, School of Medicine, Ehime University, Onsen-gun, Ehime; and* [2]*Department of Otolaryngology – Head-Neck Surgery, School of Medicine, Kumamoto University, Kumamoto, Japan*

Abstract. *Background.* Considerable inconsistencies regarding the vibratory pattern of unilateral vocal fold paralysis (UVFP) have been reported. These inconsistencies are derived from differences in several factors among patients. The purpose of this study was to assess the effects of unilateral atrophy of the vocal fold (VF).

Methods. Seven excised canine larynges were studied, three normal larynges and four unilaterally atrophied larynges. The lateral and vertical displacements were monitored simultaneously with photoglottography and a laser Doppler vibrometer.

Results. The lateral amplitude was significantly greater than the vertical amplitude in all larynges. The Lissajous trajectories in the normal larynges were shaped like a reverse crescent. In the unilaterally atrophied larynges, the lateral and vertical amplitudes on the atrophied side were significantly greater than those on the normal side. The Lissajous trajectories differed from those of the normal larynges.

Conclusion. In the absence of a prephonatory glottal gap, periodical vibration occurs in unilaterally atrophied larynges. This implies that phonosurgical procedures aiming at closure of the prephonatory glottal gap may have a beneficial effect on hoarseness in UVFP patients, although displacements of the vocal folds during vibration are not symmetrical.

Keywords: laser Doppler vibrometer, Lissajous trajectory, recurrent laryngeal nerve paralysis, vocal fold atrophy.

Introduction

There are many inconsistencies regarding the vibratory mode of unilateral vocal fold paralysis (UVFP) [1–5]. The vibratory mode is determined by several factors including the position, shape, mass and stiffness of the vocal fold. To understand the mechanism of the abnormal vocal fold vibration in UVFP, it is necessary to examine the vibratory mode of the vocal fold with a single pathological factor. The purpose of this study was to assess the effects of unilateral atrophy of the vocal fold upon its vibratory mode in excised canine larynges. We examined the vibratory mode two-dimensionally with the aid of a laser Doppler vibrometer (LDV) and photoglottography (PGG).

Address for correspondence: Joji Kobayashi MD, Department of Otolaryngology, School of Medicine, Ehime University, Shigenobu-cho, Onsen-gun, Ehime 791-0295, Japan. Tel.: +81-89-960-5366. Fax: +81-89-960-5368. E-mail: joji@m.ehime-u.ac.jp

Materials and Methods

Seven healthy dogs (11 to 14 kg) were studied. Three dogs were assigned to the normal group (dogs 1—3) and the other four (dogs 4—7) were assigned to the paralysis group. The recurrent laryngeal nerve was removed unilaterally 4 months before phonation in the paralysis group. The excised canine larynx was fixed into a hole in a wooden box with a clay compound (Fig. 1). The bilateral vocal processes were sutured together to attain the glottal closure necessary for phonation. Moisture-saturated warm air was delivered to the box. In the paralysis group, the thyroid ala of the atrophied side was pressed medially with a clay compound to obtain sufficient glottal closure for steady phonation.

Lateral displacement of the vocal fold was measured using PGG. As the length of the vocal fold did not vary during phonation in our study, lateral displacement of the vocal fold could be assessed using the PGG output. Vertical displacement (superior-inferior direction) was measured using an LDV (OFV 3000 and OFV 302, Politec, Waldbronn, Germany) placed above the wooden box (Fig. 1). The output signals from the PGG and LDV were recorded simultaneously on a data recorder for later analysis. Videostroboscopic (LS-3E, Nagashima, Tokyo, Japan) analysis was also performed to calibrate PGG output. The average maximal displacement for the three cycles was converted into an absolute value in millimeters based on the number of pixels. Lissajous trajectories were drawn in each larynx by combining the PGG and LDV output. We defined the resting position of the vocal fold, just prior to the beginning of vibration, as the starting point for drawing the trajectories.

After experimental phonation, the larynges were sectioned serially in the frontal plane and stained with elastica van Gieson stain for histological examination.

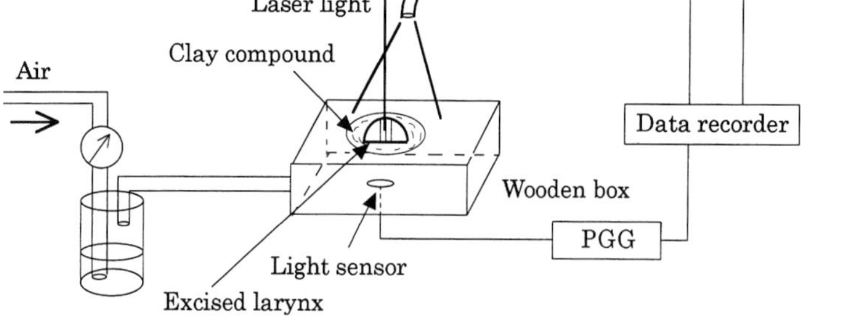

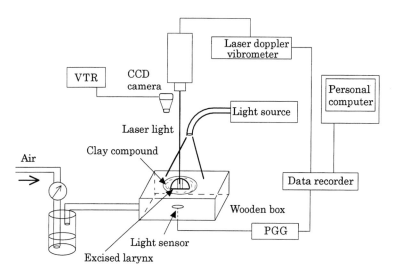

Fig. 1. The experimental set-up used to obtain PGG and LDV outputs.

Results

Normal group

Figure 2 shows the Lissajous trajectories of the vocal fold in a representative case (dog 1), for three airflow rates. The vocal fold moved upward and laterally, then moved laterally to reach the most upper lateral position, and finally moved straight back to the starting point. Thus, the trajectories were shaped like a reverse crescent. In the other larynges, the trajectories were essentially the same. The lateral amplitude was significantly greater than the vertical amplitude in all three larynges ($p < 0.05$ Wilcoxon test). As the airflow increased, the amplitude became greater in both directions.

Paralysis group

We were able to obtain steady phonation, with sufficient glottal closure, by pressing the thyroid ala medially on the atrophied side using a clay compound. Thus, the vocal fold vibrations in the unilaterally atrophied larynges were periodical and symmetric in phase. Figure 3 shows the Lissajous trajectories in a representative case (dog 4). They moved upward and laterally to reach the most upper lateral position, then moved downward and medially to reach the lowest position on the way back to the starting point. The trajectory on the atrophied side was much larger than that on the normal side. As the airflow increased, the Lissajous

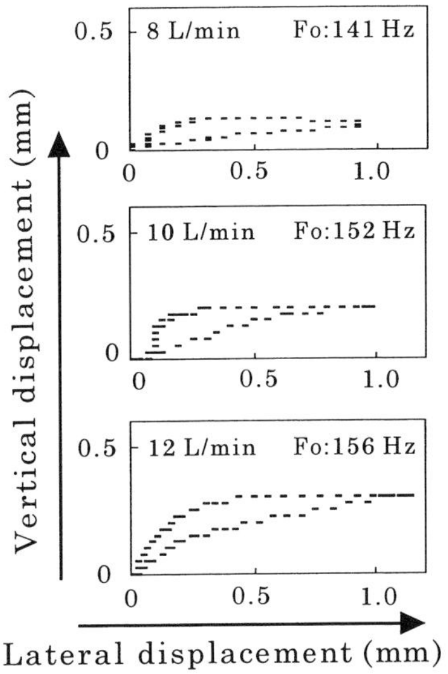

Fig. 2. Lissajous trajectories of the vocal fold in a representative case (dog 1) when the larynx was blown at three airflow rates. The horizontal and vertical axes represent lateral and vertical displacements of the vocal fold in millimeters, respectively.

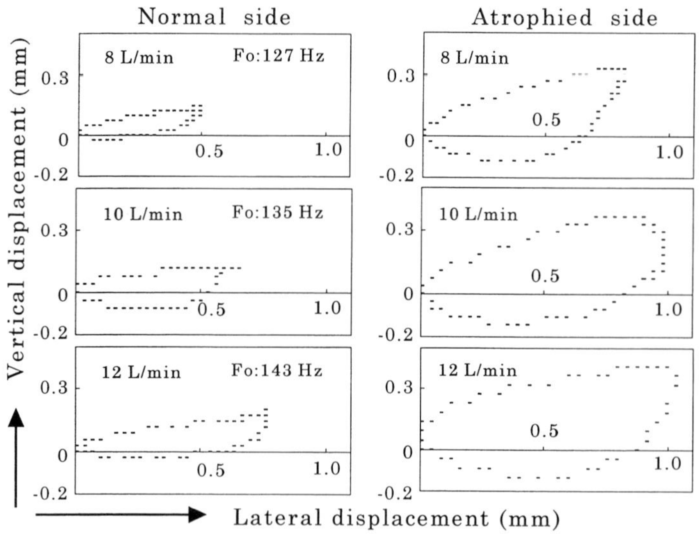

Fig. 3. Lissajous trajectories of the vocal fold in a representative case (dog 4) when the larynx was blown at three airflow rates. The horizontal and vertical axes represent lateral and vertical displacements of the vocal fold in millimeters, respectively.

trajectory became larger on both sides. The findings in the other three larynges (dogs 5—7) were similar. The lateral amplitude was significantly greater than the vertical amplitude in all four larynges ($p<0.05$, Wilcoxon test). The amplitude of the atrophied vocal fold was significantly greater than that of the normal vocal fold in the lateral and vertical directions ($p<0.05$, Wilcoxon test).

Histological examination

We observed that the muscle fibers in the thyroarytenoid muscle were thin and surrounded by fibrous tissue on the atrophied side. The lamina propria overlying the atrophic thyroarytenoid muscle was thinner than that on the normal side.

Discussion

Saito et al. [6] and Baer [7] reported the trajectories of a given point(s) on the vocal fold in excised canine larynges. Because they utilized X-ray or optical stroboscopy, they could capture only seven to 12 locations per cycle and thus, they drew Lissajous trajectories by manually connecting these locations. We drew Lissajous trajectories by combining digitized LDV and PGG outputs. We plotted between 60 and 80 locations per cycle. We followed a small medial part on the upper surface of the vocal fold, not a given point on the vocal fold.

UVFP, as a clinical entity, is the result of total or partial denervation of the RLN. Regeneration of nerve fibers may occur with or without misdirection

[8–9]. We allowed vocal fold atrophy to occur for 4 months after denervation until sacrifice. Even though partial reinnervation may have occurred, histological examination revealed the atrophic changes of the thyroarytenoid muscle. Atrophy reduces the mass and stiffness of the vocal fold and thus causes asymmetry between the vocal folds. In the atrophied larynges, the vibration was symmetrically in phase, while the amplitude of the atrophied fold was significantly greater than that of the normal fold in the lateral and vertical directions. This asymmetry in amplitude in the lateral and vertical directions may be explained by reduced stiffness of the atrophied vocal fold.

We were able to show that in the absence of a prephonatory glottal gap, a unilaterally atrophied canine larynx could produce periodical vibration with the atrophied vocal fold having a greater amplitude in the lateral and vertical directions. This implies that phonosurgical procedures aiming at closure of the prephonatory glottal gap may have a beneficial effect in UVFP patients.

References

1. Bless D, Hirano M, Feder R. Videostroboscopic evaluation of the larynx. Ear Nose Throat J 1987;66:289–296.
2. von Leden H, Moore P. Vibratory pattern of the vocal cords in unilateral laryngeal paralysis. Acta Otolaryngol 1961;53:493–506.
3. Fex S, Elmqvist D. Endemic recurrent laryngeal nerve paresis: correlation between EMG and stroboscopic findings. Acta Otolaryngol 1973;75:368–369.
4. Thompson DM, Maragos NE, Edwards BW. The study of vocal fold vibratory patterns in patient with unilateral vocal fold paralysis before and after type I thyroplasty with or without arytenoid adduction. Laryngoscope 1995;105:481–486.
5. Omori K, Kacker A, Slavit DH, Blaugrund SM. Quantitative videostroboscopic measurement of glottal gap and vocal function: an analysis of thyroplasty type I. Ann Otol Rhinol Laryngol 1996;105:280–285.
6. Saito S, Fukuda H, Isogai Y, Ono H. X-ray stroboscopy in vocal fold physiology. Tokyo: University of Tokyo Press, 1981:95–106.
7. Baer T. Observation of vocal fold vibration: measurement of excised larynges in vocal fold physiology. Tokyo: University of Tokyo Press, 1981:119–133.
8. Siribodhi C, Sundmaker W, Atkins JP, Bonner FJ. Electromyographic studies of laryngeal paralysis and regeneration of laryngeal motor nerves in dogs. Laryngoscope 1963;73:148–164.
9. Blitzer A, Jahn AF, Keidar A. Semon's law revisited: an electromyographic analysis of laryngeal synkinesis. Ann Otol Rhinol Laryngol 1996;105:764–769.

Bronchology and Bronchoesophagology: State of the Art.
H. Yoshimura et al., editors.

Neoglottis in a case of elephant-type voice reconstruction

Kiyoshi Makiyama[1], Ryuichi Kametani[1], Nahoko Shimazaki[1], Masayuki Sawashima[1], Akinori Kida[1], Seiji Niimi[2] and Motohiro Nozaki[3]

[1]Department of Otolaryngology, School of Medicine, Nihon University; [2]Research Institute of Logopedics and Phoniatrics, Faculty of Medicine, University of Tokyo; and [3]Department of Plastic and Reconstructive Surgery, School of Medicine, Tokyo Women's University, Tokyo, Japan

Abstract. In this study, we investigated neoglottic vibration in laryngectomized patients using a high-speed digital image recording system. The first case underwent total laryngectomy. The second case underwent laryngopharyngoesophagectomy with a free jejunal graft: elephant-type shunt. This technique uses a free jejunal graft to create an elephant-type shunt, aimed at improving the chance for successful voice restoration. Mucosal vibration is seen in the lumen of the jejunum. In contrast to esophageal speech, the neoglottis remains open during phonation with elephant-type shunt speech. We consider that when the expiratory air passes through the shunt to the jejunal lumen, the local mucosa is sucked by the Bernoulli effect to serve as a sound source. In patients using elephant-type shunt speech, the neoglottis may be created by an aerodynamic force, but not by muscle control. Thus, the location of the neoglottis is passively determined by the expiratory airflow and size of the jejunal lumen.

Keywords: esophageal speech, free jejunal autograft, high-speed digital imaging, total laryngectomy.

Introduction

In this study, we investigated neoglottic vibration in laryngectomized patients using a high-speed digital image recording system. The information about the location and movements of the neoglottis is essential to determine the best reconstruction material and the best surgical procedure for voice restoration in patients with head and neck cancer.

Methods

Dr Nozaki, one of our co-workers, attempted to create a shunt between the trachea and the free jejunal autograft, placed to reconstruct the missing part of the upper digestive tract in patients who have undergone combined resection of the larynx, pharynx, and cervical esophagus [1,2]. This method was named the "elephant-type" voice reconstruction. Figure 1 is a schematic drawing of elephant-type voice reconstruction. The high-speed digital imaging system was developed by the Research Institute of Logopedics and Phoniatrics, Faculty of

Address for correspondence: Kiyoshi Makiyama MD, Department of Otolaryngology, Nihon University Surugadai Hospital, 1-8-13 Kandasurugadai, Chiyoda, Tokyo 101-8309, Japan. Tel.: +81-3-3293-1711. Fax: +81-3-3294-3199. E-mail: makiyama@tokyo.email.ne.jp

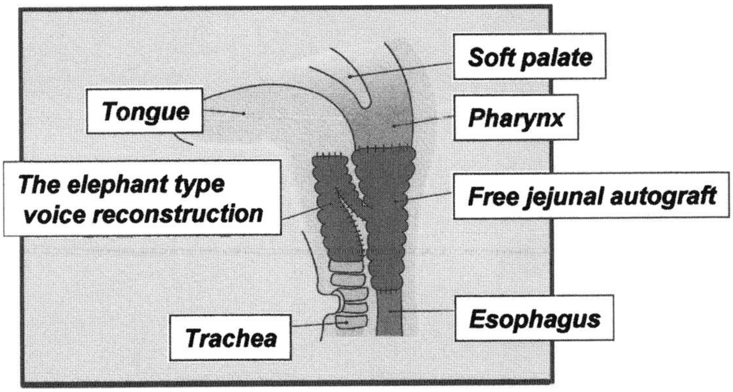

Fig. 1. A schematic drawing of elephant-type voice reconstruction.

Medicine, University of Tokyo. The present system takes 4,500 flames per second [3–5].

Results

The first case involved a 56-year-old man who underwent total laryngectomy. Figure 2 is a laryngoscopic finding in this patient during esophageal speech. In the high-speed digital imaging, the entrance portion of the esophagus was constricted circumferentially to close the lumen during phonation. Mucosal vibration started about 0.6 s after the esophageal closure. The mucosal surface of the hypopharynx protruded like a valve and vibrated.

The second case involved a 51-year-old man who underwent laryngopharyngoesophagectomy with a free jejunal graft: elephant-type shunt. Figure 3 is a laryngoscopic view of the neoglottis in this patient. In the high-speed digital imaging, mucosal vibration was seen in the lumen of the jejunum, which had a

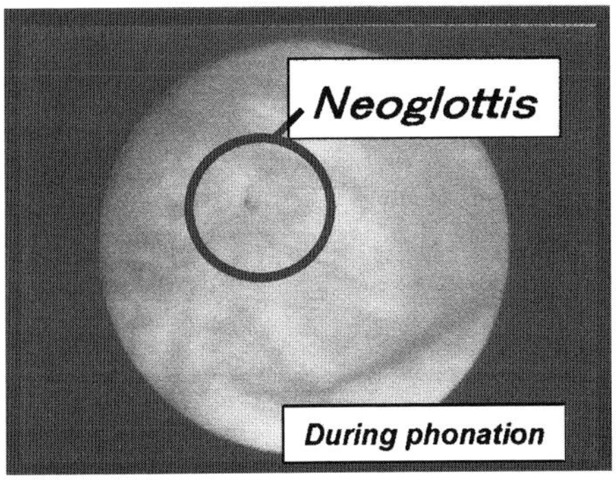

Fig. 2. A laryngoscopic finding in the case of esophageal speech.

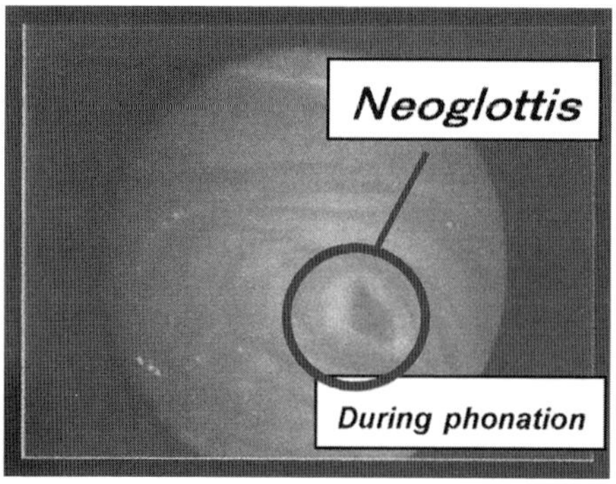

Fig. 3. A laryngoscopic finding in the case of elephant voice reconstruction.

funnel shape, and a smaller diameter at the more inferior part. The vibrating site was considered to be the neoglottis.

In contrast to esophageal speech, the neoglottis remains open during phonation with elephant-type shunt speech. We consider that when the expiratory air passes through the shunt to the jejunal lumen, the local mucosa is sucked by the Bernoulli effect to serve as a sound source.

Discussions

In patients using esophageal speech, voice control is performed by the neoglottis. Control is considered to be possible due to the preservation of the pharyngeal muscles. A voice with esophageal speech sounds close to the normal voice produced by the larynx. In patients using elephant-type shunt speech, however, the neoglottis may be created by an aerodynamic force but not by muscle control. Thus, the location of the neoglottis is determined by the expiratory airflow and size of the jejunal lumen.

References

1. Nozaki M, Sasaki K, Takeuchi M, Kida A, Sakamoto T, Takohda S. Reconstruction of neopharyngoesophagus and phonation following laryngopharyngoesophagectomy using a free intestinal graft. Head Neck Cancer 1997;23:547–552.
2. Sasaki K, Nozaki M, Ide H, Kida A, Takohda S, Kashima N, Ogawa K. Voice restoration after laryngopharyngoesophagectomy with a free jejunal graft: elephant-type shunt. J Jpn Broncho-esophagol Soc 1999;50:242–247.
3. Honda K, Kiritani S, Imagawa H, Hirose H, Hashimoto K. High-speed digital recording of vocal fold vibration using a solid-state image sensor. Ann Bull RILP 1985;47–53.
4. Imagawa H, Kiritani S, Hirose H. Further development in high-speed digital image recording system for assessment of vocal cord vibration. Ann Bull RILP 1987;9–23.
5. Kiritani S, Hirose H, Imagawa H. High-speed digital recording system for observing vocal cord vibration. Ann Bull RILP 1993;79–87.

Bronchology and Bronchoesophagology: State of the Art.
H. Yoshimura et al., editors.

Evaluation of the phonatory function after elephant-type voice reconstruction

Kiyoshi Makiyama[1], Nahoko Shimazaki[1], Akinori Kida[1], Masayuki Sawashima[1], Seiji Niimi[2] and Motohiro Nozaki[3]

[1]*Department of Otolaryngology, School of Medicine, Nihon University;* [2]*Research Institute of Logopedics and Phoniatrics, Faculty of Medicine, University of Tokyo; and* [3]*Department of Plastic and Reconstructive Surgery, School of Medicine, Tokyo Women's University, Tokyo, Japan*

Abstract. This study was conducted to investigate the neoglottis and phonatory function after elephant-type voice reconstruction using a free jejunal autograft in comparison with T-E shunts. Two patients undergoing different methods of voice restoration were investigated. The first case involved a patient with a T-E shunt of a skin flap after total laryngectomy. The second case involved a patient treated by elephant-type voice reconstruction using a jejunal autograft after combined resection of the larynx, hypopharynx, and cervical esophagus. Expiratory lung pressure during phonation was determined simultaneously along with the fundamental frequency, sound pressure level, and mean flow rate (MFR), using the phonatory function analyzer PS77E. In case 1, with the T-E shunt, both the expiratory lung pressure and MFR remained at a normal level. Airway resistance and expiratory aerodynamic power were at a high level in case 2. A phonatory efficacy index, which is the sound pressure per expiratory power quotient, was low in case 2.

Keywords: free jejunal autograft, high-speed digital imaging, mean flow rate, neoglottis, phonatory efficacy, T-E shunts.

Introduction

This study was conducted to investigate the neoglottis and phonatory function after elephant-type voice reconstruction using a free jejunal autograft in comparison with T-E shunts.

Subjects and Methods

The first case involved a patient with a T-E shunt of a skin flap after total laryngectomy. The second case involved a patient treated by elephant-type voice reconstruction using a jejunal autograft after combined resection of the larynx, hypopharynx, and cervical esophagus [1,2]. Expiratory lung pressure during phonation was determined simultaneously along with the fundamental frequency, sound pressure level, and mean flow rate (MFR), using the phonatory function analyzer NAGASHIMA PS77E [3,4].

Address for correspondence: Kiyoshi Makiyama MD, Department of Otolaryngology, Nihon University Surugadai Hospital, 1-8-13 Kandasurugadai, Chiyoda, Tokyo 101-8309, Japan. Tel.: +81-3-3293-1711. Fax: +81-3-3294-3199. E-mail: makiyama@tokyo.email.ne.jp

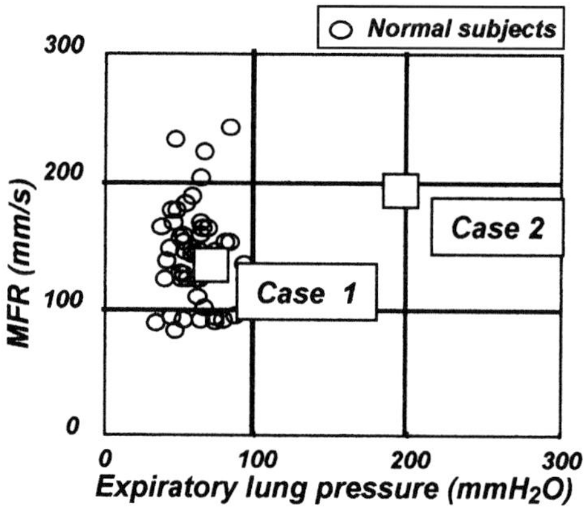

Fig. 1. The relationship between the expiratory lung pressure and mean flow rate.

Results

In Fig. 1, the horizontal axis expresses expiratory lung pressure, while the vertical axis expresses mean flow rate (MFR). The black squares represent data from the two patients, and the circles represent data from healthy male volunteers. In case 1, with the T-E shunt, both the expiratory lung pressure and MFR remained at a normal level. In case 2, with the elephant-type voice reconstruction, the pressure and MFR were at a high level. Figure 2 shows that the airway resistance, which is the expiratory lung pressure per MFR quotient, was highest in case 2. The expiratory aerodynamic power, which is the product of expiratory lung pressure and MFR, was also at a high level in case 2.

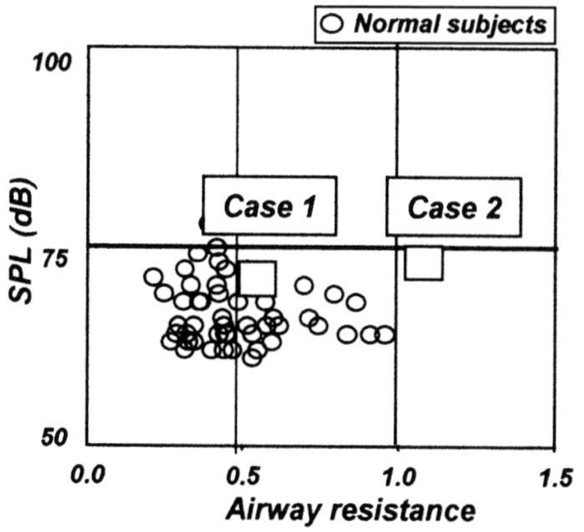

Fig. 2. The relationship between the sound pressure level and airway resistance.

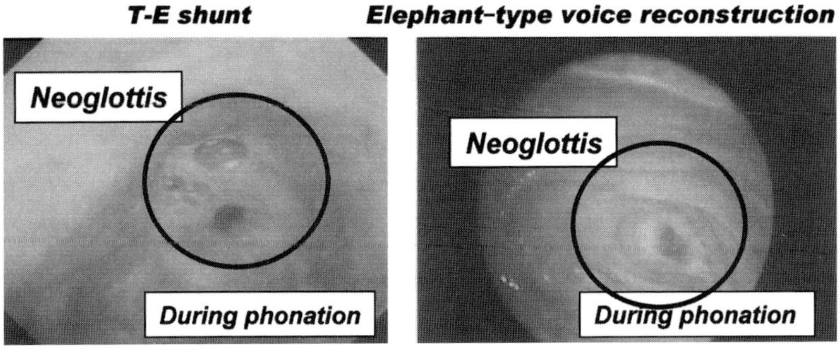

Fig. 3. Laryngoscopic findings of cases with T-E shunts and elephant-type voice reconstructions.

Discussion

Neoglottic mucosal vibration was observed using a high-speed imaging technique [5,6]. As shown in Fig. 3, the neoglottis was closed and vibrated during phonation in case 1. In case 2, the neoglottis vibrated without closure. The subglottal pressure should have been low in case 2, but why then did expiratory lung pressure show a high value? The lumen of the voice reconstruction site was narrow and possessed mucosal folds, and so airway resistance should have been high during expiration. In other words, a high expiratory lung pressure was required due to airway stenosis between the trachea and neoglottis. The voice quality of case 2 was "strained" and "breathy."

The phonatory function can be preserved by elephant-type voice reconstruction even in patients who have undergone combined resection of the larynx, pharynx, and cervical esophagus. Based on the present results, we wish to improve surgical techniques and training methods for better voice restoration.

References

1. Nozaki M, Sasaki K, Takeuchi M, Kida A, Sakamoto T, Takohda S. Reconstruction of neopharyngoesophagus and phonation following laryngopharyngoesophagectomy using a free intestinal graft. Head Neck Cancer 1997;23:547–552.
2. Sasaki K, Nozaki M, Ide H, Kida A, Takohda S, Kashima N, Ogawa K. Voice restoration after laryngopharyngoesophagectomy with a free jejunal graft: elephant-type shunt. J Jpn Broncho-esophagol Soc 1999;50:242–247.
3. Makiyama K, Makiyama Y, Kida A. Effects of glottal space during phonation on phonatory function in subjects with recurrent laryngeal nerve paralysis. Nihon Univ J Med 1997;39(1): 1–13.
4. Makiyama K, Kida A, Sawashima M. Evaluation of expiratory effort on dysphonic patients on increasing vocal intensity. Otolaryngol Head Neck Surg 1998;118(5):723–727.
5. Imagawa H, Kiritani S, Hirose H. Further development in high-speed digital image recording system for assessment of vocal cord vibration. Ann Bull RILP 1987;9–23.
6. Kiritani S, Hirose H, Imagawa H. High-speed digital recording system for observing vocal cord vibration. Ann Bull RILP 1993;79–87.

Bronchology and Bronchoesophagology: State of the Art.
H. Yoshimura et al., editors.

Control of voice intensity in tracheoesophageal phonation

Yasushi Mesuda[1], Noriko Nishizawa[1], Satoshi Fukuda[1], Makoto Takahashi[2] and Yukio Inuyama[1]

[1]*Hokkaido University School of Medicine; and* [2]*Hokkaido University School of Engineering, Sapporo, Japan*

Abstract. *Background.* It has been reported that tracheoesophageal (TE) speakers are able to modulate their voice intensity without a functioning larynx. The object of this study is to find the mechanism of their voice intensity control.

Subjects and Methods. The subjects were two TE speakers. EMG of the inferior pharyngeal constrictor (IPC) and geniohyoid muscle (GH), aerodynamic parameters and voice intensity were recorded simultaneously during steady phonation at various levels of intensity.

Results. One subject, who was examined once, revealed a positive relationship between subneoglottal pressure and voice intensity or IPC activity. The results indicated that IPC was increasingly activated against upcoming airflow. The other subject, who was examined twice, showed the same inter-relation between intensity, pressure and IPC activity, when first tested. In the second test, however, no correlation was found between these parameters. Instead, GH activity was positively related to voice intensity and efficiency. The results of the second test suggested that anterosuperior traction of the anterior wall of the pharyngoesophagus by GH was effective for modulating neoglottal efficiency.

Conclusion. The control mechanism of voice intensity in TE phonation was found to reside not only in respiratory effort, but in the moduration of the efficiency of the neoglottis itself.

Keywords: geniohyoid muscle, inferior pharyngeal constrictor, neoglottal efficiency, respiratory effort, subneoglottal pressure.

Background

In normal laryngeal speech, voice intensity is controlled by the coordination of respiratory effort along with laryngeal adjustment, which modulates glottal width, or the mass and tension of the vocal fold. It has been reported [1,2] that tracheoesophageal speakers are able to modulate their voice intensity, even without a functioning larynx. Therefore, it seems reasonable that driving power and the physical features of the vibrating source interact to control voice intensity in tracheoesophageal phonation, as well. The object of this study is to clarify the dominant factor in intensity control in tracheoesophageal phonation; is it driving power modulated by respiratory effort, the mass and tension of the neoglottis adjusted by muscle activity, or is it a combination of both.

During this study, special attention was paid to the function of the inferior

Address for correspondence: Yasushi Mesuda, Department of Otolaryngology, Hokkaido University, School of Medicine, Kita 15-Jo Nishi 7-chome, Kita-ku, Sapporo 060-8648, Japan. Tel.: +81-11-716-1161. Fax: +81-1-717-7566.

pharyngeal constrictor and the geniohyoid muscle. These two muscles have been thought to be associated with neoglottal adjustment. The inferior pharyngeal constrictor forms a protrusion in the posterior wall of the pharyngoesophageal segment after total laryngectomy and acts as a tensor of the neoglottis [3]. The geniohyoid muscle elicits an anterosuperior traction of the anterior wall of the pharyngoesophagus and is speculated to modulate the physical features of the neoglottis [4].

Methods

The subjects were two skilled tracheoesophageal speakers. One of them, subject 2, was tested twice at an interval of 2 years. The subjects were asked to repeat a set of steady phonation, ranging through three different intensity grades: soft, moderate and loud. Electromyogram of the inferior pharyngeal constrictor and geniohyoid muscle, subneoglottal pressure, flow rate and voice intensity were recorded simultaneously during phonation. 300-ms intervals, in each sustained phonation, within which the parameters were relatively stable, were sampled for processing. The averages of integrated electromyogram activities, subneoglottal pressure, flow rate and voice intensity were calculated for each sample.

The testing of the subjects was labelled as follows: testing of subject 1 is referred to as test 1; and that of subject 2, as test 2-1 and test 2-2, respectively.

Results and Summary

Comparison of the subjects' intentions to differentiate their voice intensity and the actual sound pressure monitored

In test 2-1, subject 2 was only able to change voice intensity when he made an effort to phonate loudly. Differentiation of intensity through the three grades was successfully achieved in test 1 and test 2-2.

Correlations between voice intensity and muscle activity

In test 1 and test 2-1, inferior pharyngeal constrictor activity increased as voice intensity became stronger. In test 2-2, however, no significant correlation was seen between voice intensity and inferior pharyngeal constrictor activity. Geniohyoid muscle activity was only monitored in test 1 and test 2-2. A positive correlation was seen between voice intensity and geniohyoid muscle activity in these tests.

Correlations between voice intensity and subneoglottal pressure

Test 1 and test 2-1 showed a positive relationship between voice intensity and subneoglottal pressure. Test 2-2, however, showed no significant relationship between these two parameters.

Table 1. Correlations with voice activity.

	Test 1	Test 2-1	Test 2-2
IPC activity	○	○	●
GH activity	○	—	○
Subneoglottal pressure	○	○	●
Neoglottal efficiency	○	○	○

○: positive correlation, ●: no correlation, —: not recorded.

Correlations between voice intensity and neoglottal efficiency

A positive correlation between voice intensity and neoglottal efficiency was seen in all tests.

Summary of the results mentioned so far (Table 1)

In test 1, positive correlations were found between voice intensity and both muscle activity and subneoglottal pressure. In test 2-1, inferior pharyngeal constrictor activity and subneoglottal pressure also increased with voice intensity; however, geniohyoid muscle activity was not examined. In test 2-2, only geniohyoid muscle activity increased with voice intensity. No positive correlations were found between voice intensity and inferior pharyngeal constrictor activity or subneoglottal pressure.

We then further investigated whether muscle adjustment or subneoglottal pressure was more dominant in voice intensity control.

Correlations between neoglottal efficiency and the activity of the two muscles

A positive correlation was only found between geniohyoid muscle activity and neoglottal efficiency in test 2-2. Geniohyoid muscle activity in test 1 and inferior pharyngeal constrictor activity, in all tests, were not found to influence neoglottal efficiency, in spite of positive correlations between voice intensity and muscle activity as mentioned before.

Correlations between subneoglottal pressure and muscle activity

In test 1 and test 2-1, inferior pharyngeal constrictor activity was found to increase with increased subneoglottal pressure. In test 2-2, no significant relationship was found between these parameters.

Summarizing all the results (Table 2)

In test 1 and test 2-1, muscular control of the neoglottis is not thought to control neoglottal efficiency directly, but to be associated with respiratory effort through

Table 2. What is the dominant factor in voice intensity control?

	Respiratory effort	Neoglottal adjustment
Test 1 Test 2-1	■	□
Test 2-2	–	■ (only GH)

■: dominant, □: associated, –: not significant.

activation of the inferior pharyngeal constrictor against upcoming airflow. However, in test 2-2, geniohyoid muscle activity is thought to be associated with the differentiation of voice intensity through modulation of neoglottal efficiency.

Conclusion

We found two modes of voice intensity control in tracheoesophageal phonation. In test 1 and test 2-1, respiratory effort was the dominant factor in voice intensity control, and neoglottal adjustment was thought to be associated with respiratory effort. On the other hand, in test 2-2, control of neoglottal efficiency by neoglottal adjustment was the dominant factor in voice intensity control, and respiratory effort was not significant. It was found that the mode of differentiation of voice intensity was not uniform among the subjects using tracheoesophageal phonation.

References

1. Kinishi M et al. Aerodynamic studies of laryngectomees after the Amatsu tracheoesophageal shunt operation. Ann Otol Rhinol Laryngol 1986;95:181–184.
2. Fujimoto T et al. Mechanism of neoglottic adjustment for voice variation in tracheoesophageal speech. J Otolaryngol Jpn 1994:97:1009–1018.
3. Amatsu M et al. Surgical voice reconstruction following laryngectomy. Kobe University School of Medicine, 1992.
4. Mishizawa N et al. Neoglottal adjustment in tracheoesophageal and esophageal speech. Jpn J Logop Phoniatr 1998;39:468–476.

Bronchology and Bronchoesophagology: State of the Art.
H. Yoshimura et al., editors.

Reversible swelling of the subglottic mucosa in vocal cord dysfunction

Hiroshi Ogasawara and Jun Okita
Department of Otolaryngology, Hyogo College of Medicine, Nishinomiya, Japan

Abstract. The subglottic space has never been indicated as a cause of stridor and dyspnea in vocal cord dysfunction. Four subjects showed normal openings of the glottis on inspiration, but showed slight adduction of the vocal cords without marked anterior glottic closure and a minimal decrease in the relative glottic area, and audible stridor was produced by vibration of the swollen mucosa in the subglottis on expiration. The swollen mucosa of the subglottis in one subject, showed reactivity for epinephrine, and edema with fibrous tissue infiltration of inflammatory cells.

Keywords: dyspnea, paradoxical movement, stridor, subglottis, vocal cord.

Introduction

When the vocal cords paradoxically close without the aid of an identifiable organic disease, producing obstruction and leading to stridor, the condition has been called vocal cord dysfunction (VCD) [1-2]. Adduction occurs during inspiration or in both inspiratory and expiratory phases [2]. The patient has severe dyspnea and stridor with a spasm of the false and true vocal cords. However, the subglottic space has never been indicated as a cause of stridor and dyspnea.

Case

Case 1

A 68-year-old woman had had dyspnea sensation and a cough since the age of 37. These symptoms were more intense at night, and were provocated by exercise and cold air. At the age 60, nasolaryngoscopy showed a normal position of the vocal cords on inspiration, and slight adduction of the vocal cords on expiration (Fig. 1A). Audible stridor was produced by the vibration of the swollen mucosa in the subglottis (arrow). The relative glottic area on expiration for inspiration, as described by Hurbis et al. [3], was 64% during forced respiration. When epinephrine was sprayed in the larynx, mucosal swelling in the subglottic area and audible stridor were decreased. The relative glottic area was slightly increased

Address for correspondence: Hiroshi Ogasawara, Department of Otolaryngology, Hyogo College of Medicine, 1-1 Mukogawacho, Nishinomiya, Japan. Tel.: +81-798-45-6493. Fax: +81-798-45-2855. E-mail: hogasa@hyo-med.ac.jp

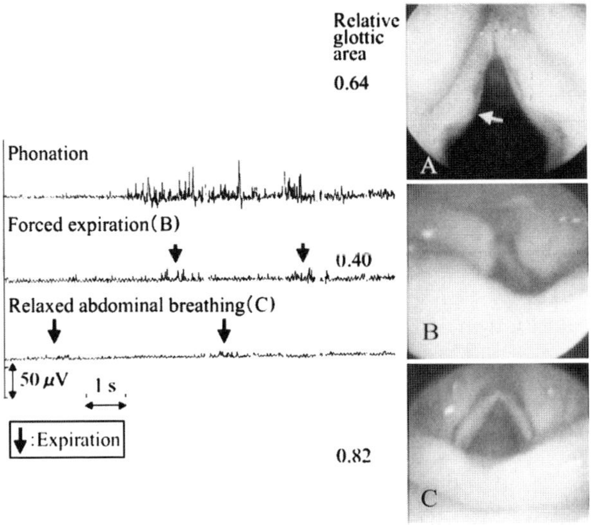

Fig. 1. The laryngoscopy and electromyogram from the lateral cricoarytenoid muscle in case 1.

from 64 to 75%. The challenge of exercise could decrease the arterial oxygen saturation from 92 to 87 with dyspnea and stridor.

At 67 years of age, the patient consented to laser therapy after receiving oral and written information. The bilateral subglottic mucosa was burnt to prevent a phonation disorder under laryngomicrosurgery. The pathology of the subglottic mucosa showed edema with fibrous tissue and infiltration of lymphocytes but not eosinophils. At 68 years of age, the patient noticed dyspnea and stridor again, but with tightly adducted true and false vocal cords on expiration (Fig. 1B), as presented previously. An electromyogram from the lateral cricoarytenoid muscle showed one-half of the evoked potential to be on forced expiration compared with phonation (Fig. 1). Relaxed abdominal breathing changed to having almost no waveform during both expiratory and inspiratory phases, and the relative glottic area recovered from 40 to 82% (Fig. 1C).

Four cases involved mild glottic obstruction as shown in Table 1. All cases

Table 1. Demographic data of patients with VCD.

Subject	Sex	Age (years)	Vocal cord adduction	Subglottis swelling	Cause	Allergy	FEV1	Flow-volume loop	Relative glottic area
1	F	68	Moderate	Moderate	Exercise	None	59	Normal	0.64
2	M	51	Mild	Moderate	Exercise	None	58	Normal	0.70
3	F	51	Mild	Moderate		Asthma	68	Normal	0.77
4	F	65	Moderate	Moderate	Stress	Asthma, nose	69	Normal	0.79

showed normal openings of the glottis on inspiration, but adduction of the vocal cords on expiration. The flow-volume loop in both expiration and inspiration was normal in the ordinary condition. Stridor was produced by the narrowing of the subglottis and the vibration of subglottic mucosa, whereas subglottic swelling and adduction of the vocal cords were mild or moderate.

Discussion

In normal subjects, the vocal cords are abducted throughout the respiratory cycle, although there may be a slight adduction at the end-expiratory phase. The histopathology of case 1 showed edema with fibrous tissue and inflammatory cells. As confirmation of glottic adduction, we performed an electromyogram, which showed that forced expiration irritated the subglottic mucosa, and caused swelling of the mucosa. Baier reported that upper-airway resistance depended on both the flow and the area of the glottis [4]. Forced expiration and glottic narrowing caused increased glottic resistance, and increased negative pressure may cause protrusion and edema of the subglottic mucosa. Despite the airway being sufficient, decreased arterial oxygen saturation and dyspnea sensation developed. The pathophysiologic mechanisms were not clear, but these data suggested that slight adduction and acute or chronic swelling of the subglottis caused stridor and dyspnea.

VCD can be precipitated by stress, exercise, cold air, upper respiratory infections and gastro-oesophageal reflux. When shortness of breath is sensed during an asthma attack or exercise, efforts are made to breathe out strongly. This state connected with the adduction of the vocal cords on expiration, causes increased tension of the laryngeal muscle. Edema of the mucosa in the subglottis increases, and causes stridor and dyspnea. In psychiatrically impaired cases, such as case 1, treatment is difficult, even though the mechanism is explained repeatedly, and treatment with relaxant therapy and voice therapy is initiated.

In summary, many asthmatics may show subglottic swelling as a cause of wheezes and dyspnea, whereas there were no typical VCD findings such as anterior vocal cord closure with a posterior diamond-shaped passage.

References

1. Rogers JH, Steel PM. Clinical records: paradoxical movement of the vocal cords as a cause of stridor. J Laryngol Otol 1978;92:157–158.
2. Wood RP, Milgrom H. Vocal cord dysfunction. J Allergy Clin Immunol 1996;98:481–485.
3. Hurbis CG, Schild JA. Laryngeal changes during exercise and exercise-induced asthma. Ann Otol Rhinol Laryngol 1991;100:34–37.
4. Baier H. Relationships among glottis opening, respiratory flow, and upper airway resistance in humans. J Appl Physiol 1977;43:603–611.

Bronchology and Bronchoesophagology: State of the Art.
H. Yoshimura et al., editors.

Autogenous fat injection for sulcus vocalis

Etsuyo Tamura, Satoshi Kitahara, Naoyuki Kohno, Taichi Furukawa and Masami Ogura
Department of Otorhinolaryngology, National Defense Medical College, Saitama, Japan

Abstract. *Background.* Although it is well known that surgical treatment for sulcus vocalis is extremely difficult, we have injected various materials into vocal folds to create new vocal fold free edges. We obtained good results by using autogenous fat as the injection material.

Methods. Two subjects with a sulcus vocalis were treated with an intracordal injection of autogenous fat harvested by suction from the abdominal wall. Voice production was evaluated prior to the injection and at intervals after the injection, using subjective, perceptual aerodynamic acoustic, and videostroboscopic assessments.

Results. The postoperative voice was significantly better than the preoperative in some parameters.

Conclusions. This is a preliminary report on fat injection for sulcus vocalis. Although the follow-up has been short, these encouraging early results and the great advantage of autogenous material for laryngeal injection warrant this preliminary report of this approach.

Keywords: dysphonia, phonosugery, vocal rehabilitation.

Introduction

The presence of a sulcus in the vocal fold may produce dysphonia, not only because of insufficient glottal closure, i.e., spindle-shaped glottal chink, but also mainly as a result of distortion or even the absence of a wave-like movement of the mucous. The treatments suggested have included vocal rehabilitation and/or surgery. Vocal rehabilitation has shown improvements through elimination of poor compensatory movements, but it is of limited aid to vocal quality. We succeeded in creating a new free edge of the vocal fold using autogenous fat injection.

Case reports

Case 1

A 67-year-old housewife has a 2-year history of the progressive weakness of her voice. During phonation, bowing and sulci of both vocal folds and a marked adduction of the bilateral ventricular folds were recognized.

Address for correspondence: Etsuyo Tamura MD, Department of Otolaryngology, National Defense Medical College, 3-2 Namiki, Tokorozawa-city, Saitama 359-8513, Japan. Tel.: +81-42-995-1686. Fax: +81-42-996-5212.

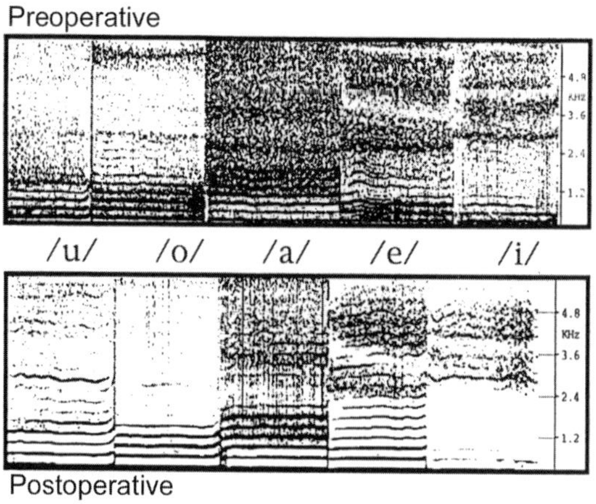

Fig. 1. Case 1. Sound spectrograms of vowels before and after injection.

Case 2

A 43-year-old office worker has noted hoarseness for 20 years. His voice quality had become worse recently.

Procedure

The procedures were performed under general anesthesia. The fat was harvested from the abdominal wall with a liposuction canula. Fat was injected through the crico-thyroid ligament with a 16-gauge needle.

Results

Subjective improvements were much better in both cases 8 weeks after injections, and videostroboscopic findings confirmed improved glottal closure during phonation, improved vibratory activity, and better symmetry. Objective voice analysis and sound spectrograms of vowels confirmed improvement in both subjects (Fig. 1 and Table 1). This was reflected in a reduction in perturbation measure

Table 1. Case 1. Summary of objective voice analysis results.

Assessment measures	Preinjection	Postinjection
GRBAS	R1A1B2S0	R1A0B1S1
M.F.R. (s)	10.1	12.5
Fo range (Hz)	273	29.4
Jitter (%)	2.19	2.26
Shimmer (%)	4.72	0.26
Harmonic noise ratio (dB)	6.04	16.4

(shimmer) and an increase in harmonic-to-noise ratio. Transglottic airflow was somewhat variable, but maximum phonation time tended to increase. However, the follow-up period for case 1 has only been 3 months as compared with 2 years for case 2, and so a longer follow-up is necessary.

Discussion

Several injectable materials have been used [1,2] on sulcus vocalis. Takayama et al. [3] and Remacle et al. [4] reported the use of a collagen injection for sulcus vocalis. Mikaelian et al. [5] reported autogenous fat injection therapy as an intervention for unilateral vocal fold paralysis. Fat is considered to be the ideal material for injection, because it is well tolerated by the body, it is the patient's own tissue, it does not become stiff, it does not appear to be extensively reabsorbed, and it can be delivered easily. We used autogenous fat to create a new free edge of the vocal fold that enabled the improvement of vibration during phonation. Therefore, we believe that autogenous fat injection can be an alternative, not only for unilateral vocal fold paralysis, but also for sulcus vocalis.

References

1. Lee ST, Niimi S. Vocal fold sulcus. J Laryngol Otol 1990;104:876–878.
2. Tanaka S, Hirano M, Tanaka Y, Fujita M. Transcutaneous intrafold injection result and its influencing factors. J Otolaryngol Jpn 1991;94:817–822.
3. Takayama E, Fukuda H, Kawaida M, Kawasaki Y, Sakoh T, Ohtsuki J, Inoue Y, Tomizawa I. Intracordal injection of atelocollagen for sulcus vocalis. J Jpn Bronchoesophagol 1990;41: 196–201.
4. Remacle M, Lowson G, Degols JC, Evrard I, Jamart J. Microsurgery of sulcus vergeture with carbon dioxide laser and injectable collagen. Ann Otol Rhinol Laryngol 2000;109:141–148.
5. Mikaelinan DO, Lowry LD, Sataloff RT. Lipoinjection for unilateral vocal cord paralysis. Laryngoscope 1991;101:465–468.

Bronchology and Bronchoesophagology: State of the Art.
H. Yoshimura et al., editors.

EGG and PGG for a high-speed digital imaging analysis of vocal fold vibration

Jun Yamanaka[1], Makito Okamoto[1], Hajime Hirose[2], Seiji Niimi[3], Shigeru Kiritani[3], Hiroshi Imagawa[3], Yoshitake Iwamoto[3] and Miyoko Ishige[3]

[1]*Department of Otolaryngology, Kitasato University School of Medicine, Sagamihara University School of Medicine;* [2]*School of Allied Health Science, Kitasato University, Sagamihara; and* [3]*Graduate School of Medicine, University of Tokyo, Tokyo, Japan*

Abstract. Simultaneous recordings of EGG, PGG and high-speed digital imaging of vocal fold vibration were made in three normal male subjects and the results were compared to evaluate the usefulness of EGG and PGG for the analysis of the vibratory pattern. Each subject was required to produce sounds of three different pitches at three different intensity levels in the recording sessions and the 27 sets of data samples were collected. For each data set, the glottal area waveform (GAW), glottal width waveform (GWW), EGG, differentiated EGG, PGG, differentiated PGG, and voice waveform were displayed in a graphic form on the same time axis and their patterns were compared. Based on the analysis of GAW and GWW, it was found that there were variations in the pattern of the closing and opening of the vocal fold margin corresponding to the differences in the type of phonation. The EGG waveform appeared to correspond well to that of the movement of the vocal fold margin in the closing phase, while this correspondence was less apparent in the opening phase. It is considered that the EGG waveform is dependent on the mode of contact between the two vocal folds and that careful observation of the EGG is useful and practical for predicting the pattern of vocal fold vibration.

Keywords: EGG, high-speed digital imaging, PGG, vocal fold vibration.

Background

Simultaneous recordings of EGG, PGG and high-speed digital imaging (HSDI) of vocal fold vibration [1] were made in three normal male subjects and the results were compared to evaluate the usefulness of EGG and PGG for the analysis of the vibratory pattern (Fig. 1).

Methods

Each subject was required to produce sounds of three different pitches at three different intensity levels in the recording sessions and the 27 sets of data samples were collected. The tasks were as follows: 1-a: low tone soft, 1-b: low tone medium, 1-c: low tone loud, 2-a: easy phonation soft, 2-b: easy phonation medium,

Address for correspondence: Jun Yamanaka MD, Kitasato University School of Medicine, 1-15-1 Kitasato, Sagamihara-shi, Kanagawa 228-8555, Japan. Tel.: +81-042-778-8111. Fax: +81-042-778-8607. E-mail: junymnk@med.kitasato-u.ac.jp

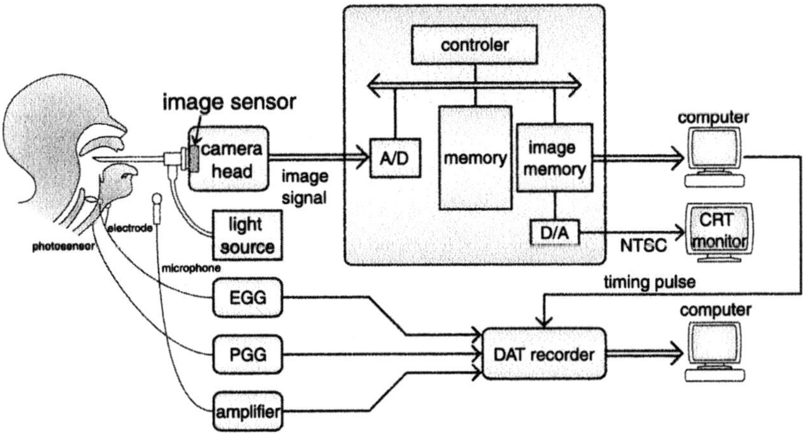

Fig. 1. Block diagram of a high-speed digital imaging system study with EGG and PGG.

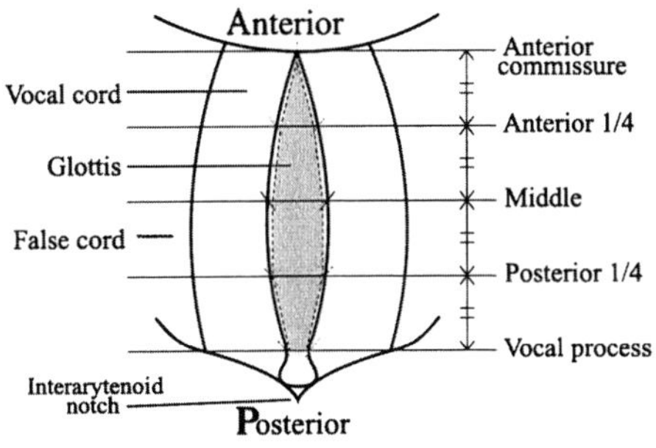

Fig. 2. The HSDI model and glottal area.

2-c: easy phonation loud, 3-a: high tone soft, 3-b: high tone medium, and 3-c: high tone loud.

For each data set, the glottal area waveform (GAW), glottal width waveform (GWW), EGG, differentiated EGG, PGG, differentiated PGG, and voice waveform were displayed in a graphic form on the same time axis and their patterns were compared.

Based on the analysis of GAW and GWW, it was found that there were variations in the pattern of the closing and opening of the vocal fold margin corresponding to the differences in the type of phonation (Fig. 2).

Results

The EGG waveform appeared to correspond well to that of the movement of the vocal fold margin in the closing phase, while this correspondence was less apparent in the opening phase (Fig. 3).

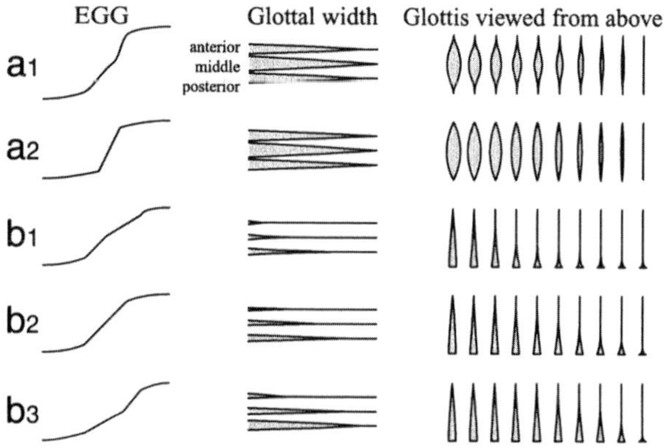

Fig. 3. Closing phase pattern models. The vertical axis of the EGG represents mV. GWW shows, in order, GWW of the anterior 1/4, middle, and posterior 1/4 of the gottal area. The vertical axis represents pixels.

Closing phase pattern models (Fig. 3, Table 1):

a1. EGG: initial gradual rise with acute incline after the notch (knee). Glottis: linear closing starts from the anterior and posterior portion followed by quick closing midportion.

a2. EGG: relatively acute rise without notch. Glottis: simultaneous closing at anterior, mid- and posterior portions.

b1. EGG: initial acute rise with gradual incline after the notch. Glottis: sudden closing from posterior portions followed by slow closing anteriorly.

b2. EGG: Similar to a2. Glottis: gradual closing from posterior portions.

b3. EGG: Similar to a1. Glottis: closing starts from posterior portions followed by quick closing anteriorly.

Opening phase pattern models (Fig. 4, Table 2):

A1. EGG: relatively acute decline without notch (knee). Glottis: linear opening

Table 1. The closing phase patterns.

Task	Subject 1	Subject 2	Subject 3
Low tone soft	a2	b1	a1
Low tone medium	a1	a1	a1
Low tone loud	a2	a2	b3
Easy phonation soft	b3	a1	b2
Easy phonation medium	a1	a2	b3
Easy phonation loud	a2	a2	b3
High tone soft	b1	b2	b1
High tone medium	a1	b2	b2
High tone loud	a2	b2	b3

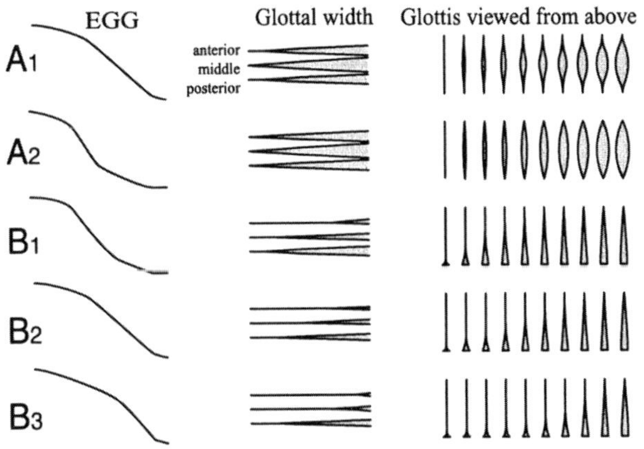

Fig. 4. Opening phase pattern models.

from the midportion.

A2. EGG: acute initial decline with gradual sloping after the notch. Glottis: simultaneous opening at anterior, mid- and posterior portions.

B1. EGG: Similar to A2. Glottis: sudden opening from posterior portions followed by slow opening anteriorly.

B2. EGG: Similar to A1. Glottis: quick linear opening from posterior portions.

B3. EGG: initial gradual decline with acute fall after the notch. Glottis: opening starts from posterior portion followed by quick opening anteriorly.

Conclusions

It is considered that the EGG waveform is dependent on the mode of contact between the two vocal folds and that careful observation of the EGG is useful and practical for predicting the pattern of vocal fold vibration.

On the other hand, it was difficult to determine the onset of the closing and

Table 2. Opening phase patterns.

Task	Subject 1	Subject 2	Subject 3
Low tone soft	B3	A1	B1/B3
Low tone medium	A1	A1	B3
Low tone loud	A1	A1	A2
Easy phonation soft	B1	A2	B1/B2
Easy phonation medium	B1	A1	A2
Easy phonation loud	B3	A1	B1
High tone soft	Unclassified	A1	B2
High tone medium	B1	A1	A1
High tone loud	B3	A1	B3

opening phases from just PGG waveform and there was a timing difference between the PGG and GAW. Although PGG seemed to be useful for judging the presence or absence of the opening phase and for the pitch measurement, it is considered to be unsuitable for a precise cycle-by-cycle analysis of the pattern of vocal fold vibration.

Reference

1. Yamanaka J. Usefulness of electroglottogram (EGG) and photoglottogram (PGG) for the analysis of vocal fold vibration — a high speed digital imaging study. J Otolaryngol Jpn 2000;103: 905–915.

Lung transplantation and bronchoscopy

©2001 Published by Elsevier Science B.V.
Bronchology and Bronchoesophagology: State of the Art.
H. Yoshimura et al., editors.

The anatomic distribution of acute cellular rejection in the allograft lung: implications for monitoring by transbronchial biopsy

Tsuyoshi Hascgawa[1], Yasunori Sohara[1], Aldo Iacono[2], Samuel A. Yousem[2] and Fuse Katsuo[1]
[1]Jichi Medical School, Kawachi, Tochigi, Japan; and [2]University of Pittsburgh Medical Center, Pittsburgh, Pennsylvania, USA

Background

Transbronchial lung biopsy (TBLB) is the technique used for routine monitoring and the diagnosis of acute cellular rejection (ACR) in the lung allograft, but the optimal anatomic site for lung biopsy has not been investigated. We examined our clinical data to clarify the distribution of ACR.

Methods

A retrospective case-series study was carried out, reviewing the pathology files and slides of TBLB performed on lung allograft recipients. Approximately 380 lung transplants and 4500 transbronchial biopsies were performed from 1984 to 1998.

Results

In 73 cases, biopsies were taken from more than one lobe. Identical grades of ACR were seen in 33 of the 73 cases (45%), and a single-grade difference was noted 34 of the 73 cases (47%). Among cases with different grades of ACR, the "upper" lobes had a higher grade in 35% of cases (14/40), and the "lower" lobes in 65% (26/40). Six cases demonstrated two or more grade differences on biopsies taken from two lobes.

Conclusions

If there are limitations on the site for bronchial biopsies, biopsies of the lower lobes appear to be more informative.

Address for correspondence: Tsuyoshi Hasegawa, Jichi Medical school, 3311-1 Yakushiji, Minami-kawachi, Kawachi, Tochigi 329-0498, Japan. Tel.: +81-258-58-7368. Fax: +81-285-44-6271.

Miscellaneous

Bronchology and Bronchoesophagology: State of the Art.
H. Yoshimura et al., editors.

Role of nasofibroscopy and acoustic nasometry in assessment of snorers

Emad K. Abdel Haleem[1], Ahmed A. Abdel Wahab[2], Montasser A. Hafez[2] and Alia M. El Shobary[3]

[1]Phoniatric Unit, and [2]ENT Department, Assiut University, Assiut; and [3]Phoniatric Unit, Ain Shams University, Cairo, Egypt

Abstract. Forty-nine adult snorers and 19 nonsnorers' upper air way tracts have been examined by video nasofibroscopy during quiet breathing conditions and modified Muller's maneuver. Nasalance scores were also measured as an index of velar function. The nasofibroscope proved to be a valid tool in identifying both the place and shape of collapse, which might be the cause of snoring and/or sleep apnea. Velar function was normal in all snorers.

Keywords: acoustic nasometry, nasofibroscopy, snoring.

Introduction

Fiberoptic nasopharyngo-laryngoscopy is a useful diagnostic tool for evaluating the airway dynamics of sleep apnea patients who are usually snorers. During this examination, the patient can be asked to perform a Muller's maneuver [1] or a modified Muller's maneuver [2] which consists of a forced inspiratory effort with the mouth and nose closed. Using this technique, many authors have tried to determine the level of obstruction in patients with sleep apnea [3–6]. The nasometer is a noninvasive, computer-based instrument designed to measure nasalance (the nasal-to-oral acoustic energy during speech) [7]. Nasalance has been found to correlate with perceived nasality [8], and thus could be used to detect disorders of nasal resonance in speech. The aim of this work is to evaluate the diagnostic value of fiberoptic video nasopharyngo-laryngoscopy when used as a routine clinical tool for the precise detection of obstruction sites in the upper airway of snorers. This will help guide the planning of the surgical intervention, documentation and monitoring of the surgical results, and to investigate the value of the nasometer as a preliminary assessment tool for velar function in snorers.

Address for correspondence: Dr Emad K. Abdel Haleem, Phoniatric Unit, ENT Department, Faculty of Medicine, Assiut, Egypt. Tel.: +20-88-341648. Fax: +20-88-333327. E-mail: emad-kamel@usa.net

Materials and Methods

Subjects

Forty-nine adult subjects (34 males and 15 females) with a mean age of 37.62 years (range: 12–58 years) presented to the Snoring Out Patients Clinic, Assiut University Hospital between October 1998 and November 1999, and 19 normal subjects (14 males and five females) with a mean age of 40.27 years (range: 19–50 years) as the control group.

Methods

Clinical examination
Anterior rhinoscopy. Using simple examination tools, both nasal cavities were examined for detection of any signs of nasal obstruction.

Oral examination.

Soft palate:	long/short/average.
Uvula:	long/long and wide-based/average.
Redundant pillars:	anterior/posterior/both.
Posterior pharyngeal wall:	bulging anteriorly/granular/contains ridges/normal.
Tonsils:	hugely enlarged/mildly enlarged/slightly enlarged/ removed.

Nasofibroscopic video examination
A Machida ENT 30 PIII fiberoptic nasofibroscope with a distal end diameter of 3 mm, a Stortz video camera (Telecam SL pal) connected to a video recorder (Panasonic AG 5700), a colour video monitor (Panasonic MT-H1480) and a video printer (Panasonic NV–MP1) were used. The continuous halogen light of a Brul and Kjaer 4914 stroboscope was used as a light source. While the subject was sitting comfortably on a chair, xylocain gel (2%) was used as a topical anaesthetic. The nasofibroscope was used to examine the upper airway starting with both nasal cavities (each one apart), naso, oro and hypopharynx, during quiet respiration, and then during the modified Muller's maneuver. The following assessment protocol was used for analysis of the recorded video for each subject by four judges (the authors: two ENT surgeons and two phoniatricians).

Nasal cavities. For documentation of clinical examination items (turbinates, mucosal appearance and colour, masses, secretions, septal deviation).

Choana:	narrow/wide.

Nasopharynx.

Adenoid mass:	none/diffuse/unequally distributed/ridges/tubal tonsils.
Muller's maneuver:	degree of collapse (in %): 0/25/50/75/100 (according to

	Utley et al. [9]), [2].
Shape of collapse:	coronal/sagittal/circular/other.

Oropharynx.

Tonsils occupy:	minimal space/25%/50%/75%/removed surgically.
Tongue base:	normal/pushes epiglottis posteriorly.
Muller's maneuver:	degree of collapse (in %): 0/25/50/75/100.
Site of collapse:	tonsillar/tongue/both.
Shape of collapse:	coronal/sagittal/other.

Hypopharynx.

Epiglottis:	normal/omega-shaped/curled/other.
Pyriforms:	normal/full.
Muller's maneuver:	degree of collapse (in %): 0/25/50/75/100.
Epiglottis:	sucked in/not.
Aryepiglottic folds:	sucked in/not.

Acoustic nasometry
Using a Kay 6200-3 Nasometer, with software version 3, every subject was asked to repeat the following speech samples while sitting comfortably on a chair applying the nasometer pick-up device, and using the face mask provided:

- /ʕali r***a***:h jelʕab korah / as an oral sound; this sentence is for detection of hypernasality.
- / m***a***m***a*** betnajm mana:l/ as a nasal sound; this loaded sentence is for detection of hyponasality.

The mean nasalance scores are measured for three repetitions of each sentence.

Results

Clinical examination

Anterior rhinoscopy
No significant correlation was found between subjects and control group as regards to signs of nasal obstruction indicated by either turbinate enlargement, septal deviation or both.

Oral examination
The soft palate has been scored clinically to be of average length in 60.6% of subjects, long in 36.4% and short in only one subject (3%), while it was scored as being average for all of the control group. The subjective clinical evaluation of uvular size showed a score of average length in 21.2% of subjects, long in 75.8%, and short in only one subject (3%), while all of the control group scored average. The pharyngeal pillars showed normal appearance in 32.4% of subjects, but were redundant in 78.7% (11.85% showed only redundant posterior pillar,

Table 1. Analysis of some nasofibroscopic findings between subjects and control group (test used: χ^2).

Item	p value	Degree of significance
Adenoid presence / shape	0.026	Significant
Nasopharynx collapse degree	0.003	Highly significant
Nasopharynx collapse shape	0.055	Nonsignificant
Tonsils size	0.144	Nonsignificant
Oropharynx collapse degree	0.001	Highly significant
Oropharynx collapse site	0.004	Highly significant
Oropharynx collapse shape	0.000	Very highly significant

55.9% showed both anterior and posterior redundant pillar). The control group showed the reverse: 84.2% had normal pillars, 15.8% showed both redundant pillars. A highly significant correlation was found between both groups ($p = 0.001$). The posterior pharyngeal wall was normal in 47% of subjects, granular in 32.4% and bulging in 20.6%, while the control group showed a normal appearance of the posterior pharyngeal wall in 73.7% and granular appearance in 26.3%. No significant correlation was found between the subjects and controls ($p = 0.061$).

Nasofibroscopic findings

The most indicative correlations of nasofibroscopic scores between subjects and the control group are summarized in Tables 1 and 2.

Acoustic nasometry

The means of the nasalance scores for both snorers and nonsnorers are shown in Table 3.

Table 2. Correlation of collapse shape between subjects and controls.

Shape of collapse	Nasopharynx (%)		Oropharynx (%)	
	Subjects	Control	Subjects	Control
Coronal	3.1	2.3	0	60
Circular	65.6	30.8	30	0
Sagittal	6.3	0	56.7	0
Irregular	3.1	0	3.3	40
p value	0.055		0.000	
Significance	Nonsignificant		Very highly significant	

Table 3. Nasal scores for snorers and nonsnorers.

Nasalance scores (mean ± SD)	Snorers (49)	Nonsnorers (19)
Oral sentence	14.67 ± 12.9	14.01 ± 6.93
Nasal sentence	52.89 ± 8.3	54.72 ± 8.59

SD: standard deviation.

Discussion

Although the data obtained from the simple clinical examination of both nasal and oral cavities were indicative for some, but not all, anatomical landmarks that are supposed to be relevant to the production of snoring, they lack objectivity and reliability. The clinical scoring of items such as soft palate length, uvular or tonsillar size, and redundant pharyngeal pillars needs a controlled study that uses multiple judges and randomized samples. Recordings carried out by nasofibroscopy were satisfactory for the rating procedure for all judges. The scores used in this study were the mean values deduced by the four judges. This "pooling" may counteract the major problem of unreliability. Although there are many inherent problems or fallacies of fiberoptic observations discussed in early research [10], they may not affect the results of the present study because both control and subject groups are examined with the same endoscope, using the same procedure. Only the lack of actual quantitative measures [6] that could be obtained from nasofibroscopic views make the trial to objectify these fibroscopic data an actual challenge. The obtained significant differences between subject and control groups are encouraging results. The presence of a highly significant difference between subjects and controls for the degree of collapse at both levels (nasopharynx and oropharynx) are indicative of the major role of the pharyngeal walls in producing upper airway narrowing. In this study the shape of collapse at both sites gave a very important indication. The sagittal shape of collapse, which was the major type found in the subject group (Table 2) means that the lateral pharyngeal walls share more in collapse production at the oropharynx but not at the nasopharynx. In comparison, a circular shape of collapse (meaning an equal degree of sharing of surrounding walls from all directions) was dominant in both subject and control groups at the nasopharyngeal level (Table 2). Collapse shape could be of great value for preoperative planning of surgical corrective procedures. Nasofibroscopy could be a feasible and useful tool as a preoperative assessment tool in cases of snoring or obstructive sleep apnea. The nasalance scores obtained from both the snorers and the control group in this study were within normal standards of the research locality [9]. No differences between both groups were found because they were matched for both age and gender. The individual data showed neither high nasalance scores on the oral speech sample (indicating the presence of hypernasality, i.e., velopharyngeal incompetence) nor low nasalance scores on the nasal speech sample (indicating the presence of hyponasality). This nasometric assessment could be used as a preliminary objective tool for evaluating velopharyngeal valve function before any surgical interference that may affect its function. This is of great value in order to detect borderline cases that are liable to develop hypernasality and/or nasal regurgitation postoperatively. The acoustic nasometer showed normal velopharyngeal valve function in snorers. It could be helpful in monitoring velar function for speech after the usual uvulo palato pharyngeal surgical procedures used to manage snoring.

References

1. Borowiecki B, Pollak CK, Weitzman ED, Rakott S, Imperato J. Study of pharyngeal airway during sleep in patients with hypersomnia obstructive sleep- apnea syndrome. Laryngoscope 1978;88:1310–1313.
2. Crumley RL, Stein M, Gamsu G, Golden J, Dermon S. Determination of obstructive site in obstructive sleep apnea. Laryngoscope 1987;97:301–308.
3. Fletcher SG, Bishop ME. Measurement of nasality with TONAR. Cleft Palate J 1973;10: 610–21.
4. Kotby MN, Abdel Haleem EK, Hegazi MA, Safe I, Zaki M. Validity of some diagnostic procedures of velopharyngeal valve incompetence. Proceedings of XV World Congress of ORL & Head and Neck Surgery, Istanbul, Turkey. 1993;576–584.
5. LaBlance GR, Steckol KF, Cooper MH. Advances in non-invasive measures of vocal acoustics. ENT J 1991;70(10):691–696.
6. Peter N, Suadicani P, Widschidtz G, Jorgensen JB. Predictive value of Muller maneuver, cephalometry and clinical features for the outcome of uvulopalatopharyngoplasty. Acta Otoloryngol (Stockholm) 1994;114:565–571.
7. Pigott RW, Makepeace AP. Some characteristics of endoscopic and radiologic systems used in elaboration of the diagnosis of v.p velopharyngeal incompetence. Br J Plast Surg 1982;35: 19–32.
8. Rojewski TE, Schuller DE, Clark RW, Schmidt HS, Potts RE. Synchronous video recording of the pharyngeal airway and polysomnograph in patients with obstructive sleep apnea. Laryngoscope 1982;92:246–249.
9. Utley DS, Shin FJ, Clerk AA, Terris DJ. A cost-effective and rational surgical approach to patients with snoring, upper airway resistance syndrome, or obstructive sleep apnea syndrome. Laryngoscope 1997;107:726–734.
10. Wilms D, Popovich J, Conway W, Fujita S, Zorick F. Anatomic abnormalities in obstructive sleep apnea. Ann Otol Rhinol Laryngol 1982;91:595–596.

Bronchology and Bronchoesophagology: State of the Art.
H. Yoshimura et al., editors.

Digital fluorography for the diagnosis of radiolucent tracheobronchial foreign bodies

Minoru Ikeda, Shuntaro Shigihara, Akihiro Ikui, Yukiko Yamauchi and Akinori Kida
Department of Otolaryngology, Nihon University School of Medicine, Tokyo, Japan

Abstract. In a total of 19 cases of radiolucent foreign bodies in the lower respiratory tract, digital subtraction fluorography (DSF) was conducted. Obstruction of the bronchial lumen was observed on DSF in 15 cases. Visualization of the bronchial lumen was indistinct in three cases. No abnormalities were observed on DSF in one case. Out of the 15 cases with obstruction on DSF, the presence of a foreign body was confirmed operatively in 11 (73%). In the remaining four cases, obstruction of the bronchus with viscous secretion or by granulation was observed fiberscopically. A foreign body was detected fiberscopically in two of the three cases in which bronchial lumen was indistinct on DSF. In the remaining one case, stenosis of the bronchial lumen due to mucosal edema was observed. Fibroscopy was performed in one case in which no abnormal findings were obtained by DSF, but the episode at the time of onset strongly suggested the presence of foreign body aspiration. However, foreign bodies or any pathological changes were not recognized. We showed that DSF was a very sensitive diagnostic procedure for radiolucent tracheobronchial foreign bodies and its stenotic changes.

Keywords: bronchial stenosis, bronchofibroscopy, digital radiography, lower respiratory tract, ventilation bronchoscopy.

Introduction

Recent developments in computer technology have resulted in improved radiological apparatus. A digital subtraction fluorography (DSF) system is one of these instruments. By using this system, it has become easier to identify the target organ vividly by converting radiological information into digital signals and processing the data as figures. This technique is now widely used as digital subtraction angiography (DSA). We conducted DSF of the lower respiratory tract by using the DSA device in order to diagnose radiolucent tracheobronchial foreign bodies in infants. We report the usefulness of DSF based on our experience. Obstruction of the bronchial lumen was observed on DSF in 15 cases. Visualization of the bronchial lumen was indistinct in three cases. No abnormalities were observed on DSF in one case. Out of the 15 cases with obstruction on DSF, the presence of a foreign body was confirmed operatively in 11 (73%). In the remaining four cases, obstruction of the bronchus with viscous secretion or by granulation was observed fiberscopically.

Address for correspondence: Minoru Ikeda MD, Department of Otolaryngology, Nihon University School of Medicine, 30-1 Oyaguchi Itabashi-ku, Tokyo 173-8610, Japan. Tel.: +81-3-3972-8111. Fax: +81-3-3972-1321. E-mail: mikeda@med.nihon-u.ac.jp

Subjects and Methods

In a total of 19 cases of radiolucent foreign bodies in the lower respiratory tract, DSF was conducted preoperatively, using Digital Subtraction Fluorography (DFP-03A, Toshiba Co.). Foreign bodies in their airways were inspected under general anesthesia. The patients age ranged from 11 months to 4 years and 7 months (mean: 1.8 ± 0.9 years).

Results

Surgical operation

In two cases in which a tracheal foreign body was diagnosed preoperatively, a ridged ventilation bronchoscope (Nagashima Co.) was initially inserted under general anesthesia, and the foreign body was extracted. In the remaining 17 cases, a tracheal tube was transorally inserted, and bronchofibroscopy was performed via the tube to inspect the foreign body. When the presence of a foreign body was confirmed, a ridged ventilation bronchoscope was inserted to retrieve it.

Results of surgery

Foreign bodies were present in 13 of the 19 cases. A foreign body was not identified, but obstruction of the bronchial lumen with viscous secretion was observed in three cases, stenosis by granulation was noted in one case, and stenosis with mucosal edema was seen in one. No abnormal findings were observed in one case.

Comparison of abnormalities on DSF and results of surgery

Obstruction of the bronchial lumen was observed on DSF in 15 cases. Visualization of the bronchial lumen was indistinct in three cases. No abnormalities were observed on DSF in one case. Out of the 15 cases with obstruction on DSF, the presence of a foreign body was confirmed operatively in 11 (73%). In the remaining four cases, obstruction of the bronchus with viscous secretion or by granulation was observed fiberscopically. A foreign body was detected fiberscopically in two of the three cases in which bronchial lumen was indistinct on DSF. In the one remaining case, stenosis of the bronchial lumen due to mucosal edema was observed. Fibroscopy was performed in one case in which no abnormal findings were obtained by DSF, but the episode at the time of onset strongly suggested the presence of foreign body aspiration. However, no foreign bodies or any pathological changes were recognized.

Sensitivity of DSF to foreign body aspiration

Among 13 cases in which the presence of a foreign body was surgically confirmed, all cases showed abnormal findings of bronchial lumen on DSF, and the sensitivity of DSF to aspirated foreign body was 100%. In those 13 cases, 11 cases showed clear obstruction of the bronchial lumen on DSF. Among the 18 cases in which stenotic changes were noted fiberscopically, DSF showed abnormal findings in all cases (100%).

Specificity of DSF to foreign body aspiration

Among the six cases in which foreign bodies were not surgically detected, the result of DSF was negative in only one case (17%), suggesting low specificity. In the remaining five of the six cases, however, even though no foreign body was observed, airway obstruction or stenosis according to viscous discharge or granulation was present. In one case in which no lesions of stenosis were shown fiberscopically, DSF showed no abnormal findings. Accordingly, when considered from the point of view of airway stenosis, the specificity of DSF was favorable (100%).

Conclusion

In pediatric cases, 60% of tracheobronchial foreign bodies were of vegetable origin, and they were radiolucent. In this study, we showed that DSF was a very useful diagnostic procedure for radiolucent tracheobronchial foreign bodies. When any abnormal findings are observed on DSF, it is almost certain that some lesions are present in the airway. However, the abnormality found on DSF is not necessarily to be a foreign body itself. In some cases, it can be explained as stenosis due to inflammation. Therefore, with respect to treatment procedure, a tracheal tube should be intubated under general anesthesia, and fibroscopy should be performed via the tube. When a foreign body is confirmed, then ventilation bronchoscopy should be performed to retrieve it. Operations within the lower respiratory air tract under ventilation bronchoscopy are not always safe and easy, especially in infants. Therefore, when this sequence is followed, the high abnormality detection rate of DSF against airway stenosis including foreign bodies is believed to enable safe and appropriate treatment of individual cases.

Bronchology and Bronchoesophagology: State of the Art.
H. Yoshimura et al., editors.

Fibrin glue application through bronchoscope in the treatment of acute bronchopleural fistula

Shigemi Ishikawa[1], Yukinobu Goto[1], Hideo Ichimura[1], Yuko Minami[1], Yukio Sato[1], Tatsuo Yamamoto[1], Masataka Onizuka[1] and Eiichi Akaogi[2]

[1]*Department of Surgery, Institute of Clinical Medicine, University of Tsukuba, Tsukuba; and* [2]*Kogashi Fukushinomori Shinryoujo, Koga, Japan*

Abstract. *Background.* Bronchopleural fistula (BPF) is one of the serious complications following pulmonary resection. It is important to prevent the development of aspiration pneumonia and empyema in treating the acute phase of BPF. The bronchoscope can play an important role not only in diagnosing but also in treating BPF.

Methods. The subjects were 36 patients who developed BPF (3.7%) following pulmonary resection for lung cancer since 1977. BPF was a complication after pneumonectomy in 13 cases, after bilobectomy in six, and after lobectomy in 17. Fibrin glue was applied through a catheter inserted into a bronchoscope in 16 cases after primary resection and in two cases after pedicled omental flap transposition.

Results. Twelve cases (67%) of BPF were closed by fibrin glue application. BPF closed without closed or open drainage of pleural cavity in seven cases. Fenestration of the chest wall and muscle flap transposition was performed in six cases of BPF in which fibrin glue was ineffective to manage acute BPF.

Conclusions. Fibrin glue application was found to be effective in managing BPF of which the fistula was less than 3 mm in diameter. Fibrin glue application to BPF through the bronchoscope may play a role in managing BPF, preventing the extension of aspiration pneumonia and empyema.

Keywords: bronchopleural fistula, bronchoscopy, fibrin glue.

Introduction

Bronchopleural fistula (BPF) is one of the serious complications following pulmonary resection. It is important to prevent the development of aspiration pneumonia and empyema in treating the acute phase of BPF. The purpose of this retrospective study is to determine the clinical efficacy of primary bronchoscopic sealing in BPF and to identify patients who may profit by avoidance of aggressive surgical intervention.

Address for correspondence: Shigemi Ishikawa MD, Department of Surgery, Institute of Clinical Medicine, University of Tsukuba, Tennoudai 1-1-1, Tsukuba, Ibaraki 305-8575, Japan. Tel.: +81-298-533210. Fax: +81-298-533097. E-mail: ishikawa@md.tsukuba.ac.jp

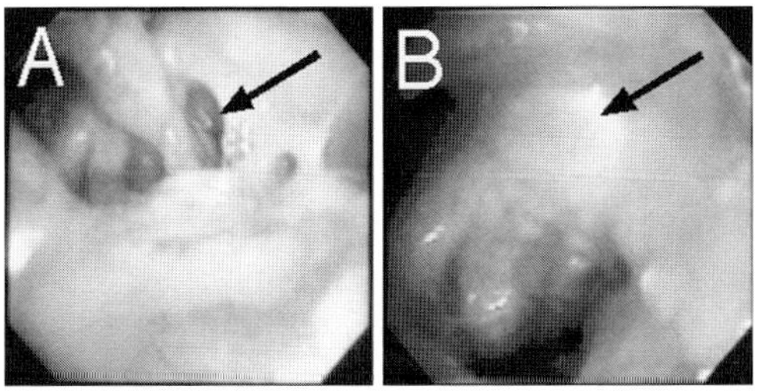

Fig. 1. A 70-year-old man had a left upper lobectomy with bronchoplasty and pulmonary arterial plasty for stage IIIA squamous cell carcinoma. **A:** BPF developed 17 days after surgery. **B:** Bronchoscopic photograph 52 days after bronchoscopic sealing with fibrin glue.

Methods

The subjects were 36 patients (3.7% of the total number of cases with resected lung cancer) who developed BPF following pulmonary resection for lung cancer between 1977 and 1999. Eighteen out of 25 BPF were treated with bronchoscopic sealing using fibrin glue since 1987. In seven cases, bronchoscopic treatment was not performed. Of these, open window drainage was performed in five cases because of progressive aspiration, and BPF closed spontaneously in two. All procedures were performed under local anesthesia with a fiberoptic bronchoscope or a video bronchoscope. The two components of fibrin glue were injected consecutively using two catheters or simultaneously using a double-lumen catheter through the operating channel of the bronchoscope.

Results

A case of bronchoscopic treatment of BPF is shown in Fig. 1. Twelve out of 18 cases of BPF (67%) closed by bronchoscopic application of fibrin glue. Of these, seven patients were cured without any chest drainage, and five patients required open or closed chest drainage. Two patients had fistula recurrence 3 weeks and 3 months after gluing. Five patients died, and four of these deaths were post-pneumonectomy. Bronchoscopic failure necessitated open window drainage in six patients. These six BPFs closed by muscle flap transposition or omentopexy. One patient died of pneumonia. The results of bronchoscopic sealing in 18 patients are shown in Table 1.

The rate of closure of BPF by fibrin glue sealing was 92% when the fistula size was less than 3 mm in diameter and 17% when it was greater than 4 mm ($p = 0.002$ by χ^2 test).

Discussion

The purpose of endoscopic sealing of BPF is to prevent progression of aspiration pneumonia and infection in the pleural cavity. Although some BPF may close

Table 1. Results of bronchoscopic treatment in 18 patients.

Result	No. of patients	Fistula size (mm)	Onset after surgery	No. of fibrin applications
Close	12	1–4 (2.1)	17–1115 (141)	1–5 (2.3)
Open	6	2–8 (4.8)[a]	10–210 (62)	1–5 (2.8)
Total	18	1–8 (3.0)	10–1115 (114)	1–5 (2.5)

Data are shown as range and mean. [a]$p = 0.001$ compared with low above by t test.

only by tube drainage, bronchoscopic treatment of BPF has been shown to be effective using several materials including fibrin glue [1,2], acrylate [2,3], human spongiosa [4] and polidocanol [5]. Bronchoscopic treatment of BPF using fibrin glue appears an efficient alternative, especially when the fistula size is small (< 3 mm) and the pleural cavity is not contaminated.

References

1. Hollaus PH, Lax F, Janakiev D, Lucciarini P, Katz E, Kreuzer A, Pridun NS. Endoscopic treatment of postoperative bronchopleural fistula: experience with 45 cases. Ann Thorac Surg 1998; 66:923–927.
2. Torre M, Chiesa G, Ravini M, Vercelloni M, Belloni PA. Endoscopic gluing of bronchopleural fistula. Ann Thorac Surg 1994;58:901–902.
3. Scappaticci E, Ardissone F, Ruffini E, Baldi S, Mancuso M. Postoperative bronchopleural fistulas: endoscopic closure in 12 patients. Ann Thorac Surg 1994;57:119–122.
4. Baumann WR, Ulmer JL, Ambrose PG, Garvey MJ, Jones DT. Closure of a bronchopleural fistula using decalcified human spongiosa and a fibrin sealant. Ann Thorac Surg 1997;64: 230–233.
5. Varoli F, Roviaro G, Grignani F, Vergani C, Maciocco M, Rebuffat C. Endoscopic treatment of bronchopleural fistula. Ann Thorac Surg 1998;65:807–809.

Bronchology and Bronchoesophagology: State of the Art.
H. Yoshimura et al., editors.

Endobronchial therapy: a decade of experience in a Singapore hospital

Alan W.K. Ng
Department of Respiratory Medicine, Tan Tock Seng Hospital, Singapore

Abstract. Endobronchial Nd:YAG laser therapy (EBLT) and tracheobronchial stenting (TBS) have revolutionised the management of central airway obstruction. Since September 1989, 281 EBLT procedures have been performed on 189 patients; 151 (80%) had symptomatic malignant obstruction of the trachea or main bronchi. Squamous cell carcinoma (55%), adenocarcinoma (13%) and large cell carcinoma (9.3%) were the most common cancers. 83% of cases were performed under general anaesthesia, the patient was ventilated through an endotracheal tube (ETT) or a rigid bronchoscope (RB). The flexible bronchoscope, passed through the ETT or RB, was used to aim the laser at the lesion. An excellent result was achieved in 71% of EBLT where relief of obstruction was accompanied by symptom relief. Improvements in FEV_1 or FVC were recorded in 37 of the 84 patients. The overall complication rate was low: there were four (1.4%) deaths within 72 h of EBLT.

67 airway stents (63 Dumon, four Wallstent) have been placed in 50 patients since October 1994. Extrinsic compression by tumour or lymph nodes was the most common indication (58%). Six patients had tracheo- or bronchoesophageal fistulas requiring stenting. Fifteen (30%) patients had stenoses of the trachea or main bronchi associated with tuberculosis. TBS provided effective and lasting relief of airway obstruction. The stents were well tolerated. The main problems encountered were granulation tissue (12%) and migration (10%).

In conclusion, the development of endobronchial therapy provides an acceptable and effective way to restore airway patency. Its availability today allows rapid and effective symptom palliation of patients with advanced malignancy and airway obstruction although in the long term, patients with advanced cancer did not do well.

Keywords: central airway obstruction, Nd:YAG laser, tracheobronchial stenting.

Introduction

Endobronchial therapy techniques have revolutionised the management of central airway obstruction in the last decade. The development of the Nd:YAG laser and airway stent have made it possible for bronchoscopic intervention to restore airway patency in these patients who are often inoperable. This paper reviews the practice of endobronchial Nd:YAG laser therapy (EBLT) and tracheobronchial stenting (TBS) in a Singapore hospital.

Address for correspondence: Alan W.K. Ng, Department of Respiratory Medicine, Tan Tock Seng Hospital, 11 Jalan Tan Tock Seng, 308433 Singapore. Fax: +65-357-7871.
E-mail: alan_ng_wk@notes.ttsh.gov.sg

Nd:YAG laser therapy

From September 1989 to December 1999, 189 patients have been treated: 281 procedures were performed. Most patients (77%) were treated in a single session. 151 of the patients had malignant disease, while 38 had benign disease. Squamous cell carcinoma (55%), adenocarcinoma (13%) and large cell carcinoma (9.3%) were the most common causes of malignant airway obstruction. Six patients with small cell carcinoma were treated; three were dyspneic, including one who required intubation. There were six patients with endobronchial metastases from extrapulmonary cancers. Five patients had airway involvement by esophageal cancer while three had thyroid cancer invading the airway.

Tuberculous stricture (11) and tracheal stenosis (8) were the most common benign lesions treated; most of these required multiple treatments.

All patients had endobronchial disease causing airway obstruction of varying degrees. In some of the patients, the laser was used to palliate haemoptysis from a bleeding endobronchial tumour. The majority of patients had inoperable disease; most had received conventional treatment modalities but with little or no response, while some had recurrent disease presenting with airway obstruction.

Nd:YAG laser therapy was performed under general anaesthesia in the majority (83%) of cases: patients were ventilated with an endotracheal tube (ETT) or a rigid bronchoscope (RB). In all cases, the flexible bronchoscope, which was passed through the ETT or RB, or transnasally when performed under local anaesthesia, was used to aim the laser beam.

The site of treatment was most commonly in the central airway (trachea, 32; left main bronchus, 53; right main bronchus, 61). In 29 procedures, a stent was also inserted to maintain airway patency. These were patients in whom there was extensive endobronchial disease, loss of cartilaginous support or in whom there was fibrosis or stricture of the airway.

The effectiveness of laser therapy was determined from assessment of symptoms, relief of airway obstruction, and where available, pulmonary function and radiological re-expansion of atelectatic lung. 71% of the procedures had an excellent result: there was improvement in symptoms following successful relief of airway obstruction. The result was fair in 18.5% while in 10.3% there was no improvement.

In 44 patients for whom pulmonary function data were available before and after EBLT, there was improvement in either FEV_1 or FVC in 37 (84%). The improvement in the mean predicted $\%FEV_1$ was from 52.4 to 65.4% while the improvement in the mean %FVC was from 61.9 to 70%.

The complication rate was low despite many patients being fairly ill. There were no intraoperative deaths; three patients had cardiac arrest during the procedure, but they were successfully resuscitated. Four patients died within 72 h of the procedure: they had extensive disease of the airways for which laser therapy was unlikely to help.

Tracheobronchial stenting

Airway stents were developed for relieving airway obstruction caused by extrinsic compression, loss of cartilaginous support, where there was residual airway tumour after laser resection, or where there was a fistula.

Between October 1994 and December 1999, 67 airway stents (63 Dumon, four Wallstent) were inserted into 50 patients. Twenty-nine patients had malignant airway obstruction; 21 had benign airway disease. The most common cause of benign airway stenosis amongst treated patients was tuberculous stenosis (30%). This was mainly seen in women. Six patients had fistulas between the esophagus and the trachea (3) or main bronchus (3) which required stenting.

The site of stent placement was the trachea (12 malignant, eight benign), left main bronchus (nine malignant, 12 benign) and right main bronchus (11 malignant, one benign). In benign disease, the most common site which required a stent was the left main bronchus. Seven patients required two stents. Symptom relief followed restoration of airway patency in all patients.

The only procedure-related complication encountered was pneumothorax (1) which was evacuated by aspiration and did not require a chest tube. Of the stent-related complications, granulation tissue (12%) and migration (10%) were the most commonly encountered. This was usually detected during check bronchoscopy and was not life-threatening. Stents were readjusted or replaced in eight patients.

As in the case of Nd:YAG laser therapy, our experience is that airway stents provide effective relief of airway obstruction: the benefit is immediate and lost lasting; the stents are well tolerated and no life-threatening complications were encountered.

Conclusion

EBLT and TBS have made a major impact in the management of central airway obstruction. Patients with advanced cancer and airway obstruction can be rapidly and effectively palliated of their distressing dyspnea by EBLT or TBS, although in the long term, these patients did not do well. These techniques may also be a reasonable alternative to surgery in cases of benign stenoses. Pulmonologists familiar with these techniques will play an important role in the management of patients with central airway obstruction.

Bronchology and Bronchoesophagology: State of the Art.
H. Yoshimura et al., editors.

Different clonal growths of multiple lung cancers from chromate-exposed workers

Kazuya Kondo[1], Toshiyuki Hirose[1], Yuji Takahashi[1], Hisashi Ishikura[1], Masaru Tsuyuguchi[2], Tomoyuki Yokose[3], Tetsurou Kodama[4] and Yasumasa Monden[1]

[1]Second Department of Surgery, School of Medicine, University of Tokushima; [2]Surgical Division, Tokushima Municipal Hospital, Tokushima; [3]Pathological Division, National Cancer Center Institute East, Kashiwa; and [4]National Cancer Center Hospital, Tokyo, Japan

Abstract. Our previous studies have demonstrated that lung cancers from chromate-exposed workers frequently show microsatellite instability (MSI) (30/38, 78.9%) compared with lung cancers from patients without chromate exposure (4/26, 15.4%). We now examined MSI in 17 lesions arising from the proximal bronchus in seven multiple lung cancer patients (double: five; triple: one; quadruple: one) with chromate exposure using six microsatellite markers (3p23, 3p21.3, 3p21.1, 5q21-22, 9p21, and 17p13.1 loci). They consisted of 16 squamous cell carcinomas including eight carcinoma-in-situ (CIS) lesions, and one small cell carcinoma. Eleven of 17 cancerous lesions (64.7%) had MSI at more than two loci. Five of eight CIS lesions (62.5%) had MSI at more than two loci. The frequency of MSI in CIS was almost the same as that in the advanced cancers. Each lesion in cases of multiple lung cancers showed more than one different MSI pattern, which is suggestive of different clonal growth. These findings demonstrate that MSI may be an early event in chromate lung carcinogenesis, and that each cancer lesion in cases of multiple lung cancers with chromate exposure shows different clonal growth.

Keywords: chromium, field cancerization, microsatellite instability, multiple lung cancer.

Introduction

Several epidemiological surveys performed in various countries have confirmed that the risk of lung cancer in chromate-exposed workers is 2.0–18.3 times higher than in the general population [1]. We have shown that exposure to chromate induces a particular mutation pattern in the p53 gene seen in human lung cancers [2]. Recently, we examined genomic instability in lung cancers from chromate-exposed workers using six microsatellite markers. The frequency of replication error (RER+) in tumors with chromate exposure (30/38, 78.9%) was significantly higher than that in tumors without chromate exposure (4/26, 15.4%). The epithelia of the aerodigestive tract in chromate-exposed workers are exposed to the chromium. They frequently had multiple lung cancers. This supports the concept of "field cancerization", where there are carcinogen-induced

Address for correspondence: Kazuya Kondo, Second Department of Surgery, School of Medicine, University of Tokushima, Tokushima 770-8503, Japan. Tel.: +81-88-633-7143. Fax: +81-88-633-7144. E-mail: kondo@clin.med.tokushima-u.ac.jp changes throughout the mucosa of the upper aerodigestive tract [3].

In this study, we try to elucidate the genetic basis for the "field cancerization" of lung cancer induced by chromium using six microsatellite markers.

Materials and Methods

Patients

Seventeen tumors and corresponding mediastinal lymph nodes without metastasis were obtained from seven chromate workers with multiple lung cancers during surgery, or at autopsy from the Second Department of Surgery, School of Medicine, University of Tokushima, National Cancer Center Hospital East and Tokushima Municipal Hospital between August 1975 and October 1997. There were five cases of double cancers, one case of triple cancers, and one case of quadruple cancers. The ages of the patients ranged from 38 to 68 years. All seven patients were male and smokers with a Brinkman index ranging from 360 to 900. They were exposed to chromate for a period of 14—33 years. The types of cancer included 16 squamous cell carcinomas and one small cell carcinoma. We used the Union International Contre le Cancer (UICC) TNM staging system to grade the cancers as follows: stage I, 15 cases including eight carcinoma-in-situ (CIS); stage IIIA, one case; stage IV, one case [4].

DNA extraction

Six serial sections were cut from formalin-fixed paraffin-embedded tissue blocks. An area representative of the tumor was identified, microdissected, and transferred into an Eppendorf reaction tube. The DNA was extracted as described previously [5]. DNA from lymph nodes without metastasis was also extracted as normal DNA.

Analysis of microsatellite instability (MSI)

We examined the MSI at six microsatellite loci containing (CA)n repeats: D3S647(3p23); D3S966(3p21.3); D3S1289(3p21.1); D5S346(5q21-q22); D9S 161(9p21); TP53(17p13.1). The PCR was performed as described previously [5]. The PCR products were diluted 10-fold in distilled water, then the second PCR was performed using 1 μl of the diluted PCR products following the same protocol. The second PCR products were diluted 10-fold, denatured, and electrophoresed on 6% polyacrylamide gels containing 8.3 M urea for 3—4 h at 40 W at room temperature.

MSI was defined by a mobility shift in the tumor DNA band compared to the normal DNA band detected. The replication error-positive (RER+) phenotype was defined as the presence of MSI at two or more loci.

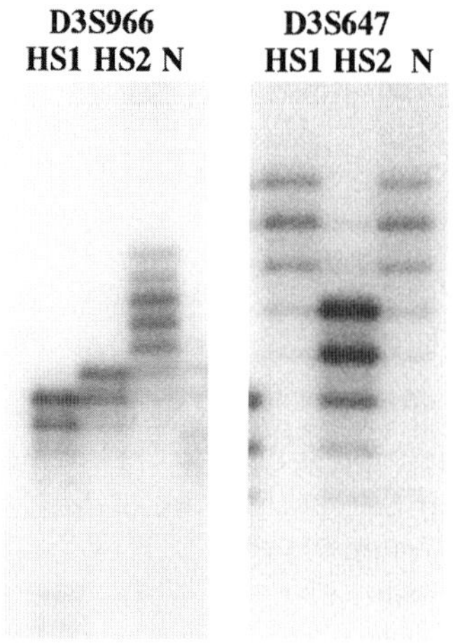

Fig. 1. MSI analysis showing MSI at D3S966 and D3S647 microsatellite marker in the two tumors of patient SH: advanced squamous cell carcinoma (SH-1) in the right B^6 bronchus and carcinoma-in-situ (SH-2) in the right B^8 bronchus. N; normal tissue.

Results and Discussion

One representative case is presented in Fig. 1. Patient SH had advanced squamous cell carcinoma (pT1N2M0, SH-1) in the right B^6 bronchus and CIS (SH-2) in the right B^8 bronchus simultaneously. For the D3S966 microsatellite marker, typings with MSI were identified by random size shifts of alleles in two tumor DNA samples (SH-1, 2) compared to normal tissue DNA. The allele shifts in each tumor DNA samples showed different patterns. For the D3S647 marker, the allele shifts in one tumor DNA sample (SH-1) were the same as those of DNA from normal tissue. The other (SH-2) shows an MSI pattern. These findings demonstrate that the two tumors have grown from different clones. It suggests that this patient had double primary cancers.

Figure 2 summarizes MSI and loss of heterozygosity (LOH) data from the analyses of 17 lesion samples from seven multiple lung cancer patients. Eleven of 17 cancers (64.7%) showed RER+. Five of eight CIS lesions (62.5%) showed RER+. This frequency is almost the same as that in more advanced lung cancers (6/9, 66.7%). Miozzo et al. reported that MSI was found not only in lung cancers (17/53, 32%) but also in normal bronchial mucosas (15/42, 36%), and suggested that much of the bronchial epithelium had been "mutagenized" as a result of exposure to carcinogens [6]. Both our and Miozzo's findings suggest that MSI is involved in the early stage of lung carcinogenesis in lung cancer-exposed chromium.

Although two tumors in patients IS and YM show MSI, random size shifts of alleles in each tumor DNA samples showed the same pattern. Other cases with MSI (90%) had different allele shifts in each tumor DNA sample. Additionally,

Sample	Histology	D3S647	D3S966	D3S1289	TP53(17P)	D5S346	D9S161	
SI-1	SQ			×	×	×	×	
SI-2	SCLC		MI	×	MI	×	MI	RER+
SI-3	SQ		MI	×		MI	MI	RER+
IS-1	SQ			MI	×	MI		RER+
IS-2	SQ,cis	MI	MI	MI	MI	MI	MI	RER+
II-1	SQ,cis	MI	MI	×	×	×		RER+
II-2	SQ,cis	MI	×	×	MI	×		RER+
II-3	SQ,cis		MI					
II-4	SQ,cis		MI	×				
YM-1	SQ		MI	MI		×	MI	RER+
YM-2	SQ,cis	MI	MI	MI	MI		MI	RER+
HS-1	SQ		MI	×				
HS-2	SQ	MI	MI	×	×	×	×	RER+
AO-1	SQ	MI	×	×	×	MI		RER+
AO-2	SQ						×	
HK-1	SQ,cis		MI	×		×		
HK-2	SQ,cis	MI	MI	×	MI	×		RER+

Multiple cancer with differences of MI patterns
Multiple cancer without differences of MI patterns

Fig. 2. Microsatellite instability patterns in multiple chromate lung cancers. SQ, squamous cell carcinoma; SCLC, small cell lung cancer; MI, microsatellite instability; X, not amplified; RER+, replication error.

each lesion showed more than one MSI pattern, which is suggestive of different clonal growth. These findings demonstrate that each lesion in cases of multiple lung cancers with chromate exposure arose from different clones. This study supports the theory of "field cancerization" induced by chromium, and our next study will be to clarify whether there are chromium-induced changes throughout the mucosa of the bronchi.

MSI analysis can increase our understanding of the biology of these lesions, and may have an impact on designing effective diagnostic strategies to distinguish between cases of multiple cancers and metastatic cancer.

References

1. IARC. IARC Monographs on the Evaluation of Carcinogenic Risk to Humans, vol 49. Lyon: IARC, 1990.
2. Kondo K et al. Mutations of the p53 gene in human lung cancer from chromate-exposed workers. Biochem Biophys Res Commun 1997;239:95–100.
3. Slaughter DP, Southwick HW, Smejkal W. "Field cancerization" in oral stratified squamous epithelium: clinical implications of multicentric origin. Cancer (Philadelphia) 1953;6:963–968.
4. Union International Contre le Cancer (UICC), Sherman CD (Chairman). 1987 Manual of Clinical Oncology, 4th edn. Berlin: Springer-Verlag, 1987.
5. Hino N, Kondo K, Miyoshi T, Uyama T, Monden Y. High frequency of p53 protein expression in thymic carcinoma but not in thymoma. Br J Cancer 1997;76:1361–1366.
6. Miozzo M et al. Microsatellite alterations in bronchial and sputum specimens of lung cancer patients. Cancer Res 1996;56:2285–2288.

Bronchology and Bronchoesophagology: State of the Art.
H. Yoshimura et al., editors.

The usefulness of bronchial biopsy for the diagnosis of smoke inhalation

K. Kumagai, M. Katagiri, N. Yanase, H. Imai, K. Soma and T. Ohwada
Department of Critical Care and Emergency Medicine, Department of Internal Medicine, Kitasato University, School of Medicine, Kanagawa, Japan

Background

Smoke inhalation injury is one of the important clinical factors of burn victims, and it influences their prognosis. Therefore, early definite diagnosis of airway injury is essential for the appropriate treatment. Generally, smoke inhalation injury is suspected on the basis of clinical signs or the circumstances of the injury, and often diagnosed by bronchoscopy [1,2]. In endoscopic examinations, the diagnosis of inhalation injury is difficult because the signs are various and nonspecific, and it is hard to evaluate the severity of the injury. Several approaches have been reported to make endoscopic examination more objective. These include the existence of the cough reflex during the bronchoscopy [2], blood gas analysis, and respiratory index, etc.

We use the histologic examination of the bronchial biopsy specimens as a support of bronchoscopy for the definite diagnosis of inhalation injury.

Study objective

To evaluate the reliability of macroscopic findings and the usefulness of bronchial biopsy, we compared these two diagnostic methods.

Study population

We studied the burn patients, who were admitted to our hospital between May 1997 and April 2000, and were suspected of having inhalation injury according to Stone's diagnostic criteria [3] (Table 1).

Methods

After local anesthesia was administered to the oropharynx, the patients under-

Address for correspondence: K. Kumagai, Department of Critical Care and Emergency Medicine, Department of Internal Medicine, Kitasato University, School of Medicine, 1-15-1 Kitasato, Sagamihara-shi, Kanagawa 228-8555, Japan. Tel.: +81-42-778-8128. Fax: +81-42-778-9778.

Table 1. Stone's criteria for the diagnosis of smoke inhalation injury.

1. Flame burns involving the face (mouth and nose)
2. Singed nasal vibrissae
3. Burn sustained in a closed space

went flexible fiberoptic bronchoscopy and biopsy of the bronchial mucosa simultaneously, as soon as possible within 48 h after injury. Two or three biopsy specimens were taken from the spur between the right upper lobe bronchus and the truncus intermedius. The results of macroscopic and histologic diagnoses were classified into three severity groups; normal, mild, and severe. We compared two diagnostic methods, and investigated the reliability of macroscopic diagnoses using histologic diagnoses as the "gold standard". All endoscopic examinations were performed by the same bronchoscopist, and the biopsy specimens were examined by the same pathologist. Informed consent was obtained from all patients or their nearest relatives before any procedures were performed.

Classification of endoscopic severity

In order to facilitate the statistical analysis, the bronchoscopist used the standardized descriptions: soot deposits, redness, edema, erosion, and paleness. Those who had no abnormal findings were defined normal. Those with soot deposit, redness and edema were defined mild. Those with erosion and paleness were defined severe, because these findings may indicate injury to deeper layers.

Classification of histopathological severity

In order to facilitate the statistical analysis, the pathologist used the standardized descriptions: edema, cell infiltration, erosion, and necrosis. Those who had no abnormal findings were defined normal. Those with edema and cell infiltration were defined mild. Those with erosion and necrosis were defined severe.

Results

There were no adverse effects associated with bronchoscopic procedures. Twenty-five patients were studied, and three cases were excluded. Too many soot deposits disturbed observation in one case, and no biopsy specimens were available in the other two cases. The results of the 22 cases included are presented in Table 2.

Comparison between macroscopic and histologic findings

We evaluated the reliability of macroscopic diagnoses using the histological conclusions as the "gold standard" (Table 3). The sensitivity and specificity of endoscopic examination were 84.2 and 66.7%, respectively. There were three false

Table 2. Results of the study (n = 22).

Case	Age	Sex	Cause	Bronchoscopic diagnosis	Histological diagnosis
N.O.	59	M	Fire	Mild	Mild
Y.F.	49	F	Self-burning	Mild	Severe
Y.K.	47	F	Fire	Severe	Severe
K.M.	46	F	Self-burning	Normal	Normal
E.F.	60	F	Fire	Mild	Severe
M.S.	31	M	Fire	Mild	Normal
E.M.	40	F	Self-burning	Normal	Mild
T.E.	24	M	Fire	Mild	Mild
N.S.	25	M	Fire	Mild	Severe
H.Y.	34	M	Self-burning	Mild	Severe
H.I.	38	M	Fire	Mild	Severe
Y.S.	37	F	Fire	Severe	Severe
M.S.	31	F	Fire	Mild	Mild
Y.T.	30	M	Accidental burning	Mild	Severe
T.N.	64	M	Gas explosion	Mild	Mild
A.S.	51	M	Self-burning	Normal	Severe
M.H.	53	M	Self-burning	Mild	Severe
H.N.	64	M	Accidental burning	Normal	Mild
M.K.	37	F	Fire	Severe	Severe
K.S.	24	M	Fire	Mild	Severe
K.M.	42	M	Accidental burning	Normal	Normal
Y.U.	31	M	Fire	Mild	Mild
Average	41.7	M/F = 14/8			

negative cases.

The macroscopic conclusion about the severity of injury was compared with the pathologist's diagnosis in each case. There was excellent agreement between macroscopic conclusions and histology in 10 cases (45.5%). The macroscopic conclusion underestimated the severity, compared to histology, in 11 cases (50.0%). The macroscopic conclusion was mild, whereas the histological conclusion was normal in one case (4.5%).

Discussion

In this study, there were 19 of 22 cases (86.3%) who were diagnosed as having inhalation injury using histological examination. The macroscopic signs of injury were present in 17 of 22 cases (77.3%), and the sensitivity and specificity of endoscopic diagnosis were 84.2 and 66.7%, respectively. Masane and colleagues reported that the sensitivity of bronchoscopy was 79%, and concluded that endoscopic examination was sensitive for the diagnosis of inhalation injury [1].

On the other hand, there are several reports stating that endoscopic diagnosis does not reflect the clinical severity of inhalation injury [4]. Because macroscopic

Table 3. Comparison between macroscopic and histologic findings.

	Histology		Total
	Mild, severe	Normal	
Bronchoscopy:			
Mild, severe	16	1	17
Normal	3	2	5
Total	19	3	22

signs of inhalation injury are various and nonspecific [1,5], the reliability of bronchoscopy depends on the bronchoscopist's experience [1,2]. That makes the endoscopic examination less objective, and marks the limits of this diagnostic method. Thus, we consider histological evidence of injury as more reliable than macroscopic findings, and think it should be used as the "gold standard" for the diagnosis of inhalation injuries.

Using bronchial biopsy simultaneously, the bronchoscopic examination will be a more reliable diagnostic method. With regard to the severity of evaluation, the endoscopic examination diagnosed one-half of the cases accurately, and tended to underestimate the severity in the rest. This can be accounted for in two ways, one, the insufficient objectivity of macroscopic diagnosis, and two, the difficulty of defining the severity. However, it remains to be questioned, whether endoscopic and histologic severity correlates with the clinical seriousness, such as the morbidity and mortality. Further investigation is necessary concerning this problem.

We conclude that the endoscopic examination showed high sensitivity for the diagnosis of inhalation injury, but was insufficient in terms of objectivity. The histologic examination of bronchial biopsy is more objective and more reliable than macroscopic findings, and is a safe, useful tool for the definite diagnosis of smoke inhalation injury.

References

1. Masanes MJ, Legendre C, Lioret N et al. Fiberoptic bronchoscopy for the early diagnosis of subglottal inhalation injury. J Trauma 1994;36:59–67.
2. Masanes MJ, Legendre C, Lioret N et al. Using bronchoscopy and biopsy to diagnose early inhalation injury. Chest 1995;107:1365–1369.
3. Stone HH, Martin JDJ, Claydon CT. Management of the pulmonary burn. Am Surg 1967;33: 616–620.
4. Hantson P, Butera R, Clemessy JL et al. Early complications and value of initial clinical and paraclinical observations in victims of smoke inhalation without burns. Chest 1997;111: 671–675.
5. Toor AH, Tomashefski JF, Kieinerman J. Respiratory tract pathology in patient with severe burns. Hum Pathol 1990;21:1212–1220.

Bronchology and Bronchoesophagology: State of the Art.
H. Yoshimura et al., editors.

Clinical analysis of press-through package (PTP) as esophageal foreign bodies

K. Manaka, S. Shigihara, S. Endo, Y. Yamada, S. Yoshida and A. Kida
Department of Otorhinolaryngology-Head Neck Surgery, Nihon University School of Medicine, Tokyo, Japan

Abstract. *Introduction.* PTP as esophageal foreign bodies, from 1981 through 1999, were reviewed at the Nihon University Itabashi Hospital.

Subjects and Results. During a 19-year period, we treated 271 esophageal foreign body cases. PTP consisted of 21.0% (57/271) of esophageal foreign bodies encountered during the same period. Ages ranged from 14 to 89 years. PTP impaction is most common in elderly patients. Our series included 19 men and 38 women. Generally, the first stricture was the most common site of lodging of an esophageal foreign body, but in this study the most common site was the second stricture. The method of retrieval must be chosen according to the condition of the patient. In 47 cases, foreign bodies were removed through rigid esophagoscopy. Nine cases were removed through flexible esophagoscopy, and only one case was removed using balloon retrieval.

Conclusion. PTP impaction is expected to increase with the rise of elderly population in our country. We urge a medical and sociological effort to be continued to prevent the occurrence of this avoidable disorder.

Keywords: flexible esophagoscopy, prevention, retrieval, rigid endoscopy.

Introduction

The press-through package (PTP) is used widespread as a packing for tablets and capsules. In Japan, PTP is a common foreign body in the esophagus. PTP as esophageal foreign bodies, from January 1981 through December 1999, were reviewed at the Nihon University Itabashi Hospital.

Patients

During a 19-year period, we treated 271 esophageal foreign body cases. The most frequent cause of esophageal impaction among adults was PTP, and among children it was coins. 57 cases of PTP were seen in this period. PTP consisted of 21.0% (57/271) of all esophageal foreign bodies encountered during the same period.

Address for correspondence: Kazue Manaka MD, Department of ORL-HNS, Nihon University School of Medicine, 30-1 Oyaguchi-kamicho, Itabashi-ku, Tokyo 173-8610, Japan. Tel.: +81-3-3972-8111. Fax: +81-3-3972-1321.

Results

Ages ranged from 14 to 89 years. Patients over 60 years of age accounted for 71.2% (40/57) of all PTP patients. PTP impaction is most common in elderly patients. Our series included 19 men and 38 women. Women showed a higher incidence of PTP than men.

Lodgement in the first stricture accounted for 42% of cases (25 cases), while lodgement in the second stricture accounted for 51% (31 cases), and lodgement in the third stricture accounted for 7% (four cases). In three of the cases, two PTP were encountered within the same patient. Generally, the first stricture was the most common site of lodgement of esophageal foreign bodies [1]. However, in this study the most common site was the second stricture. The reason why foreign bodies stuck in the lower position was due to forceful swallowing.

The method of retrieval must be chosen according to the condition of the patient. In 47 cases, foreign bodies were removed through rigid esophagoscopy. Nine cases were removed through flexible esophagoscopy and only one case was removed using balloon retrieval. There were no deaths or serious postoperative complications among these cases.

Discussion

PTP impaction is expected to increase with the rising elderly population in our country. Elderly patients are often treated with numerous drugs over prolonged periods of time for chronic diseases. Diminished visual acuity and hyposthesia of the oral cavity and pharynx are common in elderly persons [2,3]. This may account for the increasing incidence of PTP impaction in elderly patients. The reason why women showed a higher incidence was not clear, however, one questionnaire reported that more women have an inclination to separate into each tablet cutting down the package sheet into individual pieces than men do.

To prevent the occurrence of PTP impaction, it is necessary to instruct patients and their families on the proper drug usage of PTP and to warn them against the separation of PTP material. It is also recommended that pharmacy dispensaries only utilize a one-dose package (ODP) or unit dose package (UDP) system instead of PTP [4,5]. Furthermore, pharmaceutical companies should improve PTP with respect to the size, shape and material, in particular avoiding the use of shape edges on PTP sheets. PTP material which is radiopaque and which can be digested or decomposed even if swallowed by accident should be developed.

We urge a medical and sociological effort to be continued to prevent the occurrence of this avoidable disorder.

References

1. Sakawa A et al. Clinical study of esophageal foreign bodies attributable to PTP material. Auris Nasus Larynx 1997;24:411–416.

2. Wecksell A et al. Odynophagia caused by inadvertent blister pack ingestion: a case report. Otolaryngol Head Neck Surg 1995;112:747–749.
3. Yamada Y et al. Press-through package as esophageal foreign bodies. Jibi-Rinsho 1995;78 (Suppl):132–135.
4. Iwata S et al. Statistic observation of PTP foreign bodies of the esophagus and their prevention. J Jpn Bronchoesophagol Soc 1995;46:406–418.
5. Yip LWL et al. "I've got a UFO stuck in my throat!"– An interesting case of foreign body inpaction in the oesophagus. Singapore Med J 1998;39:121–123.

Bronchology and Bronchoesophagology: State of the Art.
H. Yoshimura et al., editors.

Double bronchial blockade in patients with empyema and bronchopleural fistula without drainage

Makoto Nonaka[1], Mitsutaka Kadokura[1], Daisuke Kataoka[1], Shigeru Yamamoto[1], Tadanori Kawada[1], Toshihiro Takaba[1] and Akiyoshi Hosoyamada[2]
[1]First Department of Surgery and [2]Department of Anesthesiology, Showa University, Tokyo, Japan

Abstract. Adequate pleural drainage is crucial when an empyema is complicated by bronchopleural fistula. However, there are some cases in which drainage cannot be performed. The fistula allows pleural fluid to enter the bronchial tree and the contralateral lung when the patient is placed in the lateral position for pan-pleuropneumonectomy. This can occur even if a double-lumen cuffed endobronchial tube is used. Especially, with a right-sided blockade for a left thoracotomy, the blocker may slip into the trachea as a result of traction on the lung.

To achieve double luminal occlusion, a double-lumen endobronchial tube with an endobronchial blocker was used in two patients who had a chronic left empyema and a bronchopleural fistula in whom preoperative drainage was impossible. The massive pleural effusions were drained through the endobronchial blocker during surgery in the right lateral position. Good results were obtained. We did not use this double blocking method for right thoracotomies in the left lateral position, because in our experience to date, a left-sided blocker has never slipped out.

Keywords: aspiration pneumonia, bronchopleural fistula, chest drainage, chronic empyema, double-lumen endobronchial tube, endobronchial blocker.

Introduction

Proper chest drainage is essential when an empyema is complicated by a bronchopleural fistula [1]. The drainage reduces the risk of contralateral aspiration pneumonia. The surgical treatment of chronic empyema, such as pan-pleuropneumonectomy and decortication, can be undertaken after the inflammation is controlled. However, if pleural drainage is impossible and pan-pleuropneumonectomy is indicated for empyema with bronchopleural fistula, lateral positioning can be fatal due to contralateral aspiration pneumonia. This may occur even if a double-lumen endobronchial tube (DLET) [2] is used, because the bronchial cuff can be dislodged by surgical manipulation. Especially during left thoracotomy, tube malpositioning is more likely, due to the right main bronchus being short and the safety margin being narrow with a right-sided DLET [2]. We performed left thoracic pan-pleuropneumonectomy in the right lateral position without preoperative chest drainage in two patients with empyema and a broncho-

Address for correspondence: M. Nonaka, First Department of Surgery, Showa University School of Medicine, 1-5-8 Hatanodai, Shinagawa-ku, Tokyo 142-8666, Japan. Tel.: +81-3-3784-8588. Fax: +81-3-3784-8307.

pleural fistula. An endobronchial blocker [3] was inserted into the left side of the DLET, and was fixed at the left main bronchus. This double bronchial blocking method completely prevented pus drainage from the left to the right lung.

Methods and Results

Case 1 was a 63-year-old man who had recurrent pneumonia, hemosputum, and a cough with mucopurulent sputum. Chest roentgenography revealed niveau formation in the left hemithorax. Thoracentesis revealed brown pus. A diagnosis of chronic left empyema with bronchopleural fistula was made. Chest tube insertion could not be performed because of the thick calcified peel. The left remaining lung was considered nonfunctional. A pan-pleuropneumonectomy was planned.

Case 2 was a 72-year-old man who had continuous hemoptysis. Chest roentgenography revealed niveau formation in the left hemithorax. Thoracentesis revealed bloody pus. A diagnosis of chronic left empyema with bronchopleural fistula was made. Embolization of the feeding arteries was ineffective. Chest drainage was not performed because of the risk of creating negative pressure in the empyema space, which could result in bleeding. Since the bronchiectasia in the remaining left lung was severe, neither open-window thoracostomy, decortication, nor thoracoplasty could reliably stop the hemoptysis. Pan-pleuropneumonectomy was the only therapeutic option.

To protect transbronchial spill over and crosscontamination, while the patient was in the lateral position, an endobronchial blocker was added to the DLET. Since the endobronchial blocker has a suction port and a cuff, and can be inserted into the tracheal lumen of the DLET, double blocking can be achieved. After the induction of general anesthesia in the supine and head-up position, the DLET was placed in the airway in the usual fashion (Fig. 1A) [4]. Then, the

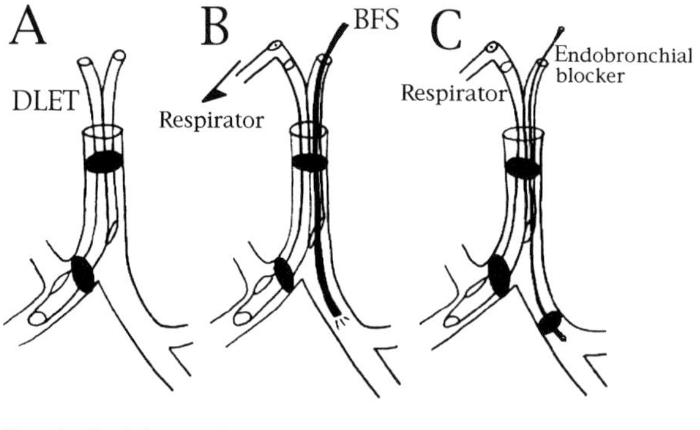

Fig. 1. Endobronchial blocker insertion via the left side of a double-lumen endobronchial tube (DLET). **A:** A standard cuffed DLET is placed in the airway. **B:** A bronchofiberscope (BFS) is passed through the left side of the DLET. The distance from the left main bronchus to the endcap of the DLET is measured. **C:** When the tip of the endobronchial blocker reaches the left main bronchus, the blocker is positioned so that the tip lies above the orifice of the left upper lobe. The cuff of the blocker is inflated. The endobronchial blocker is secured in position with the endobronchial tube.

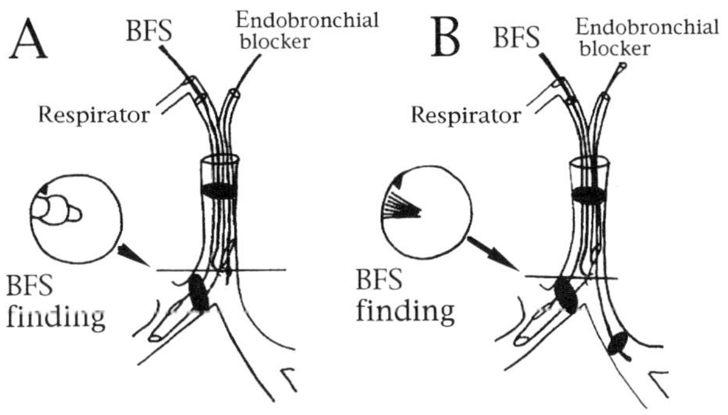

Fig. 2. **A:** Under right lung ventilation, the bronchofiberscope (BFS) is passed through the right side of the double-lumen endobronchial tube (DLET) to the level of the trachea. An endobronchial blocker is inserted through the left side of the endobronchial tube. The insertion of the endobronchial blocker is observed with the BFS through the right side of the DLET. **B:** When the tip of the endobronchial blocker reaches the left main bronchus, the blocker is positioned so that the tip is above the second carina. Then, the cuff of the blocker is inflated.

bronchofiberscope (BFS) was passed through the left side of the DLET (tracheal lumen), and the distance from the left main bronchus to the endcap of the DLET was measured (Fig. 1B). Under right lung ventilation, the BFS was inserted in the right side of the DLET (bronchial lumen) to the level of the carina (Fig. 2A). Then, the endobronchial blocker was inserted into the tracheal lumen (Fig. 2A). Insertion of the endobronchial blocker beyond the carina was confirmed using the BFS in the bronchial lumen of the DLET (Fig. 2A). When the tip of the endobronchial blocker reached the left main bronchus, the blocker was positioned so that the tip was above the second carina. Then, the cuff of the blocker was inflated (Figs. 1C and 2B). The endobronchial blocker was secured in position with the DLET. After confirmation that all of the cuffs of the endobronchial tube and the endobronchial blocker were inflated, the patient was turned to the right lateral position with continuous suction of the exudate from the left lung through the endobronchial blocker. After the patient was in the right lateral position and right lung ventilation was established, the BFS was used to confirm correct positioning of the tubes and that there was no efflux from the left to the right bronchus. The method was effective and reliable.

Via a posterolateral thoracotomy, left pan-pleuropneumonectomy was performed using right lung ventilation and low-intermittent suction of the exudate from the left lung through the endobronchial blocker. The BFS was used to confirm that there was no efflux from the left to the right bronchus during surgery. This reduced the possibility of contamination of the right lung, which may occur with a standard DLET. Just prior to resection of the left main bronchus, the endobronchial blocker was deflated and pulled back to avoid its inclusion in the incisional line. These techniques were used in both patients. Extubation was possible in the operating theater. Postoperative chest roentgenography showed no abnormalities in the right lung. There were no intraoperative or postoperative complications. These techniques effectively eliminated the preoperative symptoms. The patients were both discharged in good condition. They were still well at 30 and 10 months follow-up examinations, respectively.

Discussion

Chest drainage is a fundamental part of the treatment of patients with empyema and a bronchopleural fistula. In case 2, drainage was avoided because of the risk that negative pressure in the empyema could cause bleeding, but in case 1, open drainage may have been technically feasible in the prone or supine position via a mini-thoracotomy under epidural anesthesia. Without our double blocking method, chest drainage is performed with a high risk of bleeding from the tearing of the vascularized peel. Furthermore, the most dependent portion of the empyema space is a long reach from an anterolateral open-window thoracotomy in the supine position.

Without chest drainage, pan-pleuropneumonectomy can be performed via a posterolateral incision with the patient in the prone and head-down position. However, the intercostal spaces are narrow, and many ribs must be incised. Alternatively, the empyema can be approached through a median sternotomy or anterolateral incision with the patient in the supine position. However, in our two cases, the surgical approach to the costophrenic and costovertebral angles using these approaches would have been difficult because the most dependent portion was posterior, just above the diaphragm.

The DLET is usually effective. However, the blocker of the right main bronchus sometimes slips into the trachea. Since aspiration pneumonia of the right lung would be fatal, we believe that the double blocking method is justified in patients undergoing pan-pleuropneumonectomy in the right lateral position for a left thoracic empyema and bronchopleural fistula without preoperative chest drainage. However, as left-sided blockers have never, to our knowledge or experience, slipped out, the double blocking method is not indicated for right thoracotomy.

References

1. Navarini EA. Surgical approach to the acute empyema. In: Deslauriers J, Lacquet LK (eds) Thoraeic surgery: surgical management of pleural diseases. St Louis: The CV Mosby Company, 1990;207–219.
2. Mckenna MJ, Wilson RS, Botelho RJ. Right upper lobe obstruction with right-sided double-lumen endobronchial tubes: a comparison of two types. Anesthesiology 1988;63:734–740.
3. Gayes JM. The univent tube is the best technique for providing one-lung ventilation. J Cardiovasc Vasc Anesth 1993;7:103–107.
4. Cohen E. Is bronchoscopy necessary for insertion of double-lumen endotracheal tubes? J Bronchol 2000;7:72–77.

Bronchology and Bronchoesophagology: State of the Art.
H. Yoshimura et al., editors.

Characterization of immunoglobulin binding factor in sputum from patients with chronic airway diseases

Fumitaka Ogushi[1], Waka Ichikawa[1], Kenji Tani[1], Koji Maniwa[1], Yoichi Nakamura[1], Mitunori Sakatani[2] and Saburo Sone[1]

[1]Third Department of Internal Medicine, The University of Tokushima, School of Medicine, Tokushima; and [2]Department of Internal Medicine, National Kinki Chuo Hospital for Chest Disease. Sakai, Osaka, Japan

Abstract. *Background.* Immunoglobulin binding factor (IgBF) is known to bind immunoglobulin, to interact with anti-Fcγ-III antibodies and to be present in the lower respiratory tract of normal healthy subjects. In this study, we investigated whether IgBF existed in the respiratory tract of patients with chronic airway diseases.

Methods. IgBF was measured in the sputum from patients with chronic airway diseases and induced sputum from control subjects by enzyme-linked immunosorbent assay.

Results. IgBF concentration in the sputum of patients with chronic airway diseases (purulent: 50.2 ± 8.2 μg/ml; mucoid: 88.6 ± 12.8 μg/ml) was higher than that in induced sputum (6.3 ± 5.5 μg/ml, $p < 0.001$). IgBF level in mucoid sputum was significantly higher than that in purulent sputum ($p < 0.05$). A significant inverse correlation was shown between the IgBF level and the elastase activity in sputum, and the concentration of IgBF purified from seminal plasma was decreased by the treatment with neutrophil elastase.

Conclusion. These results demonstrated that a high level of IgBF is present in the respiratory tract of patients with chronic airway diseases and may be related to the pathogenesis of these diseases.

Keywords: chronic bronchitis, diffuse pan bronchiolitis, mucoid sputum, purulent sputum.

Introduction

Immunoglobulin binding factor (IgBF) was initially purified from human seminal plasma [1]. It has a molecular weight of 16 kDa as shown by sodium dodecyl sulfate polyacrylamide gel electrophoresis (SDS-PAGE) under reducing conditions, and 27 kDa under nonreducing conditions. There are reports that IgBF binds immunoglobulins of various species and interacts with anti-Leu-11b antibodies raised against Fc-γ-RIII [1]. Although the reduced form (a 16-kDa protein) of IgBF can bind immunoglobulin, the native form (a 27-kDa protein) cannot. Although the physiological roles of IgBF are still unknown, these results suggest that IgBF may be located in areas of the body in contact with the outer environment, and may modulate the local immune system. We have demonstrated that IgBF is present in bronchoalveolar lavage from normal subjects, and histo-

Address for correspondence: Fumitaka Ogushi MD, Third Department of Internal Medicine, University of Tokushima, School of Medicine, Kuramoto-cho 3, Tokushima 770-8503, Japan. Tel.: +81-88-633-7127. Fax: +81-88-633-2134. E-mail: fumitaka@clin.med.tokushima-u.ac.jp chemically we demonstrated IgBF immunoreactivity in mucous glands and goblet cells [2]. In the present study, to clarify the physiological role of IgBF, we investigated whether IgBF exists in the airway of patients with chronic airway diseases. For this purpose, we measured the IgBF concentration in sputum of patients with chronic airway diseases and IgBF level in mucoid sputum was compared with that in purulent sputum.

Materials and Methods

Subjects

Sputum samples were obtained from 59 chronic airway disease patients with hypersecretory diseases and from healthy subjects. All of the subjects were non-smokers or ex-smokers who had stopped smoking at least 10 years earlier. The patient group consisted of 37 patients (18 men, 19 women) with chronic bronchitis (CB), aged from 31 to 77 years, 18 patients (11 men, seven women) with bronchiectasis (BE), aged from 38 to 78 years, and four patients (one man, three women) with diffuse pan bronchiolitis (DPB), aged from 31 to 66 years. All of the patients had been expectorating over 20 ml of sputum per day. All patients with mucoid sputum were in a stable stage. On the other hand, eight (two BE patients, six CB patients) of 31 patients with purulent sputum were thought to be in an acute exacerbation stage, because they complained of increasing sputum volume, while 23 patients were in a stable stage. The control groups consisted of 28 normal healthy subjects (20 men, eight women), aged from 15 to 78 years. In this study, for convenience, the sputa were classified into two groups: mucoid (consisting of mucoid and mucopulurent sputum) and purulent sputum. Mucoid sputa were obtained from 28 patients (19 CB patients, eight BE patients and one DPB patient), and purulent sputa were obtained from 31 patients (18 CB patients, 10 BE patients and three DPB patients). Thirty-seven patients with CB, 18 patients with BE and four patients with DPB were receiving expectorants, and four patients with DPB were receiving low doses of erythromycin. Sputum from patients was collected after they gargled. Sputum from healthy subjects was induced by having the subject inhale hypertonic saline solution (3% saline).

Measurement of IgBF in the sputum

The IgBF concentration in the sputum was measured using an enzyme-linked immunosorbent assay (ELISA) which we developed [3]. This ELISA method consistently detected IgBF concentrations greater than 20 pg/ml.

Assay of elastase activity in the sputum

Elastase activity was measured by a modification of the spectrofluorometric method of Oshima et al. [12] with Suc-Ala-Pro-Ala-7-amino-methylcoumarine

(AMC) (Peptide Institute, Osaka, Japan) as the substrate. The elastase activity was expressed in units, 1 unit being defined as the amount of enzyme needed to cleave one nanomole of substrate per hour.

Results

IgBF levels in the sputum

The level of IgBF was measured in the sputum of the patients with chronic airway diseases and normal subjects. As shown in Fig. 1A, the IgBF concentration in the sputum of patients with chronic airway diseases (purulent sputum: 50.2 ± 8.2 μg/ml; mucoid sputum: 88.6 ± 12.8 μg/ml) was significantly higher than that in induced sputum of normal subjects (6.3 ± 5.5 μg/ml) ($p<0.001$). The IgBF concentrations in the mucoid sputum were significantly higher than those in the purulent sputum ($p<0.05$). The IgBF concentration in sputum, normalized to that of total protein (TP) (IgBF/TP ratio), was also significantly higher in the mucoid sputum ($p<0.001$) (Fig. 1B).

Relation between elastase activity and IgBF concentration in the sputum

To investigate the reason why the IgBF levels in the purulent sputum were lower than those in the mucoid sputum, we measured the elastase activity in the spu-

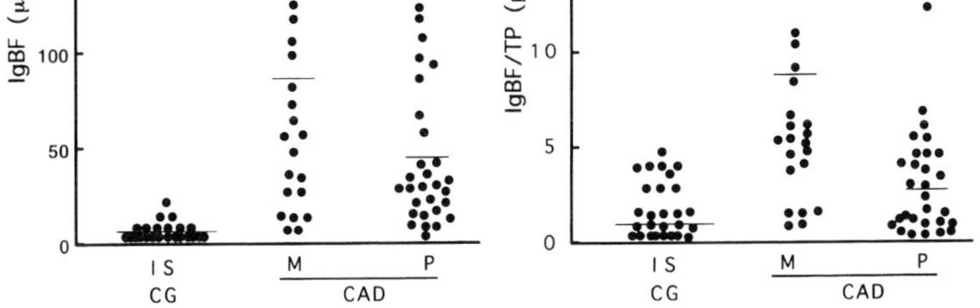

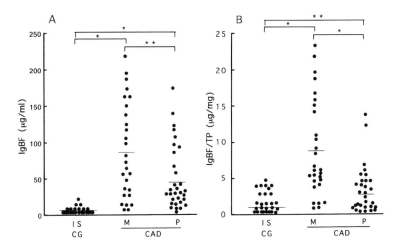

Fig. 1. Concentration of IgBF and IgBF normalized to total protein (TP) in sputum obtained from 28 healthy subjects and 59 patients with chronic airway diseases. The IgBF concentration in sputum was measured by ELISA as described in Materials and Methods. **A:** Ordinate, IgBF concentration (μg/ml); abscissa, control group (CG), chronic airway diseases group (CAD). **B:** Ordinate, IgBF/TP (μg/mg); abcissa, control group (CG), chronic airway diseases group (CAD). Horizontal bars represent mean values. IS, induced sputum; M, mucoid sputum; P, purulent sputum. IS, n = 28; M, n = 28; P, n = 31. $^{*}p<0.001$; $^{**}p<0.05$.

tum, because elastase might digest IgBF. The elastase activity in purulent sputum was significantly higher than that in mucoid sputum (1,239.2 ± 1,017.8 vs. 45.7 ± 115.1 units, $p < 0.001$). We examined the relationship between elastase activity and IgBF levels in the sputum, and found a significant correlation between elastase activity and IgBF concentration in the sputum ($r = -0.77$; $p = 0.001$). When IgBF purified from human seminal plasma was incubated with human neutrophil elastase, the IgBF concentration was decreased by the addition of elastase in a dose-dependent manner.

Discussion

To clarify the role of IgBF in respiratory diseases, we investigated the IgBF level in the sputum of chronic airway disease patients who were nonsmokers, to avoid the effect of smoking. High levels of IgBF were detected in both mucoid and purulent sputum (Fig. 1). These results may be related to the increased numbers of mucus glands and goblet cells which produce IgBF, or to an increase of another aspect of IgBF production in chronic airway diseases.

The reason why IgBF levels in the mucoid sputum were significantly higher than those in purulent sputum is not clear. Neutrophils accumulate in the lesion of bronchi due to an infection, and the elastase activity of sputum from patients with chronic airway diseases with infection was found to be increased. Since neutrophil elastase was reported to degrade immunoglobulins such as IgG and s-IgA, we measured the elastase activity in the sputum, and found an inverse correlation between IgBF level and elastase activity. Moreover, when purified seminal plasma IgBF was incubated with neutrophil elastase, the levels of IgBF was decreased. These results suggested that IgBF in purulent sputum might be digested by neutrophil elastase, and thus the concentration of IgBF in purulent sputum would be less compared with that in mucoid sputum. The physiological roles of IgBF in the respiratory tract are unknown, but IgBF probably modulates the local immune system, judging from recent reports on possible functions of IgBF, because IgBF has been shown to bind to serum immunoglobulin of several species and to interact with antibodies against Fcg receptor type III [1]. IgBF was shown to suppress pokeweed mitogen-stimulated lymphocyte blastogenesis, and had no influence and a slightly inhibitory effect on phytohemagglutinin- and concanavalin A-stimulated blastogenesis, respectively [4]. IgBF was also detected in other biological fluids such as uterine cervical fluid, suggesting that this protein may have some function related to mucus secretion and may be located in areas of the body in contact with the outer environment [3]. Recently, we found that glutathione, protein disulfide isomerase, and 20S proteosomes altered the inactive form to active form [5]. Based on these results, this native IgBF may be converted to the active monomer by a reducing enzyme or reductants present in many tissues or cells, or by processing within immunocompetent cells under certain conditions. It is likely that the increased content of IgBF in purulent and mucoid sputum of patients with chronic airway diseases reflects a role of IgBF in local areas of the lung and the regulation of the IgBF production of lung cells may be important in the treatment of chronic airway diseases.

Acknowledgements

This work was supported by a Grant-in-Aid for Scientific Research from the Ministry of Education, Science and Culture of Japan.

References

1. Kamada M, Liang Z, Koide SS. Identification of IgG and Fc-binding proteins in human seminal plasma and sperm. Arch Androl 1991;27:1–7.
2. Ogushi F, Sone S, Tani K et al. Identification and localization of immunoglobulin binding factor in bronchoalveolar lavage fluid from healthy smokers. Am J Respir Crit Care Med 1995;152: 2133–2137.
3. Kamada M, Maeda N, Maegawa M et al. Detection of immunoglobulin binding factor by enzyme-linked immunosorbent assay using monoclonal antibodies. Biochem Mol Biol Int 1994;34:837–844.
4. Maeda N, Kamada M, Daitoh T et al. Immunoglobulin binding factor in human seminal plasma: immunological function. Arch Androl 1993;31:31–36.
5. Mori H, Kamada M, Maegawa M et al. Enzymatic activation of immunoglobulin binding factor in female reproductive tract. Biochem Biophys Res Commun 1998;246:409–413.

Bronchology and Bronchoesophagology: State of the Art.
H. Yoshimura et al., editors.

Nasal and lower airway level of nitric oxide (NO) and carbon monoxide (CO) in children with ciliary dyskinesia

E. Péterffy[1], Gy. Baktai[1], Zs. Rázga[2], L. Tiszlavicz[2] and I. Horváth [3]

[1]*Pediatric Institute 'Svábhegy (Szabadsághegy)', Budapest;* [2]*Albert Szent-Györgyi Medical University, Pathological Institute, Szeged; and* [3]*Korányi National Institute of Pulmonology, Budapest, Hungary*

Abstract. *Purpose.* Recent reports suggest that the level of nasal nitric oxide (NO) is low in primary ciliary dyskinesia (PCD), however, there is no experience with nasal and/or exhaled NO and exhaled carbon monoxide (CO) in secondary ciliary dyskinesia (SCD). Therefore, we aimed to determine nasal and external NO and CO in children with histologically proven PCD and SCD.

Methods. Nasal and exhaled NO and CO were measured by Logan analyser (LR2000, UK) in three groups of children aged between 76 and 186 months: 1) PCD (n = 7), 2) SCD (n = 5), and 3) healthy controls (n = 7) (clinical evaluation).

Results. On the basis of clinical aspects and nasal NO (nNO) values the PCD group was divided into two subgroups: 1) PCD1 (n = 4): all classical features of primary ciliary dyskinesia and/or Kartagener syndrome, lower than 100 parts per billion (ppb) nNO values, and 2) PCD2 (n = 3): clinically controversial primary ciliary dyskinesia, situs solitus, higher than 100 ppb nNO values. In PCD1, NO and CO results were as follows: external NO (eNO), 2.48 ± 0.34 ppb; nNO, 39.8 ± 12.0 ppb; exhaled CO (eCO), 2.15 ± 0.33 parts per million (ppm); nasal CO (nCO), 1.01 ± 0.73 unit. In PCD2: eNO, 3.42 ± 0.55 ppb; nNO, 874.7 ± 117.1 ppb; eCO, 3.4 ± 0.94 ppm; nCO, 1.05 ± 0.40 unit. In SCD: eNO, 7.32 ± 1.64 ppb; nNO, 622.6 ± 192.8 ppb; eCO, 2.32 ± 0.25 ppm; nCO, 0.77 ± 0.22 unit. In healthy controls: eNO, 3.51 ± 0.36 ppb; nNO, 1,047.0 ± 83.0 ppb; eCO, 3.26 ± 0.15 ppm; nCO, 0.97 ± 0.07 unit. (Data are given as mean ± SEM.)

Conclusions. We found that in one subgroup of PCD patients (PCD1), nNO levels were extremely low with a moderate decrease in eNO concentration. In PCD2, nNO and eNO values were similar to those in the SCD group. Therefore, the clinical relevance of histologically proven primary ciliary dyskinesia with high nasal NO (PCD2), is the subject of further examination.

Keywords: exhaled nitric oxide (eNO), nasal nitric oxide (nNO), primary ciliary dyskinesia (PCD), quantitative analysis, secondary ciliary dyskinesia (SCD), ultrastructural examination.

Introduction

For the last few years much attention has been focused on abnormalities of ciliated cells and their association with chronic or recurrent respiratory tract diseases.

The diagnosis of ciliary dyskinesia was based on the ultrastructural examination of respiratory mucosa samples [1–3]. These samples were gained by rigid bronchoscopy in general anaesthesia. We proved primary and secondary ciliary dyskinesia by the quantitative analysis of dynein alterations of cilia [4].

Address for correspondence: Erzsébet Péterffy, Pediatric Institute "Svábhegy", Budapest, H-1535 POB 939, Hungary. Tel.: +36-1-395 4922. E-mail: pet6445@helka.iif.hu

Less than 5% normal dynein arms found in the examined cilia is the criterion of primary ciliary dyskinesia (PCD). If there is more than 5% normal dynein arms found, secondary ciliary dyskinesia (SCD) is proven.

In some cases the result of quantitative analysis did not correlate with clinical features. Therefore, we completed our examinations by measuring nasal and exhaled nitric oxide (NO) and carbon monoxide (CO) with the same patients.

Nitric oxide is produced by various cells within the respiratory tract and plays an important role in the pathophysiology of airway diseases. It is detectable in the exhaled air. The great advantage of measuring exhaled nitric oxide (eNO) is that it is completely noninvasive and can be performed repeatedly [5,6]. It can be used easily with children.

The normal eNO from lower airways and the normal nasal NO (nNO) values are 4.8 parts per billion (ppb) and 1,024 ppb, respectively, among children aged 6–17 years (by Kharitonov [6]).

Lundberg and Karadag reported that the level of nNO is low or almost absent in children with primary ciliary dyskinesia [7,8].

To our knowledge, there are no data on nNO and eNO in children with histologically proved secondary ciliary dyskinesia. Therefore, we aimed to compare the levels of nasal and exhaled NO in primary and secondary ciliary dyskinesia.

Materials and Methods

nNO was measured in the upper airways by direct nasal sampling during a breath-hold. eNO was shown in lower airways on the end-tidal plateau level. We used the Logan chemoluminescence NO analyser [6]. The tests were repeated 3 times and the mean values were calculated.

We measured 19 children aged from 6 to 16 years in three groups: seven children in PCD, five children in SCD and seven children in the healthy group were also examined. The healthy controls were defined clinically: they had no history of any respiratory diseases. The patients in the PCD and SCD groups did not receive any steroids. Results are given in Table 1.

Although histologically we had only one PCD group, the nNO values we found were divided into two subgroups.

In PCD1 where all classical features of primary ciliary dyskinesia and Kar-

Table 1. Results.

	eNO (ppb)	NNO (ppb)	eCO (ppm)	nCO (ppm)
PCD1 (n = 4)	2.48 ± 0.34	39.8 ± 12.0	2.15 ± 0.33	1.01 ± 0.73
PCD2 (n = 3)	3.42 ± 0.55	874.7 ± 117.1	3.4 ± 0.94	1.05 ± 0.40
SCD (n = 5)	7.32 ± 1.64	622.6 ± 192.8	2.32 ± 0.25	0.77 ± 0.22
Healthy (n = 7)	3.51 ± 0.36	1047 ± 83.0	3.26 ± 0.15	0.97 ± 0.07

Data are given as mean ± SEM; ppb = parts per billion, ppm = parts per million.

tagener syndrome can be recognised, nNO was found to be markedly reduced, lower than 100 ppb. The mean eNO was also significantly lower than that in the healthy children.

In PCD2 where primary ciliary dyskinesia was clinically controversial, nNO values were higher, similar to healthy or SCD children.

We simultaneously measured CO levels, but we did not find significant difference between the groups.

Summary

Setting the diagnosis of PCD may be difficult, since secondary functional and structural changes of cilia may be confused with primary disease.

This study has demonstrated that a significant subgroup of children with primary ciliary dyskinesia, PCD1, had a negligible amount of nasally derived NO and also a reduced level in their lower airways. In the other subgroup, PCD2, the NO values were similar to those in SCD and the healthy group.

The measurement of nNO may be useful as a complementary test for PCD.

The clinical relevance of histologically proven PCD with high nNO is the subject of further examination.

Acknowledgements

This study was supported by OTKA (T030340).

References

1. Jorissen M, Cassiman J-J. Relevance of the ciliary ultrastructure in primary and secondary ciliary dyskinesia: a review. Am J Rhinol 1991;5(3):91—101.
2. Schidlow Daniel V. Primary ciliary dyskinesia (the immotile cilia syndrome). Review article. Ann Allergy 1994;73:457—468.
3. Bush A, Cole P, Hariri M, Mackay I et al. Primary ciliary dyskinesia: diagnosis and standards of care. Eur Respir J 1998;12:982—988.
4. Van der Baan S, Bezemer PD, Veerman AJP, Feenstra L. Primary ciliary dyskinesia: quantitative investigation of the ciliary ultrastructure with statistical analysis. Ann Otol Rhinol Laryngol 1987;96:264—272.
5. Baraldi E, Azzolin NM, Cracco A, Zacchello F. Reference values of exhaled nitric oxide for healthy children 6—15 years old. Pediatr Pulmonol 1999;27:54—58.
6. Kharitonov S, Alving K, Barnes PJ. Exhaled and nasal nitric oxide measurements: recommendations. Eur Respir J 1997;10:1683—1693.
7. Lundberg JON, Weitzberg E, Nordvall SL, Kuylenstierna R et al. Primarily nasal origin of exhaled nitric oxide and absence in Kartagener's syndrome. Eur Respir J 1994;7:1501—1504.
8. Karadag B, James AJ, Gültekin E, Wilson NM, Bush A. Nasal and lower airway level of nitric oxide in children with primary ciliary dyskinesia. Eur Respir J 1999;13:1402—1405.

Bronchology and Bronchoesophagology: State of the Art.
H. Yoshimura et al., editors.

A 9-year review of pediatric tracheotomy

Fumiko Shishiyama, Nobuko Kawashiro, Nobuaki Tsuchihashi and Noriko Morimoto
Department of Otorhinolaryngology, National Children's Hospital, Tokyo, Japan

Abstract. We reviewed the 9-year experience at the National Children's Hospital with patients requiring tracheotomy. A total of 92 patients underwent tracheotomy. Fifty-eight patients (63%) were younger than 24 months. The patients had multiple symptoms of dyspnea. Surgical indications were divided into two groups: airway stenosis (45 patients, 49%) and ventilatory management (47 patients, 51%). Subglottic stenosis was found in 19 patients, subglottic hemangioma in eight patients, vocal cord paralysis in five patients, and tracheal stenosis in four patients. Twenty-five patients had neurologic disease, seven had cardiovascular disease, and four had chromosomal abnormalities. Follow-up time after tracheotomy ranged from 2 months to 8 years 7 months. Among the 92 patients, 52 (57%) were tracheotomized. Fifteen patients (16%) were eventually decannulated, and all of them required tracheotomy for airway stenosis. There were 15 (16%) deaths. Two deaths were attributed to the tracheotomy: accidental decannulation and tracheal bleeding. The other 13 patients died of underlying medical problems. Ten patients were unavailable for follow-up because they were transferred to other care facilities.

Keywords: airway stenosis, decannulation, dyspnea, prognosis, tracheotomized, ventilatory management.

Introduction

The number of pediatric tracheotomies performed per year has increased in recent years, reflecting the improved care provided in neonatal intensive care units or intensive care units.

We reviewed the 9-year experience at the National Children's Hospital with patients requiring tracheotomy.

Patients and Methods

The charts of patients who underwent tracheotomy at the National Children's Hospital between April 1991 and December 1999 were reviewed.

A total of 92 patients underwent tracheotomy. Forty-four patients were male, and 48 patients were female.

Their ages ranged from 2 days to 26 years 11 months, with a mean age of 4

Address for correspondence: Fumiko Shishiyama, Department of Otorhinolaryngology, National Children's Hospital, 3-35-31 Taishido, Setagaya-ku, Tokyo 154-8509, Japan. Tel.: +81-3-3414-8121. Fax: +81-3-3414-9210. E-mail: fms@mc.kcom.ne.jp

Table 1. Indication of tracheotomy.

Diagnosis	No. of patients
Airway stenosis group	45
1) Subglottic stenosis	19
2) Subglottic hemangioma	8
3) Subglottic cyst	1
4) Glottic web	2
5) Vocal cord paralysis	5
6) Laryngotracheitis	1
7) Foreign body in larynx	1
8) Tracheal stenosis	4
9) Tracheomalacia	1
10) Pierre Robin syndrome	2
11) Bronchial cleft syndrome	1
Ventilatory management group	47
1) Neuromuscular disease	25
2) Cardiovascular disease	7
3) Chromosomal abnormality	4
4) Central hypoventilation	2
5) Malignant tumor	2
6) Others	7

years 7 months and a median age of 1 year 4 months. Fifty-eight patients (63%) were younger than 24 months.

Indication of tracheotomy

The patients had multiple symptoms of dyspnea. Surgical indications were divided into two groups: airway stenosis (45 patients, 49%) and ventilatory management (47 patients, 51%) (Table 1). Though many patients were found to have airway stenosis and multiple disorders, they were classified into either group according to conditions.

Prognosis

The follow-up time after tracheotomy ranged from 2 months to 8 years 7 months. Table 2 shows the prognosis.

Among the 92 patients, 15 (16%) were eventually decannulated. All of these were patients who required tracheotomy for airway stenosis (Table 3). The duration of tracheotomy ranged from 15 days to 5 years 6 months, with a mean duration of 1 year 4 months and a median duration of 6 months. Twelve patients needed surgical treatment before decannulation, including excision of subglottic hemangioma, excision of subglottic cyst, removal of foreign body, laryngomicrosurgery, and laryngotracheoplasty (autogenous costal cartilage graft reconstruc-

Table 2. Prognosis.

	AS (n = 45)	VM (n = 47)	Total (N = 92)	%
Tracheotomized	25	27	52	57
Decannulated	15	0	15	16
Dead	3	12	15	16
Unavailable for follow-up	2	8	10	11

AS, airway stenosis; VM, ventilatory management.

Table 3. Decannulated cases.

	No. of patients
Decannulated cases	15
Subglottic stenosis	2
Subglottic hemangioma	7
Subglottic cyst	1
Laryngotracheitis	1
Foreign body of larynx	1
Tracheal stenosis	1
Pierre Robin syndrome	1
Bronchial cleft syndrome	1

tion, Y tube placement).

There were 15 deaths. Two deaths were attributed to the tracheotomy: accidental decannulation and tracheal bleeding. The other 13 patients died of underlying medical problems.

Ten patients were unavailable for follow-up, because they were transferred to other care facilities.

Conclusions

1. We reviewed the 9-year experience at the National Children's Hospital with patients undergoing tracheotomy.
2. Of the 92 patients, 48 (63%) were younger than 24 months.
3. Indications were divided into two groups: airway stenosis (45 patients, 49%) and ventilatory management (47 patients, 51%).
4. Fifteen patients (16%) were eventually decannulated. All of these were patients who required tracheotomy for airway stenosis.

Bronchology and Bronchoesophagology: State of the Art.
H. Yoshimura et al., editors.

Serum gastrointestinal (GI) hormone altering in patients with carcinoma of the lung and esophagus

Y. Yamashita[1], E. Miyahara[1], K. Shimizu[1], T. Toge[1] and T.E. Adrian[2]

[1] *Department of Surgical Oncology, Research Institute for Radiation Biology and Medicine, Hiroshima University, Hiroshima, Japan; and* [2] *Department of Biomedical Sciences, Creighton University School of Medicine, Omaha, Nebraska, USA*

Abstract. We investigated the reaction of six gastrointestinal (GI) hormones to food in patients with carcinoma of lung (n = 8) and esophagus (n = 10) compared with nine healthy controls. Gastrin, motilin, glucose-dependent insulinotropic peptide (GIP), cholecystokinin (CCK), pancreatic polypeptide (PP) and peptide YY (PYY) were measured by specific radioimmunoassay. Each hormone was evaluated by fasting level (F), incremental integrated responses (IIR60, IIR180 pmol/l/min), and total integrated responses (TIR60, TIR180 pmol/l/min) after a meal. The data were analyzed using Student's t test. In patients with lung cancer, the F value of PP was significantly higher than that in healthy controls (24.4 vs. 12.3 pmol/l, $p = 0.002$). Consequently, sensitivity is 75% (6/8) and specificity is 100% (9/9). With regard to PP and PYY, almost all parameters of IIR60, IIR180, TIR60 and TIR180 were significantly higher than in healthy controls (PP: p value = 0.00020–0.021; PYY: 0.0077–0.30). In patients with esophageal cancer, CCK was significantly lower than in healthy controls: in IIR180 ($p = 0.039$) and TIR180 ($p = 0.041$). However, the other hormones showed similar secretion levels in the patient group compared to healthy controls. GI hormone altering may provide autocrine stimulation of growth, or it may be the result of abnormal metabolism in cancer patients. PP and PYY would be useful tumor markers for lung cancer.

Keywords: esophageal cancer, gastrointestinal hormone, lung cancer, tumor marker.

Background

Serum gastrointestinal (GI) hormones have been observed in hormone-producing tumors concerning patients with carcinoma, for example pancreas tumor. Recently, serum ProGRP (gastrin-releasing peptide) was a useful tumor marker in the diagnosis of small cell lung cancer. Some GI hormones would give a better understanding of carcinogenesis and progression of the carcinomas, according to the literature. We investigated the reaction of six GI hormones to food in patients with carcinoma of the lung and the esophagus.

Address for correspondence: Yoshinori Yamashita MD, Department of Surgical Oncology, Research Institute for Radiation Biology and Medicine, Hiroshima University, 1-2-3 Kasumi, Minami-ku, Hiroshima 734-8553, Japan. Tel.: +81-82-257-5866. Fax: +81-82-256-5866.
E-mail:genge@ipc.hiroshima-u.ac.jp

Table 1. Six GI hormones released to the test meal in esophageal cancer patients.

	F (pmol/l)	TIR60 (pmol/l/60 min)	IIR60 (pmol/l/60 min)	TIR180 (pmol/l/180 min)	IIR180 (pmol/l/180 min)
Gastrin	11.9	2199	1485	6129.0	3987.0
Motilin	26.9	1866	251.5	3110.5	–1731.5
GIP	27.1	3995	2369	15689	10811
CCK	0.86	112.5[a]	60.93[a]	3659.6[b]	3504.8[b]
PP	17.8	4351	3283	11734	8530.0
PYY	13.6	906.5	90.50[a]	3069.5	621.50

[a]$p < 0.1$, [b]$p < 0.05$ vs. healthy control.

Methods

Subjects were 10 patients with esophageal cancer, and eight patients with lung cancer, and they were compared to nine healthy controls. Gastrin, motilin, glucose-dependent insulinotropic peptide (GIP), cholecystokinin (CCK), pancreatic polypeptide (PP) and peptide YY (PYY) were measured 30 min before and 5, 15, 30, 60, 120 and 180 min after a test meal, using a specific radioimmunoassay. The test meal consisted of a standard breakfast containing adequate carbohydrate, protein and fat in 600 kcal. Each hormone was evaluated by fasting level (F), incremental integrated responses (IIR60, IIR180 pmol/l/min), and total integrated responses (TIR60, TIR180 pmol/l/min) after a meal. The data were analyzed with Student's t test.

Results

In patients with esophageal cancer, CCK is significantly lower than in healthy controls in IIR180 ($p = 0.039$) and TIR180 ($p = 0.041$), as shown in Table 1. In patients with lung cancer, the F value of PP is significantly higher than that in healthy controls (24.4 vs. 12.3 pmol/l, $p = 0.002$), as shown in Table 2. Consequently, sensitivity is 75% (6/8) and specificity is 100% (9/9). With reference to

Table 2. Six GI hormones released to the test meal in lung cancer patients.

	F (pmol/l)	TIR60 (pmol/l/60 min)	IIR60 (pmol/l/60 min)	TIR180 (pmol/l/180 min)	IIR180 (pmol/l/180 min)
Gastrin	25.9	3791	2238	10383	5725.6
Motilin	41.0	3133	672.5	5217.5	–2162.5
GIP	27.1	4461	2833	15767	10884
CCK	1.12	159.3	91.06	5146.1	4941.3
PP	24.4[a]	8311[b]	6849[b]	19985[b]	15598[a]
PYY	14.5	1491[b]	620.6[a]	4610.6[a]	2000.6

[a]$p < 0.05$, [b]$p < 0.01$ vs. healthy control.

PP and PYY, almost all parameters of IIR60, IIR180, TIR60 and TIR180 were significantly higher in lung cancer patients than in healthy controls (PP: p value = 0.00020–0.021, PYY: 0.0077–0.30). However, in the patients, the other hormones showed similar secretion levels as healthy controls.

Conclusions

The abnormal reaction of CCK to food may result in some disorder of transient lower esophageal sphincter relaxation (TLESR) because it is reported that CCK plays an important role for the TLESR [1,2]. However, decreased CCK cannot explain esophageal carcinogenesis, although it may induce gastroesophageal reflux.

Pulmonary hypertrophic osteoarthropathy, so-called clubbed finger, is sometimes observed in the patients with lung cancer. Involvement of the vagal nerve has been suggested in the literature [3,4]. This can indicate that there is some relationship with PP.

GI hormone altering may provide autocrine stimulation of growth, or it may be the result of abnormal metabolism in cancer patients. PP and PYY would be useful tumor markers for lung cancer.

References

1. Dent J, Dodds WJ, Friedman RH et al. Mechanism of gastroesophageal in recumbent asymptomatic human subjects. J Clin Invest 1980;65:256.
2. Dodds WJ, Dent J, Hogan EJ et al. Mechanism of gastroesophageal in patients with reflux esophagitis. N Engl J Med 1982;307:1547.
3. Rutherford RB, Rhodes BA, Wagner HN Jr. The distribution of extremity blood flow before and after vagotomy in a patient with hypertrophic pulmonary osteoarthropathy. Dis Chest 1969;56: 19–23.
4. Yacoub MH. Vagotomy through mediastinoscopy for pulmonary osteoarthropathy. Br J Dis Chest 1966;60:144–147.

©2001 Published by Elsevier Science B.V.
Bronchology and Bronchoesophagology: State of the Art.
H. Yoshimura et al., editors.

Bronchial embolization using silicone (BEUS) for an intractable pneumothorax and the development of endobronchial Watanabe spigot (EWS)

Yoichi Watanabe, Shinobu Hosokawa, Takeshi Horiuchi, Akihiko Tamaoki, Keisuke Matsuo and Shunkichi Hiraki
Department of Pulmonary Disease, Okayama Red Cross Hospital, Okayama, Japan

Abstract. We developed bronchial embolization using silicone (BEUS) in 1989. BEUS was performed on 11 patients, of which there were six cases of intractable pneumothorax, two cases of pyothorax with bronchial fistula, one case of postoperative bronchial fistula, one case of traumatic pneumothorax with consistent bronchial bleeding, and one case of pyelobronchial fistula. BEUS was performed on nine of the 11 patients successfully. It is thought that BEUS has the possibility of providing a surer and longer bronchial blockade than conventional methods. Therefore, we developed the endobronchial Watanabe spigot (EWS), made of silicone, in collaboration with NOVATECH. BEUS with EWS was successfully performed on three patients, of which there were two cases of intractable pneumothorax and one case of gall bladder bronchial fistula.

Keywords: bronchial fistula, bronchial embolization, endobronchial Watanabe spigot, pneumothorax, silicone.

Introduction

The first report on bronchial embolization using silicone (BEUS) was made by us [1] in 1989, as a treatment for intractable bronchial fistula and pneumothorax. BEUS was thought to be more useful than conventional bronchial embolization. Under such circumstances, we developed the endobronchial Watanabe spigot (EWS), in collaboration with NOVATECH, as a bronchial filler.

Materials, Methods and Patients

Our method of utilizing BEUS is as follows. First, a determination of affected bronchi is made, using Wilson Cook's balloon catheter. A blockade of the bronchus is carried out for 20 to 30 s. If air leakage stops, then the affected bronchi exist in the peripheral area of that bronchus. After determination of the affected bronchi, embolization is performed using silicone filler under bronchofiberscopy. The silicone filler is put into the affected bronchus firmly. The method of administering BEUS with the EWS is almost the same as with a handmade

Address for correspondence: Yoichi Watanabe, Department of Pulmonary Diseases, Okayama Red Cross Hospital, 2-1-1 Aoe, Okayama 700-8607, Japan. Tel.: +81-086-222-8811. Fax: +81-086-222-8841. E-mail: ywatanabe@hi-ho.ne.jp spigot. Therapy is optional. When thought to be necessary, however, pleurodesis or other therapy is added to the treatment.

BEUS was performed, using a handmade bronchial filler, on 11 patients, of which there were six cases of intractable pneumothorax, one case of pyelobronchial fistula, one case of bronchial fistula, two cases of pyothorax with bronchial fistula, and one case of traumatic hemopneumothorax. After the development of the EWS, BEUS was performed on three patients using the EWS, which included two cases of intractable pneumothorax and one case of gall bladder-bronchial fistula.

Results

BEUS using a handmade bronchial filler was successfully performed on nine of the 11 patients. The two unsuccessful cases consisted of one case of postoperative bronchial fistula and one case of pyothorax with multiple bronchial fistula. BEUS using EWS was performed successfully in all three patients. There were no severe complications with BEUS.

Discussion

Many bronchial embolization methods have been developed as a treatment for intractable bronchial fistula and pneumothorax, however, they were not reliable enough as a bronchial blockade. The first report on BEUS was made by us in 1989. Afterwards, additional trials [2] were performed. As a result, BEUS is thought to be more useful than conventional bronchial embolization methods. We think that BEUS should be recommended in cases of peripheral bronchial fistula, intractable pneumothorax, and peripheral bronchial bleeding, etc. In such cases an operation should be avoided as far as possible, not only owing to the severe pulmonary condition, but the poor general condition, as well as other reasons. Under such circumstances, we, together with NOVATECH, developed the EWS as a bronchial filler. We designed the EWS to be easily grasped with forceps, and made studs on the surface to avoid it being expectorated by coughing. The EWS comes in three sizes. A medium-sized EWS (M) is used to embolize the subsegmental bronchus in ordinary cases. Considering the many cases of clinical trials we have carried out, we would like to confirm the usefulness of the EWS.

References

1. Watanabe Y et al. Bronchial embolization using dental impression material in a case of pyelobronchial fistula with Candida Fungemia. J Jpn Soc Bronchol 1991;13:607–610.
2. Matsuo K et al. Bronchial embolization using silicone. J Jpn Soc Bronchol 2000;22(5):333–336.

Pulmonary nodules (diagnosis and treatment)

Bronchology and Bronchoesophagology: State of the Art.
H. Yoshimura et al., editors.

Thoracoscopic and open-chest biopsy for small peripheral pulmonary nodules

Masaharu Inagaki[1], Shingo Usui[1], Naoya Funakoshi[1], Tomohiko Takabe[2] and Yoko Shinohara[2]
Departments of [1] Thoracic Surgery, and [2] Internal Medicine, Tsuchiura Kyodo General Hospital, Ibaraki, Japan

Abstract. We studied the efficiency of thoracoscopic and open-chest biopsy for indeterminate peripheral pulmonary nodules of less than 20 mm in 46 lesions in 43 patients. Bronchofiberscopic examination of 34 patients and CT-guided percutaneous needle cytology in one patient could not diagnose the nodules. Thirteen thoracoscopic biopsies and 31 open-chest biopsies revealed 12 cases of primary lung cancer and six cases metastatic lung tumors. Of 33 patients who only underwent biopsy, there were no complications experienced by the eight patients who underwent thoracoscopic biopsy, and postoperative hospital stay was shorter. There was one T4 and two N2 disease cases within the 12 patients who had primary lung cancer, and these patients' prognoses were poor. We concluded that thoracoscopic and open-chest biopsy were effective in the diagnosis of small peripheral pulmonary nodules.

Keywords: bronchofiberscopy, lung cancer, solitary peripheral pulmonary nodule, thoracoscopy.

Background

Recently partial resection of small peripheral pulmonary nodules was widely recognized to be thoracoscopically feasible [1,2]. Lung cancer screening examinations using helically computed tomography enhance the identification of ever smaller nodules [3]. We studied the efficacy of thoracoscopic and open-chest biopsy for peripheral pulmonary nodules of less than 20 mm in diameter.

Patients and Methods

Forty-three patients with 46 nodules (one patient had two nodules on the bilateral side, two patients had two nodules on the ipsilateral side) underwent thoracoscopic or open-chest biopsy for indeterminate peripheral pulmonary nodules of less than 20 mm in diameter between January 1990 and December 1997. These patients were studied in terms of their sex, age, tumor diameter, location, reason for detection, preoperative examinations, operative methods, and histology. A comparison between thoracoscopic and open-chest biopsy and a review of lung cancer patients was added. The follow-up period was until December 1999.

Address for correspondence: Masaharu Inagaki MD, Department of Thoracic Surgery, Tsuchiura Kyodo General Hospital, 11-7 Manabe shin-machi, Tsuchiura, Ibaraki 300-0053, Japan. Tel.: +81-298-23-3111. Fax: +81-298-23-1160.

Results

There were 27 male and 19 female patients with ages ranging from 38 to 84 years of age (median: 60 years). The mean size of the nodules was 12.3 mm. Twenty-eight nodules were found on the right side and 28 nodules on the lower lobe. Nodules were detected by chest roentgenograms in 39 patients (21 mass screening, 12 routine chest roentgenogram during follow-up of other disease and six during follow–up of malignant disease). Symptoms were only found in only four patients. Sputum cytology was examined in only 13 patients. There was no sputum in the other 40 patients. Frozen sectioning revealed a class 3 nodule to be adenocarcinoma and a class 4 nodule to be an inflammatory tumor.

Bronchofiberscopic examination was performed on 34 patients, which included 15 brushings, 11 curettings, 27 lavages, 10 TBLBs and 12 cultures. Of the 15 brushings, the brush instrument was only considered to roentgenologically "hit the nodule" in three nodules. These three nodules consisted of a class 1 case that was diagnosed as a metastatic nodule (breast cancer) using frozen sectioning, a class 2 case that was diagnosed as hamartoma, and a class 3 case that was diagnosed as adenocarcinoma. In one patient, CT-guided percutaneous cytology revealed a class 3 nodule which was diagnosed to be adenocarcinoma using frozen sectioning.

The thoracoscopic approach was used in 13 patients and the open-chest approach in 31 patients. The thoracoscopic approach was recently increased. There were three enucleations, 41 partial resections, one segmentectomy and one lobectomy.

There were no histological differences in diagnosis between frozen sectioning and formalin-fixed sectioning. Twelve cases of primary lung cancer, nine inflammatory tumors, eight hamartoma, six metastatic lung tumors, six tuberculoma, four intrapulmonary lymph nodes and one fungus ball were diagnosed by thoracoscopic or open-chest biopsy. Of the 12 lung cancer cases, the lobectomy and dissection of lymph nodes were added in nine patients. There were nine cases of adenocarcinoma, two of small cell carcinoma and one squamous cell carcinoma. There was one T4 (dissemination), two N2 and one M1(pm2) disease cases and these patients' prognoses were poor (Table 1).

There were eight cases of thoracoscopic biopsy and 25 cases of open-chest biopsy, except for nine lung cancer patients who had added lobectomies. In the eight cases of thoracoscopic biopsy, operation time was 122 min, operative bleeding was 76 ml, postoperative chest drainage was 2 days, hospital stay was 10 days and there were no postoperative complications. On the other hand, in the 25 cases of open-chest biopsy, operation time was 127 min, operative bleeding was 79 ml, postoperative chest drainage was 2 days, hospital stay was 24 days and postoperative complications occurred in four patients (gastric ulcer, asthma attack and two reopenings of the wound). Thoracoscopic biopsy has the clear advantages of shorter hospital stays and a lower occurrence of postoperative complications.

Table 1. Twelve cases with lung cancer.

No.	Age/ sex	Location	Operation	Histology	Added	Size (mm)	pTNM	Adu-vant	Prognosis (months)
1	75/M	R S4a	Open	sm	RML,R0	15	T1NXM0	ch	Dead (other)(54)
2	69/F	R S4b	Open	ad	RML,R2	13	T1N0M0	–	Alive (89)
3	84/F	R S6a	Open	sm	–	20	T1NXM0	–	Unknown
4	51/F	L S8	Open	ad	LLL,R2	15	T4N0M0	–	Dead (34)
5	66/M	L S3a	Open	sq	–	7	T1NXM0	–	Alive (60)
6	61/M	L S3c	Open	ad	LUL,R2	20	T1N0M0	–	Alive (59)
7	47/F	L S10	Open	ad	LLL,R2	17	T2N2M0	rad	Dead (14)
8	77/F	L S6a	Thoraco	ad	LLL,R2	18	T1N0M0	–	Alive (51)
9	64/M	R S10b	Thoraco	ad	–	15	T1NXM0	–	Dead (other) (5)
10	62/F	R S2	Open	ad	RUL,R2	19	T1N2M0	rad	Alive (rec) (39)
11	74/M	R S3a	Thoraco	ad	RUL,R2	20	T1N0M1	–	Dead (29)
12	48/F	L S1+2	Thoraco	ad	LU Seg,R2	12	T1N0M0	–	Alive (30)

Open: open-chest biopsy, Thoraco: thoracoscopic biopsy, sm: small cell carcinoma, ad: adenocarcinoma, sq: squamous cell carcinoma, RML: right middle lobectomy, LLL: left lower lobectomy, LUL: left upper lobectomy, RUL: right upper lobectomy, LU Seg: left upper segmentectomy, other: other cause, rec: recurrence, ch: chemotherapy, rad: radiation.

Conclusions

Twelve cases of primary lung cancer were diagnosed by open-chest or thoracoscopic biopsy in 43 cases of undiagnosed peripheral pulmonary nodules of less than 20 mm in diameter. Thoracoscopic biopsy has the advantages of shorter hospital stays and a lower occurrence of postoperative complications. There was one T4, two N2 and one M1 disease cases within the 12 cases of primary lung cancer, and these patients' prognoses were poor. We concluded that thoracoscopic and open-chest biopsy were effective in the diagnosis of indeterminate small peripheral pulmonary nodules.

References

1. Mack MJ, Hazelrigg SR, Landreneau RJ, Acuff TE. Thoracoscopy for the diagnosis of the indeterminate solitary pulmonary nodule. Ann Thorac Surg 1993;56:825–832.
2. Santambrogio L, Nosotti M, Bellaviti N, Mezzetti M. Videothoracoscopy versus thoracotomy for the diagnosis of the indeterminate solitary pulmonary nodule. Ann Thorac Surg 1995;59: 868–871.
3. Mori K, Sasagawa M, Moriyama N. Detection of nodular lesions in the lung using helical computed tomography: comparison of fast couch speed technique with conventional computed tomography. Jpn J Clin Oncol 1994;24:252–257.

Bronchology and Bronchoesophagology: State of the Art.
H. Yoshimura et al., editors.

VATS procedures: multiple sclerosing hemangioma resected by a two-port approach

Yusuke Kita, Hiroshi Nogimura, Hiroshi Neyatani, Ryo Kobayashi, Hutoshi Toyoda, Yoshihiko Kageyama, Satoshi Ohi, Kozo Matsushita, Yasushi Ito, Tsuyoshi Takahashi, Kazuya Suzuki and Teruhisa Kazui
First Department of Surgery, Hamamatsu University School of Medicine, Hamamatsu, Japan

Abstract. Sclerosing hemangioma of the lung is uncommon benign neoplasms of uncertain histogenesis. The histological appearance consists of distinct and well-circumscribed nodules in general. Each nodule is usually found to arise from epithelial cells, perhaps type II alveolar cells. This lesion usually appears as a solitary nodule and a plural case is rare. Two patients with multiple sclerosing hemangioma were discovered on chest X-ray examination. We performed the video-associated thoracoscopic surgery (VATS) procedure using a two-port approach and it was very useful. First, thoracoscopic examination with a rigid thoracoscope (5 mm in diameter) was performed through the port in the anterior axillary line in the sixth intercostal space. It was difficult to recognize the location of the nodules. Then we located our original port, ellipse-like in shape and about 35x15 mm in size in the cross-section, in the fifth intercostal space near the nodules. We could easily confirm the tiny nodules and the borderline of the diseases by fingers. The patients underwent the wedge resection of the lung uneventfully and were discharged. Access to the pleural cavity was achieved by making two incisions, each a length of only 4 and 0.5 cm. The two-port method can be regarded as a safe and less invasive procedure for tiny nodules, such as in our cases.

Keywords: histology, lung nodule, surfactant apoprotain A, surgery, thoracoscope.

Background

Sclerosing hemangioma is an unusual lung tumor that arises from the epithelial cells, perhaps type II alveolar cells. This disease usually appears as a solitary nodule and a pleural nodular case is rare. In 1956, Liebow and Hubbell reported the clinicopathologic properties and pathologic entity of the lung which they called sclerosing hemangioma [1]. They emphasized the scant symptoms and frequency with which these lesions were diagnosed on routine chest X-rays. They described the characteristic X-ray images as rounded, well-circumscribed growths, usually with no involvement of the surrounding pulmonary parenchyma. They also concluded that this disease was a primary proliferation of blood vessels. The term sclerosing hemangioma was applied because the histologic findings were identical to those observed in soft tissues by Gross and Wolbach [2].

Improvement in video technology and endoscopic equipment allows surgeons to opt for video-associated surgery or video-associated thoracic surgery (VATS)

Address for correspondence: Yusuke Kita MD, First Department of Surgery, Hamamatsu University School of Medicine, 3600 Handa-cho, Hamamatsu 431-3192, Japan. E-mail: kita21@aqua.ocn.ne.jp as a therapy for the diseases classically managed by open thoracotomy. Through incisions and ports, pulmonary resection is carried out with good visualization, less postoperative pain and without the need for large incisions. Thoracoscopy offered an exciting viewpoint into the pleural space without the need for a major surgical incision. An operating thoracoscope allows the wedge resection to be accomplished with only two sites of intercostal space access. A more flexible approach must be used towards VATS resection of the indeterminate pulmonary nodules.

Case 1

A 54-year-old man with a history of asthma was referred to the hospital for tiny circular shadows in the right middle lung on a chest X-ray. The results of routine blood tests, including tumor markers, were normal. Wheezing and rales were not detected on admission. A CT scan revealed three tiny nodules (6, 3 and 2 mm in diameter) in the right S3 and one of them had clear pleural indentation. We thought that the nodules were benign lung tumors, such as granulomas, intrapulmonary lymph nodes, hamartomas or sclerosing hemangiomas. The possibility of malignant tumors could not be ruled out and VATS was carried out.

Thoracoscopic examination was performed through the first port in the anterior axillary line in the sixth intercostal space. The location of the nodules was undetermined by using the thoracoscope only. We located our original port, ellipse-like in shape and about 35x15 mm in size in the cross-section, in the fifth intercostal space, secondary. The position of the second port was near the nodules. We could then confirm the nodules by fingers. The patient underwent wedge resection with autosutures and the three nodules were resected uneventfully. Histopathologically, all the nodules consisted of many vessels and papillae. Immunohistologically, tumor cells were positive for surfactant apoprotain A, which is the indicator of type II pneumocytes. The diagnosis was sclerosing hemangioma.

Case 2

A 22-year-old, previously healthy woman was hospitalized because of multiple nodular shadows in the left S4 on chest X-ray examination. She had no discomfort. Routine blood tests, including tumor markers, were normal and no rales were observed on admission. A CT scan revealed that the innumerable, various sized (10 mm or less) nodules were localized in S4. She underwent VATS, and wedge resection was performed in a similar way to that of case 1.

Histopathologically, the main nodules were composed of cavernous hemangiomas, but the small nodules, of less than 3 mm in diameter, were all solid and not demarcated well. They also did not have any blood pooling. Immunohistologically, the tumor cells in this case were also positive for surfactant apoprotain A.

Discussion

VATS wedge resection is well suited for the evaluation of the tiny multiple nodules. The initial camera site at the sixth or seventh intercostal space in the anterior to posterior axillary line offers good visualization of the hemithorax and pulmonary parenchyma. After exploration, the second access site is chosen, usually in the fourth or fifth intercostal space. These two sites align the instruments along the interlobar fissures, providing good exposure and allowing manipulation of most lateral areas of the lung and the application of the endoscopic stapler along a variety of parenchymal edges, if there is no pleural adhesion. The port should be located at an appropriate distance from the target lesion so that the jaw mechanism of the stapler can be opened and maneuvered freely. We often accomplished the wedge resection with only two sites of intercostal space access. An endoscopic forceps, 3 or 5 mm in diameter, is introduced through the second port to grasp an appropriate site along the edge of the lung. Then the endoscopic stapler is introduced through the second intercostal space site and positioned to begin the V wedge resection. The positions of the forceps and stapler are reversed to complete the V wedge resection.

A flexible approach is better used for VATS resection of the indeterminate pulmonary nodules. Careful examination of the preoperative CT scan of the chest is very important prior to deciding on the trocar placement for VATS pulmonary nodular resection [3]. Lesions deep within the substance of the parenchyma of the lung can be difficult to resect using staples alone. In these circumstances, suturing through the original port is possible.

The initial enthusiasm for VATS has been replaced by critical evaluation in comparison with the open techniques. The severity of postoperative discomfort was expected to be an advantage of VATS. All trocar sites must be inspected from the intrathorax for bleeding, as a laceration of the intercostal vessels can occur during the insertion of the trocar. Our original port was elastically soft. This can help avoid injury of intracostal vessels and nerves. VATS offers the potential benefit of reduced morbidity for patients with thoracic problems. However, the extended operating time and imprecise handling of the intrathoracic tissues diminishes the advantages of VATS. Well-planned surgical approaches to the target are an absolute necessity.

Conclusions

Proper placement of the instruments and thoracoscope is critical for accurate VATS exploration and resection of pulmonary nodules. We developed the two-port VATS procedure for treating multiple nodules, such as multiple sclerosing hemangioma. This method can be regarded as a safe and less invasive procedure.

References

1. Liebow AA, Hubbel DS. Sclerosing hemangioma (histiocytoma, xanthoma) of the lung. Cancer 1956;9:53–75.
2. Gross RE, Wolbach SB. Sclerosing hemangiomas: their relationship to dermatofibroma, histiocytoma, xanthoma and to certain pigmented lesions of the skin. Am J Pathol 1943;19:533–551.
3. Daly BDT, Faling LJ, Diehl JT et al. Computed tomography-guided minithoracotomy for the resection of small peripheral pulmonary nodules. Ann Thorac Surg 1991;51:465.

©2001 Published by Elsevier Science B.V.
Bronchology and Bronchoesophagology: State of the Art.
H. Yoshimura et al., editors.

Video-assisted thoracoscopic surgery (VATS) for small undeterminate peripheral lung nodules

Motoo Kuroki, Akihiko Takeshi, Norihisa Ohata, Kazunori Kasama and Nobuyasu Kano
Department of Surgery, Endoscopic Surgery Center, Kameda Medical Center, Chiba, Japan

Keywords: lung cancer, solitary pulmonary nodule, unexpected malignancy.

Introduction

Frequently, physicians have to deal with very small nodules discovered serendipitously by CT scans or chest X-rays performed while screening for other diseases. Early histological diagnosis is often important as lung cancer detected in its earlier stages has a much better prognosis than cancer detected at later stages. In this study, we examine VATS biopsy cases at the Kameda Medical Center and evaluate the histological results.

Materials and Methods

Kameda Medical Center carried out 54 video-assisted thoracoscopic surgery (VATS) biopsies for small lung nodules from January 1994 to November 1999. None of the nodules had a known histology prior to VATS. Twenty-four patients underwent bronchoscopic examination without definitive diagnosis prior to the operation and four patients underwent a CT-guided needle biopsy, also without a definitive diagnosis. The other patients proceeded directly to VATS resection because the nodules were too small to sample under CT-guided needle biopsy. Thirteen patients had a history of previous malignancy. Chest X-rays detected 36 of the cases and CT scans 18 cases.

Results

Postoperative pathology is as follows: 11 cases (20.4%) were primary lung cancer, consisting of 10 cases of adenocarcinoma and one case of peripheral squamous cell carcinoma, nine cases were metastatic malignancies, and the remaining 34 cases (67%) were benign lesions or postinflammatory change.

Address for correspondence: Motoo Kuroki, Department of Surgery, Endoscopic Surgery Center, Kameda Medical Center, 929 Higashi-cho, Kamoagawa, Chiba 296-8602, Japan. Tel.: +81-470-90-0011. Fax: +81-470-99-1198. E-mail: motoo@olive.ocn.ne.jp

Table 1. Age distribution according to postoperative histology.

	30 years of age	40 years of age	50 years of age	60 years of age	70 years of age
Nonmalignant	2	8	6	10	8
Primary ca.	0	0	2	6	3
Metastatic ca.	0	0	3	4	2

Of the 13 cases that had a past history of malignancy, VATS biopsies found two patients to have primary lung cancer while nine were metastatic lesions from prior malignancy and two were benign lesions. Of the 31 patients who did not have a malignancy history, nine cases were primary lung cancer and 22 were benign lesions. Patients between the ages of 30 and 49 years had no malignant lesions. After the age of 50, six cases (31%) were primary lung cancer and none were metastatic lesions.

The nodules ranged from less than 0.5 to 3.5 cm in diameter (Table 1). Only two cases were over 3 cm. There were three primary lung cancers of less than 1 cm in diameter. In those nodules less than 2 cm in diameter, there were eight cases of primary lung cancer.

The characteristics of each nodule on the CT scans were analyzed. We focused on three CT characteristics (Table 2). These were 1) fine spiculation around the nodule, 2) vessel involvement, and 3) fine opacification surrounding the nodule [1,2]. Fine spiculation appears to represent vasculature and septal structures and is often considered a malignant finding. In our series, eight of the 11 cases of primary lung cancer had fine spiculation, but six of 15 inflammatory/granulomatous cases and one of 11 benign cases also had fine spiculation. Vessel involvement was also observed both in cancer cases and benign cases. Fine opacification surrounding the nodule was more specific to primary lung cancer with five of 11 primary lung cancers having fine opacification and only one of nine metastatic cases and two of 15 inflammatory/granulomatous cases (Table 3).

Conclusion

We cannot establish absolute criteria, using CT scans or chest X-rays alone, to differentiate malignant nodules from benign ones. VATS is a procedure that allows us to obtain a histological result with reasonable morbidity and cost. The cost of this procedure is acceptable given the importance of a histologic diagnosis.

Table 2. Distribution of the nodules according to the diameter.

	< 0.5 cm	0.5 to 1.0 cm	1.0 to 1.5 cm	1.5 to 2.0 cm	2.0 cm <
Nonmalignant	8	15	5	3	3
Primary ca.	0	3	4	1	3
Metastatic ca.	0	4	2	1	1

Table 3. Characteristics of the nodules (excluding 8 intrapulmonary lymph nodes).

	Primary ca.	Metastatic ca.	Benign tumor	Inflammatory
Fine spiculation	8/11	3/9	1/11	6/15
Vessel involvement	8/11	4/9	1/11	9/15
Fine opacification	5/11	1/9	0/11	2/15

Discussion

The prognosis of lung cancer is generally poor. However, treatment results in early (stage 1) cases is frequently good. Therefore, early detection and operative therapy is important. Many diagnostic tools have been proposed for early diagnosis of solitary pulmonary nodules [3,4]. However, obtaining a definitive diagnosis of small peripheral nodules is challenging [5]. In these cases, the probability of obtaining a specific diagnosis using fluoroscopy-guided CT needle biopsy is low. The possible diagnosis of malignancy requires surgical intervention. VATS should be given priority for those patients with small pulmonary nodules where histological sampling is needed.

References

1. Shimosato Y, Melamed MR, Nettesheim P. Morphogenesis of Lung Cancer, vol 1. Boca Raton, Florida: CRC Press, 1982;92–120.
2. Groskin SA. Pulmonary neoplasm: radiologic-pathologic correlations of lung–tumor interface. In: Farrell R (eds) The Lung – Radiologic – Pathologic Correlations. St. Luis: Mosby, 1993; 361–427.
3. Khouri NF, Stitik FP et al. Transthoracic needle aspiration of benign and malignant lung lesions. Am Roentgenology 1985;144:281–288.
4. Fletcher EC, Levin DC. Flexible fiberoptic bronchoscopy and brush biopsy in the diagnosis of suspected pulmonary malignancy. West J of Med 1982;136:477–483.
5. Mack MJ, Hazelrigg SR et al. Thoracoscopy for the diagnosis of the indeterminate solitary pulmonary nodule. Ann Thorac Surg 1993;56:825–832.

Bronchology and Bronchoesophagology: State of the Art.
H. Yoshimura et al., editors.

Ultrathin bronchoscopy as a new tool in the diagnosis of peripheral lung lesions: preliminary results of a prospective evaluation

Nicolas Schoenfeld[1], Tobias Temme[1], Annette Fisseler-Eckhoff[2], Wolfgang Rahn[2], Monika Serke[1] and Robert Loddenkemper[1]
[1]Second Department of Pulmonary Medicine, and [2]Department of Pathology, Lungenklinik Heckeshorn, Berlin, Germany

Abstract. *Background.* The diagnostic yield of conventional bronchoscopy for peripheral lesions is limited because of lacking visibility beyond the segment level, and the frequent inability to reach the lesions under fluoroscopic guidance.

Methods. A 2.8-mm thin flexible bronchoscope ("babyscope," prototype BF-XP 40, Olympus Optical) was tested in 90 patients with peripheral lung lesions and with normal macroscopical findings during conventional bronchoscopy. 81 patients were diagnosed for definite.

Results. Visibility was found to go up to the 10th generation of bronchi. The lesion size varied from 1 to 9 cm. Under fluoroscopy 82 out of 90 lesions appeared to be reachable using the babyscope. In 32 out of 62 patients with malignancy, the babyscope revealed macroscopically direct or indirect signs of peripheral tumour growth. Malignancy was proven either by histology and/or cytology in 30 out of 62 patients using the babyscope. Five out of 19 benign conditions could be diagnosed, as well.

Conclusion. The babyscope is a new, and probably complementary, tool in the diagnosis of peripheral lung lesions. There is an ongoing study to obtain more precise data on specific indications for the method.

Keywords: flexible bronchoscopy, lung cancer, peripheral lung lesion, ultrathin bronchoscope.

Introduction

Flexible bronchoscopy is the most important diagnostic tool for peripheral lung lesions. However, the visible area of conventional bronchoscopes is restricted to the central bronchial system, up to the segmental level. Peripheral lesions are accessible only indirectly under fluoroscopic guidance, and depending on the size and localisation of lesions the diagnostic yield of biopsy techniques is limited.

Thin endoscopes were already in use in the bronchial system, in children [1] or in adults [2,3]. We report on our preliminary results of a prospective evaluation of a new prototype with an outer diameter of only 2.8 mm (the "babyscope").

Address for correspondence: Robert Loddenkemper MD, Lungenklinik Heckeshorn, Zum Heckeshorn 33, 14109 Berlin, Germany. Tel.: +49-30-8002-2435. Fax: +49-30-8002-2286.
E-mail: loddheck@zedat.fu-berlin.de

Methods

The prototype BF-XP4O was produced by Olympus Optical Co., Tokyo. Through the working channel of 1.2 mm, a forceps and brush can be used for biopsies, besides direct suction through the channel. All patients had normal macroscopical findings during conventional flexible bronchoscopy.

Results

Ninety patients (65 men, 25 women) were examined between August 1999 and May 2000. The size of peripheral lung lesions varied between 1 and 9 cm in diameter. In 62 patients, the final diagnosis was a malignancy. 19 were diagnosed to have a benign lesion, whereas nine patients have remained without a definite diagnosis so far. The following diagnostic methods were used in cases which could not be diagnosed using the babyscope: surgery in 16 malignant and six benign lesions, conventional bronchoscopy in four malignant cases, extrathoracic biopsy of metastases in four cases, transthoracic needle aspiration in seven malignant lesions, and a clinical course in seven benign and three malignant conditions.

Under fluoroscopic guidance 82 out of 90 peripheral lesions were reached. 32 out of 62 malignant lesions were already macroscopically suspicious, either by direct or indirect signs of tumour growth. In 30 out of 62 cases malignancy was proven using babyscope biopsies. Among the five out of 19 benign lesions, which could be diagnosed using the babyscope, there were two cases of tuberculosis, one aspergillosis, one hamartoma and one case of M. Wegener.

Among the biopsy techniques used, forceps was diagnostic in 30 out of 70 procedures, the uncoated brush in 14 out of 70 and simple suction in eight out of 73 cases (Table 1). In cases with malignancy, the forceps was positive in 27 out of 53 procedures, the brush in 14 out of 61, and suction in eight out of 81 lesions (Table 2).

Discussion

After having evaluated a first series of 90 patients in an interim analysis, the technically improved prototype of an ultrathin bronchoscope appears to be a useful and complementary tool in the diagnosis of peripheral lung lesions. The study is ongoing, which is necessary due to the variety of size, localisation and character of pulmonary lesions.

Table 1. Instruments used for sampling with the babyscope (n = 90).

Tool	Positive (n)	Negative (n)	Total
Forceps	30	40	70
Brush	14	56	70
Suction	8	73	81

Table 2. Instruments used for sampling with the babyscope in malignancy (n = 62).

Tool	Positive (n)	Negative (n)	Total
Forceps	27	26	53
Brush	14	47	61
Suction	5	51	56

First of all, we can confirm the considerably extended visibility up to the 10th generation of bronchi. In some cases, however, visibility may be impaired by hypersecretion or bleeding which cannot be cleared so easily with a conventional bronchoscope. Yet it was impressive that a considerable number of lesions could be recognized by direct vision through the babyscope, whereas conventional bronchoscopic findings were normal in all patients. We also observed a "learning curve" for the involved bronchoscopists, achieving a higher yield in the second half of patients.

Under fluoroscopic guidance, the flexible tip of the bronchoscope made it possible to reach the lesion in the vast majority of cases. Without having performed a direct comparison with conventional techniques, we have the impression that the babyscope offers a wider potential in this aspect than the conventional instrument for biopsy of peripheral lesions. However, the increased number of bronchial branches that can be inspected, obviously leads to a longer duration of the whole bronchoscopy and eventually also to the duration of fluoroscopy.

Among the instruments available for the babyscope, the flexible forceps has by far the highest yield, compared with the brush or suction, through the working channel. The failure of the brush may be due to the fact that the instrument is inserted uncoated into the channel. A suggestion for improvement was made to the brush manufacturer.

Besides the diagnostic potential for peripheral lung lesions, the babyscope may also play a role in the evaluation of poststenotic bronchi, in cases of high grade central bronchial stenoses. However, no conclusions can be drawn on that point as yet, based on our experiences so far.

References

1. Hasegawa S, Hitomi S, Murakawa M, Mori K. Development of an ultrathin fiberscope with built-in channel for bronchoscopy in infants. Chest 1996;110:1543–1546.
2. Tohda Y, Muraki M, Iwanaga T, Kubo H, Haraguchi R, Fukuoka M. Applicability of uretero-pelvic fiberscopy in the diagnosis of peripheral lung cancer. J Bronchol 1999;6:251–256.
3. Tanaka M. Advances and usefulness of ultra-thin bronchofiberscopes. Keio J Med 1996;45: 296–300.

Bronchology and Bronchoesophagology: State of the Art.
H. Yoshimura et al., editors.

Problems in the diagnosis of minor lesions in the peripheral lung field

Akira Shoji, Hiroshi Takahashi, Nobuo Ogawa and Shigeki Odagiri
Kanagawa Prefectural Cardiovascular and Respiratory Center, Yokohama, Japan

Abstract. *Background.* The number of cases in which small shadows are seen in the lung field periphery, by CT examinations, has increased. Bronchoscopic examinations are commonly found to be powerless in supporting qualitative diagnoses of small shadows, and the general impression is that, together with the spread of video-assisted thoracic surgery (VATS), the frequency with which patients are handed over to surgeons without a definitive diagnosis is increasing.

Methods. Regarding the 6-year period between 1988 and 1993 as period 1, and the 6-year period between 1994 and 1999 as period 2, we studied the cases of minor peripheral lung field shadows with unconfirmed preoperative diagnoses.

Results. In period 2, we saw an increase in the number of cases of indefinite diagnoses and the proportion of patients in whom VATS was performed. The average number of preoperative bronchoscopies and the period of observation decreased. On the basis of CT images, almost all tumors were suspected to be malignant, but this was correct in only about one-half of the cases.

Conclusions. It is expected that the number of such cases will increase as a result of the wider use of CTexaminations, and the development of new technologies for qualitative diagnosess are a matter of urgency.

Keywords: computerized tomography (CT) examinations, peripheral lung small shadows, video-assisted thoracic surgery (VATS).

Background

Recent technological advances have made fast, low-dose computerized tomography (CT) examinations possible. As a result, the use of CT in physical examinations has begun, which means that the number of cases in which small shadows (nodule and ground glass shadows) are seen in the lung field periphery has increased [1]. Modern bronchoscopic examinations are commonly found to be powerless in supporting a qualitative diagnosis of small nodule shadows, and the general impression is that, together with the spread of video-assisted thoracic surgery (VATS), the frequency with which patients are handed over to respiratory surgeons without a definitive diagnosis is increasing [2]. We have been studying these issues and have given some consideration to future problems.

Address for correspondence: Dr Akira Shoji, Division of Respiratory Disease, Kanagawa Prefectural Cardiovascular and Respiratory Center. 6-16-1 Tomioka-higashi, Kanazawa-ku, Yokohama, Kanagawa 236-0051, Japan. Tel.: +81-45-701-9581. Fax: +81-45-786-4770.

Methods

We studied 152 cases of minor peripheral lung field shadows with unconfirmed preoperative diagnoses over 12 years, 1988 to 1999, noting the frequency of the preoperative examinations, the periods of preoperative observation, the tentative preoperative diagnoses, and the proportion of postoperative diagnoses that were in agreement with these.

Results

Table 1 shows the results, and the representative cases are shown in Fig. 1. Regarding the 6-year period between 1988 and 1993 as period 1, and the 6-year period between 1994 and 1999 as period 2, we saw an increase in the number of cases of indefinite diagnoses, from 54 in period 1 to 98 in period 2. In period 2, the proportion of patients in whom VATS was performed increased. The average number of preoperative bronchoscopies decreased from 1.22 in period 1 to 0.82 in period 2, and patients who had no preoperative bronchoscopic examination increased especially, from two in period 1 to 23 in period 2, while the period of observation decreased. On the basis of the CT images, almost all tumors were suspected to be malignant, but this was correct in only about one-half of the cases. The number of cases of minor shadows increased, and when there was suspiscion of malignancy, there was a vigorous tendency for VATS to be performed at an early stage. However, about one-half of the cases were benign.

Conclusions

Contrary to the increase in the frequency of minor shadows detected in the periphery of the lung field, progress in the technique of bronchoscopic biopsy is lagging, and there is a tendency to rely on VATS for qualitative diagnoses. It is expected that the number of such cases will increase sharply as a result of the wider use of CT examinations, and that the development and dissemination of new technologies for testing, such as real-time CT-guided bronchoscopic examinations, is a matter of urgency for some institutions.

Table 1. Summary of the cases unconfirmed by preoperative diagnoses.

Period	No. of cases	Preoperative bronchoscopic examinations				Method of operation		Histological diagnosis prior to operation		Average period of observation (months)
		NP	1	2+	Average (n)	VATS	Open lung	Malignancy	Benign	
1	54	2	40	12	1.22	2	52	32	22	2.8
2	98	23	70	5	0.82	77	21	56	42	1.8

NP: not performed, 1: performed once, 2+: performed more than twice.

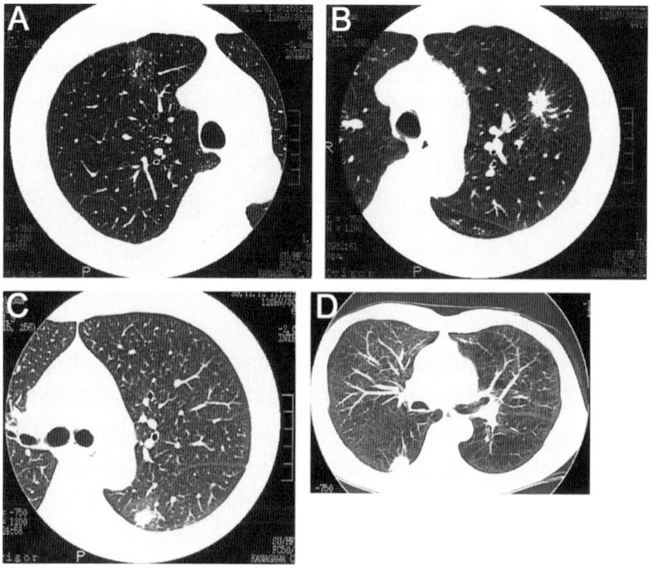

Fig. 1. Presentation of representative cases. **A:** Case 1: 69-year-old man. Reason for detection: screening CT scan. Preoperative (radiographic) diagnosis: adenocarcinoma. Bronchoscopic examination: once. Histological diagnosis (VATS): adenocarcinoma. **B:** Case 2: 55-year-old man. Reason for detection: screening chest X-ray. Preoperative (radiographic) diagnosis: adenocarcinoma. Bronchoscopic examination: once. Histological diagnosis (VATS): nodule of pneumoconiosis. **C:** Case 3: 62-year-old woman. Reason for detection: screening CT scan. Preoperative (radiographic) diagnosis: adenocarcinoma. Bronchoscopic examination: not performed. Histological diagnosis (VATS): organising pneumonia. **D:** Case 4: 72-year-old man. Reason for detection: examination CT for pulmonary emphysema. Preoperative (radiographic) diagnosis: adenocarcinoma. Bronchoscopic examination: once. Histological diagnosis (VATS): squamous cell carcinoma.

References

1. Newman L. Larger debate underlines spiral CT screening for lung cancer. J Natl Cancer Inst 2000;92:592–594.
2. Petrakis IE, Katsamouris A, Vassilakis SJ, Vrachassotakis N, Drossitis I, Chalkiadakis G. Video-assisted thoracoscopic surgery in the diagnosis of lung disease. The Cretin experience. Ann Chir Gynaecol 2000;89:24–27.

©2001 Published by Elsevier Science B.V.
Bronchology and Bronchoesophagology: State of the Art.
H. Yoshimura et al., editors.

Fine needle aspiration biopsy of pulmonary hamartoma

Marjeta Tercelj-Zorman[1], Izidor Kern[2] and Janez Erzen[1]
[1]Center for Respiratory Diseases, Clinical Center, Ljubljana; and [2]Hospital Golnik, Clinic for Respiratory Diseases, Golnik, Slovenia

Keywords: chest, coin lesion, cytology.

Introduction

Hamartoma is a benign pulmonary tumor, usually asymptomatic and discovered accidentally. When endobronchial, it may cause coughing or postobstructive pneumonia.

Study design

Thirty-nine consecutive cases of pulmonary harmartoma (PH), admitted to our hospital between 1989 and 1999, were reviewed with the objective of evaluating the usefulness of fine needle aspiration biopsy (FNAB) in the diagnosis of PH.

Materials and Methods

There were 39 patients (10 females and 29 males) aged between 32 and 75 years old, and 18 of them were smokers. All patients underwent chest X-ray and bronchoscopy, and 21 had a CT scan. Bronchoscopy with biopsy showed PH in four patients; 35 went on to FNAB.

The chest X-rays showed all lesions to be single, peripheral, nondiagnostic, and 1 to 3, 5 cm in size. The FNAB needles were 22 guage and 10 to 15 cm in length. Arch fluoroscopy was used.

Results

Out of 35 patients, FNAB was diagnostic for PH in 15, suspicious in six, and nondiagnostic in 14. Fourteen out of the 15 patients with FNAB diagnosis of PH were not subjected to surgery, but followed up for 1 to 10 years. Only one of these 14 showed evidence of slow growth during this time. No new (secondary) PH was discovered in these patients. Twenty-three patients were operated on and

Address for correspondence: Marjeta Tercelj-Zorman MD, Center for Respiratory Diseases, University Hospital, Zaloska 7, 1000 Ljubljana, Slovenia. Tel.: +386-1-300-67-32. Fax: +386-1-300-67-36.
E-mail: marjeta.tercelj@kclj.si

the diagnosis of PH was confirmed. Their follow-ups showed no recurrent tumors. Twenty-five tumors were in the right lung, 14 in right lower lobe, while only 10 were in the left lung; five in upper and five in lower lobe.

Conclusion

FNAB yielded reliable cytological guidance in our study of PH. There were no false positives for the malignancy diagnoses made. The sensitivity of FNAB was 60%. Therefore, when FNAB showed PH, surgery could safely be omitted. There was no recurrence after surgery and only one of 14 tumors left under observation showed signs of slow growth during the follow-up period of 1 to 10 years (mean time: 5.3 years).

Bronchology and Bronchoesophagology: State of the Art.
H. Yoshimura et al., editors.

Bronchoscopic microsample probe assessment for the diagnosis of small peripheral lung cancer

Masazumi Watanabe[1], Akitoshi Ishizaka[2], Hayanori Horiguchi[1], Makoto Sawafuji[1], Masafumi Kawamura[1], Hirohisa Horinouchi[1] and Koichi Kobayashi[1]
[1]*Keio University School of Medicine; and* [2]*Tokyo Electric Power Company Hospital, Tokyo, Japan*

Abstract. *Background.* Making a pathological diagnosis before surgery in patients with small lung nodules, found by high-resolution CT scans, is still difficult. We applied a newly developed microsampling probe to measure tumor markers in epithelial lining fluid (ELF), recovered from tumor surrounding tissues, in order to test its clinical utility.

Methods. In patients with peripheral lung adenocarcinoma, ELF from tumor tissue and/or surrounding tissue, within 1 cm of the tumor, was collected using a microsampling probe under bronchoscopy. The concentrations of three tumor markers, CEA, CYFRA and SLX, in the ELF were measured.

Results. The concentrations of CEA and CYFRA were higher in the ELF obtained from tumor surrounding tissues (2.71 ng/mg, 7.23 ng/mg; n = 6) than in the ELF obtained from the contralateral side of the lung cancer (0.08 ng/mg, 0.1 ng/mg; n = 51) or the control patients (0.18 ng/mg, 0.40 ng/mg; n = 6). Although the concentration in serum was lower than the cut-off level, the concentration in ELF was higher in these lung cancer patients. Meanwhile, the concentration of SLX (10.52 U/mg) in the tumor surrounding tissues showed similar levels compared to the contralateral side (6.68 U/mg) and control group (5.81 U/mg).

Conclusions. CEA and CYFRA in ELF may play an interesting role in the diagnosis of lung adenocarcinoma. Microsampling probe assessment may supplement pathological diagnosis in patients with small peripheral lung cancer.

Keywords: CEA, CYFRA, epithelial lining fluid, SLX, tumor markers.

Introduction

Recently, many cases of small lung nodules have been found using new imaging methods, such as high-resolution CT scanning. Pathological diagnosis before surgery is still difficult in such cases, even using bronchoscopic or percutaneous biopsy guided by a CT scan. We developed a new, less invasive bronchoscopic microsampling probe to assess new biochemical substances in epithelial lining fluid (ELF). In the present study, we applied the probe to measure tumor markers in order to test its clinical utility in patients with small peripheral lung cancer.

Address for correspondence address: Masazumi Watanabe, Department of Surgery, School of Medicine, Keio University, 35 Shinanomachi, Shinjuku, Tokyo 160-8582, Japan. Tel.: +81-3-5363-3806. Fax: +81-3-5363-3493. E-mail: masazumi@med.keio.ac.jp

Materials and Methods

In six patients with peripheral lung adenocarcinoma in whom the tumor diameters were less than 3 cm, ELF from tumor tissue and/or from surrounding tissue, within 1 cm of tumor, was collected using a microsampling probe (Olympus, Tokyo, Japan). The probe was inserted into the lungs through a 3.2-mm diameter channel of the bronchoscope. The probe consisted of an outer polyethylene sheath, with a 2.8-mm diameter, and an inner 1.2-mm cotton probe attached to a stainless steel guide wire. Concentrations of three tumor markers, carcinoembryonic antigen (CEA), cytokeratin fragment 19 (CYFRA), and sialyl SSEA-1 (SLX), in ELF were measured using the ELISA method. Values were corrected using the measured weight of the recovered ELF. Concentrations of tumor markers in ELF from patients with benign diseases were measured as a control. Concentrations in serum were also measured in patients with lung cancer.

Results

The mean concentrations of the three tumor markers recovered from ELF and serum are shown in Table 1. The concentrations of CEA and CYFRA were higher in ELF obtained from tumor surrounding tissues than in both ELF obtained from the contralateral side of the lung cancer and from control patients. On the other hand, the concentration of SLX in tumor surrounding tissues showed similar levels compared to the contralateral side or control group. It was suggested that the concentrations of CEA and CYFRA in ELF were more specific than that of SLX in the present study for diagnosing lung cancer. Moreover, although serum concentration was lower than the cut-off level, the ELF concentration was higher in these lung cancer patients.

Table 1. Concentration of tumor markers in the epthelial lining fluid and serum in lung cancer patients.

	CEA (ng/mg)	CYFRA (ng/mg)	SLX (U/mg)
ELF:			
Lung cancer (n = 6)	2.31	7.32	10.52
Another side (n = 51)[a]	0.08	0.10	6.68
Control patients (n = 6)	0.18	0.40	5.81
Serum:			
Lung cancer (n = 6)	8.4	1.30	32.6
Cut-off value	5.0	2.0	38.0

[a]Another side: ELF recovered from the contralateral lung in lung cancer patients.

Conclusions

These results suggest that tumor markers produced in cancer tissue diffuse into the surrounding area, and that microsampling probe assessment can detect them even if the probe does not hit the tumor directly. Several investigators have failed to detect tumor markers in bronchoalveolar lavage fluid in lung cancer patients [1–3]. The microsampling method may have the potential to detect tumor markers more specifically than bronchoalveolar lavage. CYFRA and CEA values in ELF may play an interesting role in the diagnosis of primary lung adenocarcinoma. Microsampling probe assessment under bronchoscopy may supplement pathological diagnosis in patients with small peripheral lung cancer.

References

1. Trevisani L, Putinati S, Sartori S, Abbasciano V, Bagni B. Cytokeratin tumor marker levels in bronchial washing in the diagnosis of lung cancer. Chest 1996;109:104–108.
2. Zaleska J, Pirozynski M, Kwiek S, Sakowicz A, Rowinska-Zakrzewska E. CEA, NSE and SCC Ag in bronchial lavage in patients with lung cancer. Rocz Akacl Med Bialymst 1997;42(Suppl 1):179–189.
3. Cremades MJ, Menendez R, Pastor A, Llopis R, Aznar J. Diagnostic value of cytokeratin fragment 19 (CYFRA 21-1) in bronchoalveolar lavage fluid in lung cancer. Respir Med 1998;92: 766–771.

Rare diseases

Bronchology and Bronchoesophagology: State of the Art.
H. Yoshimura et al., editors.

Complications in Hutchinson-Gilford syndrome related to the narrow upper airway and esophagus

M. Dedovic[1], Dj. Zdravkoavic[1], G. Dragutinovic[2], G. Vukomanovic[1] and T. Vukomanovic[2]
[1]*Centre of Public Health New Belgrade; and* [2]*Magnetic Center, University of Belgrade, Belgrade, Yugoslavia*

Abstract. A 12-year-old boy suffering from the extremely rare Hutchinson-Gilford syndrome (progeria) is presented. This syndrome is recognizable in the first 6 months after birth. It is characterized by a rare craniofacial dysostosis and failure to thrive, dyscephaly with a “bird-like face”, a large, poorly ossified skull with decreased ossification in sutural areas, a pinched nose, and a small mandible with crowded teeth that protrude late. The skin is dry and thin and nails are brittle and short (reflecting shortening and lysis of the underlying distal phalanges and cartilages). Hypertension, cardiomegaly and atheroma are also present.

Complications in the syndrome are related to the narrow upper airway and associated with the craniofacial configuration and progressive early chondro-osteolysis. Severe complications may include pulmonary infection, respiratory embarrassment, obstructive sleep apnea (which is correlated with tracheomalation), increased secretion of fibronecetin and collagen, and probably hyaluronic acid (HA) in urine.

Keywords: esophagus, Hutchinson-Gilford progeria syndrome, narrow upper airway.

Introduction

The Hutchinson-Gilford progeria (H-G) syndrome is a well-delineated malformation syndrome of somewhat variable severity. The cause is unknown, and although no mutations are known to extend the maximal human life span, there are a number of mutations that shorten life span. The basic mutation underlying this disease is not known. Progeria patients excrete an excessive amount of glycosoaminoglycan (GAG) and hyaluronic acid (HA). Abnormalities in basal metabolism and bioinactive growth hormone raise the possibility that one or several genes affect the aging process.

Failure to thrive in infancy is accompanied by striking clinical features. Patients with this disease generally appear normal at birth, but by 1 year of age can already display many features of the syndrome. Widespread losses of subcutaneous fat results in the veins over the scalp becoming particularly noticeable. The skin appears aged and pigmented age spots are present. The median age of death is 12 years. The most common cause of death is myocardial infarction or congestive heart failure caused by atherosclerosis.

Address for correspondence: M. Dedovic, Center of Public Health New Belgrade, Bulevar Arsenija Carnojevica 173/15, Belgrade, Yugoslavia. Tel.: +381-11-555-775.

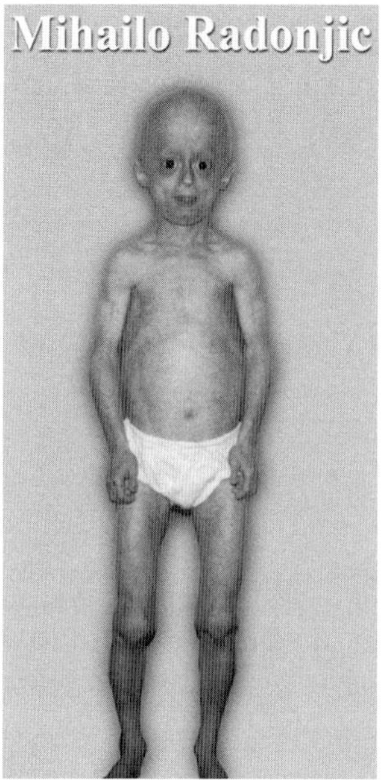

Fig. 1. Front view of a 12-year-old patient. Note the small mandible, frontal prominence, hypotrichosis, microstomia, irregular brownish-yellow skin pigmentation, coxa valga, bowing of knees, and tibia with further signs of deterioration.

Clinical report

The patient, born on 6 December 1987, was the second child of young, healthy, nonconsanguineous parents; the family history was unremarkable and the older sister is healthy. The mother had noted that fetal movements were slightly weaker than that in her first pregnancy. The infant was born at term with a weight of

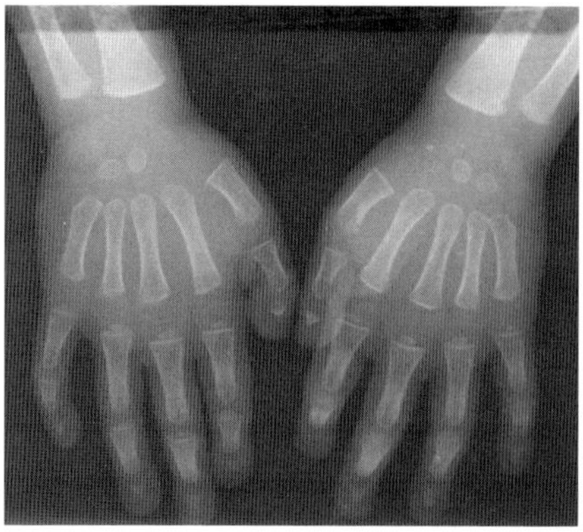

Fig. 2. Hand radiograph demonstrates lytic changes on distal phalanges.

3,400 g, a length of 53 cm, the circumference of the head (CH) of 36 cm, and an Apgar score of 9/10. A left clavicle fracture and cephalhematoma on the right side were also noted. Early postneonatal development was normal. At the age of 4 months the problems started. For example, thickened, shiny skin formed on the abdominal, tibial and gluteal regions. At this time the patient had a weight of 5,600 g, a CH of 41 cm, and a fontanelle of 2.5 × 3.5 cm. There was the occasional "setting-sun sign" sign and a positive Babinski. Routine FBC, biochemistry, and thyroid function tests were normal. Forty-six XY chromosomes were present, the urinary metabolic screen was normal, lipids, cholesterol, triglycerides were normal, and HDL was low-to-normal.

In spite of vigorous antioxidation therapy at the end of the year 2000 (when the patient was 13 years of age), there was a failure to thrive, such as 6 years previously. The patient had a weight of 12.5 kg, height 104 cm, "bird–like" facies, generalized microstomia, a short tongue, the first set of teeth were still present, and a small mandible; the head was in general hydrocephalic; there was exophtalmia; subcutaneous tissue was atrophic; hypoplastic nails; decreased mobility of joints (knees and hands) (see Fig. 1). Cholesteatoma presented after an ear infection and hearing changes (presbycusis). Bone age lagged behind, with lytic changes on the terminal phalanx (Fig. 2), hypoplastic clavicles and scapulas (Fig. 3). A US study documented ventricular septal defect (VSD), intermittent but corrected hypertension (23/15.5). Transaminases were mildly elevated, bilirubin was normal and HbsAg negative. Mentally the patient is above normal.

Radiographs of the head and chest showed unusually slender bones. A lateral view of the face showed a markedly increased neurosomatic ratio, thin calvaria, and a very hypoplastic mandible. An MRI study documented an unusually narrow oesophagus. Poor feeding in H-G is one of the first problems. Pulmonary infiltration was not present in this examination.

Respiratory difficulties had not been present since birth. The patient had never had problems breathing through his nose. At the age of 11 years, he was admitted with an impressive fracture of the occipital bone and although osteolysis was not the cause of the fracture, it probably was an additional factor. His mandible, especially the processus condyloideus, showed signs of osteoporosis (Fig. 4) and osteolysis with displaced mandible (Fig. 5), and some effaced mandibular angle

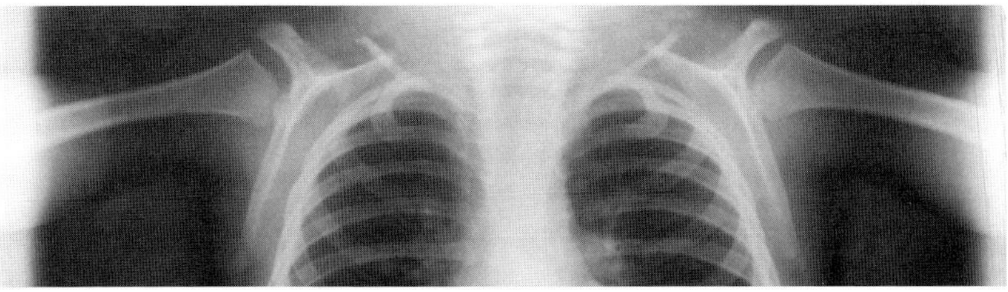

Fig. 3. Anteroposterior toracic radiograph showing slender bones with loss of outer clavicle.

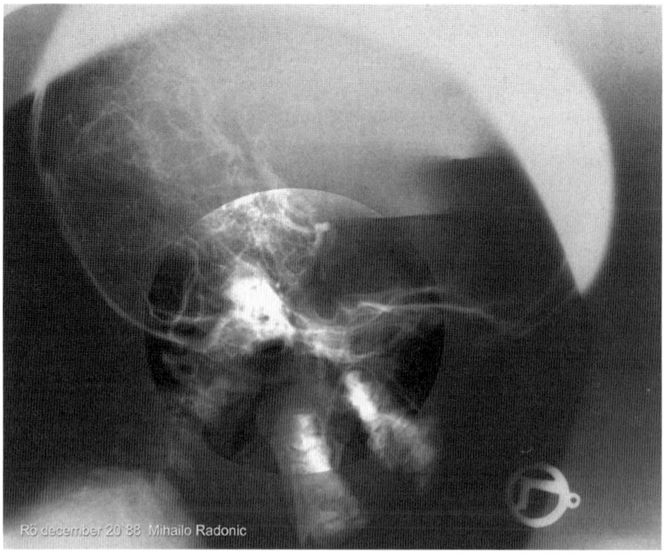

Fig. 4. Lateral radiograph of skull shows signs of osteoperosis, and the hypoplastic mandible with gracile processus condyloideus.

(Fig. 6). His heart gradually became enlarged. From the age of 8 years, spasm of the bronchi stems became almost continuous with every infection and had a long duration, in spite of vigorous symptomatic therapy. The cardiothoracic ratio increased from 0.50, at 4 years, to 0.63, at 13 years (Fig. 7), during which time his hemoglobin concentration rose to 154 g/l and problems with hypertension developed. Further, stiffening of finger joints, elbow and knee joint enlargement, and coxa valga resulted in a poor condition.

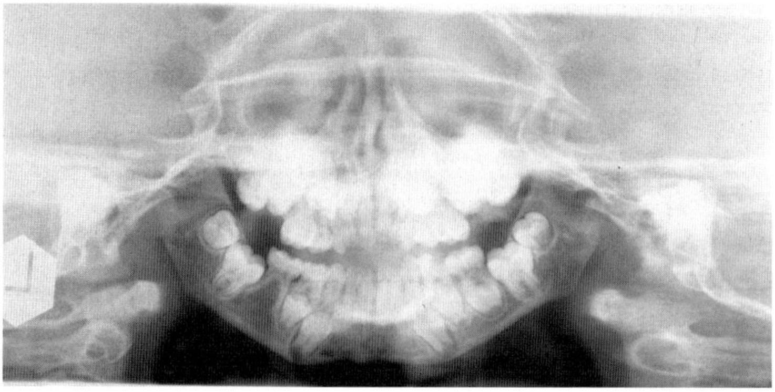

Fig. 5. Anter oposterior mandible radiograph demonstrates osteolysis with displaced mandible and some effaced mandibular angles.

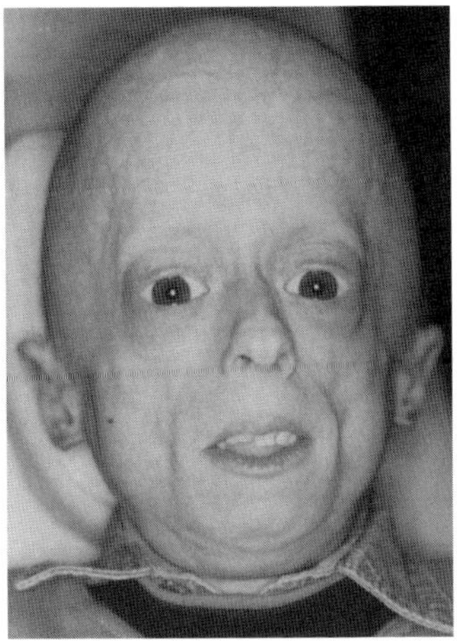

Fig. 6. Patient at 12 years of age with micrognathia and effaced mandibular angles.

Discussion

In view of the very hypoplastic mandible [1,2], distinctive changes with resorption and replacement by fibrous tissue [2], osteoporosis [3] of all bones and cartilages, especially caput of the processus condyloideus with a displaced mandible and some effaced mandibular angle (Schema 1), which are a constant finding in latter phases of H-G syndrome, one might expect upper airway obstruction and cor

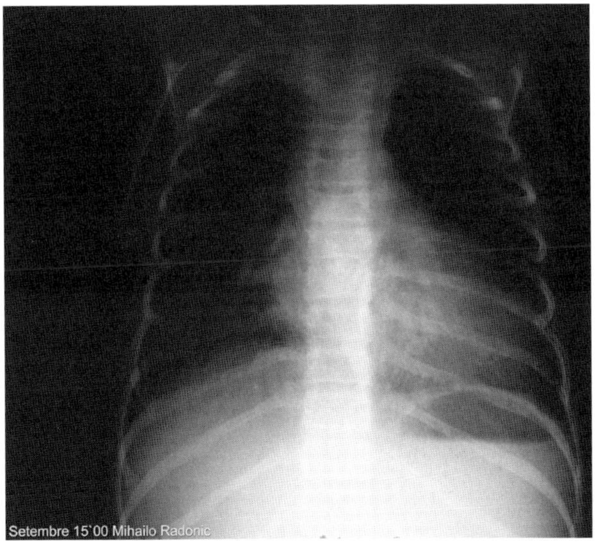

Fig. 7. Anteroposterior chest radiograph shows increased cardiothoracic ratio.

pulmonale to be the rule. Perhaps a reasonable explanation is that the tongue in H-G syndrome may also be shorter, thus providing some protection from the dangers of micrognathia. In any event, potential life-threatening respiratory problems can occur in the H-G syndrome, as well.

This is an additional factor to all basic genetic abnormalities (widespread atherosclerosis [2,4], with interstitial fibrosis of the heart [4], malnutrition [2], high level of basal metabolic rates [2], hyaluronuria [5,6], low amino acid concentration in blood [3], osteoporosis [3], osteolysis [2]), and may help to further evaluate (expected) patients with this syndrome.

The clinician needs to be aware of such complications and must evaluate the source of obstruction.

References

1. Sweeney JK, Weis SA. Hyaluronic acid in progeria and the aged phenotype. Gerontology 1992; 38:139–152.
2. Brown WT. Progeria: a human-disease model of accelerating aging. Am J Clin Nutr 1992;55: S1222–1224.
3. Styables GI, Morley WN. Hutchinson-Gilford syndrome. J Royal Soc Med 1994;87:243–244.
4. Baker PB, Baba N, Boesel CP. Cardiovascular abnormalities in progeria. Arch Pathol Lab Med 1981;105:385–386.
5. Kieras FJ, Brown WT, Houck GE, Yebrower M. Elevation of urinary hyaluronic acid in Werner syndrome and progeria. Biochem Med Metab Biol 1985;36:276–282.
6. Zebrower M, Kieras FJ, Brown WT. Urinary hyaluronic acid elevation in Hutchinson-Gilford progeria syndrome. Mech Ageing Dev 1986;35:39–46.

Bronchology and Bronchoesophagology: State of the Art.
H. Yoshimura et al., editors.

A case of relapsing polychondritis with severe tracheal stenosis

Hiroya Iwatake, Isao Kato, Kouichiro K. Tsutsumi, Hideo Tomisawa, Sigenori Nobukiyo and Izumi Koizuka
Department of Otolaryngology, St. Marianna University, School of Medicine, Kawasaki, Japan

Abstract. Relapsing polychondritis (RP) is an uncommon disease manifested by recurrent episodes of progressive inflammation of cartilaginous structures. In the literature, laryngotracheal involvement was found in about 50 to 70% of reported cases and occasionally results in acute airway obstruction. We report a case of RP with severe tracheal stenosis that had been treated by expandable metallic stents placement.

A 58-year-old male was hospitalized with a high fever and inspiratory difficulty. A tracheostomy was performed electively and a silicone T-tube was placed. A diagnosis of RP was made based on the biopsy of auricular and tracheal cartilage. After that, expandable metallic stents were placed at the trachea and bilateral main bronchus, because he had progressive dyspnea. The airway lumen was satisfactory dilated and the dyspnea disappeared completely. However, 18 months later, a sudden massive hemorrhage occurred through the tracheostoma, and he died of respiratory failure. Autopsy findings showed tracheo-innominate artery fistula. We discussed management of RP with severe tracheal stenosis.

Keywords: expandable metallic stents, tracheo-innominate artery fistula, tracheobronchial stenosis.

Introduction

Relapsing polychondritis (RP) is an uncommon disease manifested by recurrent episodes of progressive inflammation of cartilaginous structures. Although the etiology and pathogenesis remain uncertain, current evidence suggests that autoimmune mechanisms may be involved [1]. In the literature, laryngotracheal involvement was found in about 50% of reported cases and occasionally results in acute airway obstruction [2]. We present a case of tracheo-innominate artery fistula that occurred after long-term placement of Gianturco expandable metallic stents in RP with severe tracheal stenosis.

Case report

A 58-year-old male had a high fever and inspiratory difficulty in February 1995. On admission to another hospital, steroids therapy resulted in rapid improvement. However, his respiratory condition worsened again over the next 2 weeks and he was then referred to our hospital. Physical examination revealed

Address for correspondence: Hioya Iwatake, Department of Otolaryngology, St. Marianna University School of Medicine, 2-16-1 Sugao, Miyamae-ku, Kawasaki, Kanagawa 216-8511, Japan. Tel.: +81-4-4977-8111. Fax: +81-4-4976-8748. E-mail: iwatake@marianna-u.ac.jp hoarseness, stridor and saddle deformity of the nose. A chest X-ray and CT scan demonstrated subglottic and tracheal stenosis in expiration with a diffuse thickened tracheal wall and focal calcification. Fiberscopy revealed epiglottis deformity and vocal cord movement was impaired bilaterally. The portion of the trachea was collapsed and extended over 4 to 5 cm in length, which ended at 3 cm above the main carina. Then, a tracheostomy was performed electively and a silicone T-tube was inserted. A diagnosis of RP was made based on the biopsy of auricular and tracheal cartilages and clinical features; such as auricular chondritis and saddle nose deformity.

After 18 months, he was readmitted with severe dyspnea. Fiberscopy revealed severe stenosis of the tracheobronchial systems. On 23 June 1997, Gianturco expandable metallic stents were inserted under local anesthesia using a combined endoscopic and fluoroscopic control. Stents of 12 mm in diameter were placed in the bilateral main bronchus and a stent of 15 mm in diameter was placed in the distal trachea. The dyspnea and the results of the blood gas analysis showed marked improvement after the procedure. Six weeks after insertion, he showed no respiratory symptoms, and fiberscopy revealed epithelialization of the stent wires. Seventeen months after insertion, he had stridor on exertion and hemoptysis. On 24 November 1998, a massive hemorrhage occurred suddenly through the tracheostoma. He was diagnosed as having tracheo-innominate artery fistula. Unfortunately, he died of respiratory failure 7 days after the hemorrhage. Autopsy confirmed a fistula between the innominate artery and trachea at a level of 3 cm below the tracheostoma. Histopathological findings showed loss of basophilic staining of the cartilage matrix, infiltration of inflammation cells and cartilage destruction with replacement by fibrous tissue.

Discussion

RP is a rare multisystem disorder of unknown cause, characterized by recurrent inflammation and destruction of cartilages. Tracheal and bronchial obstruction is often seen as a complication of pulmonary infections due to impaired clearance of secretions. It is reported that almost 50% of patients with RP died from these complications [3]. Therefore, the management of tracheobronchial stenosis is the key to RP.

The placement of Gianturco expandable metallic stents can result in improved severe airway obstruction. This stent is a cylindrical structure made of stainless steel wire bent in a zigzag pattern and compressed into an introducer sheath to allow expansion when it is released in the airway. This stent has some significant advantages, as follows:

1. It does not interfere with the mucociliary function.
2. It does not block the ventilation of another bronchus, because of the spaces between the wires.

On the other hand, the disadvantages are as follows:

1. It is not effective in terms of intraluminal tumor invasion or granulation tissue, because the tumor or granulation tissue can grow between the wires.
2. It cannot be removed endoscopically.

Several studies have reported that the Gianturco expandable metallic stent is noninvasive and improves the quality of life in patients with terminal cancer [4,5]. Other studies have reported that the Gianturco expandable metallic stent is an effective therapeutic approach to tracheal stenosis in patients with RP [6,7]. In our case, respiratory symptoms of RP were improved by Gianturco expandable metallic stents. However, tracheo-innominate artery fistula occurred, caused by stent wire deterioration, after long-term placement. We think that the use of Gianturco expandable metallic stents should not be indicated for the management of benign tracheobronchial obstruction such as RP or long-term placement. Recently, some authors reported that other types of stents (Wallstent [8] or Palmatz stent [9]) are a safe, effective and noninvasive procedure for RP. Further studies are required to determine the ideal type of tracheal stent and the optimal timing to place it to extend long-term morbidity. Longer follow-up evaluations and greater clinical experience are needed to answer these important questions.

References

1. Foidart JM et al. Antibodies to Type II collagen in relapsing polychondritis. N Engl J Med 1978; 8:820–824.
2. McAdam LP et al. Relapsing polychondritis: prospective study of 23 patients and a review of the literature. Medicine 1976;55:193–215.
3. Dolan DL et al. Relapsing polychondritis. Analytical literature review and studies on pathogenesis. Am J Med 1966;41:285–299.
4. Sawada S et al. Malignant tracheobronchial obstructive lesion: treatment with Gianturco expandable metallic stents. Radiology 1993;188:205–208.
5. Egan AM et al. Expandable metallic stents for tracheobronchial obstruction. Clin Radiol 1994; 49:162–165.
6. Jeremy P et al. Role of Gianturco expandable metallic stent in the management of tracheobronchial obstruction. Cardiovasc Intervent Radiol 1992;15:375–381.
7. John AD et al. Use of metallic stent in relapsing polychondritis. Chest 1994;105:864–867.
8. Faul JL et al. Endobronchial stenting for severe airway obstruction in relapsing polychondritis. Chest 1999;116:825–827.
9. Sarodia BD et al. Management of airway manifestations of relapsing polychondritis: case reports and review of literature. Chest 1999;116:1669–1675.

Bronchology and Bronchoesophagology: State of the Art.
H. Yoshimura et al., editors.

A case of endobronchial bronchus-associated lymphoid tissue lymphoma that responded to radiotherapy

Akihiko Kitami, Takashi Suzuki, Yoshito Kamio and Shuichi Suzuki
Department of Thoracic and Cardiovascular Surgery, Showa University Fujigaoka Hospital, Yokohama, Japan

Abstract. A 66-year-old male was admitted for the evaluation of an abnormal chest radiograph. A chest roentgenogram revealed an abnormal shadow in the right hilum. Bronchoscopy on admission revealed that the right lower lobe bronchus was severely narrowed by an irregular mucosal lesion. Microscopic examination of the transbronchial biopsy specimen showed the mucosal and submucosal tissue to be diffusely infiltrated, mainly by lymphocytes composed of small lymphocytes, centrocyte-like cells. B cell origin was suggested by a positive L-26 stain. Based on these findings, we diagnosed primary endobronchial lymphoma of bronchus-associated lymphoid tissue (BALT). The patient underwent radiation therapy of the right hilum at doses of 4000 cGy, delivered over 4 weeks, and has been in complete remission for 9 months. Radiotherapy was effective for endobronchial BALT lymphoma.

Keywords: BALT lymphoma, endobronchial, radiotherapy.

Introduction

In 1963, Saltzstein attempted to establish histologic criteria to distinguish malignant from benign lymphocytic pulmonary infiltrates, and termed the benign lymphocytic proliferation as pseudolymphoma [1]. Recently, many studies have shown that, what was previously described as pseudolymphoma, is actually a heterogeneous disease group, which includes nodular lymphoid hyperplasia and low-grade B cell lymphoma, arising from the bronchus-associated lymphoid tissue (BALT) [2,3]. Because BALT lymphoma is a rare neoplasm, the standard therapy for BALT lymphoma is unestablished. We present a case of endobronchial BALT lymphoma that responded to radiotherapy.

Case report

A 66-year-old man was admitted to Showa University Fujigaoka Hospital for the evaluation of an abnormal chest radiograph. Four months earlier, he presented progressive dyspnea on exertion, a productive cough, and a 3-kg loss of weight over 3 months. He had a history of smoking half a pack/day for 10 years, but had quit 20 years ago.

Address for correspondence: Akihiko Kitami, Showa University Fujigaoka Hospital, 1-30 Fujigaoka, Aoba-ku, Yokohama 227-8518, Japan. Tel.: +81-88-45-971-1151. Fax: +81-88-45-971-7125.

On examination the patient was in no respiratory distress. He was afebrile. Laboratory studies on admission revealed elevated serum lactic dehydrogenase (548 U/l) and ferritin levels (491 ng/ml). Other blood chemistry, a complete blood count, and blood gas analysis were normal. The interleukin-2 receptor antibody, which is a marker of lymphoma, and other tumor markers, such as the squamous cell carcinoma-related antigen and the carcinoembryonic antigen, were normal. Chest radiography showed an infiltrative shadow in the right hilum. Computed tomography (CT) of the chest showed a mass around the inferior lobe bronchus and obstructive pneumonia in the right S6 area (Fig. 1). Flexible bronchoscopy revealed an irregularity in the right inferior bronchus and a marked narrowing of the right B6 bronchus (Fig. 2A). Histopathology from the biopsy of the endobronchial mass showed centrocyte-like lymphocytes infiltrating the bronchial epithelium to form lymphoepithelial lesions (Fig. 3). Immunohistochemically, lymphocytes were positive for the B-cell marker L26 antigen, and negative for the T-cell marker UCHL-1 antigen. From these findings, the patient was diagnosed with BALT lymphoma. The patient received 40-Gy Linac irradiation of the right hilum over a period of 4 weeks. Bronchoscopic examination after radiation therapy showed normal findings of the right inferior lobe bronchus, and the biopsy of the mucosa revealed normal findings too (Fig. 2B). The patient has remained asymptomatic, and repeat bronchoscopy 9 months after the initial diagnosis did not show any recurrence.

Discussion

Bienenstock et al. introduced the term "bronchus-associated lymphoid tissue" (BALT) as an analogue to the well-defined "gut-associated lymphoid tissue" (GALT), the best known example of which is Peyer's patches [4]. BALT lymphomas are indolent neoplasms, characterized by a prolonged clinical course and persistent disease, generally with a lung tumor.

An endobronchial BALT lymphoma, in the present case, is extremely rare. As BALT lymphoma is a rare neoplasm, a standard therapy for BALT lymphoma

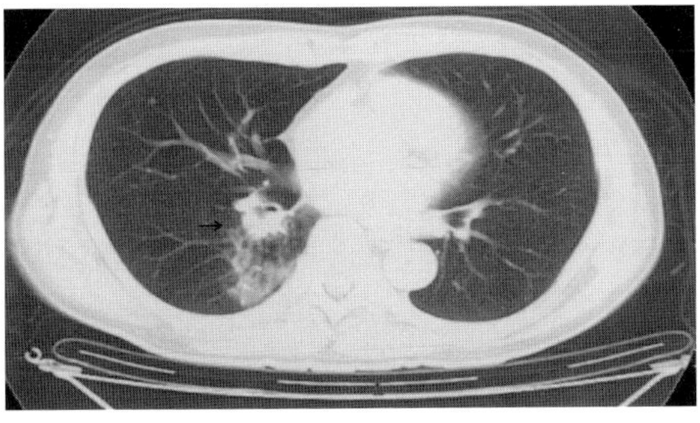

Fig. 1. Chest CT findings on admission, showing a mass around the inferior lobe bronchus (arrow) and obstructive pneumonia in the right S6 area.

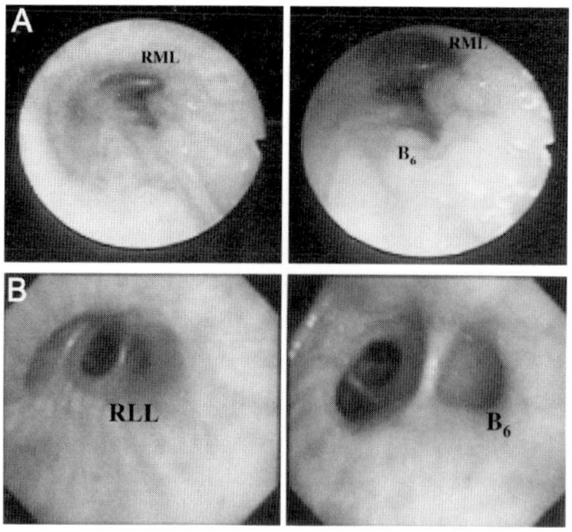

Fig. 2. **A:** Bronchoscopic findings on admission, showing the irregular mucosal lesion and the marked narrowing of the right inferior lobe bronchus. **B:** Bronchoscopic findings after radiotherapy, showing the normal mucosa of the right inferior lobe bronchus.

has not yet been established. An operation is probably suitable for pulmonary peripheral lesions. We think that wedge or partial resection of the lung is adequate for this condition, because BALT lymphoma is a low-grade malignancy, and seldom metastasizes to hilar or mediastinal lymph nodes. However, the operation for an endobronchial BALT lymphoma, like in the present case, is a problem, because as the endoscopic bronchial mucosal pathological change has diffused, it is difficult to determine the proper cutting line of the bronchus. Chemotherapy may be a useful treatment in some cases. We treated another case of BALT lymphoma in the trachea, in which we obtained a complete response after CHOP-E therapy, although the patient died of interstitial pneumonia 11 months after the therapy [5]. As we questioned the need for the systemic admini-

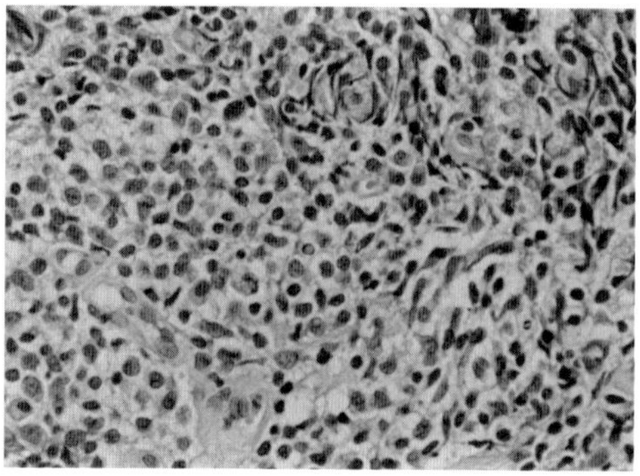

Fig. 3. Photomicrograph of bronchoscopic biopsy specimen, showing centrocyte-like lymphocytes infiltrating the bronchial epithelium to form a lymphoepithelial lesion (hematoxylin and eosin; × 400).

stration of anticancer drugs for low-grade malignant lymphoma, like BALT lymphoma, and for the above reasons, we chose radiotherapy in this case.

Further accumulation of clinical experience with this disease is necessary to determine a treatment protocol.

Conclusion

We presented a case of bronchus-associated lymphoid tissue lymphoma in the right lower lobe bronchus. Radiotherapy was effective in the treatment of endobronchial BALT lymphoma.

References

1. Saltzstein SL. Pulmonary malignant lymphomas and pseudolymphomas: classification, therapy and prognosis. Cancer 1963;16:928–955.
2. Herbert A, Wright DH, Issacson P. Primary malignant lymphoma of lung: histopathologic and immunologic evaluation of nine cases. Hum Pathol 1984;15:415–422.
3. Addies B, Hyjek E, Isaacson P. Primary pulmonary lymphoma: a reappraisal of its histogenesis and its relationship to pseudolymphoma and lymphoid interstitial pneumonia. Histopathology 1988;13:1–17.
4. Bienenstock J, Johnston N, Perey DYE. Bronchial lymphoid tissue: I, morphologic characteristics. Lab Invest 1973;28:686–692.
5. Suzuki T, Akizawa T, Suzuki H. Primary tracheal mucosa-associated lymphoid tissue lymphoma accompanying lung cancer. JJTCVS 2000;(In press).

Bronchology and Bronchoesophagology: State of the Art.
H. Yoshimura et al., editors.

Lower respiratory tract involvement of Rosai-Dorfman Disease

J. Kozielski[1], J. Kamiski[1], D. Ziora[1], M. Misioek[2] and A. Gabriel[3]
Departments of [1]Pneumonology, [2]Laryngology and [3]Patomorphology, Silesian School of Medicine, Zabrze, Poland

Abstract. Rosai-Dorfman Syndrome, known as sinus histiocytosis with massive lymphadenopathy, is a disorder characterised by the presence of tissue infiltrates formed by cells with the ability of cytophagocytosis. The involvement of organs, other than lymph nodes, in the course of Rosai-Dorfman Syndrome is possible. A case of a young patient with Rosai-Dorfman Syndrome is described. Apart from the enlargement of the cervical lymph nodes, lesions in the lower respiratory tract were also noted. After the treatment was administered, the lesions within the respiratory tract diminished significantly.

Keywords: changes in bronchial tree, histiocytosis, lymphadenopathy, Rosai-Dorfman Syndrome.

Rosai-Dorfman Syndrome, known as sinus histiocytosis with massive lymphadenopathy (SHML), is a disorder characterised by the presence of tissue infiltrates formed by cells with the ability of cytophagocytosis. Rosai and Dorfman first described it in 1969 [1].

The disease is characterised by pronounced cytophagocytosis of histiocytes, mostly infiltrating within the sinuses of the lymph nodes [2,3]. The disease is described as a systemic, proliferative disorder with a favourable prognosis. Apart from the enlargement of lymph nodes, mainly cervical ones, the presence of infiltrates within the organs is also noted. The lesions are accompanied by subfebrile states, malaise, and weight loss. Sedimentation rate is usually accelerated, and anaemia and leucopenia with neutrophilia also occur [1,4—7].

There are also cases of death noted in the course of Rosai-Dorfman Syndrome, resulting from complications, mainly infections [8,9]. They, however, happen very rarely. The disease is a self-limited disorder with a tendency for spontaneous resolution [1]. The origin of Rosai-Dorfman Disease is undetermined, although the herpes virus is supposed to participate in it.[10].

Case Report

A case involving a 26-year-old male patient, who is a physical worker and nonsmoker, is presented. The patient was admitted to the department of physiopneumonolgy at the Silesian Medical University in February 1999, in order to diagnose the cause of cervical lymph-node enlargement, with suspected

Address for correspondence: J. Kozielski, Department of Pneumonology, Silesian School of Medicine, Koziolka 1, Zabrze 41-803, Poland. Tel.: +48-32-271-5608. Fax: +48-32-274-5664.

tuberculosis as the possible cause-factor. The patient complained mainly of severe, intensive, rest dyspnea. Symptoms of left ear otitis, including bleeding, were also present.

The patient had not faced any health problems, except for the recurrent sinusitis and otitis since early childhood, till June 1996, when another incidence of otitis was present, but, for the first time accompanied by the enlargement of cervical lymph nodes and dyspnea. The patient was hospitalised in September 1996. A computed tomography of the neck and mediastinum was performed revealing the presence of numerous enlarged lymph nodes of pathologic structure, with features of decomposition within them. The nodes within the neck were seen to compress the trachea and to dislocate it to the right side. A biopsy of bone marrow was performed but an unequivocal diagnosis was not established. Numerous biopsies of lymph nodes were performed, but no final diagnosis, from any of the results of the histological examinations of the nodes, was reached. Mostly on the grounds of clinical presentation, the diagnosis of Non-Hodgkin Lymphoma was then suggested in October 1999. As the patient's status was deteriorating and the dyspnea was increasing, it was decided to commence chemotherapy in December 1999. Since then, the patient was administered seven cycles of treatment with doxorubicin, cyclophosphamide, pretension, and vincristine (CHOP), every 21 days. Improvement in clinical status and a decrease in the sizes of the nodes was achieved. Treatment was completed in July 1997.

On admission to the department of physiopneumonology in February 1999, cervical supraclavicular and axillary, palpable, painless, movable lymph nodes of 3 to 5 cm in diameter were found. Tracheal stridor was stated in the physical examination. Functional tests of the respiratory system revealed the presence of meaningful disorders within the flow-volume loop, with the reduction of airflow, particularly in its inspiratory phase. All the results of laboratory blood and urine tests were found to be within the normal range. Any of the mycobacteria species, both in sputum and in bronchoalveolar lavage, were cultured at any of disease's stages. A computed tomography of the neck and thorax revealed the presence of pathological, nodular lesions within the trachea and the main bronchi, narrowing their inside measurements. Few lymph nodes of up to 2 cm in diameter were found within the mediastinum. Numerous infiltrations, with partial decomposition inside, were visualised within the head and neck skin tissue and muscles. In the bronchofiberoscopy, the slit-like narrowing of the trachea, of approximately 3 cm in length, was found, and then sampled, directly under the glottis (Figs. 1 and 2). A change was found in the membrane in the main bronchi (Figs. 3 and 4). The consultant laryngologist, in face of increasing dyspnea, performed tracheostomy and sampled the subglottic lesions too. A diagnosis of Rosai-Dorfman Disease was suggested on the ground of histological examination of both samples. The pathologist examining the supraclavicular lymph node, sampled on admission to the department, established the same histological diagnosis.

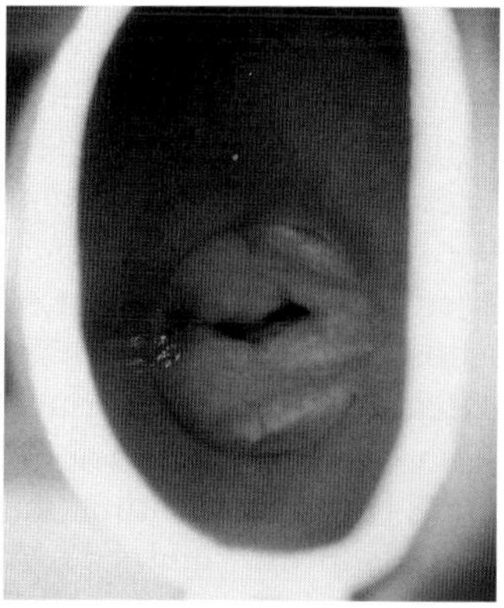

Fig. 1. The lesions observed in trachea during directoscopy.

The involved lymph nodes were characterised by the presence of capsular fibrosis, as well as fibrosis of the pericapsular adipose tissue. Conspicuous dilatations of all the sinuses and a compression of multiplication centers within the sinuses effaced the architecture of the lymph nodes. Lymphostasis within the sinuses was noted, as well as a mixed population of cells, including leukocytes with polymorphism and a predominant number of histiocytes with polymorphism and cytophagocytosis. Histiocytes had an acid-fast, vacuolated cytoplasm (Fig. 5). There were distinct nucleoli within nuclei. Some histiocytes contained vacuoles within the cytoplasm, with lymphocytes, erythrocytes and neutrophil leukocytes. Numerous plasma cells, lymphocytes and histiocytes with deposits of fat were seen within the pulp (Fig. 6). Large histiocytes phagocytize lymphocytes seen in vacuoles, and represent an active emperipolesis (Fig. 7) [1,3,5,11].

Considering the clinical presentation and the results of the histological examinations, the diagnosis of Rosai-Dorfman Disease was established. Treatment consisting of 30 mg of prednisone and 150 mg of cyclophosphamide was administered on 5 March 1999. Bronchofiberoscopy, carried out a month later

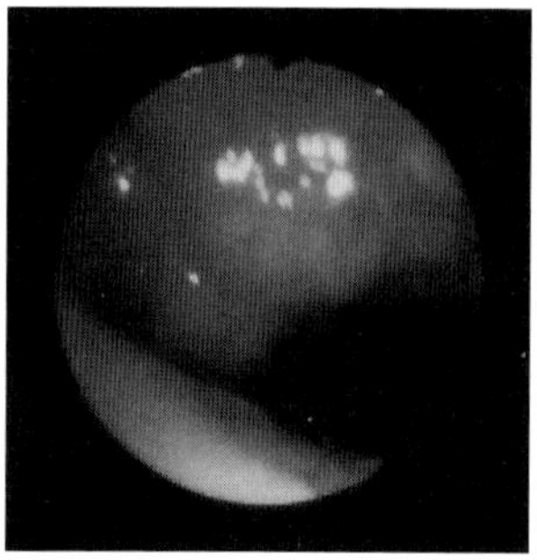

Fig. 2. The lesions observed in trachea under the vocal cords.

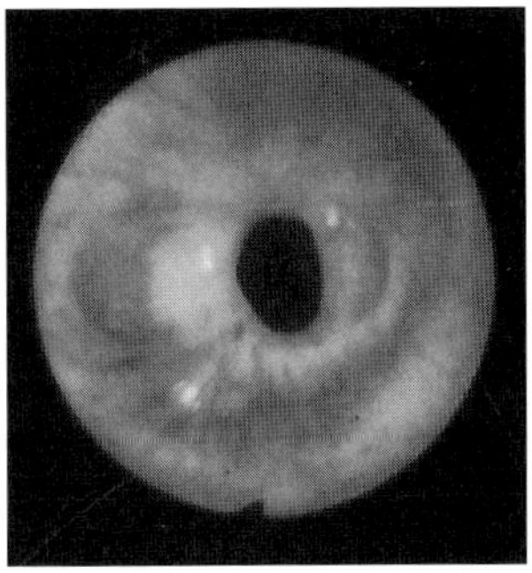

Fig. 3. Small, convex lesions of mucous membrane in the bronchi.

(bronchofiberoscope was put through tracheostomy tube), revealed regression in size and range, of the previously stated lesions, and was accompanied by the complete regression of the dyspnea. The size of the enlarged lymph nodes started to decrease gradually. Another bronchofiberoscopy was performed after a month, and further regression was confirmed. The patient was discharged from the department on the 5 May 1999 with the recommendation of continuing the treatment and having periodical outpatient visits. On discharge, the patient presented no complaints, and the lymph nodes were hardly palpable, but it was decided to leave the tracheostomy tube at place, in case of the recurrence of dyspnea.

The patient was readmitted to the department on 15 September 1999. His clinical status was excellent and he presented with no complaints. The tracheostomy tube was removed. Bronchofiberoscopy was performed, revealing no hypertrophy-like lesions. Treatment was complete.

Discussion

Cellular infiltration in Rosai–Dorfman Disease is not only found within lymph nodes, mainly cervical ones, but in other organs as well. The extranodal presenta-

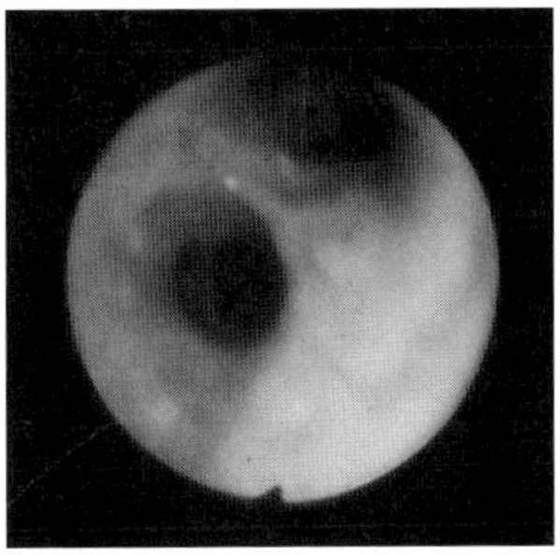

Fig. 4. Small, convex lesions of mucous membrane in the bronchi.

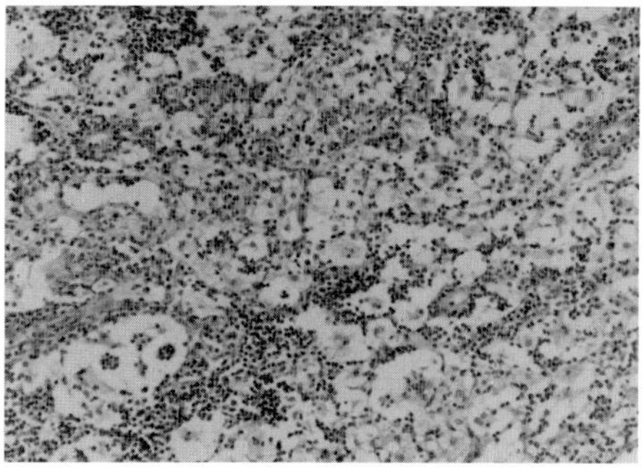

Fig. 5. Infiltration of histiocytes in the lymph node tissue (× 200).

tion of Rosai–Dorfman Disease was noted in 43% of patients with the disease [7,8,12,13]. The involvement of skin, subcutaneous tissue, the skeletal system, appendages, the central nervous system and central respiratory system were presented. Green et al. presented information about the involvement of mammary glands without any nodular involvement. The course of the disease was asymptomatic [12].

Older patients are predisposed to extranodular presentation of the disease, whereas the presentation within cervical lymph nodes occurs mainly in younger patients. The extranodular presentation is usually improperly diagnosed, mainly as lymphoma or as a fibrohistiocytic neoplasm [4,7,13].

Lymphadenopathy may be combined with the involvement of lesions within the upper respiratory tract, mucous membrane and submucosa of the nasal cavity, paranasal sinuses and trachea [8].

In chest roentgenograms of 21 patients, there were no abnormalities detected in 11 of the patients, while in the other cases, lymphadenopathy was stated within the hyli or mediastinum. The lesions were situated both unilaterally and bilaterally, including three patients with focal pulmonary consolidations, situated in different lobes of the right lung [1].

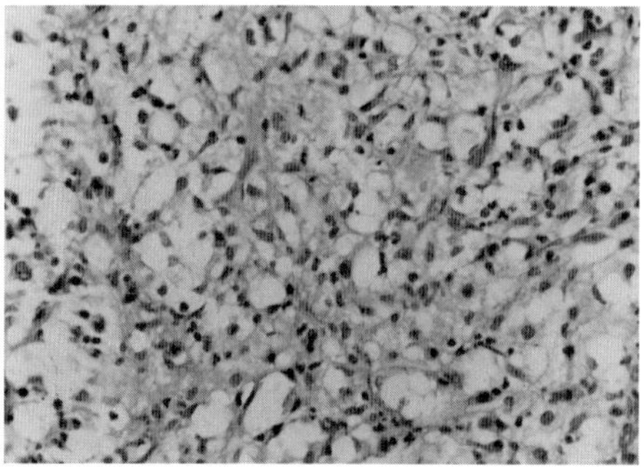

Fig. 6. Numerous, fat-loaded histiocytes (× 400).

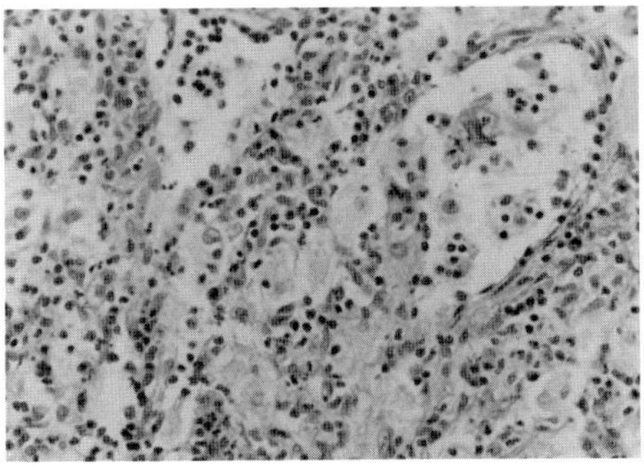

Fig. 7. Active emperipolesis (× 400).

Infiltrations in Rosai-Dorfman Disease are mostly to be found within mucous membrane and submucosa of the upper respiratory tract. A case involving a 10-year-old boy who died in the course of the Rosai-Dorfman Disease, due to a pseudomonas aeruginosa infection, is also known. Lesions within the nasal cavity, trachea and bronchi were found in the patient's autopsy [8].

The presence of systemic symptoms in the course of the disease may result from the presence of some monokinins (TNF-α, IL1, IL6) in damaged tissues.[14].

Diagnosis is based on the recognition of typical polyclonal histiocytes. Numerous authors have presented histologic features of the Rosai-Dorfman Disease [1,3]. On the grounds of histochemical examination, the cells found in this syndrome, can be said to represent functionally activated macrophages. Immunohistochemical staining for S-100 is the most valuable tool for conformation of diagnosis [7,12].

Sinus histiocytosis is a histologic feature also observed in the course of other neoplasms, for example lymphoma [15]. The presence of this kind of histological presentation in lymph nodes in the course of carcinoma of the larynx has a positive prognostic value.[16].

The prognosis in Rosai-Dorfman Disease is favourable. The administration of glicocorticoids, cytostatic agents and interferon-α, in cases with a severe course, have significantly improved prognoses [4,11].

References

1. Rosai J, Dorfman RF. Sinus histiocytosis with massive lymphadenopathy: a pseudolymphomatous benign disorder. Cancer 1972;30:1174–1188.
2. Alvarez-Alegret R, Martinez-Tello A, Ramirez T, Gallego P, Martinez D, Garcia-Julian G. Sinus histiocytosis with massive lymphadenopathy (Rosai-Dorfman Disease): diagnosis with fine-needle aspiration in a case with nodal and nasal involvement. Diagn Cytopathol 1995;13(4): 333–335.
3. Lopez P, Estes ML. Immunohistochemical characterization of the histiocystes in sinus histiocytosis with massive lymphadenopathy: analysis of an extranodal case. Hum Pathol 1989;20:

711–715.
4. Hicke A, Wieczorek M, Olejnik I. Zespó Rosai-Dorfmana u 17 letniego chopca jako problem diagnostyczny limfadenopatii. Acta Heamatologica Polonica 1995;26(4).
5. Lampert F, Lennert K. Sinus histiocytosis with massive lymphadenopathy. Fifteen new cases. Cancer 1976;37:783–789.
6. Madyk J, Lipski M, Stawowska B. Rzadka choroba wzów chonnych — sinus histiocytosis with massive lymphadenopathy. Polski Tygodnik Lekarski 1983;T XXXVIII.
7. Montgomery EA, Meis JM, Frizzera G. Rosai-Dorfman Disease of soft tissue. Am J Surg Pathol 1992;16(2):122–129.
8. Foucar E, Rosai J, Dorfman RF. Sinus histiocytosis with massive lymphadenopathy. An analysis of 14 deaths occurring in patient registry. Cancer 1984;54:1834–1840.
9. Zagdaska J, Krakówka P, Polowiec Z. Zatokowa histiocytoza z uogólnionym powikszeniem wzów chonnych — choroba Rosai i Dorfmana. Pneumonol Alergol Pol 1992;60(1–2):55–62.
10. Luppi M, Barozzi P, Garber R, Maiorana A, Bonacorsi G, Artusi T, Trovato R, Marasca R, Torelli G. Expression of human herpesvirus-6 antigens in benign and malignant lymphoproliferative diseases. Am J Pathol 1998;153(3):815–823.
11. Löhr HF, Gödderz W, Wölfe T, Heike M, Knuth A, Meyer zum Büschenfelde K-H, Dippold W. Long-term survival in a patient with Rosai-Dorfman Disease treated with interferon-α. Eur J Cancer 1995;31A(13/14):2427–2428.
12. Green I, Dorfman RF, Path FRC, Rosai J. Breast involvement by extranodal Rosai-Dorfman Disease: report of seven cases. Am J Surg Pathol 1997;21(6):664–668.
13. Saenz-Santamaria MC, Reed JA, Ochs RL, McNutt NS. Asymptomatic nodules on the chest. Cutaneous sinus histiocytosis (CSH) (cutaneous Rosai-Dorfman Disease). Arch Dermatol 1997;133(2):233,236.
14. Foss HD, Herbst H, Araujo I, Hummel M, Berg E, Schmitt-Graff A, Stein H. Monokine expression in Langerhans' cell histiocytosis and sinus histiocytosis with massive lymphadenopathy (Rosai-Dorfman Disease). J Pathol 1996;179(1):60–65.
15. Maia DM, Dorfman RF. Focal changes of sinus histiocytosis with massive lymphadenopathy (Rasai-Dorfman disease) associated with nodular lymphocyte predominant Hodkin's disease. Hum Pathol 1995;26(12):1378–1382.
16. Patt BS, Close LG, Vuitch F. Prognostic significance of sinus histiocytosis in metastatic laryngeal cancer. Laryngoscope 1993;103.

Sleep apnea syndrome

Bronchology and Bronchoesophagology: State of the Art.
H. Yoshimura et al., editors.

Overnight monitoring of patients with OSAS while sleeping in the led position

Yasutaka Akita, Tadao Nishimura, Nobuhiro Shibata, Kenji Kawakatsu, Chikaya Hattori, Munenori Hayakawa, Youichi Nishimura and Mikio Yagisawa
Department of Otolaryngology, Fujita Health University, Second Affiliated Hospital, Nagoya, Japan

Abstract. We studied 12 adult men who were diagnosed as having obstructive sleep apnea syndrome based on overnight monitoring, and who were subsequently monitored after led position on hospital day 2. The results obtained after led position were compared with those obtained in the natural sleeping position. After led position, the proportion of total sleep time spent in the lateral position had increased, the apnea hypopnea index improved, and the desaturation rate and lowest oxygen saturation values indicated improvement of hypoxia. It is concluded that the led position is a useful conservative treatment for obstructive sleep apnea syndrome and that it alleviates respiratory disorders. The technique is very effective for patients with a medium to low apnea hypopnea index, and in those with mild obesity.

Keywords: apnea hypopnea index, conservative treatment for OSAS, respiratory disorders, sleeping position.

Introduction

Sleeping in the lateral position is reported to be an effective therapy for patients with obstructive sleep apnea syndrome (OSAS). However, little work has been done on the method that should be used to maintain the lateral position or on the outcome of sleeping in this position. We investigated the effect of leading the body position on OSAS using overnight monitoring.

We studied 12 adult men who were diagnosed as having OSAS based on overnight monitoring, and who were subsequently monitored after led position on hospital day 2. Their mean age was 44.8 years. The results obtained after led position were compared with those obtained in the natural sleeping position.

Methods

On hospital day 1, patients were assessed in their natural sleeping posision; in other words, without any restrictions on the body position. On hospital day 2, the patients who were diagnosed as having OSAS underwent overnight monitor-

Address for correspondence: Yasutaka Akita, Department of Otolaryngology, Fujita Health University, Second Affiliated Hospital, 3-6-10 Otoubashi, Nakagawa-ku, Nagoya, Aichi 454-8509, Japan. Tel.: +81-52-321-8171. Fax: +81-52-331-6843.

ing in the led position. This was achieved by placing a soft ball against the patients back to maintain the lateral position for as long as possible. A soft ball was placed in a stocking, and tape was wrapped around the stocking on either side of the ball to stop it from moving. The ball was placed against the patients back and attached to the patients nightwear with safety pins. Then, the stocking was wrapped around the patient's waist and tied at the front. We called this condition the "led position".

Results

The proportion of the total sleeping time spent in the lateral position was compared before and after led position (Fig. 1). There was a significant increase in the time spent in the lateral position after the led position in all of the patients, with the increase being around two-fold on average.

Comparison of the apnea hypopnea index (AHI) before and after showed a significant improvement in all of the patients, with the value decreasing by about 50% on average (Fig. 2). The AHI improved by less than 50% in three patients and was unchanged in two patients. Four patients had a high index value and four were severely obese, with a body mass index of 30 or higher. It is, therefore, concluded that sleeping in the lateral position is very effective in patients with a medium to low AHI, or with mild obesity.

The desaturation rate (DR) decreased significantly after led position in all of the patients (Fig. 3), indicating improvement of hypoxia. The value was reduced by 50% on average.

The led position also resulted in a significant change in the lowest oxygen saturation (L-SaO_2) (Fig. 4). This indicated improvement of hypoxia, as was also shown by the change in DR.

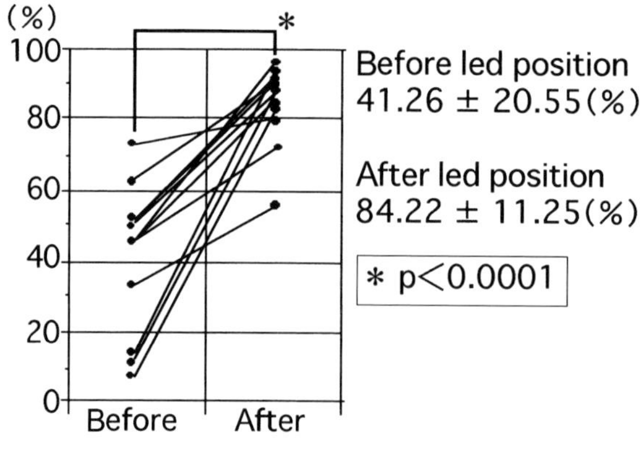

Fig. 1. The proportion of the total sleeping time spent in the lateral position.

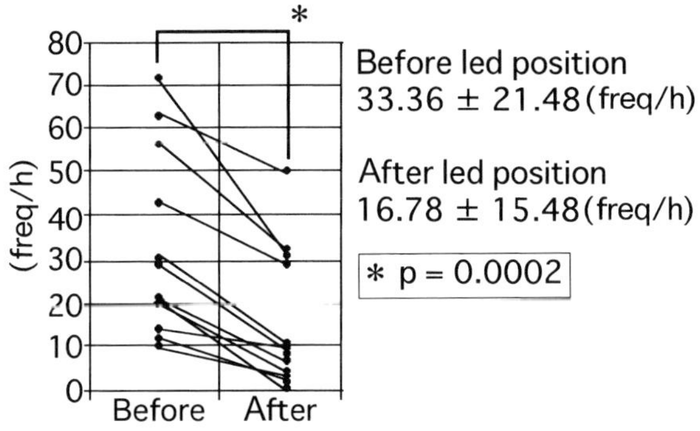

Fig. 2. The apnea hypopnea index (AHI).

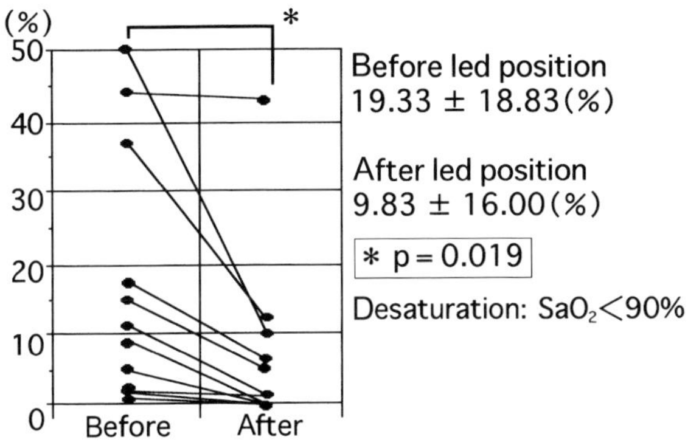

Fig. 3. The desaturation rate (DR).

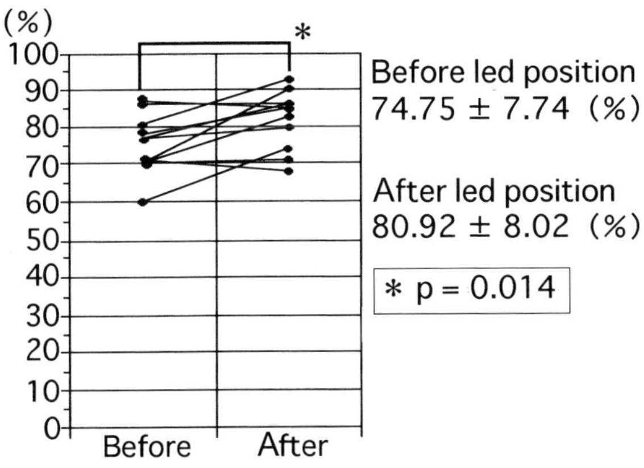

Fig. 4. The lowest oxygen saturation (L-SaO_2).

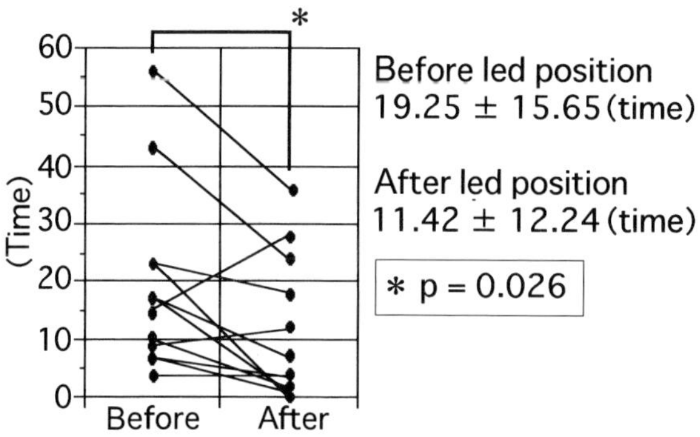

Fig. 5. The frequency of body movement during sleep.

The frequency of body movement during sleep was significantly reduced after led position (Fig. 5). This was also thought to be related to a decrease in the severity of respiratory disorders when the patient was sleeping in the led position.

Conclusions

Our results can be summarized as follows:

1. Twelve adult men, diagnosed as having OSAS based on overnight monitoring, were assessed after led position, and the results were compared with those obtained in the patients' natural sleeping positions.
2. After led position, the proportion of total sleep time spent in the lateral position was increased, the AHI improved, and the DR and L-SaO_2 values indicated improvement of hypoxia.
3. It is concluded that led position is a useful conservative treatment for OSAS, and that it alleviates respiratory disorders. The technique is very effective for patients with a medium to low AHI, and in those with mild obesity.

Stenting

Bronchology and Bronchoesophagology: State of the Art.
H. Yoshimura et al., editors.

Bacterial biofilm formation on airway stents

Y. Hosokawa[1], M. Yamaguti[1], Y. Gon[2], S. Sawada[1] and T. Horie[2]
[1]Department of Internal Medicine, Nihon University at Nerima Hikarigaoka Hospital; and [2]First Department of Internal Medicine, Nihon University School of Medicine, Tokyo, Japan

Abstract. Recently, a report concerning the improvement of QOL after the insertion of various stents for tracheobronchial stenosis in a case of terminal lung cancer was seen. However, there are very few reports about the infections caused by stenting. On the other hand, severe infections of bacteria biofilm are a problem that come along with the development of medical devices made to be installed inside the body. We report on this issue because we observed six extendable metallic stents (EMS) that were analysed using a scanning electron microscope on their detainment at autopsy and bacteria biofilm was confirmed on the surfaces of all of them. These EMS were collected from four lung cancer patients who had EMSs inserted into their stenotic lesions.

Keywords: airway stents, biofilm, scanning electron microscope.

Introduction

Bacterial biofilm formation (BBF) is one of the major reasons for the occurrence of infections and it persists at various sites in the human body, especially in association with medical devices. BBF should be taken into consideration in terms of bronchial stents as well, in care of poststenting. We report BBF on the surface of an expandable metallic stent (EMS) in autopsy, confirmed using a scanning electron microscope.

Methods

A deceased subject with bronchial stenosis was observed, and the EMS was recovered at the time of the autopsy. In this case, the EMS had been inserted because of lung cancer. The characteristics of the subjects are indicated in Table 1.

The recovered EMS was observed using a scanning electron microscope (HITACHI S-4000), after primary fixation by 2% glutaraldehyde (in 0.1 M PBS, pH 7.4, 4°C, 120 min), and secondary fixation by 2% osmic acid (in 0.1 M PBS, pH 7.4, 4°C, 90 min).

Address for correspondence: Y. Hosokawa, Department of Internal Medicine, Nihon University, Nerima Hikarigaoka Hospital, 2-11-1 Hikarigaoka, Nerima-ku, Tokyo 179-0072, Japan. Tel.: +81-3-3979-3611. Fax: +81-3-3979-3868.

Table 1. Patient and stent characteristics.

Age/sex	Patho	Site	Recovered stent	Survival (days)
41/M	Ad	Rt main	2 (stent in stent)	218
54/M	SqCC	Lt main	2 (second stent)	243
70/M	SqCC	Rt main	1	34
81/M	SqCC	Rt main	1	794

Ad: adenocarcinoma, SqCC: squamous cell carcinoma, Rt main: right main bronchus, Lt main: left main bronchus.

Results (Figs. 1—3)

As for the difference in degree, a membrane structure entity was observed on the surface of the EMS. Coccus, bacillus, and fungus had formed a lump, and an attached entity was observed on the surface. The structure of their circumferences suggested BBF.

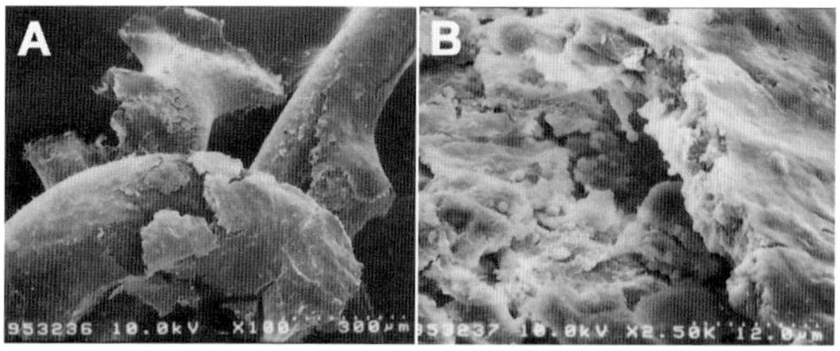

Fig. 1. **A:** A membrane structure is covering almost the entire surface of the EMS. **B:** The center of the image from Fig. 1A is magnified. The membrane structure itself is confirmed as the cluster of the coccus.

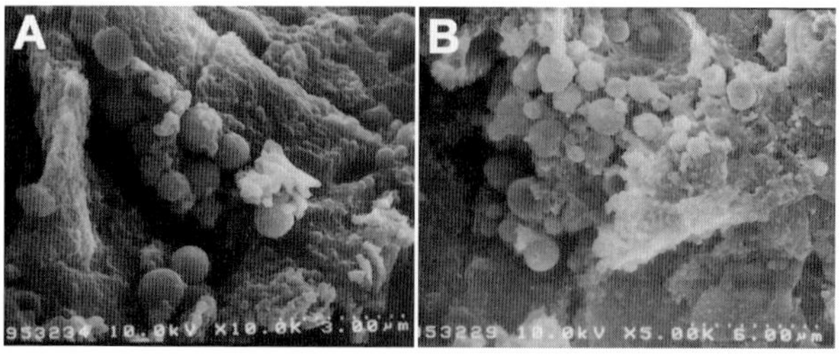

Fig. 2. **A:** The lump of the cluster. An attachment has been created, consisting of a convexo-concave, bacterial body surface, which is agglutinated to the mutuality and forms the membrane structure. It is the plasty of the biofilm. **B:** The plasty of the biofilm from the coccus is remarkable in this example, as shown in the Fig. 2A and 2B.

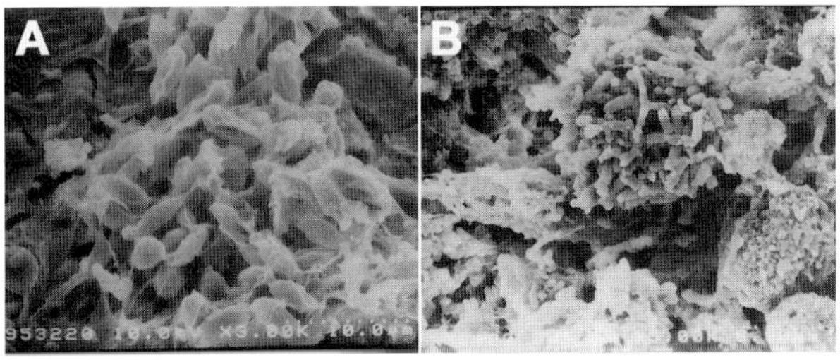

Fig. 3. **A:** Though most of the bacteria, which has already been observed in one example, are coccuses, there is also a cluster of rods. The cluster is agglutinated in the same way as the coccus, and the membrane structure was partly formed here. **B:** The cluster of fungus can be recognized in the same way as the coccus and rods, in the section at the bottom of the figure.

Conclusions

EMSs are used in the respiratory tract, and are suggested, in the same way as other medical devices that are inserted into the body, to be susceptible to BBF as well.

Reference

1. Reid G. Biofilms in infectious disease and on medical devices. Antimicrob Agents 1999;11; 223–226.

©2001 Published by Elsevier Science B.V.
Bronchology and Bronchoesophagology: State of the Art.
H. Yoshimura et al., editors.

Long-term follow-up of three cases after stenting for tracheobronchial stenosis of malignant tumor

Teruhiko Imai[1], Yuko Nishimoto[1], Hajime Ohishi[1], Hideaki Otsuji[1], Hitoshi Yoshimura[1], Hideo Uchida[1], Munehiro Maeda[3], Kouichi Maeda[2], Kaoru Hamada[2], Kazuya Fukuoka[2], Masahiro Sakamoto[2], Yukinori Okamoto[2] and Nobuhiro Narita[2]

[1]Departments of Oncoradiology and Radiology, and [2]2nd Department of Internal Medicine, Nara Medical University, Kashihara; and [3]Department of Radiology, Osaka University, Osaka, Japan

Introduction

Central airway obstruction is a cause of morbidity in patients with lung cancer. Expandable metallic stent (EMS) placement is effective in removing dyspnea immediately. Radiation therapy and/or chemotherapy after stenting can lead to better quality of life and longer survival. Three cases are reported in this study, of which it was possible to do a long-term follow-up with various palliative therapies after stenting.

Case reports

Case 1

A 43-year-old woman with squamous cell carcinoma of the trachea. She began to feel dyspnea and suffered a loss of consciousness lasting a few seconds, and was transported to our hospital. An emergency EMS was placed at the site of severe stenosis in the upper to middle trachea caused by the tumor. Histological diagnosis was squamous cell carcinoma. After chemoradiotherapy, the stent was buried under the mucosa in fiberscopic findings (Fig. 1A). Seven years and 9 months after stenting, granulation was observed to be half of the size of the tracheal lumen (Fig. 1B). Laser ablation, endobronchial ethanol injection and heat probe coagulation (HPT) were performed. The size of granulation decreased, but increased again after 1 week. Steroid therapy was performed and it reduced the symptoms. This case has now been followed up for 10 years after stenting.

Address for correspondence: Teruhiko Imai, Department of Oncoradiology, Nara Medical University, 840 Shijyou-cho, Kashihara city, Nara 634-8522, Japan. Tel.: +81-744-29-8908. Fax: +81-744-25-3434. E-mail: timai@naramed-u.ac.jp

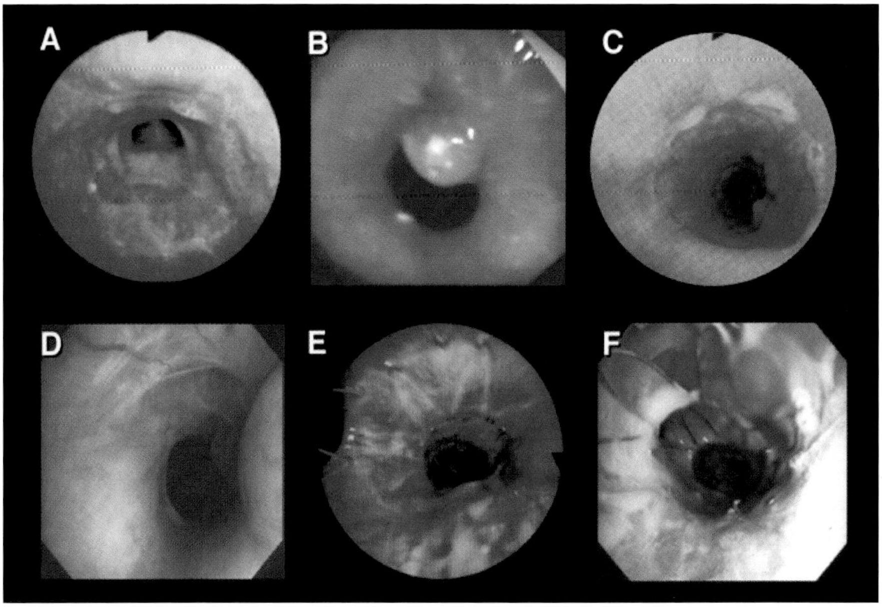

Fig. 1. **A:** Case 1: fiberscopic findings after chemoradiotherapy (middle trachea). **B:** Case 1: 7 years and 9 months after stenting (upper trachea). **C:** Case 2: after radiotherapy (trachea). **D:** Case 2: the latest fiberscopic findings (upper trachea). **E:** Case 3: after radiotherapy (Rt main br.). **F:** Case 3: after laser ablation and 192 Ir HDR therapy (trachea).

Case 2

A 48-year-old woman with adenoid cystic carcinoma of the trachea. An EMS was inserted into the tracheal stenosis near the tumor. Histological diagnosis was adenoidcystic carcinoma. Fiberscopic findings after radiotherapy, consisting of 70 Gy, showed the tumor was much reduced (Fig. 1C). After stenting, granulation occurred at the oral side of the stent. Laser ablation, endobronchial ethanol injection, and HPT were performed at 5 months, 1 year, 2 years, 3 years, and 4 years after stenting. Five years after stenting, tracheal stenosis recurred at the upper side of the stent due to the granulation. Laser ablation was planned, but symptoms improved with steroid therapy. Eight years and 3 months after stenting, the latest fiberscopic findings showed disappearance of granulation at the upper side of stent (Fig. 1D).

Case 3

A 55-year-old woman with adenoid cystic carcinoma of the right main bronchus. The right main bronchus was stenotic due to adenocarcinoma. An EMS was inserted from the middle of the trachea to the right main bronchus and radiotherapy, consisting of 60 Gy, was performed. After therapy the tumor was reduced and the right main bronchus was patent in the fiberscopic findings (Fig. 1E). Four years and 11 months after stenting the tumor recurred and stent-in-stent placement was performed. At this time the histological diagnosis was corrected to adenoidcystic carcinoma. Five years and 7 months after initial stenting, the tumor recurred again. Laser ablation was performed, but the effectiveness was insufficient, so endobronchial brachytherapy with a high-dose-rate after-loading of 192 Ir was performed. Six years and 6 months after initial stenting, endobronchial brachytherapy with 192 Ir HDR was added. After therapy the tumor decreased and the lower trachea and right main bronchus were patent (Fig. 1F). The case is still being followed up.

Discussion

By the time symptoms appear, the stenosis caused by a tumor is already severe. The expandable metallic stent is an effective means of restoring airway patency [1]. Metallic stents have been used for palliating dyspnea caused by central airway stenosis. However, longer survival can be expected after stenting, chemo- and/or radiotherapy and brachytherapy as shown in the three cases in this follow-up study.

There are problems after metallic stent placement: lower airway infection, stent breakage, granular formation and tumor growth through the stent. In the three cases in this study there was one case of mild pneumonia and one of partial stent deformation, but neither caused problems in terms of survival. The biggest problems in the study were granular formation and tumor growth through the stent. Laser ablation, endobronchial ethanol injection and HPT have been found to be effective in controlling granulation. In this study, steroid therapy was particularly effective in two cases. In case 1 there was a complete response to therapy by the tumor, so a retrievable stent would have been very useful.

Conclusion

1. Symptoms and quality of life improved after stenting and made it possible to perform chemo- and/or radiotherapy.
2. Endobronchial therapies and brachytherapy were useful for granular formation and tumor recurrence after stenting and survival time was extended.
3. Steroid therapy was effective in controlling granular formation.
4. In cases of complete remission a retrievable stent would be very useful.

Reference

1. Tojo T, Imai T, Sasaki Y et al. Improvement of mucociliary transport system four years after metal stent insertion in trachea. Evaluation by aerosol inhalation cine-scintigraphy. J Bronchol 1999;6:35–38.

Bronchology and Bronchoesophagology: State of the Art.
H. Yoshimura et al., editors.

Endoscopic treatment of esophago-pleural fistula via a covered expandable metallic stent

Akitoshi Kinoshita[1], Shunji Nagai[1], Yukihiro Kaneko[1], Mitsuhiko Osumi[1], Kosei Miyashita[1], Hiroharu Tsuji[1], Mikio Oka[2] and Shigeru Kohno[2]
[1]Nagasaki-Chuo National Hospital, Omura; and [2]Nagasaki University School of Medicine, Nagasaki, Japan

Abstract. Esophago-pleural (E-P) fistula, without primary esophageal lesions, is a rare clinical event. Many therapies, including surgical treatment, have been performed in these cases, however, the efficacy of these therapies is not sufficient. Here, we report a successful case of E-P fistula, that was treated with endoscopy using a covered expandable metallic stent (EMS), subsequent to chemotherapy for lung cancer. A 53-year-old man, who had received a right pneumonectomy, due to squamous cell carcinoma of the right lung 5 years ago, was admitted to our hospital for further examination of the left axillar lymphadenopathy. He was diagnosed as having a recurrence of lung cancer accompanied by mediastinal and left axillar lymph node involvement. The lymph nodes regressed following the first chemotherapy treatment, which consisted of carboplatin and docetaxel. He was complaining of a high fever and a pain in the right side of his chest on day 6 of the second chemotherapy treatment. Chest X-ray and a CT scan demonstrated a high air-fluid level in the right thoracic cavity. Esophagography and endoscopy revealed an E-P fistula. Although various conservative therapies were not so effective, the insertion of a covered EMS into the esophagus via endoscopy was successful in our present case. The covered EMS method should be considered in cases of E-P fistula when conservative therapy is not effective.

Keywords: chemotherapy, lung cancer, pneumonectomy, thoracic drainage.

Introduction

Esophago-pleural (E-P) fistula, without primary esophageal lesions, is a rare clinical event. Many therapies, including surgical treatment, have been performed in these cases, however, the efficacy of these therapies is not sufficient. Here, we report a successful case of E-P fistula, that was treated with endoscopy using a covered expandable metallic stent (EMS), subsequent to chemotherapy for lung cancer.

Case report

A 53-year-old man, who received a right pneumonectomy due to squamous cell carcinoma of the right lung 5 years ago. The postoperative stage of the lung can-

Address for correspondence: Akitoshi Kinoshita MD, Department of Respiratory Medicine, Nagasaki-Chuo National Hospital, 2-1001-1 Kubara, Omura 856-8562, Japan. Tel.: +81-957-52-3121. Fax: +81-957-54-0292. E-mail: akitosik@nmc.hosp.go.jp

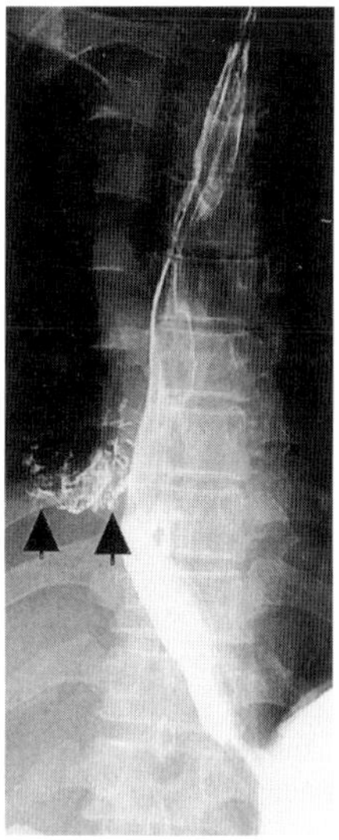

Fig. 1.

cer was pT4N2M0 (IIIB), and one course of postoperative chemotherapy (carboplatin and vindesine) and thoracic radiotherapy (56 Gy) were performed.

The patient recognized a tumor at the left axilla, 4 months ago. The tumor gradually increased in size (approx. 5 cm). He was admitted to our hospital for the further examination of the left axillar lymphadenopathy. He was diagnosed as having a recurrence of lung cancer, accompanied by mediastinal and left axil-

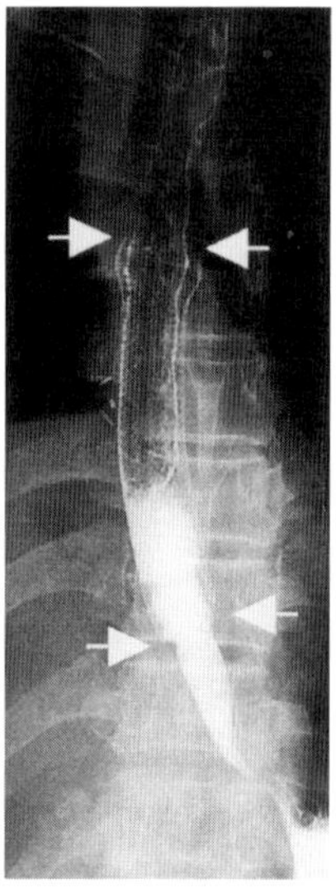

Fig. 2.

Table 1. Summary of esophago-pleural fistula without primary esophageal lesions.

Underlying disease	No.	Ope	Pn (right/left)
Lung cancer	22[a]	22[a]	18[a]/4
Malignant mesothelioma	3	3	3/0
Pulmonary tuberculosis	8	7	3/3
Empyema	4	4	3/0
Other pulmonary lesions	3	3	3/0
Total	40	39	30/7

[a]Present case, as well as other cases in the reported 39 cases. Ope: resection of the lung, Pn: pneumonectomy.

lar lymph node involvement. He was treated with systemic chemotherapy, which consisted of carboplatin and docetaxel. The lymph nodes regressed after the first chemotherapy treatment.

The patient complained of a high fever and pain in the right side of his chest on day 6 of the second chemotherapy treatment. Chest X-ray and a CT scan demonstrated a high air-fluid level in the right thoracic cavity. Esophagography and endoscopy revealed an E-P fistula (Fig. 1). Although various conservative therapies (thoracic drainage, etc.) were not so effective, a covered EMS was successfully inserted into the esophagus via endoscopy in our present case (Fig. 2). The patient became able to eat satisfactorily.

Table 2. Therapy and outcome of 39 reprted cases of E-P fistula without primary esophageal lesions.

Therapy:	
Conservative	12
OWT	4
TP	2
RB	3
ES	4
ES+OWT	2
ES+TP	11
ET+TP	1
Outcome:	
Improved	31
Dead:	7
Cancer	2
Operation	4
Pneumonia (postoperative)	1
Unknown	1

ES: esophageal suture; ET: esophageal transection; OWT: open window thoracotomy; RB: retrosternal bypass; TP: thoracoplasty.

Discussion

Although there are many causes of E-P fistula, most of them are primary esophageal lesions (esophageal cancer, etc.). Only 39 cases of E-P fistula, without primary esophageal lesions, have been reported in English literature (Medline, 1965–1999) (Table 1). In those cases with pulmonary or pleural lesions, three-quarters of them occurred after a right pneumonectomy. The therapy and outcome of the 39 cases are shown in Table 2. Operations were performed in 27 cases, and conservative treatment was carried out in 12 cases. Covered EMS was not used in any of the 39 cases.

Covered EMS is a useful method for extending an esophageal lumen (e.g., stenosis in conjunction with esophageal cancer), or closing a foramen of the esophageal wall (e.g., esophago-tracheal fistula, due to invasion of esophageal cancer). The covered EMS was used successfully to treat the present case. In conclusion, the covered EMS method should be considered in cases of E-P fistula when conservative therapy is not effective.

Bronchology and Bronchoesophagology: State of the Art.
H. Yoshimura et al., editors.

A convenient technique for inserting a Dumon stent into the trachea

Yoshiaki Minakata[1], Masanori Nakanishi[1], Hirotaka Nakanishi[1], Yugo Nagai[2] and Susumu Yukawa[1]
[1]Third Department of Internal Medicine, and [2]Department of Endoscopy, Wakayama Medical College, Wakayama, Japan

Abstract. *Background.* For the treatment of airway stenosis, one of the most effective procedures is the placement of a Dumon stent. However, the insertion of the stent requires general anesthesia and is complicated. The object of this study is to develop a convenient technique for inserting a Dumon stent in the trachea.

Methods. The stent was set in the top of the standard tracheal intubation tube, which has a slit, and could be released easily when the tied thread was pulled out. The tracheal tube was intubated in the usual manner and its position was adjusted under X-ray, then the thread was pulled and the tracheal tube was released. In this way, the stent was placed in the anticipated position.

Cases. We applied this technique to two cases who had a tracheoesophageal fistula or tracheal stenosis by malignant tumor. The insertion was easily and successfully performed without any trouble, and it took only a few minutes.

Conclusions. This technique is convenient and very useful for inserting a Dumon stent in the trachea, and could be helpful for physicians.

Keywords: Dumon stent, insertion technique, tracheal stenosis, tracheoesophageal fistula.

Introduction

One of the most effective procedures for airway stenosis is the placement of a stent in the stenotic airway. Recently, a silicone Dumon stent has started to be widely used [1,2], because it can be removed easily when the stenosis is improved by other treatment. It can also be used for tracheoesophageal fistula [3]. On the other hand, the weak point of a Dumon stent is its complicated procedure of placement. Usually it requires general anesthesia and a rigid bronchofiberscope. To solve this problem, we developed a convenient technique for inserting a Dumon stent in the trachea using common instruments which are present in any clinic.

Address for correspondence: Yoshiaki Minakata, Third Department of Internal Medicine, Wakayama Medical College, 811-1 Kimiidera, Wakayama 641-0012, Japan. Tel.: +81-73-441-0619. Fax: +81-73-446-2877. E-mail: minakaty@wakayama-med.ac.jp

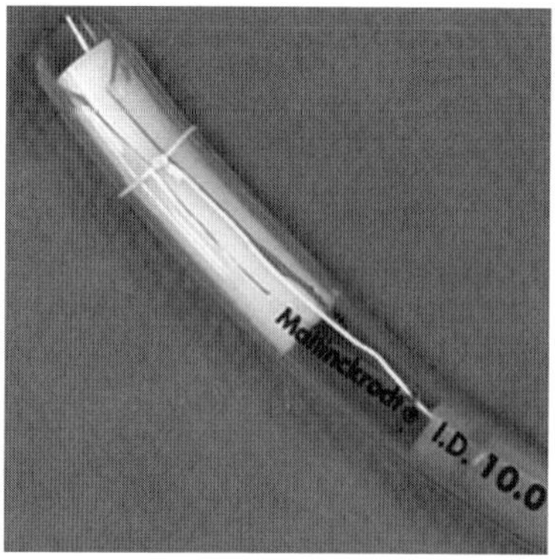

Fig. 1. A Dumon stent is set in the top of the outer tube, which is tied with thread and easily untied when the other end of the thread is pulled.

Methods

The prepared instruments were: 1) an intratracheal intubation tube (inner diameter: 10 mm) as an outer tube, 2) an intratracheal intubation tube (inner diameter: 6 mm) as an inner tube, 3) a silk thread, 4) a positional marker which was originally prepared with needles, and 5) a Dumon stent. The length of the outer tube was shortened to about 28 cm. A slit (5 cm in length) was made at the top of the tube, and a hole (2 mm in diameter) at the end of the slit. A Dumon stent which is coated with lidocaine gel, was set in the top of the outer tube. Then the top of it was tied with thread so that it will untie easily when the other end of the thread, which comes out of the inner tube, was pulled (Figs. 1 and 2A). As a procedure, the position was decided under X-ray by using the positional marker which was put on the chest wall. After the outer tube, including a Dumon stent, was intubated in the usual manner for tracheal intubation, the thread was pulled and untied. The outer tube was pulled keeping the inner tube in the same position, and the stent was thus placed at the anticipated position.

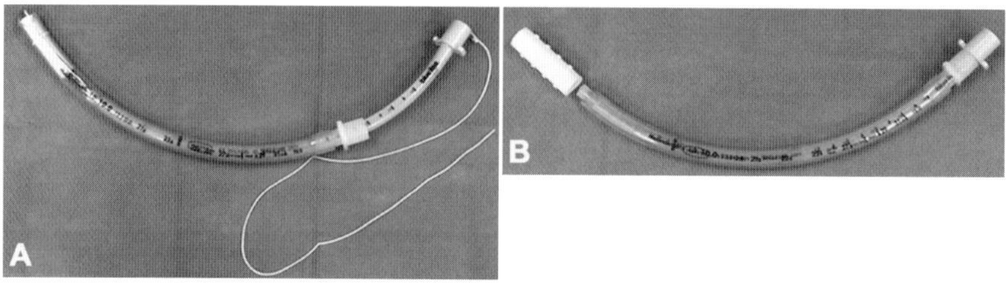

Fig. 2. Before (**A**) and after (**B**) stenting.

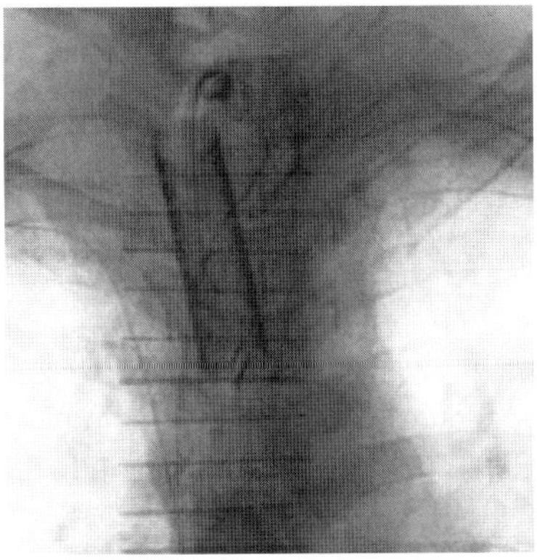

Fig. 3. A Dumon stent was inserted into the patient with tracheoesophageal fistula.

Cases

A 53-year-old man was diagnosed as having esophageal cancer and had received chemo-radiotherapy, but recurrence created a tracheoesophageal fistula. After an esophageal stenting, a Dumon stent was inserted in the trachea using the new technique (Fig. 3). It can be done very easily without any trouble, and it took only a few minutes.

A 48-year-old man came to our hospital because he had had a cough for a few weeks and felt dyspnea. Bronchoscopic findings showed tracheal stenosis from squamous cell lung cancer. A Dumon stent was easily inserted using the technique. As the chemo-radiotherapy improved the stenosis, the Dumon stent was removed.

Discussion

A Dumon stent is useful for the treatment of airway stenosis [1,2] or tracheobronchial fistula [3]. However, it requires a rigid bronchoscope under general anesthesia, and this makes physicians hesitant to use a Dumon stent. Many techniques have been tried in order to insert Dumon stents without a rigid bronchoscope [4,5], but they still have some problems. Our new technique is an improvement of Umemoto's method [4]. The first improved point is that the stent is in the top of the outer tube so that it can be released out of the outer tube easily. The second improvement is that the outer tube is pulled instead of pushing the inner tube when the stent is released. The third improvement is that the top of the outer tube is tied with thread which unties easily when the other end of the thread is pulled. This makes intubation easy and does not injure vocal cords. This newly developed technique does not require general anesthesia or a rigid bronchoscope, and takes only a few minutes, like the insertion of a metallic stent. The required instruments are things that are commonly used in a clinic. Actually, in cases of severe stenosis or easy bleeding conditions, it may be better to use a rigid bronchoscope and coagulate or open the airway by laser treatment before inserting the stent. However, in a case of tracheoesophageal fistula or relatively mild stenosis, this technique could be helpful for physicians.

References

1. Dumon JF. A dedicated tracheobronchial stent. Chest 1990;97:328–332.
2. Bolliger CT, Probst R, Tschopp K, Soler M, Perruchoud AP. Silicone stents in the management of inoperable tracheobronchial stenosis. Indication and limitations. Chest 1993;104:1653–1659.
3. Belleguic C, Lena H, Briens E, Desrues B, Bretagne JF, Delaval P, Kernec J. Tracheobronchial stenting in patients with esophageal cancer involving the central airways. Endoscopy 1999;31: 232–236.
4. Umemoto M, Saitoh Y, Imamura H, Yonezu S. Placement of a Dumon stent with special tracheal tube and fiberscope. J Jpn Soc Bronchol 1996;18:607–611.
5. Ohi M, Murashima S, Seta H, Nomoto Y, Syouji K, Takano K, Nakagawa T, Namikawa S. A Case of broncheal stenosis indwelling Dumon stent using flexible fiberscope and balloon catheter. J Jpn Soc Bronchol 1994;16:614–618.

Bronchology and Bronchoesophagology: State of the Art.
H. Yoshimura et al., editors.

Development of a flowchart for the treatment of tracheobronchial stenosis

Masanori Nakanishi[1], Takeshi Nishimoto[1], Hirotaka Nakanishi[1], Yoshiaki Minakata[1], Yugo Nagai[2] and Susumu Yukawa[1]
[1]Third Department of Internal Medicine, and [2]Department of Endoscopy, Wakayama Medical College, Wakayama, Japan

Abstract. *Background.* Many kinds of stents have been used for the treatment of airway stenosis, however, it is difficult to decide which one is best for each case.

Methods and Results. We considered characteristics of silicone and metallic stents, and made a flowchart for the treatment of tracheobronchial stenosis. The flowchart shows that when the stenosis is expected to improve, we should insert a silicone stent. When a silicone stent migrates or the stenosis is not expected to improve, we should choose a metallic stent. When the stent is obstructed by granulation or tumor ingrowth, microwaves should be used for cauterization. We applied this flowchart to two clinical cases.

Cases. In the first case, a Dumon stent was inserted in the trachea and removed after chemoradiotherapy. In the second case, as a Dumon stent migrated, a Gianturco Z stent was inserted in the left main bronchus. Then the granulation was cauterized by microwaves.

Conclusions. This flowchart could be useful for the treatment of airway stenosis.

Keywords: demerit, merit, metallic stent, selection, silicone stent.

Background

There are several kinds of treatment available for the improvement of airway stenosis, including metallic stenting, silicone stenting, microwaves, YAG laser, etc. However, the choice of the treatment depends on each doctor, and there has been no guideline for treatment selection.

Methods and Results

To choose the treatment for airway stenosis, especially for the selection of a stent, we considered the pros and cons of silicone and metallic stents (Table 1). We then made a flowchart for the treatment of tracheobronchial stenosis on the basis of the patient's condition (Fig. 1). According to this flowchart, we inserted a stent in two clinical cases, obtaining good results.

Address for correspondence: Masanori Nakanishi, Third Department of Internal Medicine, Wakayama Medical College, 811-1 Kimiidera, Wakayama 641-0012, Japan. Tel.: +81-73-441-0619. Fax: +81-73-446-2877.

Table 1. Characteristics of stents.

Stent type	Merits	Demerits
Silicone stent (Dumon stent)	Removable	Migration Expectration Rigid bronchoscope neccessary
Metallic stent (Gianturco Z stent)	Easy insertion Strong expansion	Granulation/tumor ingrowth Not removable

Case 1

A 48-year-old man was admitted to the hospital in June 1999 due to hoarseness and a cough. He then felt dyspnea day by day. It was difficult to find an abnormal shadow on chest X-ray, but the computed tomography (CT) showed a tumor shadow at the upper mediastinum. On endoscope, the tumor narrowed the trachea. Histological diagnosis was squamous cell carcinoma. We inserted a Dumon stent because the stenosis was expected to improve and the stent to be removed after chemo-radiotherapy. When we inserted it, we employed a convenient insertion technique without using a rigid bronchoscope. We could remove the stent after chemo-radiotherapy.

Case 2

An 84-year-old man was admitted to the hospital in December 1998 because of a traffic accident. After an operation for the injury of his cervical vertebrae, he

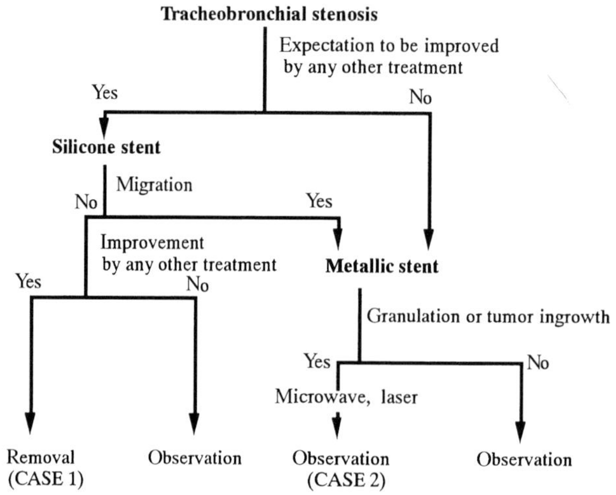

Fig. 1. Flowchart for the treatment of tracheobronchial stenosis. In case 1, the Dumon stent was removed after chemo-radiotherapy. In case 2, as the Dumon stent migrated, a Gianturco Z stent was inserted. Then the granulation was cauterized by microwave.

had sudden dyspnea. Chest X-ray showed an atelectasis of the left lower lobe and a shift of the mediastinum to the left. Computed tomography (CT) showed a stenosis of the left main bronchus. We diagnosed it as traumatic bronchial stenosis and inserted a Dumon stent because we anticipated its later removal. However, the Dumon stent migrated after a while, and we exchanged it with a Gianturco Z stent. Ten days later, chest X-ray showed an atelectasis of the left lower lobe again. On endoscope, the stent was obstructed by granulation. The granulation was cauterized by microwaves.

Discussion

Many kinds of stents have been used for the treatment of airway stenosis. At present, the Dumon stent is most widely used, however, it is not ideal [1]. The merit of a Dumon stent is that it is removable. However, it involves potential difficulty of sputum drainage and migration, and requires general anesthesia and rigid bronchoscopy for insertion [2–4]. A metallic stent is easy to insert and may not require general anesthesia or rigid bronchoscopy. Because they are very hard to reposition or remove, metallic stents should be chosen very carefully [5,6]. On the flowchart, we first choose a silicone stent for airway stenosis, but if the stenosis is not expected to improve, or the stent migrates, we choose a metallic stent. When the stent is obstructed by granulation or tumor ingrowth, microwaves or a laser are used for cauterization. In both cases, we chose a silicone stent at first, because the stenosis was expected to improve and the stent to be removed. In case 1, the stent did not migrate and was removed as expected. In case 2, as the Dumon stent migrated, we exchanged it for a Gianturco Z stent. We are going to treat tracheobronchial stenosis using this flowchart.

Conclusion

We developed a flowchart for the treatment of tracheobronchial stenosis, especially for the selection of a stent. We applied this flowchart to two clinical cases with good results.

References

1. Dumon JF. A dedicated tracheobronchial stent. Chest 1990;97:328–332.
2. Nomori H, Horio H. Use of silicone stents for tracheobronchial stenosis due to tumors. Nippon Kyoubu Geka Gakkai Zasshi 1997;45:666–669.
3. Noppen M, Meysman M, Claes I, D'Haese J, Vincken W. Screw-thread vs Dumon endoprosthesis in the management of tracheal stenosis. Chest 1999;115:532–535.
4. Kim H. Stenting therapy for stenosing airway disease. Respirology 1998;3:221–228.
5. Rafanan AL, Mehta AC. Stenting of the tracheobronchial tree. Radiol Clin North Am 2000;38: 395–478.
6. Hind CR, Donnelly RJ. Expandable metal stents for tracheal obstruction: permanent or temporary? A cautionary tale. Thorax 1992;47:757–758.

Bronchology and Bronchoesophagology: State of the Art.
H. Yoshimura et al., editors.

Complications of Dumon and Nitinol stents for lung and esophageal cancer patients with tracheal and bronchial stenosis

Seiichi Nobuyama, Tsutomu Yoneda, Atsusi Kamitani, Tomoya Kawaguchi and Masaaki Kawahara
National Kinki Central Hospital for Chest Diseases, Sakai, Osaka, Japan

Abstract. Dumon Stents and Nitinol Stents have been widely used for tracheal and endobronchial airway stenosis caused by malignant tumors. We examined and compared the complications of these two types of stents. Although Dumon stents caused hypersecretion and chest discomfort more often than Nitinol stents, when these two side effects are effectively controlled, the use of Dumon stents is preferable.

Keywords: airway stenosis, Dumon stent, esophageal cancer, lung cancer, Nitinol stent.

Introduction

There has been considerable progress during the last decade in endoscopic treatment of central airway stenosis. Bronchoscopic stent implantation has been reported to be a useful treatment for tracheal and endobronchial airway stenosis due to malignant tumors [1,2]. Because both Dumon and Nitinol stents have been widely used, but there remains controversy as to which is superior, we examined and compared the complications of these two types of stents.

Results

Ten Dumon stents were inserted into 10 patents (eight lung cancer patients and two esophageal cancer patients), and nine Nitinol stents into five patients (four lung cancer patients and one esophageal cancer patient). Two patients required a second stent. The most frequent complications of Dumon stents were hypersecretion (90%, 9/10), chest oppression (50%, 5/10) and bronchoesophageal fistula esophageal stenosis (10%, 1/10). There was no tumor protrusion in patients with the Dumon stents. In the nine Nitinol stent cases, the major complications were hypersecretion (67%, 6/9), bronchoesophageal fistula (11%, 1/9) and migration (11%, 1/9). Tumor protrusions were found in three patients (33%, 3/9) with Nitinol stents. There were no treatment-related deaths.

Address for correspondence: Seiichi Nobuyama, National Kinki Central Hospital for Chest Disease, Nagasone-cho 1180, Sakai, Osaka 591-8555, Japan. Tel.: +81-722-52-3021. Fax: +81-722-50-4034. E-mail: nobuyama@rr.iij4u.or.jp

Conclusion

Dumon stents caused hypersecretion and chest discomfort more often than Nitinol stents, but there was no tumor protrusion. Conversely, Nitinol stents caused less hypersecretion and granuloma formation than Dumon stents, but with Nitinal stents tumor protrusion and fistula caused complications. Additionally, Nitinol stents proved difficult to remove. Therefore, we concluded that when hypersecretion and chest discomfort is controlled, the use of Dumon stents is preferable.

References

1. Colt HG, Dumon J-F. Airway stents, present and future. Clin Chest Med 1995;16(3):465–478.
2. Dumon J-F, Cavaliere S. Tracheobronchial Stents. Proceedings in Rigid Bronchoscopy Meeting in Marseille: 1994;13–18.
3. Miyazawa T, Doi M, Fukuhara N et al. Kouseikikanshikyou ni yoru stent chiryou. J Jpn Soc Bronchol 1994;16(8):874–878.

Bronchology and Bronchoesophagology: State of the Art.
H. Yoshimura et al., editors.

New bioabsorbable tracheal stent – comparison of tissue reaction in experimental rabbit model; poly-L-lactide and silicone stent

Yukihito Saito, Kenichiro Minami, Yoshihisa Nakao, Masashi Kobayashi, Hideyasu Omiya, Hiroji Imamura and Akiharu Okamura
Department of Thoracic and Cardiovascular Surgery, Kansai Medical University, Moriguchi, Japan

Abstract. We tested the tissue reactions of a bioabsorbable stent, made of poly-L-lactic acid (PLLA), within the normal airway, and compared them with those of a stent made of silicone. The bioabsorbable knitted airway stent, made of PLLA wire, was implanted in New Zealand white rabbits; silicone stents served as the control. Light and electron microscopic studies showed that the ciliated cell layer was spared between the mesh holes of knitted PLLA stent. In this study, the PLLA stent showed biocompatibility good enough to make it a promising material for an airway stent.

Keywords: bioabsorbable material, PLLA, silicone, tracheal stent.

Purpose

Treatment of tracheobronchial stenosis is problematic. Conservative methods include stenting the stenotic area using stents made of silicone or metallic materials, but an ideal stent has not yet been developed [1–3]. Bioabsorbable airway stents offer benefits; the extraction of the device is unnecessary, and the airway preserves its normal function after stent resorption. The purpose of this study was to examine the suitability of poly-L-lactic acid (PLLA) as a material for an airway stent.

Materials and Methods

The bioabsorbable knitted airway stent, made of PLLA wire was implanted in New Zealand white rabbits; silicone stents served as controls. Silicone stents were group A (Fig. 1) and PLLA stents were group B (Fig. 2). The mean weight of the animals was 3.1 kg in each group. PLLA tracheal stents were made of 170 μm PLLA wire with an outer diameter of 5 mm and a length of 12 mm. The silicone stents were tubes 0.7-mm thick with a 6-mm outer diameter and a length of 12 mm. The rabbits were anesthetized using halothane inhalation. The animals maintained spontaneous breathing without intubation. The operation procedure

Address for correspondence: Yukihito Saito MD, Department of Thoracic and Cardiovascular Surgery, Kansai Medical University, 10-15 Fumizonocho, Moriguchi 570-8507, Japan. Tel.: +81-6-6992-1001. Fax: +81-6-6994-7022. E-mail: saitoy@takii.kmu.ac.jp

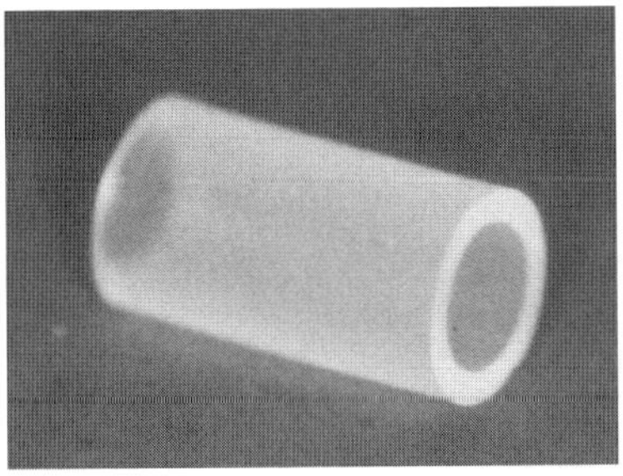

Fig. 1. Silicone stent (group A). Configuration: 0.7 mm thick, 6-mm outer diameter, 12 mm in length.

is as follows; First, the midline of the cervical trachea was prepared for the implantation of the stent. The trachea was opened transversely between cartilage rings for two-thirds of its circumference. Second, the stent was implanted intra-tracheally and fixed with a 5—0 polypropylene suture, and the tracheotomy was closed. This study was evaluated by bronchoscopic and histologic examination. The cervical trachea was excised and divided into two pieces, one for light microscopic studies and the other for scanning electron microscopic studies, after the mean follow-up of 2 months in group A, and 2 to 5 months in group B was carried out. At the time of sacrifice, a bronchoscopic examination of the rabbit-implanted stents was made for each group.

Results

In group A, three animals died within 2 months of implantation and three animals had stridor at the time of sacrifice. After 2 months follow-up, obstructive material was visible inside the stent. Mucosal swelling at both ends of the stents was also observed. Although silicone stents are widely used, they have certain disadvantages. They interfere with normal airway mucociliary functions, which can result in the accumulation of secretions inside the stent and the obstruction of its lumen.

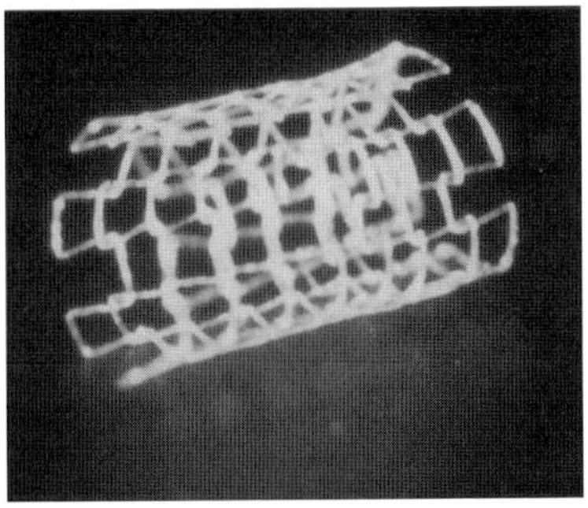

Fig. 2. PLLA stent (group B). Configuration: 5-mm outer diameter, 12 mm in length.

On the other hand, in group B, one animal died 3 weeks after implantation due to anorexia. The autopsy of this animal revealed that the bronchial lumen was not stenosed. After 2 months follow-up of the remaining animals, the bronchial lumen was fully open with slight sputum at the edge of the PLLA stent. The PLLA stents of 2 months kept their mechanical strength. After 5 months follow-up, a part of the stent had been absorbed.

Histologic examination of group A showed marked regression of ciliated cells under the stent. In some areas, the epithelium had disappeared. Epithelial erosion and chronic lymphocytic inflammation were shown in the submucosa 2 months after implantation. In group B, the ciliated epithelium was preserved and numerous capillary blood vessels were observed in the submucosa. Scanning electron microscopic study in group A showed marked regression of ciliated cells under the silicone stent, 2 months after implantation. In group B, the ciliated cells had been preserved between the mesh holes of the knitted PLLA stent at the times of 2 and 5 months follow-up.

Conclusion

We tested the tissue reactions of a bioabsorbable stent, made of PLLA, within the normal airway, and compared them to those of a stent made of silicone. Light and electron microscopic studies showed that the ciliated cell layer was spared between the mesh holes of the knitted PLLA stent. In this study, the PLLA stent showed biocompatibility good enough to make it a promising material for an airway stent.

References

1. Wallace MJ, Charnsangavej C, Ogawa K, Carrasco CH, Wright KC, McKenna R, McMurtrey M, Gianturco C. Tracheobronchial tree: expandable metallic stents used in experimental and clinical applications. Radiology 1986;152:309–312.
2. Dumon JF, Meric B, Cavaliere S. Indwelling tracheobronchial prosthesis. Chest 1988;94:68S.
3. Dumon JF. A dedicated tracheobronchial stent. Chest 1990;97:328–332.

Surgery

Bronchology and Bronchoesophagology: State of the Art.
H. Yoshimura et al., editors.

Tracheobronchoplasty for primary lung cancer: results and complications

Shuhei Inoue, Shozo Fujino, Keiichi Kontani, Satoru Sawai, Yuji Suzumura, Jun Hanaoka and Minako Fujita
Second Department of Surgery, Shiga University of Medical Science, Seta, Otsu, Shiga, Japan

Abstract. *Background.* We reviewed the results and complications of thirty-six patients (33 males, three females; mean age: 63 years) who underwent tracheobronchoplasty for primary lung cancer between 1978 and 1998. We compared the first half period in 18 cases (group I) with the latter half period in 18 cases (group II).

Results. There were one tracheal resection and 17 sleeve lobectomies in group I, while there were two sleeve pneumonectomies and 16 sleeve lobectomies in group II. The mean operative times and blood losses were 417.7 min, and 1110 ml in group I, and 395 min, and 520 ml in group II, respectively. The anastomotic sites were covered with soft tissues in 21 cases. The 5-year-survival rate was 40.4% in group I and 64.2% in group II. There were five postoperative deaths (two in group I and three in group II) from ARDS, acute myocardial infarction, broncho-pulmonary artery fistel, renal failure and pneumonia (18.9%).

Conclusion. Our experience suggests that operative time and blood loss were decreased in group II, but that the operative mortality was still higher than that of patients who underwent standard operations.

Keywords: bronchoplasty, complication, lung cancer, sleeve resection.

Background

Tracheobronchoplasty either with or without lung resection has become a routine procedure for the treatment of lung cancer while preserving the functioning lung tissue [1,2]. We herein report the results and complications of 36 cases of tracheobronchoplasty procedures for primary lung cancer.

Materials and Methods

We reviewed the results and complications of thirty-six patients (33 males, three females; mean age: 63 years) who underwent tracheobronchoplasty for primary lung cancer between 1978 and 1998. We compared the first half of the period in 18 patients (group I) with the latter half of the period in 18 patients (group II).

Address for correspondence: Shuhei Inoue, Second Department of Surgery, Shiga University of Medical Science, Seta, Otsu, Shiga 520-2192, Japan. Tel.: +81-77-548-2244. Fax: +81-77-544-2901. E-mail: shuhei@belle.shiga-med.ac.jp

Table 1. Patient characteristics.

	Former period (n = 18) October 1978–December 1991		Latter period (n = 18) January 1992–December 1998	
	No.	%	No.	%
Histology:				
Squamous	13	72.2	13	72.2
Adenocarcinoma	3	16.7	3	16.7
Adenoid cystic carcinoma	1	5.6	1	5.6
Adenosquamous	1	5.6	0	0
Small cell carcinoma	0	0	1	5.6
p-stage:				
IA	1	5.6	3	16.7
IB	6	33.3	1	5.6
IIB	2	11.1	6	33.3
IIIA	6	33.3	2	11.1
IIIB	1	5.6	5	27.8
IV	2	11.1	1	5.6

Results

Staging and histology

Histologic characteristics for both groups are in Table 1. There were 26 cases of squamous cell carcinoma (72.2%), six of adenocarcinoma (16.7%), two of adenoid cystic carcinoma (5.6%), one of adenosquamous carcinoma (2.8%), and one of small cell carcinoma (2.8%). There were four of postoperative pathologic stage IA (11.1%), seven of stage IB (19.4%), eight of stage IIB (22.2%), eight of stage IIIA (22.2%), six of stage IIIB (16.7%), and three of stage IV (8.3%).

Type of resection for both groups (Table 2)

Tracheal resection was performed in one patient (2.8%), sleeve pneumonectomy in two (5.6%), sleeve lobectomy in 25 (69.4%), and wedge lobectomy in eight (22.2%). Wrapping of the anastomosis was performed in 21 patients (58.3%), and recently, the intercostal pedicle flap has been used in many cases [3]. Durations of operations were 417.7 min in group I and 395 min in group II. Intraoperative blood loss was 1110 ml in group I and 520 ml in group II.

Mortality

The 30-day-mortality rate was two (5.6%) in both groups. The causes of death were acute myocardial infarction, on day 2, and ARDS. Early mortality occurred in three patients (8.5%), and the causes of death were cerebral bleeding, bronchovascular fistula and pneumonia.

Table 2. Types of resection.

	Former period (n = 18) October 1978—December 1991		Latter period (n = 18) January 1992—December 1998	
	No.	%	No.	%
Operative methods:				
Tracheal resection	1	5.6	0	0
Sleeve pneumonectomy	0	0	2	11.1
Sleeve lobectomy	10	55.6	15	83.3
Wedge lobectomy	7	38.9	1	5.6
Wrapping of the anastomosis:				
Intercostal muscle	3	16.7	16	88.9
Mediastinal pleura	0	0	1	5.6
Fat tissue	1	5.6	0	0
Operation time (min)	417.7		395.0	
Blood loss (ml)	1110		520	
Mortality	2	11.1	3	16.7
5-year-suvival rate (%)	40.4		64.2	

Survival (Figs. 1 and 2)

The overall 5-year-survival rate was 50.6%. The latter period (group II, 64.2%) showed a significantly better prognosis than group I (40.4%). Survival according to postoperative staging is given in Fig. 2.

Discussion

In the last decade, a review of the results of lung cancer treated by bronchoplasty has been reported by Tedder et al. [4]. In this large series, the complications

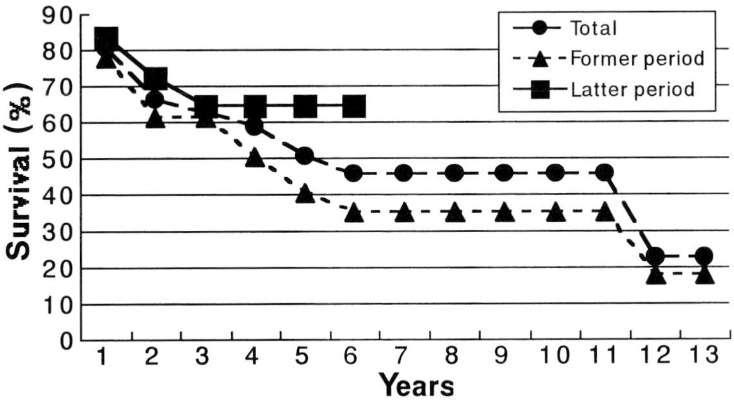

Fig. 1. Actuarial survival after operation.

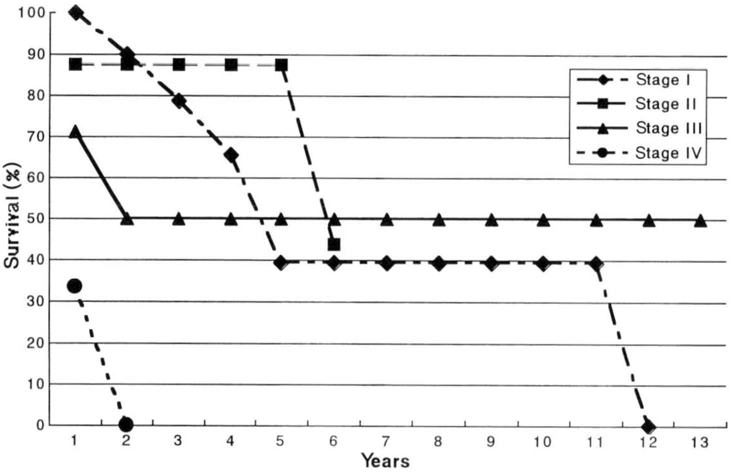

Fig. 2. Actuarial survival after operation by stage.

included local recurrence (10.3%), 30-day mortality (7.5%), pneumonia (6.7%), atelectasis (5.4%), benign stricture (5.0%), bronchopleural fistula (3.5%), empyema (2.8%), bronchovascular fistula (2.6%), and pulmonary embolism (1.9%). The 5-year-survival rates for stage I, II, and III were 63%, 37%, and 21%, respectively.

The 30-day-mortality and stage-II and stage-III survival rates in the present series were better than those in this review, but were still higher than those of patients who underwent standard operations. Based on these results, we suggest that highly attentive pre- and postoperative management is necessary to reduce the complications.

Conclusions

Our experience suggests that operative time and blood loss were decreased in group II, but that the operative mortality was still higher than that of patients who underwent standard operations.

References

1. Paulson DL, Urschel HC, McNamara JJ, Shaw RR. Bronchoplastic procedures for bronchogenic carcinoma. J Thorac Cardiovasc Surg 1970;59:38—47.
2. Jensik RJ, Faber LP, Milloy FJ, Amato JJ. Sleeve lobectomy for carcinoma. J Thorac Cardiovasc Surg 1972;64:400—412.
3. Rendina EA, Venuta F, Ricci P, Fadda GF, Bognolo DA, Ricci C, Rocci P. Protection and revascularization of bronchial anastomoses by the intercostal pedicle flap. J Thorac Cardiovasc Surg 1994;107:1251—1254.
4. Tedder M, Anstadt M, Tedder S, Lowe JM. Current morbidity, mortality, and survival after bronchoplastic procedures for malignancy. Ann Thorac Surg 1992;54:387—391.

Bronchology and Bronchoesophagology: State of the Art.
H. Yoshimura et al., editors.

Tracheo-carinal resection for bronchogenic carcinoma

Makoto Saito, Norihiko Ikeda, Masaharu Nomura, Toshimitsu Hiyoshi, Haruhiko Nakamura, Norihiko Kawate, Chimori Konaka and Harubumi Kato
Department of Surgery, Tokyo Medical University, Tokyo, Japan

Abstract. Tracheo-carinal resection was performed in 15 cases of bronchogenic carcinoma during a 10-year period. The mean age of patients was 59 years, with ages ranging from 40 to 70 years. There were 12 males and three females. The tumor was located on the right side in seven cases, on the left side in two cases, on the trachea in four cases and on the carina in two cases. The histological examination showed squamous cell carcinoma in seven cases, adenocarcinoma in four cases and adenoid cystic carcinoma in four cases. The staging revealed T4N2M0 stage IIIB in five cases, T4N3M0 stage IIIB in one case, T4N0M0 stage IIIB in three cases and T3N2M0 stage IIIA in two cases. The remaining four cases had primary tracheal carcinoma. The surgical methods were as follows: sleeve pneumonectomy in five cases, wedge carinal resection with pulmonary resection in three cases, carinal resection in two cases and tracheal resection in five cases. The site of bronchial anastomosis was overlapped by thymus in seven cases. The 30-day-mortality rate in tracheo-carinal resection was 7% (one patient). Eight patients died of disease and the remaining seven patients are still alive without any evidence of recurrence. All patients underwent tracheal resection and remained alive for the follow-up period, ranging from 22 to 180 months, although two of five cases had adenoid cystic carcinoma, histologically. The 5-year-survival rate was 50%. These outcomes were almost equal to those of surgical cases in the same stage.

Keywords: bronchogenic carcinoma, tracheo-bronchoplasty, tracheo-carinal resection.

Introduction

Tracheo-carinal resection and reconstruction for bronchogenic carcinoma has been used in cases of extended disease of tracheal tumors or the carinal invasion of tumors [1,2]. On the other hand, this technique may make it possible to preserve the pulmonary function, such as in a case of sleeve lobectomy to avoid pneumonectomy. Although a general consensus, concerning tracheo-carinal resection and reconstruction, has not yet been obtained, this technique has contributed to the surgical treatment of bronchogenic carcinoma, and the survival of the patients undergoing nonsurgical treatment is extremely limited.

We present our experiences concerning the tracheo-carinal resection of bronchogenic carcinoma and discuss the validity of present approaches.

Address for correspondence: Makoto Saito MD, Department of Surgery, Tokyo Medical University, 6-7-1 Nishishinjuku, Shinjuku-ku, Tokyo 160-0023, Japan. Tel.: +81-3-3342-6111. Fax: +81-3-3349-0326. E-mail: cbe97310@pop06.odn.ne.jp

Patients and Methods

Table 1 shows the clinical characteristics of eight tracheo-bronchoplasty cases from 1981 to 1995. In these cases, tracheo-bronchoplasty was performed without the overlapping of the bronchial anastomosis. Five cases were male and three female. The majority of tumors were squamous cell carcinoma (three cases) and adenoidcystic carcinoma (three cases), followed by adenocarcinoma (two cases). There were four tracheal carcinomas and three bronchogenic carcinomas. Surgical procedures included right sleeve pneumonectomy in two cases, tracheal resection in four cases, carinal resection in one case and sleeve upper lobectomy with partial carinal resection in one case. TNM staging, adjuvant therapy and the surgical outcome are shown in Table 1.

Table 2 shows the clinical characteristics of seven tracheo-bronchoplasty cases from 1991 to 1999. In these cases, tracheo-bronchoplasty was performed with thymopexy of bronchial anastomosis. Five cases were male and two female. The majority of tumors were squamous cell carcinoma (five cases), followed by adenocarcinoma (two cases). There were one tracheal and six bronchogenic carcinomas. Surgical procedures included right sleeve pneumonectomy in two cases, left sleeve pneumonectomy in one case, tracheal resection in one case, carinal resection in one case and sleeve upper lobectomy with partial carinal resection in one case. TNM staging, adjuvant therapy and the surgical outcome are shown in Table 2.

Results

Eight patients died of disease and the remaining seven patients are still alive without any evidence of recurrence. All patients underwent tracheal resection and remained alive for the follow-up period, ranging from 22 to 180 months, although two of the five cases had adenoid cystic carcinoma, histologically. The overall 5-year-survival rate of patients with tracheo-carinal resection using the Kaplan-Meyer method was 50%.

In the group without overlapping, major complications of bronchial anastomosis were seen in two cases (cases 3 and 5). Dehiscence of bronchial anastomosis occurring in those two cases resulted in empyema and respiratory failure. Local tumor recurrence was seen in one case (case 4), 12 months after surgery, and resulted in broncho-pulmonary artery fistula. Distant tumor recurrence was seen in both lungs in one case (case 6) and the patient died of disease.

In the group with thymopexy, no major complications of bronchial anastomosis were seen. Minor complications of bronchial anastomosis were seen in one case (case 2), who showed minor leakage from bronchial anastomosis, but it was cured after nonsurgical treatment. Distant tumor recurrence was seen in two cases (cases 3 and 4) and they died of disease.

Table 3 shows morbidity, mortality and outcome, according to the overlapping method of bronchial anastomosis. The group without overlapping showed dehis-

Table 1. Tracheo-carinal resection for bronchogenic carcinoma without overlapping of bronchial anastomosis.

Case	Age	Sex	TNM	Stage	Hist.	Op. day	Op. method	Adjuvant	Overlapping	Prognosis (months)	Survival	Cause of death
1	40	M	Tr.	Tr.	AdCys	1981/01	Tr. res.	—	No	180	A	
2	43	F	Tr.	Tr.	AdCys	1986/08	Tr. res.	Rad.	No	70	A	
3	62	F	420	IIIB	AdCys	1987/10	Carina	YAG	No	7	D	Resp. failure
4	57	M	320	IIIA	AD	1987/10	RtSlU+WdCa	Chem/Rad	No	12	D	B-PA fistula
5	54	M	430	IIIB	SQ	1990/02	RtSlPn	YAG	No	0.5	D	Resp. failure
6	42	M	420	IIIB	AD	1993/08	RtSlPn	—	No	4	D	Resp. failure
7	70	M	Tr.	Tr.	SQ	1994/02	Tr. res.	PDT	No	32	A	
8	68	F	Tr.	Tr.	SQ	1995/03	Tr. res.	—	No	22	A	

Table 2. Tracheo-carinal resection for bronchogenic carcinoma with thymopexy of bronchial anastomosis.

Case	Age	Sex	TNM	Stage	Hist.	Op. Day	Op. Method	Adjuvant	Overlapping	Prognosis (months)	Suvival	Cause of death
9	65	F	420	IIIB	SQ	1991/06	RtSlPn	Chem	Thymus	65	D	Apoplexy
10	65	M	400	IIIB	SQ	1992/09	Carina	—	Thymus	70	D	Other ca.
11	57	M	420	IIIB	AD	1992/10	RtWdPn	Chem	Thymus	16	D	Cancer
12	52	F	420	IIIB	AD	1994/10	RtSlPn	Chem	Thymus	4	D	Cancer
13	61	M	Tr.	Tr.-	SQ	1995/01	Tr. res.	Rad	Thymus	64	A	
14	57	M	320	IIIA	SQ	1995/03	RtSlU+WdCa	Rd	Thymus	66	A	
15	68	M	410	IIIB	SQ	1999/11	LtSlPn	Chem	Thymus	6	A	

Table 3. Tracheo-carinal resection for bronchogenic carcinoma.

Overlapping	No	Ycs
No. of cases	8	7
Complications:		
Dehiscence	2	none
Pyothorax	2	1
Respiratory failure	3	none
Death within 1 month	1	none
Outcome:		
5-year-survival rate	33%	67%
MST	47 m	33 m

cence in two cases, pyothorax in two cases, respiratory failure in three cases and death within 1 month after surgery in one case, while the group with thymopexy, showed pyothorax in only one case and no hospital death. The 5-year-survival rate was 33% in the group without overlapping and 67% in the group with thymopexy. These outcomes were almost equal to those of surgical cases in the same stage.

Conclusions

1. Fifteen cases of tracheo-carinal resection for bronchogenic carcinoma were discussed.
2. The validity of this procedure was almost acceptable.
3. Thymopexy was effective in preventing early respiratory complications.

References

1. Grillo HC. Caranal reconstruction. Ann Thorac Surg 1982;34:356–373.
2. Roviaro GC, Varoli F, Rebuffat et al. Tracheal sleeve pneumonectomy for bronchogenic carcinoma. J Thorac Cardiovasc Surg 1994;107:13–18.

©2001 Published by Elsevier Science B.V.
Bronchology and Bronchoesophagology: State of the Art.
H. Yoshimura et al., editors.

Two cases of atypical bronchoplasty in order to avoid pneumonectomy

Noriaki Tsubota, Masahiro Yoshimura, Morihito Okada, Toshihiko Sakamoto and Hidhito Matsuoka
General Thoracic Surgery, Hyogo Medical Center, Hyogo, Japan

Introduction

Pneumonectomy is a kind of disease. A thoracic surgeon should make every effort to avoid this painful postoperative condition, if possible [1,2]. We present two cases of lung cancer treated successfully by atypical reconstruction of the airway.

Case 1

A 59-year-old man with repeated pneumonia was transferred for further examination. Bronchofiberscopy revealed a polypoid tumor obstructing the orifice of the superior bronchus (Fig. 1) and a small lesion at the angle between the right upper bronchus and the intermediate bronchus (Fig. 2). The patient could not tolerate major resection on the right side, because he had had a curative operation on the left lower lobe for cancer 2 years before. In 1999, thoracotomy was performed. The operative schema is shown in Fig. 3. The tense and suppurative superior segment was removed. The distal resection line was started at the basal bronchus posteriorly, and advanced medially and obliquely upward, saving the middle lobe and basal segment accompanied by the bronchi in a connecting fashion. The proximal resection line was started at distal part of the membranous part of the main bronchus, toward the upper bronchus in a deep wedge form. Frozen section, on both stumps, of the bronchus showed negative for cancer. The distal stump of the middle lobe bronchus was anastomosed to the upper bronchus, and the same was done with that of the basal bronchus to the main bronchus. Early bronchofiberscopic findings at the anastomotic line were acceptable (Fig. 4). The postoperative course was uneventful. The patient remains well, and has a good quality of life.

Address for correspondence: Noriaki Tsubota MD, General Thoracic Surgery, Hyogo Medical Center, 13-70 Kitaoji, Akashi, Hyogo 673-8558, Japan. Tel.: +81-78-929-1151. Fax: +81-78-929-2380.
E-mail: n-tsubo@sanynet.ne.jp

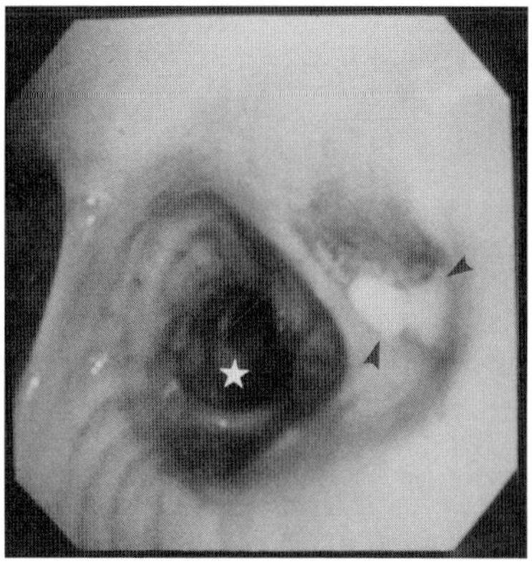

Fig. 1. Case 1: preoperative bronchofiberscopic finding. Arrows: tumor obstructing the superior bronchus, *: basal bronchus.

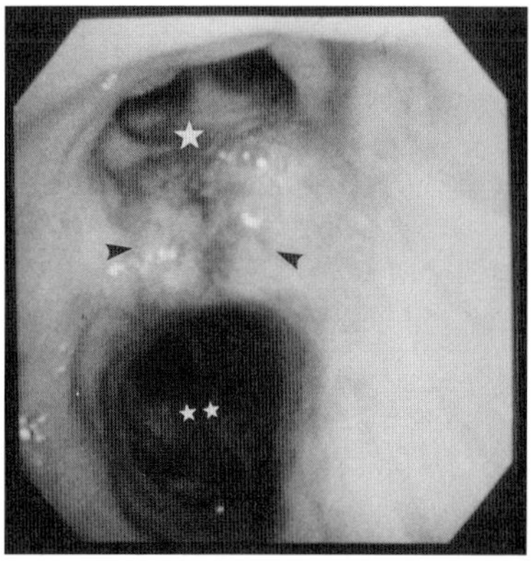

Fig. 2. Case 1: preoperative bronchofiberscopic finding. Arrows: tumor, *: right upper bronchus, **: intermediate bronchus.

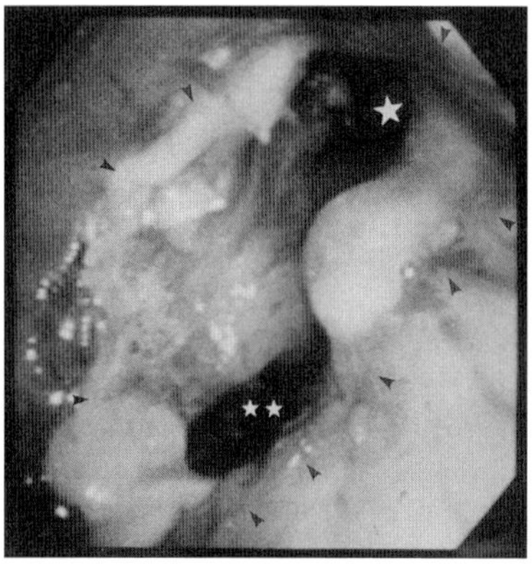

Fig. 3. Case 1: bronchofiberscopic finding, 15 days after operation. Arrows: anastomotic line, *: middle lobe bronchus, **: basal bronchus.

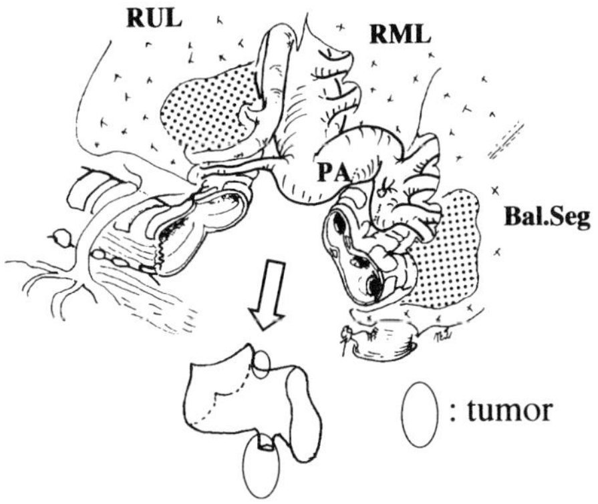

Fig. 4. Case 1: resection of the superior segment including the intermediate bronchus and distal half of the second spur. Anastomosis between the right main and basal bronchus, and between the right upper and middle lobe bronchus.

Case 2

A 71-year-old man was admitted because of a cough and sputum. Bronchoscopy revealed intimal change around the orifice of both the middle lobe bronchus and superior segmental bronchus of the lower lobe. The biopsy yielded the diagnosis of squamous cell carcinoma. In 1996, thoracotomy was performed. The middle lobe and superior segment, accompanied with their bronchi in a connecting fashion, were removed through the pulmonary artery. The bronchus was reconstructed between the proximal end of the intermediate bronchus and the basal bronchus, using 3-0 absorbable interrupted sutures (Fig. 5). The postoperative course was uneventful. The patient is in good condition, 4 years after the operation, with no signs of recurrence.

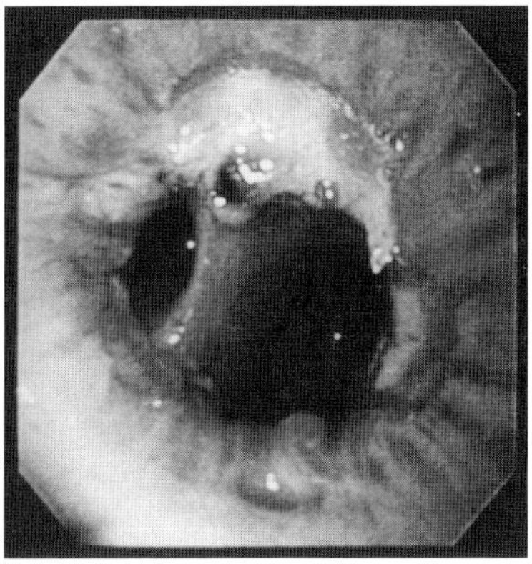

Fig. 5. Case 2: resection of the middle lobe and superior segment. Anastomosis between the intermediate and basal bronchus.

Discussion

Over the last 15 years, we have performed bronchial reconstruction in 170 of 1313 patients with lung cancer [3]. Several unusual reconstructions were completed and succeeded in preserving the lung function, and obtaining good survival without affecting the outcome. We named this type of reconstruction "extended bronchoplasty" [4]. The types are as follows: type A: anastomosis between the right main bronchus and the lower or basal bronchus, with upper and middle lobectomy with or without superior segmentectomy, type B: anastomosis between the left main bronchus and the basal segmental bronchus, with upper lobectomy and superior segmentectomy, accompanied by vascular reconstruction or not, and type C: anastomosis between the left main bronchus and the upper segmental bronchus, with lower lobectomy and lingulectomy, accompanied by vascular reconstruction or not [4]. The two cases reported here do not belong to type A, B or C, and anstomoses are unusual.

There may be a great difference in the postoperative quality of life if pneumonectomy can be avoided, even though the preserved segments are few [5]. Surgeons should reconsider the choice of pneumonectomy for interlobar tumors invading another lobe around the hilum or for separate lesions, as described here, especially in cases of N0 or N1 squamous cell carcinoma.

References

1. Rocco PM, Antowiak Jg, Takita H, Urschel JD. Long-term outcome after pneumonectomy for nonsmall cell lung cancer. J Surg Onchol 1996;61:278–280.
2. Shield TW, Humphery EW, Higgins GA, Keehn RJ. Long-term survivors after resection of lung cancer. J Thorac Cardiovasc Surg 1978;76:439–445.
3. Tsubota N, Yoshimura M, Miyamoto Y, Murotani A, Matoba Y. One hundred one cases of bronchoplasty for lung cancer. Surg Today 1994;24:978–981.
4. Okada M, Tsubota N, Yoshimura M, Miyamoto Y, Matsuoka H, Satake S, Yamagishi H. Extended sleeve lobectomy for lung cancer: the avoidance of pneumonectomy. J Thorac Cardiovasc Surg 1999;118:710–714.
5. Okada M, Yamagishi H, Satake S, Matsuoka H, Miyamoto M, Yoshimura M, Tsubota N. Survival related to lymph node involvement in lung cancer after sleeve lobectomy compared with pneumonectomy. J Thorac Cardiovasc Surg 2000;119:814–819.

Bronchology and Bronchoesophagology: State of the Art.
H. Yoshimura et al., editors.

Reinforcement of bronchial stump with latissimus dorsi muscle

Yuji Shiraishi, Yutsuki Nakajima, Keiichiro Takasuna, Naoya Katsuragi and Satoko Yoshida
Section of Chest Surgery, Fukujuji Hospital, Kiyose, Tokyo, Japan

Abstract. *Background.* Bronchopleural fistula (BPF) after lung surgery is still a serious complication. To prevent this dreadful complication, we recently started to use liberal amounts of latissimus dorsi muscle to reinforce the bronchial stump in high-risk patients.

Methods. This study investigates the outcome of nine patients to whom the latissimus dorsi muscle reinforcement was applied during 1999.

Results. There were seven males and two females, with ages ranging from 43 to 74 years. The indications for surgery were multidrug-resistant tuberculosis in three patients, aspergillosis in two, lung cancer in two, empyema in one, and Mycobacterium avium complex in one. Performed resectional procedures included two extrapleural pneumonectomies (one on the right, one on the left), three pneumonectomies (two in the right, one on the left), and four upper lobectomies (two on the right, two on the left). The bronchial stump was closed using the stapling (eight patients) or the suture (one patient) technique. The follow-up was completed on 30 April 2000. None of the patients have developed BPF so far. A complication related to the mobilization of the muscle was a subcutaneous seroma, which was successfully treated with aspiration.

Conclusions. In conclusion, the reinforcement of the bronchial stump with latissimus dorsi muscle is helpful in preventing a BPF, especially for patients undergoing a pulmonary resection for infectious lung diseases.

Keywords: bronchopleural fistula, muscle transposition, postoperative complication.

Introduction

Bronchopleural fistula (BPF) after pulmonary resection is still one of the most serious postoperative complications encountered. Moreover, it has been reported that the incidence of BPF is higher in surgery for infectious lung diseases than in that of malignant lung diseases [1,2]. To prevent BPF, the reinforcement of the bronchial stump with various kinds of tissues, including pericardial fat pads, intercostal muscles, extrathoracic muscles [3], and omentum has been advocated. Among those, we have been using liberal amounts of latissimus dorsi muscle, because the use of this muscle has several advantages. First, it is a bulky muscle. Second, it can be harvested through the same incision as the thoracotomy incision. Finally, it can be used to reduce the residual space, which is often encountered after pulmonary resection for infectious lung diseases.

Address for correspondence: Yuji Shiraishi MD, Section of Chest Surgery, Fukujuji Hospital, 3-1-24 Matsuyama, Kiyose, Tokyo 204-8522, Japan. Tel.: +81-424-91-4111. Fax: +81-424-92-4765.
E-mail: yujishi@mvb.biglobe.ne.jp

Patients and Methods

Between January 1999 and December 1999, nine patients who underwent a pulmonary resection had the bronchial stump reinforced with latissimus dorsi muscle. These patients formed 9% of the total amount of patients who underwent a major pulmonary resection, such as pneumonectomy, lobectomy, and segmentectomy during the same period. The incidences of BPF, morbidity and mortality were examined. A follow-up was completed on 30 April 2000.

There were seven males and two females with a mean age of 60 years (range: 43 to 74 years). Indications for surgery included multidrug-resistant tuberculosis in three patients, aspergillosis in two, lung cancer in two, empyema in one, and mycobacterium avium complex in one. Resectional procedures included two extrapleural pneumonectomies (one on the right and one on the left), three pneumonectomies (two on the right and one on the left), and four upper lobectomies (two on the right and two on the left). The bronchial stump was closed using the stapling technique in eight patients, and with the suturing technique in the remaining patient. A total flap of latissimus dorsi muscle was used in four patients, and a partial flap was used in the remaining four patients. In the four patients in whom the total flap was used, a subcutaneous drain was inserted to prevent a subcutaneous seroma. The drain was removed when daily drainage became less than 50 cc.

Results

There were no operative mortalities. None of the patients have developed BPF so far. One patient had a postoperative empyema due to wound dehiscence. However, this patient did not have BPF. Thoracoplasty was not necessary in four patients who underwent an upper lobectomy. Subcutaneous seroma occurred in six patients. However, the seroma was successfully treated with aspiration.

Conclusions

In conclusion, the reinforcement of the bronchial stump with latissimus dorsi muscle is helpful in preventing postoperative BPF. The use of this muscle is also useful in order to reduce the residual space after an upper lobectomy, and avoid thoracoplasty. Therefore, this technique is recommended, especially for patients who are undergoing a pulmonary resection for an infectious lung diseases.

References

1. Shiraishi Y, Nakajima Y, Koyama A, Takasuna K, Katsuragi N, Yoshida S. Morbidity and mortality after 94 extrapleural pneumonectomies for empyema. Ann Thorac Surg (In press).
2. Massard G, Dabbagh A, Wihlm JM et al. Pneumonectomy for chronic infection is a high-risk procedure. Ann Thorac Surg 1996;62:1033–1038.

3. Pairolero PC, Arnold PG, Piehler JM. Intrathoracic transposition of extrathoracic skeletal muscle. J Thorac Cardiovasc Surg 1983;86:809–817.

Bronchology and Bronchoesophagology: State of the Art.
H. Yoshimura et al., editors.

Two cases of closure of congenital tracheoesophageal fistula using a muscle flap

Takashi Suzuki[1], Yoshito Kamio[1], Shuichi Suzuki[1], Akihiko Kitami[1] and Yutaka Sanada[2]

Departments of [1]Thoracic and Cardiovascular Surgery, and [2]Surgery, Showa University Fujigaoka Hospital, Yokohama, Japan

Abstract. *Background.* When treating congenital tracheoesophageal fistula, the prevention of its recurrence along with its closure is very important.

Methods. We used two types of muscle flaps for two different types of congenital tracheoesophageal fistula. For the patient with Gross-E type, the muscle flap was obtained from the right sternohyoid muscle after closing the fistula. For the patient of Gross-C type, who had undergone two surgeries in the previous hospital, we adopted a right rectus abdominis muscle flap, as the muscular tissues surrounding the thorax were fragile due to the previous two thoracotomies.

Results: Both patients were able to endure the postoperative course and were discharged. No recurrence has occurred.

Conclusion: We successfully treated two cases of congenital tracheoesophageal fistula by the effective addition of pedicled muscle flaps. The two muscles chosen, although different types, seemed appropriate for these cases.

Keywords: rectus abdominis muscle flap, recurrence of tracheoesophageal fistula, sternohyoid muscle flap.

Introduction

When treating congenital tracheoesophageal fistula, surgical closure of the fistula is essential. Furthermore, the prevention of its recurrence is also an important issue. The most appropriate surgery should be performed according to each individual patient's needs, judging from the characteristics of the type of congenital tracheoesophageal fistula and previous therapy.

Patients

We treated two cases of congenital tracheoesophageal fistula. The first case was a 16-year-old male who had a tracheoesophageal fistula of the Gross-E type; the shape of the fistula was H-type. The H-type fistula, characteristic of this type, was located at the cervical trachea [1]. He had a history of frequent vomiting after birth. An anomaly of the esophagus was suspected, however, neither atresia nor

Address for correspondence: T. Suzuki MD, Department of Thoracic and Cardiovascular Surgery, Showa University Fujigaoka Hospital, 1-30 Fujigaoka, Aoba-ku, Yokohama 227-8501, Japan. Tel.: +81-45-971-1151. Fax: +81-45-971-7125.

fistula was found. He complained of heartburn when he was 16 years of age. His physician performed esophagography and suspected the existence of the cervical fistula. After admission, bronchoscopy revealed a fistula at the membranous portion of the cervical trachea, and esophagoscopy showed a fistula at the level of the cervical trachea. CT showed a dilated esophagus and a suspect fistula. The length of the fistula was thought to be very short. Surgery was started with the patient in the supine position. A collar incision was performed. After dissecting a wide area between the trachea and the esophagus, the fistula was proved to be longer than expected. After cutting the fistula, the esophagus and trachea were sutured separately using absorbable threads. As the two suture lines faced each other, the recurrence of the fistula was a possible complication. In order to prevent the direct contact of the suture lines, a muscle flap was placed between the suture lines. The muscle flap was obtained from the right sternohyoid muscle. Postoperative MRI showed that the flap did not compress the trachea or esophagus. The second case was a 25-year-old male, who had a history of a Gross-C type tracheoesophageal fistula. Although he had undergone two previous surgeries for closure of the fistula and anastomosis of the esophagus at another hospital, the fistula recurred. Three-dimensional CT showed that the fistula was longer than in the first case. Bronchoscopy also revealed a fistula just proximal to the carina. We chose a right thoracotomy. After transecting the fistula, each stump was sutured separately using absorbable threads. To prevent recurrence of the fistula, a muscle flap was required to interpose between the two stumps. We adopted a right rectus abdominis muscle flap, as the muscular tissues surrounding the thorax were fragile due to the previous thoracotomies.

The first patient was discharged uneventfully. Although the second patient suffered from sepsis caused by an intravenous catheter, he recovered without any trouble from his trachea or esophagus. His fistula had not recurred 2 years postoperatively.

Discussion

Recurrent tracheoesophageal fistula is a major complication of surgical therapy for congenital tracheoesophageal fistula [2]. Pedicled flaps using an intercostal muscle [3], a latissimus dorsi muscle [4], a pectoralis major muscle [5], and a pericardial flap interposition [6] have been reported to prevent recurrence. We successfully treated two cases of congenital tracheoesophageal fistula using another pedicle muscle flap, namely a sternohyoid muscle flap for a cervical fistula of Gross-E type and a rectus abdominis muscle flap for the Gross-C type patient who had undergone two previous thoracotomies. The two muscles chosen, although different types, seemed appropriate for each case.

Acknowledgements

We received no financial aid from any companies or grants.

References

1. Reynolds M. Congenital anomalies of the esophagus. A. Esophageal atresia, tracheoesophageal fistulae, and congenital laryngotracheal clefts. In: Shields TW, LoCicero J III, Ponn RB (eds) General Thoracic Surgery, 5th edition. Philadelphia: Lippincott Williams & Wilkins, 2000; 1785–1795.
2. Vos A, Ekkelkamp S. Congenital tracheoesophageal fistula: preventing recurrence. J Pediatr Surg 1996;31:936–938.
3. Gustafson RA, Hrabovsky EE. Intercostal muscle and myo-osseous flaps in difficult pediatric thoracic problems. J Pediatr Surg 1982;17:541–545.
4. Fujita H, Kawahara K, Yoshimatsu H, Nakamura K. Surgical treatment of recurrent tracheoesophageal fistula using a latissimus dorsi pedicled muscle flap—report of a case. Jpn J Surg 1989;19:78–81.
5. Siu KF, Wei WI, Lam KH, Wong J. Use of the pectoralis major muscle flap for repair of a tracheoesophageal fistula. Am J Surg 1985;150:617–619.
6. Wheatley MJ, Coran AG. Pericardial flap interposition for the definitive management of recurrent tracheoesophageal fistula. J Pediatr Surg 1992;27:1122–1125.

Thoracoscopy

Bronchology and Bronchoesophagology: State of the Art.
H. Yoshimura et al., editors.

Diagnostic thoracoscopy performed under local anesthesia for tuberculous pleurisy

Atsushi Nakamura, Takashi Kato, Masayoshi Hosoda, Yasuo Yamada and Makoto Itoh
The First Department of Internal Medicine, Nagoya City University, Medical School, Nagoya, Japan

Abstract. To evaluate the usefulness of thoracoscopy in the diagnosis of tuberculous pleurisy compared with conventional methods, we studied 27 cases of tuberculous pleurisy based on clinical features, diagnostic processes and thoracoscopic findings. Furthermore, we investigated the changes in the thoracoscopic findings and the diagnostic accuracy in the clinical course of the disease. There were some afebrile cases and some with neoplasm. Some showed atypical laboratory and/or thoracentated data for tuberculous pleurisy. Mycobacterium tuberculosis was not detected by either smear of sputum or thoracentated fluids in any of the examined cases, and was only cultured in two specimens of sputum and thoracentated fluid each. Thoracoscopy increased the number of diagnosed cases from only four, with conventional methods, to 20. Thoracoscopic findings, observed in most of the diagnosed cases, showed white plaque, small miliary nodules and/or redness of pleura, which are specific to tuberculosis. The earlier the thoracoscopy was performed, the more these specific findings were observed. We conclude that thoracoscopy is useful in the diagnosis of tuberculous pleurisy and should be performed in the early stages of tuberculous pleurisy.

Keywords: Mycobacterium tuberculosis, redness of pleura, small miliary nodules, thoracentesis, white plaque.

Background

It is difficult to diagnose tuberculous pleurisy with conventional methods because the presentation of bacteriological or histological evidences is required. Although it has been demonstrated by many investigators that thoracoscopy is useful in the diagnosis of intrathoracic diseases [1], few studies about cases of tuberculous pleurisy diagnosed by thoracoscopy have been reported.

To evaluate the usefulness of thoracoscopy in the diagnosis of tuberculous pleurisy compared with conventional methods, we studied 27 cases of tuberculous pleurisy based on clinical features, diagnostic processes and thoracoscopic findings. Furthermore, we investigated the changes in the thoracoscopic findings and the diagnostic accuracy in the clinical course of the disease.

Address for correspondence: Atsushi Nakamura, The First Department of Internal Medicine, Nagoya City University, Medical School, 1 Kawasumi, Mizuho-cho, Mizuho-ku, Nagoya, Aichi 467-8601, Japan. Tel.: +81-52-853-8211. Fax: +81-52-852-0952. E-mail: anakamur@med.nagoya-cu.ac.jp

Objects and Methods

Twenty-seven cases of tuberculous pleurisy, who underwent thoracoscopy, were studied. There were 22 males and five females, and their ages ranged from 28 to 84 years (mean: 63.1 years). Six cases of afebrile patients were contained in this. Their underlying diseases were as follows: chronic liver injury (6), diabetes mellitus (5), neoplasm (5: lung cancer, hepatocellular carcinoma, uterus cancer, malignant lymphoma, pharyngeal cancer), chronic respiratory diseases (3: old tuberculosis 2, fibrosis 1), ischemic heart disease (1), chronic pancreatitis (1), and old peritonitis (1).

Tuberculous pleurisy was diagnosed in cases showing positive bacterial examinations or specific histological findings of biopsy specimens (D group). Suspected cases (S group) were those of pleurisy who satisfied three or more of the below mentioned criteria: 1) positive purified protein derivertive (PPD) skin test, 2) positive inflammatory reactions, 3) lymphocyte predominant pleural effusion, 4) high level of adenosinedeaminase (ADA) of pleural effusion, and 5) negative tumor markers of pleural effusion.

Thoracoscopy was performed using a flexible bronchoscope through a sheath for percutaneous transhepatic cholangioscopy under local anesthesia [2].

We studied four points, as follows: 1) analysis of data with conventional diagnostic methods, 2) comparison of diagnostic accuracy between conventional methods and thoracoscopy, 3) correlation between thoracoscopic findings and diagnosis, and 4) changes in thoracoscopic findings in the clinical course of the disease.

Results

Analysis of data with conventional diagnostic methods

Atypical laboratory data for tuberculous pleurisy

The PPD skin test was negative in six of 25 examined cases, the CRP was negative (< 1.0) in three of 27, and the ESR was negative (< 20) in two of 26. M. tuberculosis was not detected by smear of sputum in any of the 21 examined cases, and was not cultured in 19 of the 21. In five of seven examined cases, percutaneous needle pleural biopsy showed nonspecific findings.

Atypical data of thoracentated fluids for tuberculous pleurisy

Neutrophil-predominant thoracentated fluids were observed in four of 25 examined cases. Low ADA (< 40) in six out of 27 cases, and high values of tumor markers were observed as follows: CEA ($\geqslant 10$) in none of 24, SCC ($\geqslant 1.6$) in six of 15, and NSE ($\geqslant 10$) in four of 12. M. tuberculosis was not detected by smear of thoracentated fluids in any of the 26 examined cases, containing nine cases who were also negative using PCR. M. tuberculosis was not cultured in 24 of 26 cases.

Table 1. Thoracoscopic findings of diagnosed and suspected cases.

	Diagnosed cases (n = 20)	Suspected cases (n = 7)
White plaque	4 (20%)	0 (0%)
Nodule	16 (80%)	1 (14%)
Redness	4 (20%)	0 (0%)
Pleural thickening	7 (35%)	4 (57%)
Fibrinous tissue	10 (50%)	4 (57%)
Adhesion	10 (50%)	4 (57%)

Comparison of diagnostic accuracy between conventional methods and thoracoscopy

The number of cases in the D group changed from four, using conventional methods, which contained two cases diagnosed by the positive culture of M. tuberculosis, to 20 using thoracoscopy. The number of cases in the S group decreased from 17, using conventional methods, to seven using thoracoscopy, and the number of nonspecific cases decreased from five, using conventional methods, to none using thoracoscopy.

Correlation between thoracoscopic findings and diagnosis

The thoracoscopic findings of the D and S groups are shown in Table 1. Most diagnosed cases showed white plaque, small miliary nodules and/or redness of pleura, which is specific to tuberculosis [3].

Changes in the thoracoscopic findings in the clinical course of the disease

The correlation between the thoracoscopic findings and the intervals from onset to the day of thoracoscopy are shown in Table 2. The earlier the thoracoscopy was performed, the more typical findings were observed.

Table 2. Correlation between thoracoscopic findings and intervals from onset to the day of thoracoscopy.

	≤ 1 W		≤ 2 W		≤ 3 W		≤ 1 M		≤ 2 M		> 2 M	
	D	S	D	S	D	S	D	S	D	S	D	S
White plaque	1		1				2					
Nodule	2		8	1	3		2				1	
Redness			2				1				1	
Pleural thickening	1	1	2	1	1	1	1	1	1		1	
Fibrinous tissue	2	1	5	2	1		1	1			1	
Adhesion	1		4	1	1	1	2	2	1		1	

Conclusions

1. We have reported in this paper six afebrile cases and five cases with neoplasm, who were suspected to have malignant pleural effusion.
2. Only four cases were diagnosed using conventional methods. In two of four cases, besides, a positive culture of M. tuberculosis was revealed after thoracoscopy.
3. Thoracoscopy increased the number of D group cases from four to 20.
4. Thoracoscopic findings, observed in most of the D group, consisted of white plaque, small miliary nodules and/or redness of pleura, which is specific to tuberculosis.
5. The earlier the thoracoscopy was performed, the more typical the findings, as desribed above, were.
6. We conclude that thoracoscopy is useful in the diagnosis of tuberculous pleurisy, and that it should be performed in the early stages of tuberculous pleurisy.

References

1. Wilsher ML, Veale AG. Medical thoracoscopy in the diagnosis of unexplained pleural effusion. Respirology 1998;3:77–80.
2. Nakamura A. Clinical study of thoracoscopy with bronchoscopy and seath for percutaneous transhepatic cholangiography. J Nagoya City Univ Med Assoc 1995;46:355–368.
3. Suzuki H, Tanaka K, Tonozuka H, Akizawa T, Narushima M, Osakabe Y, Nakagami K, Satomi T, Noguchi E. Clinical study of tuberculous pleuritis, diagnosed by thoracoscopy using flexible fiberoptic bronchoscope. J Thoracic Dis 1993;31:139–145.

Bronchology and Bronchoesophagology: State of the Art.
H. Yoshimura et al., editors.

Video-assisted thoracoscopic surgery for metastatic lung tumors

Yoshifumi Sano, Motoi Aoe, Hiroshi Date, Akio Ando and Nobuyoshi Shimizu
Department of Surgery II, Okayama University Medical School, Okayama, Japan

Abstract. It has been controversial to adopt video-assisted thoracoscopic surgery (VATS) for pulmonary metastases. We report on a retrospective review of patients who underwent pulmonary metastasectomy with VATS.

From 1992 to 1999, 55 patients (59 procedures) underwent surgical resection for pulmonary metastases at our institution. Twenty-seven patients (28 procedures) underwent metastasectomy with VATS, while 28 patients (31 procedures) had traditional thoracotomy. All of the procedures with VATS were complete resection without perioperative deaths and major complications. The mean disease-free interval (DFI) was 42.5 months. In 66.7% of the patients lung metastases were from epithelial tumors, in 11.1% from sarcomas. Prior to the surgical resection, we adopted CT-guided markers in eight out of 24 procedures. Most of the patients underwent partial resection (85.7%). Single metastases accounted for 60.7% and multiple metastases for 39.3%. The average size of those lesions was 1.8 cm in diameter. The 5-year actuarial survival of the VATS lung metastasectomy patients was 50%.

In conclusion, all of the VATS procedures were complete resection without perioperative deaths and major complications. VATS lung metastasectomy can be achieved as a minimally invasive technique with a relatively good prognosis. VATS should be considered the preferred approach for selected cases.

Keywords: lung metastasis, minimally invasive surgery, VATS.

Background

Surgical resection of pulmonary metastases has been accepted as appropriate therapy in selected cases including "complete control of the primary tumor", "ability to resect all metastatic disease", "absence of extrathoracic metastases", "lack of better alternative therapy", and "sufficient cardiopulmonary reserve for the planned resection" [1]. It has remained controversial to adopt video-assisted thoracoscopic surgery (VATS) for pulmonary metastases, particularly for therapeutic metastasectomy [2,3]. We report on a retrospective review of patients who underwent pulmonary metastasectomy with VATS.

Address for correspondence: Yoshifumi Sano, Department of Surgery II, Okayama University Medical School, 2-5-1 Shikata-cho, Okayama 700-8558, Japan. Tel.: +81-86-235-7265. Fax: +81-86-235-7269. E-mail: ysano@hospital.okayama-u.ac.jp

Patients and Methods

From December 1992 to December 1999, 55 patients (59 procedures) underwent surgical resection for pulmonary metastases at Okayama University Hospital. Of these cases, 27 patients (28 procedures) underwent metastasectomy with VATS, while 28 patients (31 procedures) underwent traditional thoracotomy. The mean age of the patients who underwent VATS metastasectomy was 54.0 years, with ages ranging from 18 to 76 years for the 15 male and 12 female patients. The disease-free interval (DFI) was calculated from the day of resection of the primary tumor to the day of initial pulmonary metastasectomy. The survival after VATS metastasectomy was calculated with the Kaplan-Meier method.

Results

All of the surgical resections of metastatic lung tumors with VATS were complete resection without perioperative deaths and major complications. One case switched to the postero-lateral thoracotomy because of severe pleural adhesion. Four out of 27 patients (14.8%) underwent metastasectomy twice in 10 to 77 months because of the recurrence of lung metastatic lesions (epithelial tumors in two, sarcomas in two). In all of the patients, the mean DFI was 42.5 months, with a range of 2 to 120 months. In 66.7% of patients lung metastases were from epithelial tumors, in 11.1% from sarcomas, in 7.4% from germ cell tumors, and in 14.8% from other types. Malignant melanoma was not found in this patient population.

Prior to the surgical resection, we adopted CT-guided markers in eight (33.3%) out of 24 VATS partial resections for identifying tiny peripheral lesions. Most of the patients underwent partial resection (85.7%), whereas only three (10.7%) and one (3.6%) of the patients underwent lobectomy and segmentectomy, respectively. The average number of lung metastatic lesions that were resected was 2.2, with a maximum of 12. Single metastases accounted for 60.7% and multiple metastases for 39.3%. The average size of those lesions was 1.8 cm in diameter, with a range of 0.5 to 4.0 cm. The average duration of the operation was 2 h and 7 min (range: 0:30–5:15), and blood transfusion was not required for all of these patients.

Figure 1 shows the actuarial survival after surgical resection of lung metastatic lesions with VATS. The 5-year actuarial survival of all of the patients was 50%.

Discussion

Surgical resection of pulmonary metastases has been considered a standard therapeutic option in selected cases. Recently, Pastorino et al. [4] reported that resectability, DFI, and the number of metastases were the most significant factors for obtaining a good prognosis after surgical resection of pulmonary metastases. In this study, all of the surgical resection of metastatic pulmonary metastases

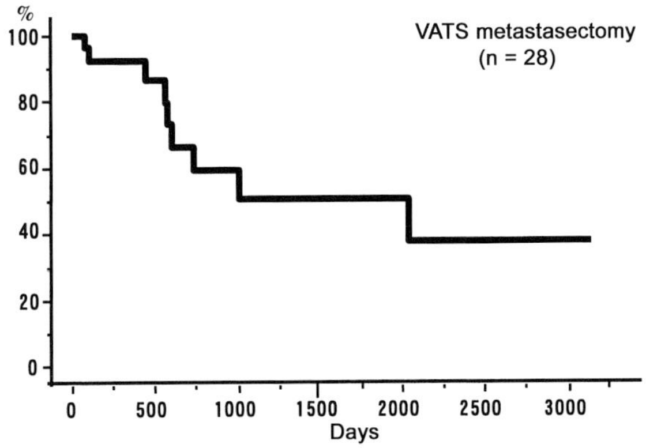

Fig. 1. Survival after the surgical resection for metastatic lung tumors (Kaplan-Meier's method).

with VATS were complete resection without perioperative deaths and major complications. Recently, we have been able to obtain more accurate information about intrathoracic nodules with high-resolution helical CT scanning. In addition, to avoid incomplete resection, we have adopted VATS for surgical resection of pulmonary metastases in selected cases such as when single or fewer, and smaller lesions were involved. Furthermore, preoperative CT-guided marking was very useful for detecting tiny pulmonary nodules, and it made the VATS procedure more effective to resect all the lesions.

Conclusions

We have reviewed 28 procedures of resection for lung metastases to determine the clinical characteristics and efficacy of VATS for metastasectomy. All of these procedures were complete resection without perioperative deaths and major complications.

VATS lung metastasectomy can be achieved as a minimally invasive technique with a relatively good prognosis. VATS should be considered the preferred approach for selected cases.

References

1. Rusch VW. Pulmonary metastasectomy: current indications. Chest 1995;107:322S–331S.
2. Dowling RD, Landreneau RJ, Miller DL. Video-assisted thoracoscopic surgery for resection of lung metastases. Chest 1998;113:2S–5S.
3. Lin JC, Wiechmann RJ, Szwerc MF, Hazelrigg SR, Ferson PF, Naunheim KS, Keenan RJ, Yim AP, Rendina E, DeGiacomo T, Coloni GF, Venuta F, Macherey RS, Bartley S, Landreneau RJ. Diagnostic and therapeutic video-assisted thoracic surgery resection of pulmonary metastases. Surgery 1999;126:636–642.
4. Pastorino U, Buyse M, Friedel G, Ginsberg RJ, Girard P, Goldstraw P, Johnston M, McCormack P, Pass H, Putnum JB Jr. Long-term results of lung metastasectomy: prognostic analyses based on 5206 cases. J Thorac Cardiovasc Surg 1997;113:37–49.

Bronchology and Bronchoesophagology: State of the Art.
H. Yoshimura et al., editors.

Video-assisted space-reducing surgery for pulmonary aspergilloma in abnormal air space of the lung

H. Yamamoto[1], M. Kanzaki[1], S. Sasano[2], T. Obara[2] and T. Isikura[2]
[1] *Tokyo Metropolitan Fuchu Hospital; and* [2] *Tokyo Woman's Medical College, Tokyo, Japan*

Abstract. Space-reducing surgery (SRS) was performed on the patients with pulmonary aspergilloma in abnormal air space of the lung in order to minimize operative mortality and morbidity. Since 1988, SRS has been applied to 36 patients for whom pulmonary resection seemed to be difficult and dangerous, in order to remove fungus and reduce the space. Triplet of thoracoplasty, cavernoplasty and pedicled muscle plombage with direct closure of the drainage bronchus is the author's standard treatment modality, and this was applied to 13 patients. We applied video-assisted thoracic surgery (VATS) to several recent patients to get a better outcome. No operative mortality existed in the SRS group. Out of 36 SRSs, 29 cases (80.6%) were successful. Out of 13 patients to whom the triplet was applied, 12 (92.3%) were successful. SRS for the patients with pulmonary aspergilloma is safe and acceptable, particularly in cases of low lung function, heavy pleural adhesion and severe complications. VATS was helpful for tight closure of the drainage bronchus.

Keywords: cavernoplasty, pedicled muscle plombage, thoracoplasty.

Introduction

Space-reducing surgery (SRS) was performed for the patients with pulmonary aspergilloma in abnormal air space of the lung, such as open negative cavity or emphysematous bulla, in order to minimize operative mortality and morbidity. Video-assisted thoracic surgery (VATS) was applied recently to achieve a better outcome.

Methods

Since 1988, 51 patients with pulmonary aspergilloma have been operated on. Pulmonary resection was performed for 15 patients and SRS was performed on 36 patients for whom pulmonary resection seemed difficult and dangerous, in order to remove the fungus mass and reduce the cavity space. Triplet of thoracoplasty, cavernoplasty and pedicled muscle plombage with closure of the drainage bronchus is the author's standard treatment modality, which was performed on 13 patients. Moreover, we applied video-assisted SRS (VASRS) to two recent patients.

Address for correspondence: Hiroshi Yamamoto, 3-7-24 Ohsawa, Mitaka City, Tokyo 181-0015, Japan. Tel./Fax: +81-42-233-6364. E-mail: yamahiro@tokyo.interq.or.jp

Table 1.

	Success rate (%)
Resection	93.3
SRS	80.6
Triplet	92.3

Results

One operative death occurred in the pulmonary resection group, but none occurred in the SRS group. Out of 36 patients who received SRS, 29 (80.6%) were successful. Out of 13 patients to whom the author's triplet operation was applied, 12 (92.3%) were successful (Table 1). Failure was due to the recurrence of fungus and bacterial infection in the residual cavity in three patients and acute respiratory failure in one patient.

Example

A 67-year-old man had previously had left upper division segmentectomy for pulmonary tuberculosis 35 years ago. The chest radiographs showed a fungus ball in the cavity on the left lung apex, where it was thought to be the superior segment of the remaining left lower lobe (S6).

A fifth rib resection was performed to get into the cavity, which was opened through the same rib bed. Initial inspection of the inside of the cavity was carried out by inserting the thoracoscope into it. The crushing of the fungus mass with the finger and scraping it out with a curette was carried out. The fourth, third and sixth ribs were resected to reduce the cavity.

The dome of the cavity was carved in the vertical direction along its posterior margin so that it became very easy to completely close the drainage bronchus

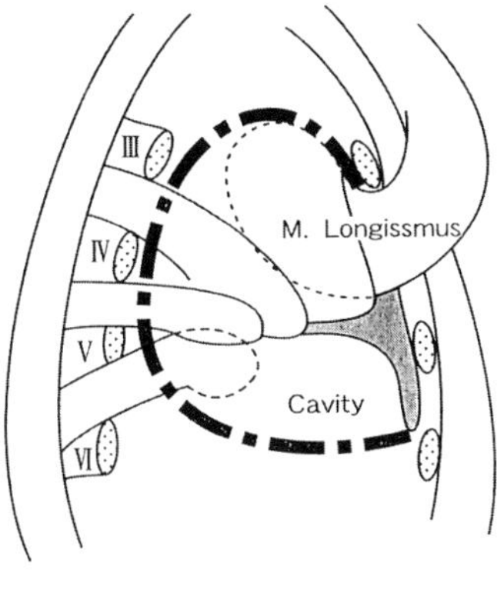

Fig. 1. Triplet of thoracoplasty, muscle plombage and cavernoplasty.

and to drop the dome toward the bottom of the cavity. Introducing VATS became very useful in observing the orifice of the drainage bronchus, which was sutured with several nylon threads.

Following thoracoplasty and cavernoplasty, muscle transposition was performed to complete SRS. The longest muscle of the chest (M. longissimus thoracis) was selected as a pedicled muscle flap for this particular patient because it is so big and long that it could plug the remaining cavity. The upper and lower half of the dome of the cavity were sutured to its bottom, respectively. The intercostal muscles were used to cover the suture lines in order to secure air tightness of the cavity (Fig. 1). Reduction in vital capacity after the operation in this particular patient was only 60 ml.

Conclusions

SRS for patients with pulmonary aspergilloma is a safe and minimally invasive procedure, particularly for patients with poor lung function, heavy pleural adhesion and severe complications. By applying VATS, the success rate of SRS is expected to rise even higher.

Thyroid cancer

Bronchology and Bronchoesophagology: State of the Art.
H. Yoshimura et al., editors.

End-to-end anastomosis of the trachea in thyroid cancer with tracheal invasion

Isao Kato, Hiroya Iwatake, Kouichiro Tsutsumi and Izumi Koizuka
Department of Otolaryngology, St. Marianna University School of Medicine, Kawasaki, Japan

Abstract. In 10 patients with tracheal invasion of thyroid cancer, tracheal resection was followed by end-to-end anastomosis. In order to achieve anastomosis without overextension, suprahyoid laryngeal release and blunt dissection of the lower trachea with the lateral bundle remaining safe, are mandatory in this operation.

Keywords: end-to-end anastomosis, suprahyoid laryngeal release, thyroid cancer.

Introduction

The aim of the present study is to confirm the efficacy and safety of end-to-end anastomosis of the trachea, following segmental resection of the trachea in thyroid cancer with tracheal invasion.

Operative procedure

Patients

Ten patients were operated on for thyroid cancer with tracheal invasion in our hospital. The 10 patients, including eight women and two men, ranged between 51 and 70 years of age. All patients were operated on using end-to-end anastomosis, following tracheal resection combined with suprahyoid laryngeal release.

A representative case (case 10)

The patient was a 77-year-old man who was admitted to the hospital complaining of hoarseness and dysphagia. Fiberscopy revealed left recurrent laryngeal plasy. The left thyroid lobe was enlarged, and hard on palpation. The enlarged lymph node was palpated in the left supraclavicular area.

Address for correspondence: Isao Kato, Department of Otolaryngology, St. Marianna University School of Medicine, 2-16-1 Sugao, Miyamae, Kawasaki 216-8511, Japan. Tel.: +81-4-4977-8111. Fax: +81-4-4976-8748.

Laryngeal tomography

Laryngeal tomography before and after the operation demonstrated stenosis and compression of the trachea.

The operation

Horizontal parallel incisions were made through the platysma. The first transverse collar incision was made across the base of the neck, about one finger-width above the clavicles. The second was made at the hyoid bone, with the two skin incisions meeting underneath the flap.

Tracheal resection

After modified neck dissection, a #11 blade knife was used to cut the intercartilaginous ligament. The incision was extended along the ligament, using scissors, to the membranous portion of the trachea. Then, the endotracheal tube was removed from the mouth, and inserted directly into the trachea via the lower cut-end of the trachea. The tumor and the involved trachea were totally resected. The distal segment of the trachea was manually ablated up to the carina, with the lateral bundle of the trachea remaining safe.

There are two kinds of release techniques for the larynx, i.e., the infrahyoid [1], and the supra technique [2]. The latter is much more simple and takes less time to perform.

End-to-end anastomosis

First, the membranous portion was sutured, with knots tied on the outside. The endotracheal tube was removed and the oral tube was inserted. The anterior and lateral sutures of the trachea were then performed. The anastomosis site was sutured with stainless steel wire, as the postoperative landmark. Finally, the leakage of air from the anastomotic site was confirmed by pouring saline solution on it.

Comments

All patients were operated on using end-to-end anastomosis, following tracheal resection combined with suprahyoid laryngeal release [2]. There were no complications recognized in any of the cases, except for one who showed recurrent thyroid cancer with unilateral recurrent palsy, that resulted in bilateral palsy. Thus, this operation is a safe and stable technique for the resection of the trachea in less than six tracheal segments.

References

1. Dedo HH. Laryngeal release and sleeve restetion for tracheal stenosis. Rhinol laryngol 1969;78: 225, 285–295.
2. Montgomery WM. Saprahyoid release for tracheal anastomosis. Arch Otolaryngol 1974;29: 225–260.

Bronchology and Bronchoesophagology: State of the Art.
H. Yoshimura et al., editors.

Resection and reconstruction of trachea for advanced thyroid carcinoma

Shunsuke Niki, Masaru Tsuyuguchi and Sinichi Yamasaki
Department of Surgery, Tokushima Municipal Hospital, Tokushima, Japan

Abstract. A retrospective analysis of 25 patients, who underwent tracheal resection and reconstruction for differentiated thyroid carcinoma invading trachea, was performed to evaluate the indication and efficacy of the procedure. The patients included eight men and 17 women. Sixteen circumferential sleeve resections, seven partial resections and one total laryngectomy were performed. The mean of the resected tracheal rings was 3.7 ± 1.5 rings (range: 2 to 7). There were two minor anastomotic leakages of the trachea, however, they were improved conservatively. Eighteen of 25 patients are alive without recurrence, four are alive with metastasis (2 lung metastases, 2 lymph node metastases), one died of thyroid carcinoma with undifferentiated transformation, and two died of other causes without evidence of recurrence. The 5 and 10-year-survival rates were 91.2 and 82.9%. There was no recurrence to the trachea. Whenever feasible, tracheal resection and reconstruction, for patients with tracheal invasion by differentiated thyroid carcinoma, should be performed. Complete resection and local curability is the key to a favorable outcome.

Keywords: tracheal invasion, tracheal reconstruction, tracheal resection.

Introduction

Differentiated thyroid carcinoma has a relatively good prognosis. However, once it has invaded the trachea, it causes a life-threatening airway hemorrhage and respiratory distress. As Yamasaki [1] has reported before, we performed tracheal resection and reconstruction in such cases, in order to achieve local curability. In this paper, we add new cases and report our recent data.

Patients and Methods

From 1885 to 1999, 25 patients with primary well-differentiated thyroid carcinoma invading trachea, were resected at Tokushima Municipal Hospital. All patients were adapted to tracheal resection and reviewed for this study. The types of tracheal resection used were a circumferential sleeve resection and a partial resection (membranous part was preserved). Anastomosis was performed using continuous suture on the posterior wall (membranous part), and interrupted

Address for correspondence: Shunsuke Niki, Department of Surgery, Tokushima Municipal Hospital, 2-34 Kita-Johsanjima-cho, Tokushima-shi, Tokushima 770-0812, Japan. Tel.: +81-88-622-5121. Fax: +81-88-656-6204.

suture on the anterior wall (cartilage part) with coated VICRYL after the tracheal mobilization by the mediastinal release technique.

Results

There were eight men and 17 women with a mean age of 56.7 ± 15.0 years. The size of the tumors were 32.5 ± 16.8 mm. Histological types consisted of onc follicular and 24 papillary carcinomas. Preoperative evaluation of tracheal invasion was diagnosed in 15 patients (ultrasonography: 11/25, bronchoscopy: 7/11). Ten were diagnosed by findings during the operation. There were 16 circumferential sleeve resections, eight partial resections and one total laryngectomy. The mean of the resected tracheal rings was 3.7 ± 1.5 rings. Morbidities derived from tracheal resection were two anastomotic airway leakages and two edemas in the vocal cord. Eighteen patients are alive without recurrence, four are alive with recurrence. One died of thyroid carcinoma with undifferentiated transformation. Two died of other causes, with no evidence of recurrence. The 5 and 10-year-survival rates were 91.2% and 82.9% (Kaplan-Meyer method).

Discussion

Recently, reports on tracheal resection and reconstruction for advanced thyroid carcinoma invading trachea have increased [2,3]. Some reports [4,5] recommended the shaving off procedure for minimal tracheal invasion, but local recurrence occurred in 15.4% in Nishida's study [5]. This technique may leave tumors and reoperation is very difficult when local recurrence occurs. Tsumori [6] stated that tumors invading the trachea had a higher malignant potential. Therefore, tracheal resection, even for minimal tracheal invasion, should be performed to achieve the complete resection of the tumor.

In order to decide the range of tracheal resection, preoperative assessments using computed tomography and bronchoscopy were useful [7]. However, some patients were found to have tracheal invasion during the operation. We determined the resection line at points one ring proximal and distal to the macroscopic finding of the adventitial invasion during operation. Surgical margins of the resected trachea were negative in all patients on postoperative histological examinations.

In the present study, two patients who underwent resection of five rings of trachea had airway leakages, however, they were improved conservatively and there was no anastomotic stenosis. Cuttings of the trachea were thought to cause the anastomotic leakage in these cases. The removal of any tension at the site of anastomosis is important to prevent cutting. The mediastinal release technique, using blunt dissection of the tracheal carina, is necessary to loosen the tension in cases where more than 5-rings of trachea are being resected. We use uninterrupted suture on the posterior wall under general anesthesia using HFJV in order to prevent cutting.

In the present series, none of the patients have had local recurrence of the trachea. There were two cases of lung metastasis and two cases of lymph node metastasis, but they had a relatively good quality of life. If the local disease was controlled, prognosis was comparatively good. The 5 and 10-year-survival rates were 91.2 and 82.9%. Ishihara [2] stated similar results, i.e., that the 5 and 10-year-survival rates were 78.1%.

Whenever feasible, tracheal resection and reconstruction, for patients with well-differentiated thyroid carcinoma invading trachea, should be performed. In cases of minimal tracheal invasion, we consider tracheal resection to be a valid surgical method due to its low morbidity, no local recurrence and easy postoperative management.

References

1. Yamasaki S, Tsuyuguchi M. Thyroidol Clin Exp 1998;10:283–287.
2. Ishihara T, Tobayashi K, Kikuchi K et al. Surgical treatment of advanced thyroid carcinoma invading the trachea. J Thorac Cardiovasc Surg 1991;102:717–720.
3. Grillo HC, Zannini P. Resectional management of airway invasion by thyroid cancer. Ann Thorac Surg 1982;42:287–298.
4. Julich MC, Thomas VM. The surgical management of laryngotracheal invasion by well-differentiated papillary thyroid carcinoma. Arch Otolaryngol Head Neck Surg 1997;123:484–490.
5. Nishida T, Nakao K, Hajime M. Differentiated thyroid carcinoma with airway invasion: Indication for tracheal resection based on the extent of cancer invasion. J Thorac Cardiovasc Surg 1997;114:84–91.
6. Tsumori T, Nakao K, Kawashima T et al. Clinicopathologic study of thyroid carcinoma infiltrating the trachea. Cancer 1985;56:2843.
7. Nakao K, Miyata M, Kawashima T et al. Radical operation for thyroid carcinoma invading the trachea. Arch Surg 1984;119:1046.

Bronchology and Bronchoesophagology: State of the Art.
H. Yoshimura et al., editors.

Possible enhancement *p53* gene therapy for undifferentiated thyroid carcinomas

Ichiro Ota[1], Katsunari Yane[1], Hiroshi Miyahara[1], Mie Emoto[1], Ken Ohnishii[2], Akihisa Takahashi[2], Hiroshi Hosoi[1] and Takeo Ohnishi[2]
Departments of [1]Otorhinolaryngology, and [2]Biology, Nara Medical University, Kashihara, Nara, Japan

Abstract. The present studies were designed to evaluate the therapeutic effects of excessive wild-type p53 introduction on *p53*-mutant undifferentiated thyroid carcinoma cells by colony formation assay and analyses of apoptosis, using 8305c cells tranfected with pC53-143 vector with a temperature-sensitive (ts) mutant of *p53*, 8305c/ts cells, and 8305c/*neo* cells, transfected with pCMV-Neo-Bam vector, as the control. Ts-p53 functions as a mutant and a wild-type at nonpermissive (37°C) and permissive (32°C) temperatures, respectively.

8305c/ts cells at 32°C (8305c/ts32 cells) were chemo- and radio-sensitive compared with 8305c/ts cells at 37°C (8305c/ts37 cells). Apoptosis was induced in the 8305c/ts32 cells, but not in 8305c/ts37 cells, using CDDP treatment or X-ray irradiation.

These results suggest that *p53*-mutant thyroid carcinomas may benefit from the combination of *p53* gene therapy before chemo- or radiotherapy.

Keywords: gene therapy, p53, undifferentiated thyroid carcinoma.

Background

Undifferentiated thyroid carcinomas are usually associated with a poor prognosis, with most patients dying within a few months. The *p53* gene, perhaps the most well-known tumor suppressor gene, plays a pivotal role in a pathway that controls cell growth and proliferation. The absence of the p53 pathway is a common feature in a large number of tumors, suggesting that it may be central to the pathogenesis of human cancers. Recently, the *p53* mutation has been reported to act as part of an important process as a factor of anaplastic change in differentiated thyroid carcinomas [1,2], suggesting that the mutation can result in the resistance of cancer therapy, such as chemo- and radiotherapy. A recent study reported that p53-defective thyroid carcinomas may benefit from the combination of p53 gene therapy and radiotherapy [3]. The purpose of this study is to evaluate chemo- and radiotherapeutic effects of excessive wild-type *p53* introduction in *p53*-mutant undifferentiated thyroid carcinoma cells.

Address for correspondence: Ichiro Ota, Department of Otorhinolaryngology, Nara Medical University, 840 Shijo-cho, Kashihara, Nara 634-8522, Japan. Tel.: +81-744-22-3051, ext. 2334. Fax: +81-744-24-6844. E-mail: iota@naramed-u.ac.jp

Materials and Methods

The cell used in this study is a human undifferentiated thyroid carcinoma-derived cell line, with a 8305c bearing and a point mutation at codon 273 in the p53 gene. We performed a clonogenic assay for cisplatin (CDDP), X-ray sensitivity, Hoechst 33342 staining, and agarose gel electrophoresis for analyses of apoptosis, using 8305c cells tranfected with pC53-SCX3 vector with a temperature-sensitive (ts) mutant of *p53*, 8305c/ts cells, and 8305c/*neo* cells, transfected with pCMV-Neo-Bam vector, as the control. Ts-p53 protein functions as a mutant and a wild-type at nonpermissive (37°C) and permissive (32°C) temperatures, respectively. We aimed to overexpress wild-type p53 in mutant-p53 thyroid carcinoma cells at 32°C.

Results

To evaluate the effectiveness of wild-type p53 or mutant p53 gene expression against the thyroid carcinoma cells, we first performed clonogenic assay for CDDP and X-ray sensitivity. 8305c/ts cells at 32°C, 8305c/ts32 cells, were CDDP- and X-ray-sensitive compared with 8305c/ts cells at 37°C, 8305c/ts37 cells. 8305c/ts32 cells showed wild-type p53 overexpression. 8305c/ts32 cells were more sensitive at a 10%-survival dose, which is about 2 times more than 8305c/ts37 cells (Fig. 1). These results suggested that these differences in sensitivities might be involved in wild-type p53-induced apoptosis after CDDP treatment or radiation. Next we performed the time-course about the frequency of apoptosis after treatment of CDDP or X-ray irradiation in 8305c/ts32 cells and 8305c/ts37 cells using Hoechst 33342 staining. In 8305c/ts32 cells, the frequency increased after the CDDP treatment or irradiation, while in 8305c/ts37 cells the frequency did not (Fig. 2). In addition, in 8305c/ts32 cells, we were able to observe the DNA ladder by means of agarose gel electrophoresis

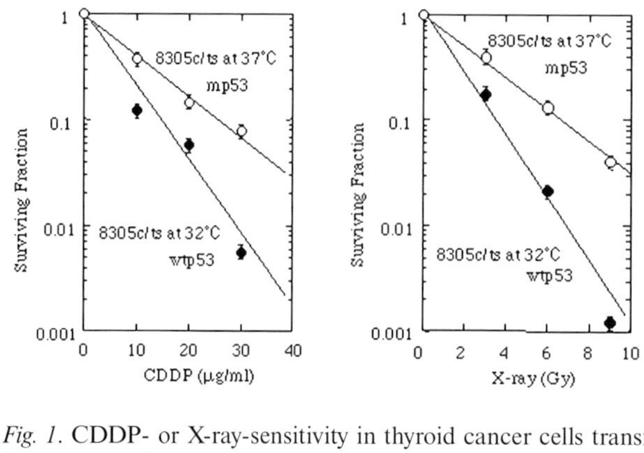

Fig. 1. CDDP- or X-ray-sensitivity in thyroid cancer cells transfected with the temperature-sensitive (ts) mutant *p53* gene.

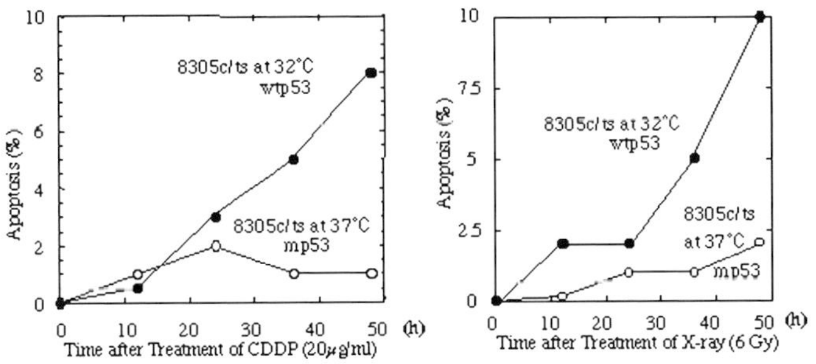

Fig. 2. p53-induced apoptosis in thyroid cancer cells transfected with the ts mutant *p53* gene after CDDP treatment. Hoechst 33342 staining study.

after the CDDP treatment, but not in 8305c/ts37 cells. These results suggested that p53-induced apoptosis in the 8305c/ts32 cells, but not in 8305c/ts37 cells, was induced by CDDP treatment or X-ray irradiation.

Conclusions

We have demonstrated that excessive wild-type p53 expression enhanced CDDP- and X-ray-sensitivities in human undifferentiated thyroid carcinoma cells. These results suggest that *p53*-mutant thyroid carcinomas could be effectively killed by the combination of *p53* gene therapy before chemo- or radiotherapy.

References

1. Ito T, Seyama T, Mizuno T, Tsuyama N, Hayashi T, Hayashi Y, Dohi K, Nakamura N, Akiyama M. Unique association of p53 mutations with undifferentiated but not with differentiated carcinomas of the thyroid gland. Cancer Res 1992;52:1369–1371.
2. Fagin JA, Matsuo K, Karmakar A, Chen DL, Tang SH, Koeffler HP. High prevalence of mutations of the p53 gene in poorly differentiated human thyroid carcinomas. J Clin Invest 1993;91: 179–184.
3. Narimatsu M, Nagayama Y, Akino K, Yasuda M, Yamamoto T, Yang TT, Ohtsuru A, Namba H, Yamashita S, Ayabe H, Niwa M. Therapeutic usefulness of wild-type p53 gene introduction in a p53-null anaplastic thyroid carcinoma cell line. J Clin Endocrinol Metab 1998;83:3668–3672.

Bronchology and Bronchoesophagology: State of the Art.
H. Yoshimura et al., editors.

Surgical treatment of thyroid carcinoma invading the trachea or esophagus

Tadayuki Oka, Masashi Muraoka, Takeshi Nagayasu, Shinji Akamine, Noriaki Itoyanagi and Hiroyoshi Ayabe
First Department of Surgery, Nagasaki University School of Medicine, Nagasaki, Japan

Abstract. *Background.* This retrospective study was undertaken to evaluate preoperative diagnosis and the significance of operation for thyroid carcinoma invading the trachea or esophagus.

Methods. Sixteen patients with thyroid carcinoma invading the trachea or esophagus were included in this study.

Results. The histological types were papillary adenocarcinoma in 11 patients, follicular adenocarcinoma in three, and anaplastic carcinoma in two. In 10 out of 12 patients, tracheal invasion was identified by fiberoptic bronchoscopy, with a sensitivity of 83%. However, CT only had 46% sensitivity. The overall sensitivities of esophagoscopy, esophagogram and CT for preoperative diagnosis of esophageal invasion were 67, 50, and 29%, respectively. Total laryngectomy and terminal tracheostomy were performed in five patients. Reconstruction of the trachea was performed using end-to-end anastomosis in 11 patients. In nine of these patients, esophageal invasion was recognized and combined resections of the trachea and esophagus were carried out. Postoperative complications of airway reconstruction consisted of tracheal anastomotic insufficiency in two patients, stenosis at the anastomotic site in one patient, and tracheo-esophageal fistula in one patient. The 5-year-survival rate in patients undergoing complete resection was 83.3%. There was no recurrence in the trachea and esophagus in this group.

Conclusions. Patients with locally advanced thyroid carcinoma invading the trachea or esophagus could be expected to have a good prognosis after combined resection of these organs.

Keywords: esophageal invasion, thyroid carcinoma, tracheal invasion.

Introduction

Invasion of the trachea or esophagus by thyroid carcinoma is uncommon [1]. This retrospective study was undertaken to evaluate preoperative diagnosis and the significance of operation for thyroid carcinoma invading these organs.

Patients and Methods

From January 1970 to May 2000, 16 patients with thyroid carcinoma invading the trachea or esophagus underwent operation. There were five males and 11 females, with a median age of 66 years. Nine patients were primary cases and

Address for correspondence: Tadayuki Oka MD, First Department of Surgery, Nagasaki University School of Medicine, 1-7-1 Sakamoto, Nagasaki 852-8501, Japan. Tel.: +81-95-849-7304. Fax: +81-95-849-7306. E-mail: oka@alpha.med.nagasaki-u.ac.jp seven were recurrent cases. A second operation was performed in four patients, and a third, fifth and sixth operation was done in one patient, respectively. Emergency operations were carried out in two patients, due to very severe dyspnea associated with SVC syndrome.

Results

The histological types were papillary adenocarcinoma in 11 patients, and follicular adenocarcinoma in three. Two patients had anaplastic carcinoma, and one of them showed a transformation from papillary adenocarcinoma during a 12-year history after the initial treatment. The other one underwent an emergency operation for primary carcinoma because of severe dyspnea caused by the stenotic trachea.

Fourteen patients had a cervical mass, 10 had dyspnea, five had dysphagia and two showed SVC syndrome.

For preoperative assessment of tracheal invasion, fiberoptic bronchoscopy and a computed tomographic scan (CT) were performed in 12 and 11 patients, respectively. In ten out of 12 patients, tracheal invasion was identified by fiberoptic bronchoscopy, with a sensitivity of 83%. However, CT only had 46% sensitivity. In two patients, tracheal invasion could not be identified, the invasions were made by the metastatic lymph nodes, not by primary tumor, and they were limited to the submucosal layer. The overall sensitivities of esophagoscopy, esophagogram and CT, for the preoperative diagnosis of esophageal invasion, were 67, 50, and 29%, respectively.

For primary cases, total thyroidectomy was usually carried out, but subtotal resection was performed in three cases in which a tumor and metastatic lymph nodes were localized unilaterally. Total laryngectomy was performed in five patients with airway invasion. Eleven patients underwent tracheal resection and reconstruction of the airway. The extension of tracheal resection varied from two to 13 tracheal rings. Tracheo-tracheal anastomosis was performed in eight patients, cricoid cartilago-tracheal anastomosis in two, and thyroid cartilago-tracheal anastomosis in one. The anastomoses were wrapped with the pedicled omental flap in three patients with nine and 13 tracheal ring resection.

Esophageal involvement was treated by the removal of the invaded muscular layer, sparing the submucosal layer in five patients. Sleeve resection was performed in three patients in whom the esophageal mucosal invasions were diagnosed preoperatively.

Postoperative complications occurred in 12 patients, and the morbidity rate was 75%. Tracheal anastomotic insufficiency occurred in two patients, esophago-tracheal fistula in one, and bilateral recurrent nerve paralysis in four, respectively.

We experienced one operative death, caused by tracheal anastomotic insufficiency. The mortality rate was 18.8%. The 5-year-survival rate of all patients, excluding the operative death, was 79.5%. The 5-year-survival rate of patients undergoing complete resection was 83.3%. There was no recurrence in

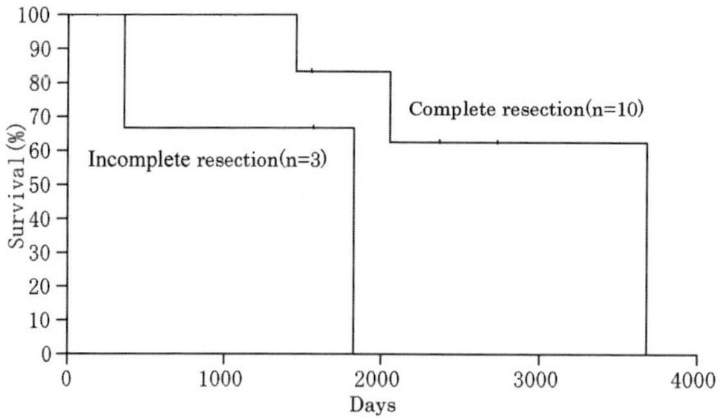

Fig. 1. Survival curves of the complete resection and incomplete resection groups (complete resection vs. incomplete resection: $p = 0.11$).

the trachea and esophagus in this group. There were no 5-year survivors in the incomplete resection group (Fig. 1).

Discussion

Airway invasion could be diagnosed with high sensitivity by fiberoptic bronchoscopy [2], although accurate diagnosis of the invasion could not be obtained by CT. CT usually shows only morphological changes, such as compressed tracheal walls, and the absence of the fat plane between the trachea and tumor. It might be difficult to identify a small invasion through CT. Therefore, fiberoptic bronchoscopy should be performed on patients in whom some suspicious findings of tracheal invasion are shown by CT. In six of eight patients with esophageal invasion, the involvement was limited to the adventitia or muscular layer. Thus, it might be difficult to make accurate diagnoses of esophageal invasion using esophagoscopy or CT preoperatively.

Melliere et al. [3] reported that a good prognosis of thyroid carcinoma with tracheal or esophageal involvement could be obtained by combined resection of these organs. Although there was one operative death in our early experience, a 5-year-survival rate excessive of 80% could be expected for patients undergoing complete resection. The longest survivor has been followed up for 28 years since the first operation.

Conclusion

Patients with locally advanced thyroid carcinoma invading the airway or esophagus can be expected to have a good prognosis after the combined resection of these organs. Airway reconstruction should be performed whenever technically feasible.

References

1. Lydiatt DD, Markin RS, Orgen FP. Tracheal invasion by thyroid carcinoma. Ear Nose Throat J 1990;69:145–149.
2. Hanamura N, Miyagawa S, Sugenoya A. Clinical study on surgical treatment of thyroid carcinoma infiltrating the trachea, larynx and esophagus. Endocrine Surg 1987;4:95–99.
3. Melliere DJM, Yahia NEB, Becquemin JP, Lange F, Boulahdour H. Thyroid carcinoma with tracheal or esophageal involvement: limited or maximal surgery? Surgery 1993;113:166–172.

Bronchology and Bronchoesophagology: State of the Art.
H. Yoshimura et al., editors.

The follow-up period to carefully observe patients with thyroid papillary carcinoma

Shinichi Takagita, Hiroyuki Kitamura, Yuka Iwahashi, Yasutaka Kawata, Masakazu Miyazaki and Tomoko Tateya
Department of Otolaryngology, Tenri Hospital, Tenri, Nara, Japan

Abstract. *Background.* Thyroid papillary carcinoma is a slow-growing disease. It is difficult to determine how long we must pay particular attention to the patients after initial treatment. We will clarify this period in this paper.

Methods. We studied the follow-up results of 183 patients who underwent surgical treatment between 1977 and 1987 at Tenri Hospital.

Results. Thirty-eight cases experienced recurrence and nine died of the carcinoma. The mean initial recurrence time was 8.9 years in the survival group and 1.9 in the death group. All of the patients who died had an initial recurrence within 4 years. The patients, whose initial recurrence occurred after 4 years survived.

Conclusions. It is necessary to maintain careful observation for at least 4 years. We consider that such measures can prevent a patient's death, if they do not have any recurrence within 4 years.

Keywords: follow-up, recurrence, thyroid papillary carcinoma.

Background

Thyroid papillary carcinoma is a slow-growing disease and has a good prognosis [1,2]. Therefore, we need to observe the patients with this carcinoma after initial treatment for a long time. It is difficult to determine how long we must pay particular attention to the patients before we see the onset of recurrence. Actually, we could not find any papers to describe this period of time. In order to clarify this period, we studied the follow-up results of patients with this disease in our hospital.

Materials and Methods

A total of 209 patients with papillary carcinoma were treated, between 1977 and 1987, in our hospital. Our study included 183 of these patients. Those living were observed over 11 years. Those who died, the causes and the dates of their deaths are clear. A total of 158 of the subjects were females and 25 were males. Their ages ranged from 15 to 84 years, and the mean age was 51.2 years. The mean follow-up period after an initial operation was 14.5 years. Referring to the

Address for correspondence: Shinichi Takagita, Department of Otolaryngology, Tenri Hospital, 200 Mishima-cho, Tenri-city, Nara 632-8552, Japan. Tel.: +81-743-63-5611. Fax: +81-743-62-5576.

subjects' clinical records, we examined the survival rate, nonrecurrence rate and some relationships between the time of recurrence and mortality.

Results

The 20-year-survival rate of all patients was 80.2%. The 20-year cause-specific survival rate was 94.4%. Nine of 160 patients died of papillary carcinoma. The 20-year-nonrecurrence rate was 74.5%, and the recurrence rate was 25.5%. The carcinoma recurred in 38 of 183 patients.

The longest interval between an initial treatment and an initial recurrence was 18.3 years. The mean recurrence time of the survival group was 8.9 ± 4.9 years, and the mean recurrence time of the death group was 1.9 ± 0.9. The difference between them was significant ($p < 0.001$). Furthermore, all of the patients who died had an initial recurrence within 4 years after surgery, and the patients, whose initial recurrence occurred after 4 years, survived. Based on these observations, patients without any recurrence within 4 years can avoid death.

In the survival group, there were five patients who had an initial recurrence within 4 years. We compared the ages, and the stage of the disease between these five living patients and the death group. In the death group, seven of the nine were older than 60. However, four of the five survivors were younger than 60. Although in the death group the ratio of pT4 was 77.8%, the ratio was 20% in the survival group. In the death group, the ratio of the patients with clinically positive nodes was 88.9%. In the survival group, the ratio was 40%.

Discussion

Although the recurrence rate was not low in patients with thyroid papillary carcinoma, most of them lived. A significant number of patients with papillary carcinoma were able to survive even with some recurrences. However, the patients with early initial recurrences had a poor prognosis. Among patients, especially older patients and patients with carcinoma that has extra thyroidal extension and/or clinically positive nodes, death seems likely. In recent years, several risk factors have been identified that influence prognosis [3–5]. Age, extra thyroidal extension and gross nodal metastasis are some of the risk factors. Not only these risk factors, but the period between initial treatment and the first recurrence are important.

We found one patient that had an initial recurrence more than 18 years after initial treatment. It goes without saying that we should observe the patients for a long time. We cannot cease to observe patients during their lifetime. However, it is necessary to maintain particularly careful observation for at least 4 years. We consider that such measures can prevent a patient's death in the short term, if they do not have any recurrence within 4 years.

References

1. Wanabo HJ, Andrews W, Keiser DL. Thyroid cancer: some basic consideration. CA 1983;33: 87–97.
2. Balan KK, Raouf AH, Critchley M. Outcome of 249 patients attending a nuclear medicine department with well differentiated thyroid cancer; a 23 year review. Br J Radiol 1994;67: 283–291.
3. Pasieka JK et al. Addition of nuclear DNA content to the AMES risk-group classification for papillary thyroid cancer. Surgery 1992;12:1154–1159.
4. Hay ID et al. Predicting outcome in papillary thyroid carcinoma: development of a reliable prognostic scoring system in a cohort of 1778 patients surgically treated at one institution during 1940 through 1989. Surgery 1993;114:1050–1057.
5. Noguchi S et al. Classification of papillary cancer of the thyroid based on prognosis. World J Surg 1994;18:552–557.

Ultrasound

Bronchology and Bronchoesophagology: State of the Art.
H. Yoshimura et al., editors.

Evaluation of bronchial wall and peribronchial nodal involvement of tumors by EBUS

Masayuki Baba[1], Yasuo Sekine[1], Hidehisa Hoshino[1], Yukiko Haga[1], Mizuto Otsuji[1], Makoto Suzuki[1], Kiyoshi Shibuya[1], Toshihiko Iizasa[1], Yukio Saitoh[1], Akira Iyoda[2], Tetuya Toyozaki[2] and Takehiko Fujisawa[1]
Departments of [1]Surgery, and [2]Pathology, Institute of Pulmonary Cancer Research, Chiba University School of Medicine, Chiba, Japan

Abstract. *Background.* The ability of endobronchial ultrasonography (EBUS) to image the bronchial wall invasion and peribronchial node involvement in bronchial or lung cancers was demonstrated.
Methods. Thirty-two patients with endobronchial tumor-findings (31 mucosal and one submucosal invasion) associated with malignant tumors (30 primary and two metastatic) were involved. EBUS was performed using mainly the thin ultrasonic probe UM-BS20-26R (20 MHz). Paying attention to the continuity of the cartilage layer, bronchial wall invasion was estimated in the EBUS images. The assessment of peribronchial nodal metastasis by EBUS in eight primary cancers were also compared with that by CT. Peribronchial nodes were considered to be involved when the short axis was 10 mm or more and/or the shape was round.
Results. The accuracy of EBUS imaging was 100% for extramural (n = 19), cartilage (n = 17), and submucosal (n = 25) invasions, and 96.9% for mucosal (n = 26) invasion. In six peribronchial lymph node stations of eight patients, including two hilar, one interlobar or three segmental nodes, which were confirmed as involved histologically, four (66.7%) were assessed as positive by EBUS although one (16.7%) was judged by CT ($p = 0.078$).
Conclusions. EBUS appears to be useful for judging the depth of tumor invasion in the bronchial walls, and for estimating peribronchial node involvement.

Keywords: bronchial wall invasion, bronchial cancer, endobronchial ultrasonography, lung cancer, nodal involvement.

Introduction

The development of miniature ultrasonic probes has enabled us to perform EBUS, and the bronchial wall structure, using EBUS, has been reported [1–3]. The ability of EBUS to image the bronchial wall invasion and peribronchial lymph node involvement in malignant bronchial tumors was demonstrated in this study.

Address for correspondence: Takehiko Fujisawa MD, Department of Surgery, Institute of Pulmonary Cancer Research, Chiba University School of Medicine, 1-8-1 Inohana, Chuo-ku, Chiba 260-8670, Japan. Tel.: +81-43-222-7171, ext. 5464. Fax: +81-43-226-2172.
E-mail: fujisawa@med.m.chba-u.ac.jp

Materials and Methods

Thirty-two patients with bronchial or lung cancers, including 30 primary bronchial cancers and two metastatic lung cancers, who underwent lobectomy, pneumonectomy or forceps biopsy at Chiba University Hospital from 1997 to April, 2000, were included in this study. The patients comprised of three females and 29 males, with a mean age of 63.6 years (range: 16 to 78 years). The ultrasonic processor Olympus EU-M30 and the miniature probe Olympus UM-BS20-26R (20MHz radial scanner; outer diameter: 2.6 mm, with latex balloon sheath) were used. The miniature probe was introduced to the bronchial lumen via the channel of the Olympus fiberoptic bronchoscope BF-XT30. The newly developed built-in ultrasonic probe Olympus XBF-UM30 (mounted in the fiberoptic bronchoscope, 20MHz radial scanner; outer diameter: 6.7 mm) was also used. Endobronchial findings consisted of 31 mucosal invasions, including 17 nodular, eight polypoid, six thickened types and one submucosal invasion. Bronchoscopy was performed in all patients, followed by EBUS under local or general anesthesia. Paying attention to the continuity of the cartilage layer, bronchial wall invasion was estimated in the EBUS images. In eight out of 30 primary lung cancers, the ability of EBUS to assess the peribronchial nodal involvement was estimated in comparison with the diagnosis using CT. Lymph nodes, imaged by EBUS, were considered to be involved when their short axes were 10 mm or more and/or they were round in shape.

Results

The ability of the EBUS to evaluate bronchial-wall invasion was studied according to the invasion level where the EBUS were performed. In the extramural level, tumor tissue was confirmed histologically in 19 out of 32 sites, and all sites were imaged precisely by EBUS (Fig. 1). In the cartilage level, tumor tissue was confirmed histologically in 17 out of 32 sites, and all sites were imaged precisely by EBUS. In the submucosal level, tumor tissue was confirmed histologically in 25 out of 32 sites, and all sites were imaged precisely by EBUS. In the mucosal level, tumor tissues were confirmed histologically in 26 out of 32 sites, and 25 sites were imaged precisely by EBUS. Superficial spread of a squamous cell carcinoma was not imaged as invasion by EBUS, because the first hyperechoic layer was thicker than epithelium. Accuracy of EBUS in the extramural, cartilage, submucosal and mucosal levels were 100%, 100%, 100%, and 96.9%, respectively.

The ability of EBUS to image the peribronchial lymph node was also compared with that of CT. A total of six peribronchial nodes, including two hilar, one interlobar and three segmental nodes were diagnosed as involved by histology. Involved lymph nodes revealed homogeneous strong hypoechoity. Two (33.3%) of six involved nodes were recognized by CT, and only one (16.7%) of six was imaged as large, of which the short axis was 10 mm. Nevertheless, all of the six involved nodes were recognized, and four (66.7%) of six involved nodes were

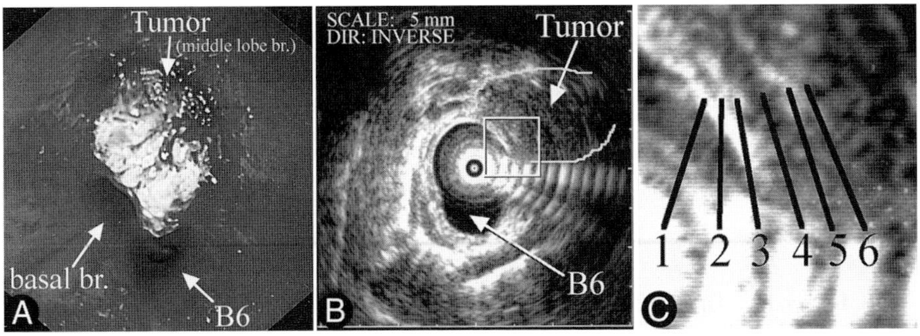

Fig. 1. **A:** Bronchoscopic image of the right intermediate bronchus, after Nd:YAG laser irradiation in a 15-year-old male, showed a polypoid tumor (carcinoid) covered with necrotic tissue, which was obstructing the middle lobe bronchus. **B:** EBUS image at the right lower lobe bronchus imaged the six-layered structure of the bronchial wall, connected with the hypoechoic area which corresponded with the tumor. **C:** Magnified view of the rectangular area in B. The numerals indicate the layers corresponding to our criteria (shown in the text). The cartilage layer and a hyperechoic layer corresponding to the adventitia were imaged, and the tumor was judged not to be invading the right basal bronchus at this site.

imaged as large by EBUS. The diagnostic rate using EBUS was 66.7%, which was better than the 16.7% using CT, and the χ^2 test revealed that the difference between two values was statistically fair ($p = 0.078$).

Discussion

We used our understanding of normal bronchial wall structure, that was established by in vitro experimental ultrasonography in saline [2], for assessing the invasion level. Ultrasonography of the normal bronchial wall is revealed as a six-layered structure by EBUS. The first, third and fifth layers were hyperechoic, due to the interface echo, the second and fourth layers were hypoechoic, and the sixth layer was slightly hyperechoic. The first and second layers correlate with the epithelium, lamina propria, and the smooth muscle and extramuscle layers. The third and fourth layers correspond with cartilage, and the fifth and sixth layers correspond with the adventitia. Using the cartilage layer as a reference point, the remainder of the bronchial wall anatomy was evaluated precisely in this study. For assessing nodal involvement, EBUS is revealed to have some advantages over CT. EBUS enables us to image the peribronchial lymph node easier and more precisely than CT, because EBUS can scan right-angled surfaces to the longitudinal axis of the bronchus. In addition to the size, EBUS enables us to estimate the ultrasonic intensity of the lymph node, which reflects the nature of the tissue. Further investigations may develop new criteria for the qualitative diagnosis of the tumor.

EBUS appears to be useful for judging the depth of tumor invasion in the bronchial wall, and for estimating peribronchial nodal involvement.

Acknowledgements

This work was supported in part by the Grant-in-aid for Scientific Research (C)(2) #10671240 from the Japanese Ministry of Education, Science, Sports and Culture.

References

1. Lam S, Becker HD. Thoracic endoscopy: future diagnostic procedures. Chest Surg Clin North Am 1996;6:363–379.
2. Baba M, Fujisawa T, Yasukawa T et al. Ultrasonography (EUS) can describe the structure of the bronchial wall. 10th World Congress for Bronchology and Bronchoesophagology (Program and abstracts) 1998;100.
3. Krimoto N, Murayama M, Yoshioka S et al. Assessment of usefulness of endobronchial ultrasonography in determination of depth of tracheobronchial invasion. Chest 1999;115:1500–1506.

Bronchology and Bronchoesophagology: State of the Art.
H. Yoshimura et al., editors.

Feasibility of endobronchial ultrasonography (EBUS): preliminary results of Italian experience

Franco Falcone, Flavio Fois, Marco Patelli, Daniele Grosso, Venerino Poletti, Luigi Tosto and Luigi Lazzari
Thoracic Diseases Department, Bellaria-Maggiore Hospital, Bologna, Italy

Abstract. EBUS allows high-definition images of the tracheobroncial tree and the surrounding structures, that are impossible to obtain through other methods. The water-filled balloon method ensures a good coupling between the ultrasonic transducer and the bronchial wall, and it is also possible to use an ultrasonic fiberscope with a transducer at the tip. The quality of images, using the balloon probe, is very high up until the depth of 2.5 cm, although the ultrasonic fiberscope allows a depth of 5 cm. Side examination and the penetration of cancer lesions are the ultimate goals of EBUS, and were well-tolerated under topical anesthesia in 93.6% of cases.

Keywords: endobronchial ultrasonography, ultrasonic fiberscope, ultrasonic catheter, ultrasound-assisted biopsy.

Introduction

Endobronchial ultrasonography (EBUS) is generally performed by inserting ultrasound transducers into the bronchial tree, which rotate in catheters pushed through the working channel of the fiberscope to the side of examination [1–3]. This method provides a radial scan of the surrounding anatomical structures. The quality of images is related to the ultrasonic coupling between the transducer and the bronchial mucosa. We evaluated this technique, particularly, during bronchoscopy under topical anesthesia.

Materials and Methods

Between January 1999 and February 2000, we performed 70 EBUS examinations in 61 subjects (mean age: 63,54 years), of which there were 50 males (mean age: 64.2 years) and 11 females (mean age: 59.5 years). Fifty-two subjects had neoplastic diseases and nine had non-neoplastic lesions. EBUS was performed, using a 2.6-mm diameter Olympus balloon catheter (MAJ-551R), and 20MHz Olympus echo probe (UM-B20-26R), in 57 cases, and a 1.8-mm diameter 20MHz Olympus probe (UM-S20-20R) with Olympus EU-M30 echo processor, in six cases. The ultrasound transducer at the tip of catheter generates a 360° radial

Address for correspondence: Franco Falcone, Divisione di Pneumotisiatria, Ospedale Bellaria-Maggiore, Via Altura 3, 40139 Bologna, Italy. Tel.: +39-051-6225322. Fax: +39-051-6225272.
E-mail: franco.falcone@ausl.bologna.it or ffalcone@qubisoft.it

scan of the surrounding area by rotating. The balloon catheter was pushed through an at least 2.8 mm diameter working channel fiberscope, to the side of examination, and the surrounding air was removed by inflating the balloon with saline to ensure a 360° ultrasonic coupling and to generate a complete circular image. The probe without a balloon needs at least a 2.0-mm diameter working channel, and allows a good 360° coupling in a less than 2- to 3-mm diameter bronchi. Without complete circular contact, the images are only defined in parts of the 360°. In seven cases, EBUS was carried out using a 6.4-mm diameter, new ultrasonic fiberscope prototype (Olympus XBF-UM30 with EU-M30 Olympus processor) with a rotating transducer at the tip that allows a 300° scanning area. A balloon camera can be inflated around the tip, using saline, up until a diameter of 15 mm, and allows a good ultrasonic coupling at the side of contact. Sixty-two examinations were performed under topical anesthesia (1% lidocaine 10 cc) according to our conventional technique (50 using the balloon probe, six using the thinner probe, and six using the new ultrasonic fiberscope prototype); eight were performed under general anesthesia (intravenous propofol 100–200 mg) through a rigid endoscope during endobronchial therapy or a follow-up control session (seven using the balloon catheter, and one using the new prototype). During topical anesthesia, we used a supply of 2 to 4 l/min, and evaluated the patient's tolerance score, as follows: 1: complete tolerance, 2: partial with cough or bleeding, 3: partial with lack of ventilatory function or hypoxia, and 4: no tolerance. We also evaluated the length of EBUS as a percentage of the time of bronchoscopy. We first evaluated the goal of EBUS, to achieve intelligible echographic images, to achieve images of specific structures, and to be able to carry out a specific diagnostic echo-assisted procedure. EBUS's results were scored as: A: achievement of intelligible images, B: achievement of intelligible images of structures that we study, C: to carry out a diagnostic echo-assisted procedure using achieved images, D: achievement of useful sample from procedure, and E: achievement of diagnostic sample from procedure. During EBUS with probes, we performed echo-assisted transbronchial needle aspiration (TBNA) in 35 cases. Endoscopic and ultrasound images were mixed on the same monitor by a TV mixer. To create hardware copy, the CV-240 Olympus video processor was linked to a BF-1T240 Olympus videoendoscope or an Olympus fiberscope through the Olympus OCV-200 video converter. All examinations were recorded by a video tape (Panasonic S-VHS MD-380) for later analysis and computer storage.

Results

The length of EBUS ranges from 5 to 15 min, and from 20 to 60% of endoscopy time. EBUS under topical anesthesia had an interesting tolerance scores: 1: 59 cases (93.6%), 2: two cases (one cough and one bleeding, 3.2%), and 3: two cases (hypoxia, 3.2%). As for patients whom EBUS was performed under topical anesthesia, we have never experienced such patient as having had to discontinue

EBUS procedures by some reason. To perform EBUS, we have to obstruct the patients' main bronchus for 20 to 100 s and have to move the balloon back and forth in the main bronchus with the balloon remaining inflated. The new ultrasonic fiberscope was inserted through the nose (four cases) or mouth (two cases) and EBUS tolerance scores were: 1: five cases (71%), and 2: two cases (cough and minimal mucosal bleeding, 29%). The balloon probe ensures a complete circular coupling between the transducer and bronchial wall. In trachea, we can inflate the ballon up until a diameter of 19 to 20 mm, but the balloon allows good contact without complete obstruction being necessary, simply by pushing on the wall. The optimal sonic waves focus on the wall was 10 to 14 mm, and allowed an image depth of 1.5 to 2.5 cm (image diameter: 3 to 5 cm.). A 360° coupling allows a completely defined circular image, but in particular cases (bronchial lavage or bleeding and endobronchial tumor), the probe without a balloon also allows a 360° scan in 4- to 5-mm diameter bronchi. The coupling of the probe without balloon in peripheral airways was enough to obtain good images of cancer, fibrosis, pleurisy or pneumonia and it improves with BAL. The new ultrasonic fiberscope generates a very high resolution image with a depth of 3 to 4.5 cm (6- to 9-cm diameter) at the side of contact.

The results of 63 EBUS examinations using probes were: AB: eight cases (12.7%), ABCD: 14 cases (22.2%), without a diagnostic TBNA sample, and ABCDE: 41 cases (65.1%), with 21 diagnostic TBNA (56% of TBNA). TBNA was carried out in lymph nodes with very small diameters (maximum: 5 mm). In four XBF cases, we studied the depth of local tumors, and in three cases we performed a diagnostic biopsy of peribronchial tumors (two cases) and lymph nodes (one case). The bronchial wall had a recognizable layer-echo-structure, and it was possible to evaluate the depth of invasion of tumors and follow up the local lesions in eight cases with 3- to 4-mm diameter lymph nodes that were recognizable.

Discussion

The EBUS technique allows very high resolution ultrasound images that are impossible to obtain with other methods. The use of EBUS is limited due to the difficulty of transmitting an echo signal to the bronchial wall with air interposition, however, the balloon method [4] allows good coupling between the transducer and bronchial wall. The new ultrasonic fiberscope prototype allows good contact, without obstructing the bronchi, simply by pushing the tip of the fiberscope onto the mucosa. By using probes, without a balloon, it is easy to explore the peripheral bronchi and surrounding lesions. We always obtain useful ultrasound images, and in 48 EBUS examinations (68.6%) this method provided diagnostic results.

Becker demonstrated characteristics of the layer structure of the bronchial wall [4], and Kurimoto [5] correlated the histopathologic findings of submucosal tissue with a specific ultrasound irregularity of the layers, demonstrating tumor invasion. In eight cases, we followed up endobronchial therapy and local tumors,

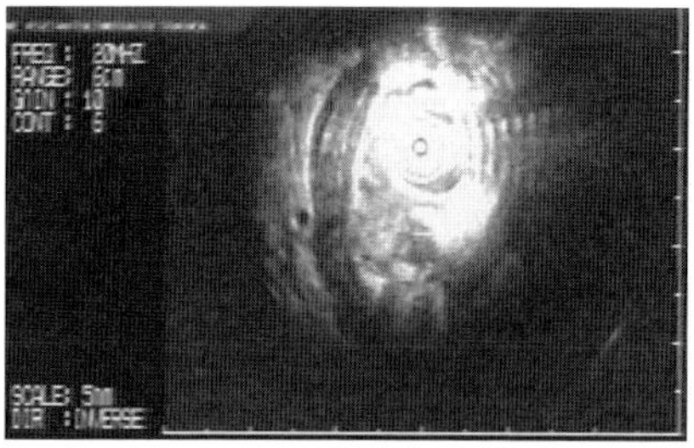

Fig. 1. Cancer of 10 mm in diameter near oesophagus with penetration of submucosa.

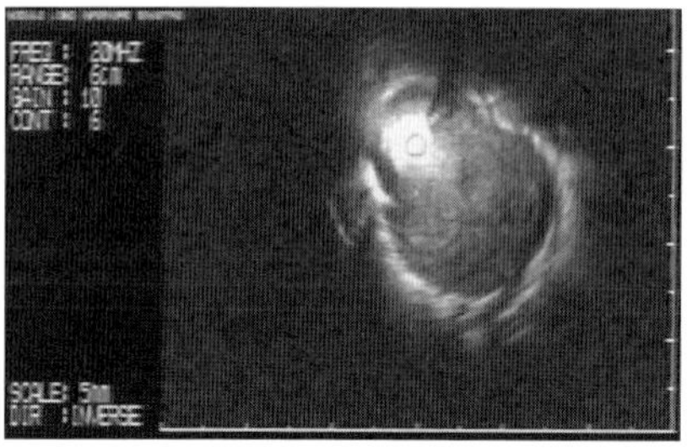

Fig. 2. Ultrasound probe near to a 2 × 2.5 cm cancer nodule.

using EBUS to evaluate the depth of the lesion (Fig. 1). Peripheral neoplastic nodules had an echo-recognizable structure in comparison with the normal surrounding lung tissue (Fig. 2). The echo image is the marker of the tumor in the inner bronchus, and can be used to suggest where to direct the biopsy forceps or needle. Outside of the trachea, radial images are different from usual CT or NMR slices, and in depth learning of marker structures in the oesophagus is required to be able to identify the surrounding anatomical structures. The EBUS learning curve requires only 6 months in order to have gained enough skill to understand what you are seeing.

References

1. Hurter T, Hanrath P. Endobronchial sonography: feasibility and preliminary results. Thorax 1992;47:565–567.
2. Goldberg B, Steiner R, Liu Ji-Bin, Merton D, Articolo G, Cohn J, Gottlieb J, McComb B, Spirn P. US-assisted bronchoscopy with use of miniature transducer-containing catheters. Radiology 1994;190:233–237.
3. Shannon J, Bude R, Orens J, Becker F, Whyte R, Rubin J, Quint L, Martinez F. Endobronchial ultrasound-guided needle aspiration of mediastinal adenopathy. Am J Respir Crit Care Med 1996;153:1424–1430.
4. Becker HD. Endobronchialer Ultrashall – eine neue Perspektive in der Bronchologie. Endoskopie Heute 1995;1:55–56.
5. Kurimoto N, Murayama M, Yoshioka S, Nishisaka T, Inai K, Dohi K. Assessment of usefulness of endobronchial ultrasonography in determination of depth of tracheobronchial tumor invasion. Chest 1999;115:1500–1506.

Bronchology and Bronchoesophagology: State of the Art.
H. Yoshimura et al., editors.

Assessment of the usefulness of endobronchial ultrasonography (balloon probe) in the determination of the depth of tracheobronchial tumor invasion

Noriaki Kurimoto[1], Koji Hayashi[1] and Masaki Murayama[2]
[1]*Department of Surgery, National Hiroshima Hospital, Higashi-Hiroshima City; and* [2]*Department of Surgery, Iwakuni Minami Hospital, Iwakuni City, Japan*

Abstract. *Purpose.* We reported that the cartilaginous portions are depicted to have five layers, and the membranous portion three, using the 20-MHz probe, and that we diagnosed 23 out of 24 cases of resected tracheobronchial tumors in water correctly. The purpose of this study was to assess the usefulness of EBUS (balloon probe) in the determination of depth tumor invasion in clinical cases.

Methods. We compared EBUS images and histopathologic findings of resected specimens. The probe is a miniature probe (20 MHz, radial type, UM-BS20-26R, OLYMPUS).

Results. In our 26 clinical lung cancer cases, depth of tumor invasion using the ultrasonograms and the histopathologic findings was the same in 23 of the 26 lesions (88.5%). We had three cases where the EBUS findings did not correlate with the histopathologic findings. In one case, the tumor had invaded the adventitia, whereas I diagnosed it beyond the adventitia. The depth of tumor invasion in the other two cases was carcinoma in situ. We are not able to detect carcinoma in situ on EBUS, because the tumor is included in the first hyperechoic marginal echo.

Conclusion. This method, using the balloon probe, allows visualization of the laminar structures of the trachea and bronchial wall.

Keywords: balloon probe, depth of tumor invasion, endobronchial ultrasonography.

Introduction

In previous reports, the bronchial wall was visualized as having three [2] and seven layers [3]. We reported that ultrasonograms, obtained at 20 MHz, showed five layers in the cartilaginous portion and intrapulmonary bronchi, and three layers in the membranous portion, based on comparisons of ultrasonographic determinations and histopathologic findings [1].

We performed the needle-puncture experiment and compared the ultrasonographic determinations of tumor invasion from 24 resected lung cancer specimens with histopathologic findings.

In this study, we compared the preoperative ultrasonographic determinations of tumor invasion, using the balloon probe, from 26 lung cancer cases with histopathologic findings.

Address for correspondence: Noriaki Kurimoto MD, Department of Surgery, National Hiroshima Hospital, 513 Jike, Saijyoucyou, Higashi-Hiroshima City, Hiroshima 739-0041, Japan. Tel.: +81-824-23-2176. Fax: +81-824-22-4675.

We will assess the usefulness of endobronchial ultrasonography in the determination of thc dcpth of tumor invasion of trachcobronchial wall.

Materials

The clinical cases of determination of depth of invasion involved 26 lung cancer cases that were determined utilizing high-frequency ultrasonography (balloon probe) between August 1994 and December 1999. The objective was to determine the accuracy of high-frequency ultrasound-determined depth diagnosis when compared with histopathological findings after sectioning the entire specimen.

Methods

While the bronchoscopy was performed, the ultrasonic probe was inserted into the bronchus, the balloon inflated with water, the tumor scanned, the ultrasonographic findings recorded, and the depth of tumor invasion determined.

After fixing the surgical specimen in formalin, sections were cut at 1-mm intervals, perpendicular to the long axis of the bronchi. The ultrasonographic determinations of tumor invasion and corresponding histopathologic findings were compared.

Equipment

The thinner ultrasonic probe was a 20-MHz, radial mechanical type (UM-BS20-26R, Olympus). We used this probe with a Balloon sheath (MAJ-643R, Olympus).

Laminar structures of the tracheobronchial wall (Fig. 1)

Conducting the needle-puncture experiment on the 45 specimens, yielded the following results. The cartilaginous portion of the extrapulmonary bronchi and

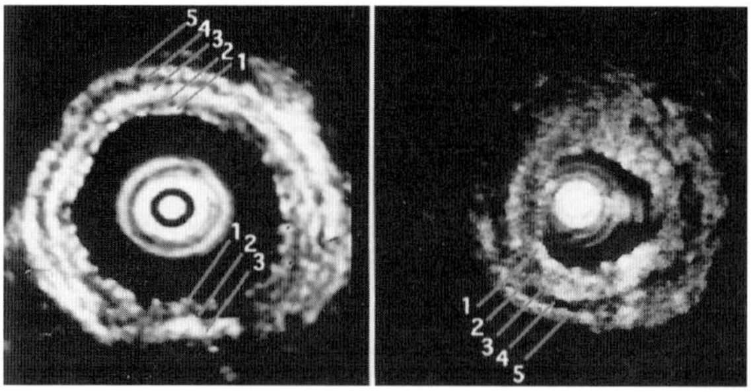

Fig. 1. Laminar structures of the tracheobronchial wall. Left: extra-pulmonary bronchus. Right: intra-pulmonary bronchus.

the intrapulmonary bronchi were visualized as having five layers. Starting on the luminal side, the first layer (hyperechoic) is a marginal echo, the second layer (hypoechoic) is submucosal tissue, the third layer (hyperechoic) is the marginal echo on the inside of the bronchial cartilage, the fourth layer (hypoechoic) is bronchial cartilage, and the fifth layer (hyperechoic) is the marginal echo on the outside of the bronchial cartilage. In the membranous portion of the extrapulmonary bronchi, the first layer (hyperechoic) is an interface echo, the second layer (hypoechoic) is smooth muscle, and the third layer (hyperechoic) is the adventitia.

Results (Table 1)

Comparison of the preoperative ultrasonograms and histopathological findings in 26 lesions showed that the findings were the same in 23 lesions (88.5%) (Fig. 2).

Table 1. Comparison of preoperative EBUS and histological findings.

No.	Histology	Location	Depth by US	Depth on patho.	Cartilage	Comparison US and patho.
1	Squamous	Lt B6	Not visualized	Ca. in situ	○	×
2	Squamous	Lt Ba-b	Not visualized	Ca. in situ	○	×
3	Adeno.	Intermediate	SM	sm	○	○
4	Squamous	Lt upper	SM	sm	○	○
5	Cartinoid	Rt upper	SM	sm	○	○
6	Squamous	Intermediate	C	c	○	○
7	Squamous	Intermediate	A	a	○	○
8	Squamous	Rt B2	A	a	○	○
9	Mucoepidermoid	Rt lower	A	a	○	○
10	Squamous	Rt upper	Ai	a	○	×
11	Squamous	Rt lower	Ai	ai	○	○
12	Squamous	Rt lower	Ai	ai	○	○
13	Squamous	Intermediate	Ai	ai	○	○
14	Squamous	Rt upper	Ai	ai	○	○
15	Squamous	Lt upper	Ai	ai	○	○
16	Adeno.	Rt main	Ai	ai	○	○
17	Adeno.	Rt lower	Ai	ai	○	○
18	Adeno.	Rt B3	Ai	ai	○	○
19	Squamous	Lt upper	Ai	ai	○	○
20	Squamous	Lt upper	Ai	ai	○	○
21	Squamous	Lt B1+2-B3	Ai	ai	○	○
22	Adeno.	Intermediate	Ai	ai	○	○
23	Squamous	Rt B6	Ai	ai	○	○
24	Cartinoid	Rt B6	Ai	ai	○	○
25	Squamous	Lt upper	Ai	ai	○	○
26	Squamous	Lt main-lower	Ai	ai	○	○

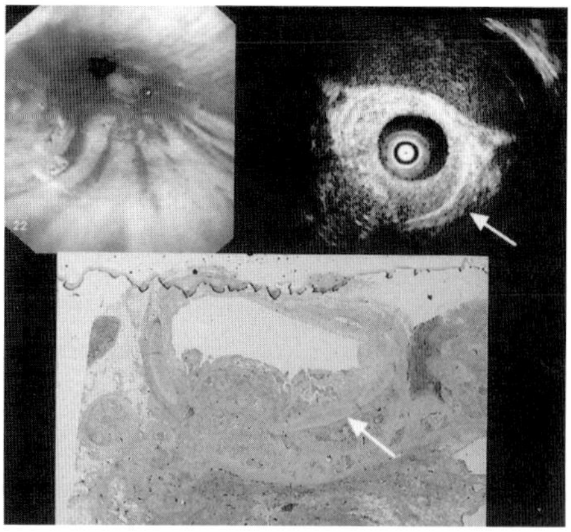

Fig. 2. A representative case. A squamous cell carcinoma was found at the intermediate trunk. On EBUS using a balloon, the tumor was judged to have invaded beyond the bronchial wall. The layers, indicated on the ultrasonogram (top arrow), corresponded with the cartilage, indicated in the histopathological findings (bottom arrow), and so the depth diagnoses using ultrasonography and histopathological findings coincided.

We had three lesions (11.5%) where the depth of tumor invasion according to EBUS findings did not agree with the histopathological findings. In one case, the tumor had invaded the adventitia, however, we diagnosed it to have invaded beyond the adventitia (Fig. 3). The depth of tumor invasion in the other two cases

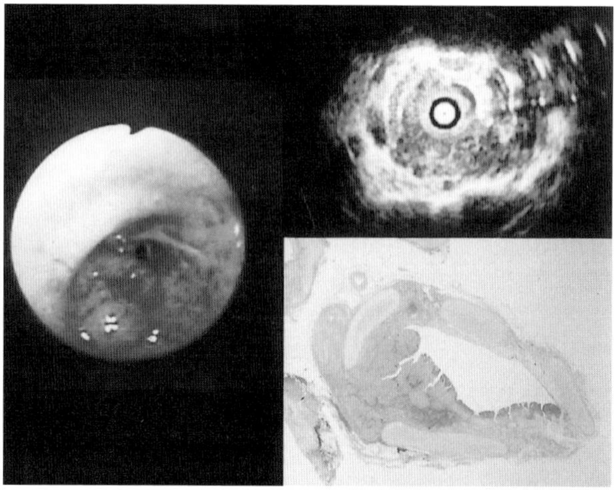

Fig. 3. A representative case. A squamous cell carcinoma was found at the right upper bronchus. On EBUS using a balloon, this hypoechoic tumor was judged to have invaded beyond the cartilage, and we could not follow the 5th layer around the tumor. On the ultrasonogram the depth of tumor invasion was judged to be beyond the adventitia. Histopathologically this tumor was observed to have invaded the adventitia, but not beyond the adventitia, and thus the depth of invasion had been overestimated.

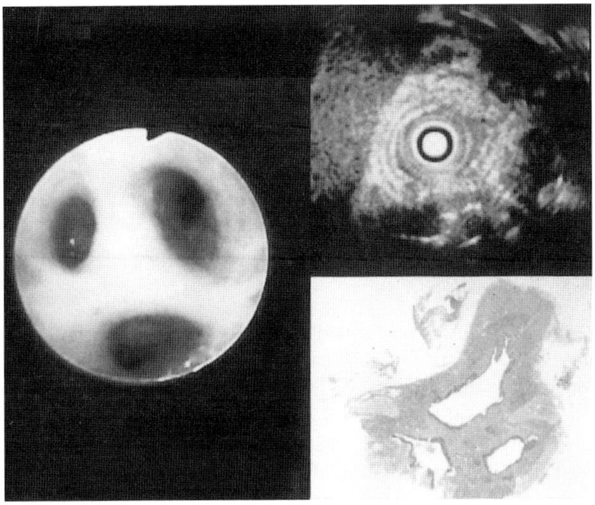

Fig. 4. A representative case. A squamous cell carcinoma was found at the left B6. On the bronchoscopic findings, the spurs of B6a, b, and c were dull. On the EBUS image using a balloon, the layers of the bronchial wall were normal. Histopathologically this tumor was carcinoma in situ. We believe, due to the needle-puncture experiment and the principle of the marginal echo, that the 1st layer carcinoma in situ, located from the mucosa through to the internal portion of the submucosa, is hidden behind the 1st layer on the EBUS image.

could not be determined, and was shown to be carcinoma in situ on histopathological findings (Fig. 4).

From this study, we are able to detect the cartilage on EBUS images in all cases. We are not, however, able to detect carcinoma in situ on EBUS, because the tumor is included in the 1st hyperechoic marginal echo.

Conclusion

Endobronchial ultrasonography allows the visualization of the laminar structure of the trachea and bronchial wall, which is impossible with other diagnostic imaging methods.

References

1. Kurimoto N, Murayama M, Yoshioka S et al. Assessment of the usefulness of endobronchial ultrasonography in determination of depth of tracheobronchial tumor invasion. Chest 1999; 115:1500–1506.
2. Hurtur Th, Hanrath P. Endobronchial sonography: feasibility and preliminary results. Thorax 1992;47:565–567.
3. Becker H. Endobronchialer Ultraschall-eine neue Perspektive in der Bronchologie. Ultraschall Med 1996;17:106–112.

Bronchology and Bronchoesophagology: State of the Art.
H. Yoshimura et al., editors.

Utility of endobronchial ultrasonography in the diagnosis of pulmonary nodular lesions

Keisuke Matsuo, Akihiko Tamaoki, Yoichi Watanabe and Shunkichi Hiraki
Department of Respiratory Medicine, Okayama Red Cross Hospital, Okayama, Japan

Abstract. Endobronchial ultrasonography (EBUS) was performed in 63 patients, which included 44 neoplastic lesions, 14 non-neoplastic lesions and five undiagnosed lesions. EBUS images were obtained in 46 cases (73%), and out of 37 lung cancer patients, EBUS images were obtained in 29 cases (78.4%). Although these rates were not very high, EBUS was still thought to be useful in detecting the affected bronchus because there were some cases in which we could not detect the affected bronchus without EBUS. These EBUS images also allowed us to obtain very useful information, enabling us to distinguish neoplastic lesions from non-neoplastic lesions. In neoplastic lesions, like in lung cancer, EBUS images tended to produce the following features: the margin of the lesion was continuous and the internal echo pattern was rough, like a sand-scattered pattern, and high echoic spots, that represent the bronchus, were rarely seen.

Keywords: endobronchial ultrasonography, nodular lesion, peripheral lung, bronchofiber.

Background

Endoscopic ultrasonography (EBUS) is sometimes performed to inspect the level of cancer invasion or peribronchial lymphadenopathy in the central bronchus [1,2]. In our hospital EBUS was performed on pulmonary nodular lesions in the peripheral lung field, in the last 2 years, to examine the utility of EBUS in the diagnosis of pulmonary nodular lesions, especially concerning the following two points: detecting the affected bronchus, and the differential diagnosis, for example, neoplastic or not. We examined the utility of EBUS and report on it.

Methods and Patients

After the routine work of bronchial brushing with a bronchofiberscope, an EBUS probe (20 MHz radial probe, UM-3R, OLYMPUS) was inserted into the target bronchus. After the examination of the EBUS image, biopsy and bronchial washing were performed.

There were 63 cases, which included 44 neoplastic cases (37 lung cancer, four metastatic lung tumor, one MALT lymphoma, one sclerosing hemangioma, and one hamartoma), 14 non-neoplastic cases (four organising pneumonia, two

Address for correspondence: Keisuke Matsuo, Department of Respiratory Medicine, Okayama Red Cross Hospital, 2-1-1 Aoe, Okayama 700-8607, Japan. Tel.: +81-86-222-8811. Fax: +81-86-222-8841. E-mail: ksk-1@fk9.so-net.ne.jp pneumonia, two atypical mycobacteriosis, two tuberculosis, one aspergillosis, one pulmonary abscess, one BOOP, and one amyloidoma) and five undiagnosed cases.

Results

EBUS images of the lesions were obtained in 46 out of 63 cases (73%). In 37 lung cancer patients, the images were obtained in 29 cases (78.4%). In these 29 lung cancer cases, 26 cases (89.7%) were diagnosed by bronchofiberscopy. Regarding the utility in detecting the affected bronchus, the results were not very good, but there were some cases in which it seemed that the EBUS probe missed the tumor under X-ray monitoring, but that only the EBUS image could prove that the bronchus was involved in the tumor.

We were able to acquire very useful information from EBUS images to distinguish neoplastic disease from non-neoplastic disease. In neoplastic lesions, the margin of the lesion was continuous (93.8%), and high echoic spots, which represent the bronchus, were rarely observed (5.9%). Also, the internal echo pattern was shown to be rough, like scattered sand (94.4%). On the other hand, in non-neoplastic lesions, the margin was not continuous (37.5%) and a high echoic spot was often seen, that ran through the lesion along the EBUS probe (100%). The internal echo pattern was not usually rough (37.5%). If the lesion had a necrotic part or an abscess, the internal echo showed a low echoic pattern.

Conclusion

The utility of EBUS was studied in cases with pulmonary nodular lesions. There were some cases in which detecting the affected bronchus was impossible without EBUS. Very useful findings were obtained by EBUS to help distinguish neoplastic from non-neoplastic lesions. If the margin of the lesion is continuous, the internal echo pattern is rough, and high echoic spots can be seen through the lesion, we can diagnose with high accuracy that the lesion is neoplastic disease.

References

1. Ono R et al. Bronchoscopic ultrasonography in the diagnosis of the lung cancer. Jpn J Clin Oncol 1993;23:34–40.
2. Kurimoto N et al. Clinical application of endobronchial ultrasound in the diagnosis of bronchial and peri-bronchial diseases. Jpn J Clin Radiol 1997;42:143–150.

Bronchology and Bronchoesophagology: State of the Art.
H. Yoshimura et al., editors.

Endoscopic assessment with the combination of AFB and EBUS for intraluminal lung cancer

Yuka Miyazu[1], Teruomi Miyazawa[1], Noriaki Kurimoto[2] and Yasuo Iwamoto[1]
[1]*Department of Pulmonary Medicine, Hiroshima City Hospital, Hiroshima; and* [2]*Department of Surgery, The National Hiroshima Hospital, Hiroshima, Japan*

Abstract. *Purpose.* We conducted a clinical trial to determine the utility of assessment using a combination of autofluorescence endoscopy (AFB) and endobronchial ultrasound (EBUS) in patients with intraluminal lung cancer.

Methods. We performed conventional white light bronchoscopy following AFB in 92 patients, and 131 lesions suspected of cancer were taken for biopsy. Later, if an endobronchial tumor was detected, EBUS was performed.

Results. We were able to detect 49 lesions (metaplasia, 20; dysplasia, two; carcinoma in situ, three; invasive carcinoma, 24) using WLB and AFB, and 17 lesions were only detected owing to the additional use of AFB (metaplasia, 11; dysplasia, two; carcinoma in situ, two; invasive carcinoma, two). Eleven patients were selected for EBUS, to be evaluated for the depth of tumor invasion into the bronchial wall. In four patients with early cancer, which were restricted within the cartilage, complete remission was achieved after photodynamic therapy. Five of seven patients with invasive cancer, that was protruding beyond the cartilage, were considered candidates for surgery, and two patients for chemo-radiotherapy. These patients were treated successfully.

Conclusions. Assessment using a combination of AFB and EBUS, when used as an adjunct to WLB, proved to be useful in deciding on a clinical course of action.

Keywords: carcinoma in situ, early lung cancer, endobronchial ultrasound, fluorescence bronchoscopy, photodynamic therapy.

Background

The addition of autofluorescence endoscopy (AFB) to white light bronchoscopy (WLB) is said to enable the detection of precancerous lesions, and assess the extent of staging in endobronchial cancers. With the improvement of diagnosis of early lung cancers, various endobronchial therapies have been achieved [1]. However, the success of endobronchial therapies is strongly influenced by the depth of the tumor invasion into the bronchial wall, or extra bronchial invasion, specifically when treated by photodynamic therapy. The EBUS can broaden the view beyond the bronchial surface, and recently the possibility of evaluating the depth of tumor invasion into the bronchial wall, by EBUS, has also been realized [2].

Address for correspondence: Teruomi Miyazawa MD, Department of Pulmonary Medicine, Hiroshima City Hospital, 7-33 Moto-Machi, Naka-ku, Hiroshima 730-0011, Japan. Tel.: +81-82-221-2291. Fax: +81-82-223-1447.

This clinical trial was to determine the efficacy of the combination assessment using autofluorescence bronchoscopy and endobronchial ultrasound.

Methods

At first we evaluated the tumor using conventional WLB and the CT scan. Then, autofluorescence bronchoscopy: LIFE (laser-induced autofluorescence bronchoscopy) or SAFE (the system of fluorescence bronchoscopy) was performed. Overall, 67 biopsies using LIFE and 64 biopsies with SAFE were taken. Later, if endobronchial cancers were detected, and they were small, and suspected as fitting the criteria of early stage lung cancer, the lesions were selected for EBUS to evaluate the depth of tumor invasion into the bronchial wall. According to the depth of tumor invasion, we divided these lesions into two levels: whether they were within the cartilage or beyond the cartilage. If the lesion was limited within the cartilage, it seemed suitable for endobronchial therapy.

Results

We detected 30 lesions (metaplasia, 17; moderate dysplasia, one; CIS, one; invasive carcinoma, 11) using WLB plus LIFE, and were only able to detect 12 lesions owing to the addition of LIFE (metaplasia, nine; CIS, one; moderate dysplasia, one; invasive carcinoma, one). We detected 19 lesions (metaplasia, three; moderate dysplasia, one; CIS, two; invasive carcinoma, 13) using WLB plus SAFE, and were only able to detect four lesions owing to the addition of SAFE (metaplasia, two; CIS, one; invasive carcinoma, one).

Later, eleven patients were selected for EBUS to evaluate the depth of tumor invasion.

In the images obtained by the EBUS, the hypoechoic layer between the hyperechoic layers indicating the cartilage, can often be clearly observed, and we consider following these layers to be the key to the correct determination of the depth of tumor invasion. We also consider it important as to whether the lesion has remained within the cartilage or beyond the cartilage, and determined the therapeutic course of action based on those assessments.

Four patients with early cancer lesions which were restricted within the cartilage, in whom images by EBUS showed an intact normal cartilage layer, could be observed as continuous and were considered candidates for PDT. Five of seven patients with invasive cancer, in whom images by EBUS showed the tumor to extend beyond the cartilage, were considered candidates for surgery. The two remaining patients with invasive cancer, who were considered to be high-risk surgical candidates, were treated with chemo-radiotherapy.

These patients were treated successfully. Histopathological findings confirmed the evaluations of EBUS in three patients after surgical resection.

Conclusion

We performed AFB to detect and localize precancerous lesions and cancers, and EBUS to evaluate the depth of tumor invasion. When we can detect such lesions, we can evaluate the depth of tumor invasion using EBUS, and if the lesions remain within the cartilage, we consider those patients to be good candidates for PDT and they can be treated more successfully than with conventional methods, i.e., by CT or WLB. Currently, this clinical approach has become a valuable additional diagnostic procedure within our institution, as we have found it very useful in making decisions regarding therapy, such as PDT, surgery or chemoradiotherapy.

References

1. Lam S, Becker DH. Future diagnostic procedures. Chest Surg Clin North Am 1996;6:363–380.
2. Kurimoto N, Murayama M, Yoshioka S. Assessment of usefulness of endobronchial urtrasonography in tracheobrinchial tumor invasion. Chest 1999;115:1500–1506.

Bronchology and Bronchoesophagology: State of the Art.
H. Yoshimura et al., editors.

Diagnosis of local invasion of lung cancer by endobronchial ultrasonography (EBUS)

Mitsumasa Ogawara, Masaaki Kawahara, Shigeto Hosoe, Sinji Atagi and Tomoya Kawaguchi
National Kinki-Central Hospital for Chest Diseases, Sakai, Osaka, Japan

Abstract. For the purpose of staging and the determination of a treatment method, we assessed the local invasion of lung cancer in 23 patients (pts) using EBUS. EBUS showed endobronchial tumors, local invasions and lymphadenopathy. EBUS proved to be a useful method of diagnosis for endobronchial lung cancer, local invasion of lung cancer and hilar or mediastinal lymphadenopathy.

Keywords: bronchofiberscopy, early lung cancer, endobronchial cancer, locally advanced cancer.

Introduction

In spite of advances in CT scans and bronchofiberscopy, it is still difficult to diagnose local invasion of lung cancer precisely. EBUS is a newly developed method, which has revealed that normal bronchial walls exhibit a five-layer structure and that tumors are shown in a hypoechoic form [1,2]. For the purpose of staging and the decision about treatment methods, we examined local invasion of endobronchial lung cancer, invasion of lung cancer into the mediastinum, trachea or great vessels, and hilar or mediastinal lymphadenopathy using EBUS.

Methods

We used 20 MHz, radial mechanical-type ultrasound probes (model, UM-3R, XUM-B20-26R or UM-BS20-26R, Olympus, Tokyo, Japan) with a balloon sheath through a bronchofiberscope and an ultrasound unit (EU-M30, Olympus).

Results

The following patients were examined: five endobronchial lung cancer pts with seven lesions; four pts after photodynamic therapy (PDT); four pts suspected to have tracheal invasion; two pts suspected to have mediastinal invasion and two large vessel invasion; and five pts suspected to have hilar or mediastinal lymphadenopathy.

Address for correspondence: Mitsumasa Ogawara, National Kinki-Central Hospital for Chest Diseases, Nagasone-cho 1180, Sakai 591-8555, Japan. Tel.: +81-722-52-3021. Fax: +81-722-50-4034. E-mail: ogawaram@kinchu.hosp.go.jp

Table 1. Central type early lung cancer.

Case	Bronchus	Bronchoscopy	EBUS	Biopsy	Treatment
1	LB^3	+	+	+	Operation
	RB^2	+	–	+	PDT
	RB^3	+	–	+	PDT
2	RB^2	+	+	+	PDT
3	RB^{8b}	+	+	+	–
4	RB^2	+	–	+	PDT
5	Lbasal	+	+	+	Operation

Four of seven endobronchial lesions were observed using EBUS (Table 1). Of the four pts examined after PDT, no tumors were detected (negative cytology). Of the five pts with advanced lung cancer, operated on locally, the findings using EBUS were consistent with the results of the histopathologies. Positive cytology using transbronchial needle aspiration (TBNA) was obtained in three of five lymphadenopathy pts. EBUS was useful in avoiding vessels in TBNA.

Discussion

These results suggest that EBUS is useful in the diagnosis of the local progression of central type early lung cancer, local invasion of lung cancer and hilar or mediastinal lymphadenopathy, and aids in the determination of appropriate therapy.

Acknowledgement

This study was partly supported by a grant from the Japanese Ministry of Health and Welfare.

References

1. Kurimoto N, Murayama M, Yoshioka S, Nishisaka T, Inai K, Dohi K. Assessment of usefulness of endobronchial ultrasonography in determination of depth of tracheobronchial tumor invasion. Chest 1999;115:1500–1506.
2. Takemoto T, Kawahara M, Ogawara M, Yamamoto S, Ueno K, Mori T, Furuse K. The experience of ultrasound guided fiberoptic bronchoscopy for diagnosis of tumor depth and invasion to mediastinum. J Bronchol (In press).

©2001 Published by Elsevier Science B.V.
Bronchology and Bronchoesophagology: State of the Art.
H. Yoshimura et al., editors.

Layer structure of central airway viewed using endobronchial ultrasonography (EBUS)

Taeko Shirakawa[1], Fujiho Tanaka[2] and Heinrich D. Becker[3]

[1]Division of Pulmonology, Internal Medicine, National Saishunso Hospital; [2]Division of Pulmonology, Internal Medicine, Kumamoto City Hospital, Kumamoto, Japan; and [3]Department of Interdisciplinary Endoscopy, Thoraxklinik-Heidelberg, Heidelberg, Germany

Abstract. *Background.* The aim of this study was to clarify the ultrasonographic layer structure of the central airway, especially its outer part.

Methods. The postmortem trachea (n = 6) were prepared for observation of the whole structure with 1) surrounding loose connective tissue (A), 2) the loose connective tissue removed (B), and 3) the external fibroelastic connective tissue (adventitia) removed (C). Sonographic findings using EBUS were compared with those of histology.

Results. A was described as having seven layers surrounded by a hazy structure. B was also described as having seven layers, but without the hazy structure. C was expressed as having five layers, lacking the outer two layers. In comparison with histological findings, the first and second layer of EBUS were considered to coincide with the mucosa and submucosa, the third, fourth and fifth layer, with cartilage, and sixth and seventh layer, with adventitia.

Conclusions. The sonographic structure of the central airway, described using EBUS, contains seven layers, which are congruent to that of histological findings.

Keywords: central airway wall, trachea, ultrasonographic layer structure.

Introduction

Through the use of endobronchial ultrasonography (EBUS) the multilayer structure of the central airway wall can be clearly analyzed. Especially concerning the identification of mucosal invasion by endoluminal tumors and the infiltration of the outer wall by adjacent tumors, EBUS is superior compared to all other methods. However, there is controversy about the sonographic layer structure. Some investigators say that it consists of five layers [1], while others found six or seven layers [2,3]. Differences occur in the interpretation of the outer layers. With respect to operability or endoscopic therapy, it is essential to know the exact normal sonographic structure.

Therefore, the purpose of this study is to clarify the sonographic layer structure of the central airway wall using EBUS by comparison to histology. For simplicity, we excluded the membranous part.

Address for correspondence: Taeko Shirakawa, Division of Pulmonology, Internal Medicine, National Saishunso Hospital, 2659 Suya, Nishigoshi-machi, Kikuchi-gun, Kumamoto 861-1196, Japan. Tel.: +81-96-242-1000. Fax: +81-96-242-2619. E-mail: taeko@aminet.or.jp

Materials and Methods

For in vitro experiments, we examined fixated postmortem tracheas (n = 5). One unfixated trachea was also applied. Tracheas were cut transversely into the segments of about 3 cm in length. Of these, we prepared three different kinds of specimens: A: whole structure with adjacent loose connective tissue containing fat tissue, B: loose connective tissue removed, C: external fibroelastic connective tissue also removed, after which cartilage appeared directly.

For the investigation, we used an Olympus 20-MHz probe with balloon catheter sheath. A 30-MHz probe was also applied for the examination of the unfixated trachea. Each material was totally immersed into water during ultrasonographic observation. Afterwards the EBUS images were compared to the histology (HE stain), respectively.

Results

In each of the five fixated tracheas, in the image of A, seven layers with adjacent hazy structures were described. In the image B, there were also seven layers but without the hazy structure, and in C, five layers, lacking the outer two layers were observed. However, in those fixated materials, the identification of the layer structure, especially of outer layers, was not so easy.

Therefore, we applied an unfixated trachea for the same evaluation. We could then identify seven layers much easier and much more clearly. Furthermore, with a 30-MHz probe and a 2-cm image range, the layer structure could be observed beautifully.

In Fig. 1, the higher magnification of the US images using the 30-MHz probe and corresponding histology of unfixated trachea are demonstrated. In material A, seven layers can be seen, representing mucosa, submucosa, cartilage, with its inner and outer perichondrium, and external fibroelastic connective tissue. Outside one can see an adjacent hazy structure, which is the loose connective tissue. Material B also has seven layers, just like material A. In material C, only five layers can been seen, lacking the outer two layers.

Through these observations, it became obvious that an ultrasonic image of the wall of the trachea can be described as having a seven-layer structure, which corresponds to the anatomical structures, and the sixth and seventh layers correspond to the external fibroelastic connective tissue, i.e., 1st and 2nd layer: mucosa and submucosa, 3rd, 4th, 5th layer: cartilage, and 6th and 7th layer: external fibroelastic connective tissue (adventitia).

Conclusions

The layer structure of postmortem trachea was investigated in vitro using endobronchial ultrasonography (EBUS).

The ultrasonic image of the tracheal wall could be confirmed as having a

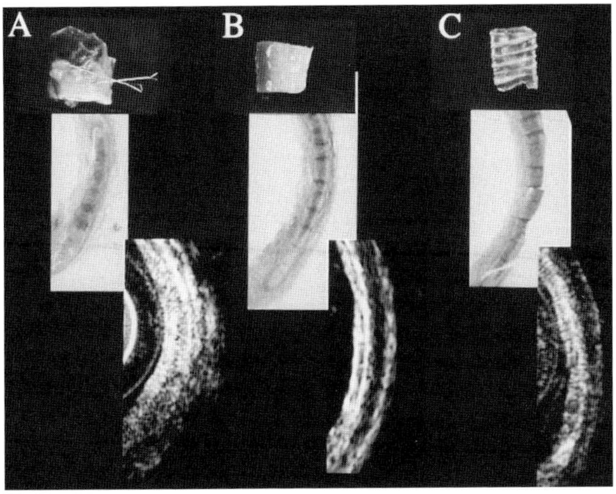

Fig. 1. Postmortem trachea. **A:** Whole structure with adjacent loose connective tissue containing fat tissue. **B:** After removal of loose connective tissue. **C:** After additional removal of external fibroelastic connective tissue, after which cartilage appeared directly. Upper images: macroscopic views, middle images: histology (HE stain) of the unfixated material, and lower images: the corresponding EBUS images using 30-MHz probe, with image range of 2 cm. In A, seven layers can be seen, from inside to outside, high-low-high-low-high-low-high, representing mucosa, submucosa, cartilage with its inner and outer perichondrium and external fibroelastic connective tissue. Outside one can see an adjacent hazy structure which is the loose connective tissue. Material B also has seven layers just like material A. In material C, only five layers can be seen, lacking the outer two layers.

seven-layer structure. After the removal of the external fibroelastic connective tissue (adventitia), five layers remained.

The ultrasonographic layers correspond to the histology.

References

1. Kurimoto N, Murayama M, Yoshioka S et al. Assessment of usefulness of endobronchial ultrasonography in determination of depth of tracheobronchial tumor invasion. Chest 1999;115: 1500–1506.
2. Becker HD. Endobronchialer ultraschall – eine neue Perspektive in der Bronchologie. Ultraschall Med 1996;17:106–112.
3. Becker HD, Herth F. Endobronchial ultrasound of the airway and the mediastinum. In: Bolliger CT, Mathur PN (eds) Interventional Bronchoscopy. Basel: Karger, 2000;30:80–93.

Index of authors

Keyword index